The Pathology of Cardiac Transplantation

Ornella Leone • Annalisa Angelini
Patrick Bruneval • Luciano Potena
Editors

The Pathology of Cardiac Transplantation

A Clinical and Pathological Perspective

Springer

Editors
Ornella Leone
Cardiovascular and Cardiac Transplant Pathology Program
Department of Pathology
Sant'Orsola-Malpighi University Hospital
Bologna
Italy

Annalisa Angelini
Pathology of Cardiac Transplantation and Regenerative Medicine Unit
Department of Cardiac
Thoracic and Vascular Sciences
University of Padua
Padua
Italy

Patrick Bruneval
Department of Pathology
Hôpital Européen Georges Pompidou
Paris
France

Luciano Potena
Heart Failure and Heart Transplant Program, Cardiology Unit
Sant'Orsola-Malpighi University Hospital
Bologna
Italy

Endorsed by the Association for European Cardiovascular Pathology

ISBN 978-3-319-46384-1 ISBN 978-3-319-46386-5 (eBook)
DOI 10.1007/978-3-319-46386-5

Library of Congress Control Number: 2016960043

Printed on acid-free paper

This Springer imprint is published by Springer Nature
The registered company is Springer International Publishing AG
The registered company address is Gewerbestrasse 11, 6330 Cham, Switzerland

To all those who generously donate their organs, to patients on the waiting list and to all transplanted patients

And to all the health professionals, too numerous to mention by name, who with their hard and dedicated work make transplantation possible

Foreword

Nearly 50 years have elapsed since Christian Barnard in Cape Town accomplished what was considered a breakthrough in medicine and cardiac surgery, namely treatment of terminal congestive cardiac failure with the replacement of the whole heart.

Richard Lower and Norman Shumway had previously done fundamental experimental work on large animals at Stanford and deserve a great part of the merit for this achievement, but the brilliant young surgeon from South Africa had the nerve to do it directly with humans. However, at that time, the barrier of immunologic tolerance was not yet resolved, and the first transplants were complicated by severe cellular rejection and graft failure. The Stanford team continued with the experimental work and in the 1980s, with the discovery and clinical application of cyclosporine, which could control T-cell immune reaction, cardiac transplantation entered into clinical practice worldwide with striking success (approximately 95 % hospital survival, 75 % still alive at 10 years follow-up).

Why was heart transplantation the dawn of contemporary cardiovascular pathology? For several reasons, well documented in the *Treatise of Pathology of Cardiac Transplantation* by Leone et al.

With transplantation, cardiac pathologists started to play a key role in diagnosis and prognosis for live patients, in close collaboration with clinicians. They moved from the anatomical to the surgical theater, from the mortuary table to the operating table, restoring health. The days were over when the cardiac pathologist only witnessed the natural end of the human body or clinical failure and when the meaning and mission of his job was "… *mors gaudet succurrere vitae*" (… death's joy in helping future lives). He became a guardian of life.

On that memorable night of November 14, 1985, in Padua, Prof. Vincenzo Gallucci carried out the first cardiac transplantation in Italy and, for the first time, I held in my hands a still beating heart, a specimen from a living patient. It was a turning point in my career. A series of successful transplantations followed, requiring weekly rejection monitoring through endomyocardial biopsy. My mind flies back to the memory of Margaret Billingham, the teacher and mentor of generations of cardiovascular pathologists in cardiac transplant centers worldwide.

In the arena of cardiac transplantation, the pathologist plays several key roles:

(a) Before operation, with diagnostic endomyocardial biopsy, to establish cause of morbidity leading to heart failure so severe as to require the extreme option of heart replacement.

(b) During operation, with manipulation and sampling of the cardiac specimens for precise diagnosis and molecular investigation.
(c) After operation, in the follow-up, with periodic endomyocardial biopsies for rejection monitoring and, in case of fatal outcome, with the usual necropsy to ascertain causes and mechanisms of failure (early multiorgan failure, recurrent acute rejection, infections, lympho-proliferative disorders, late allograft rejection). For all of us it has been a unique training experience, from gross anatomy and light or electron microscopy to infective or genetic molecular pathology.

Previously unknown diseases were discovered in the "gymnasium" of cardiac transplantation. For instance, primary restrictive cardiomyopathy with severe diastolic ventricular impairment and congestive heart failure, known as the "paradox of small heart requiring transplantation". It was eventually discovered to be genetically determined sarcomere disease.

This book has been very well orchestrated and written by a team of international experts, including pathologists, clinicians, surgeons, and immunologists. To the best of my knowledge, this is the first comprehensive treatise in the field. All the issues regarding the discipline of cardiac transplantation are covered: epidemiology of congestive cardiac failure, indication to transplant including diagnostic endomyocardial biopsy, donation and graft preservation, graft failure, immunology of cellular and humoral rejection, infective and neoplastic complications, and chronic rejection as allograft vasculopathy. Last but not least, artificial support for a failing heart with ventricular assistance devices as a bridge to transplant or destination therapy.

This book looks wonderful, enriched with beautiful illustrations, a true encyclopedia of cardiac transplantation. Let me express my congratulations to the Editors, who have been the conductors of a concert of eminent scholars in the field.

Pathology and pathologists are back again in the core of cardiovascular medicine.

Gaetano Thiene, MD,
Honorary FRCP London,
Professor of Pathology,
University of Padua,
Padua,
Italy

Preface

Today heart transplantation is an acknowledged therapy for the treatment of end-stage heart failure and is still the gold standard procedure for a selected group of patients with terminal heart failure: the 5-year survival rate is an impressive 71.7 %.

The major limiting factor is donor shortage. In addition, in recent years, the heart donor pool has had a more complex profile due to the presence of older donors with co-morbidities and the progressive shift from young and healthy trauma victims to brain death donors, which may cause adverse haemodynamic cardiac events. The decreasing number of donor hearts and the growing number of heart failure patients contribute to the substantial mortality rate in waiting list patients. Over the past two decades, this shortfall has exacerbated the need to extend criteria for organ acceptability by considering marginal/higher-risk donors, including older donors, as they represent a potential immediate increase in the number of suitable hearts.

After the pioneering era of the first heart transplantation in 1967, it became clear that this new and complex medical context called for a multidisciplinary work-up model where the various specialists involved can work closely together in standardizing diagnostic and therapeutic strategies or in research and specialist training. There was also work to be done in familiarizing the public with the very idea of heart donation.

The cardiovascular pathologist is part of this multidisciplinary team and works closely together with clinicians and surgeons and other specialists throughout the entire transplant process, thus emerging from the isolation in which the pathologists often find themselves.

This book has the backing of the Association for European Cardiovascular Pathology (AECVP) (www.aecvp.org), which was founded in 2001 as a development of the European School for Cardiovascular Pathology, founded in 1994.

AECVP aims to bring together "those in Europe actively involved in cardiovascular pathology and provides a platform to serve as a liaison between pathologists, cardiologists and surgeons as well as basic science researchers in the field of cardiovascular diseases". Its purpose is to be "instrumental in coordinating many aspects of cardiovascular pathology in Europe, such as quality control studies in the diagnostic field and in the implementation of multicentre studies in the cardiovascular pathology arena" and to "put much emphasis on mutual postgraduate education programs".

The AECVP developed a close liaison with the European Society of Pathology and participates as companion society in the annual European

Congress of Pathology meetings. AECVP regularly collaborates with the sister North American Society for Cardiovascular Pathology (SCVP) and other European scientific societies, such as the European Society of Cardiology, International Academy of Forensic Medicine and European Association for Cardio-Thoracic Surgery.

In 2008, the Association initiated a Cardiac Transplant Working Group to highlight the fact that heart transplant pathology lies within the wider discipline of cardiovascular pathology. This led to the development of a European Heart Transplant Network (whose membership currently stands at 50), in order to create an effective liaison with pathologists working in cardiac transplantation, to compare experience and exchange information on local practice and organization, as well as to develop educational programmes, reproducibility studies and online collaborative projects on cardiac transplant pathology. The European Transplant Group also collaborates with the International Society for Heart and Lung Transplantation (ISHLT) and its Pathology Council, with the Banff Foundation for Allograft Pathology and with the European Society for Solid Organ Transplantation (ESOT) and its Cardio-Thoracic Section (ECCTA), in order to develop guidelines and multicenter studies.

The book was conceived with the purpose of focusing on pathology issues in cardiac transplantation in a clinical perspective, with emphasis on the value of multidisciplinary team-work and collaborative research. Its intention is to provide a scientific framework with a comprehensive review of the chronological phases of the transplant process, up-to-date pathological protocols and classification schemes and a step-by-step approach to guide the reader. The principal points are the need for constant dialogue between the pathologist and the clinician and the need to build on what we have achieved and to continue working together to illuminate the grey areas that remain.

Bologna, Italy — Ornella Leone
Padua, Italy — Annalisa Angelini
Paris, France — Patrick Bruneval
Bologna, Italy — Luciano Potena

Acknowledgements

Special thanks go to Morag MacCuish for checking the language and style.

A big thank you to all the technicians who have collected valuable photographic material for many years.

Contents

Contributors

Valentina Agostini, MD Department of Pathology, Sant'Orsola-Malpighi University Hospital, Bologna, Italy

Annalisa Angelini, MD Pathology of Cardiac Transplantation and Regenerative Medicine Unit, Department of Cardiac, Thoracic and Vascular Sciences, University of Padua, Padua, Italy

Klaus Aumayr, MD Clinical Institute for Pathology, Medical University of Vienna, Vienna, Austria

Jonida Bejko, MD, PhD Division of Cardiac Surgery, Department of Cardiac, Thoracic and Vascular Sciences, University of Padua, Padua, Italy

Gerald J. Berry, MD Department of Pathology, Stanford Medical Center, Stanford, CA, USA

Patrick Bruneval, MD Department of Pathology, Hôpital Européen Georges Pompidou, Paris, France

Margaret Burke, MB, FRCPath Department of Histopathology, Harefield Hospital, Royal Brompton and Harefield NHS Trust, London, UK

Brian A. Clarke, MD Division of Cardiology, Department of Medicine, Dalhousie University and the QE II Health Science Center, Halifax, NS, Canada

Julien Coussement, MD Division of Infectious Diseases, CUB-Erasme, Université Libre de Bruxelles, Brussels, Belgium

Maria Crespo-Leiro, MD, PhD, FESC, FHFA Unidad de Insuficiencia Cardiaca Avanzada y Trasplante Cardiaco, Servicio de Cardiología, Complexo Hospitalario Universitario A Coruña e Instituto de Investigación Biomédica (INIBIC) A Coruña, A Coruña, Spain

Carlo Dal Lin, MD Cardiology Unit, Department of Cardiac, Thoracic and Vascular Sciences, University of Padua, Padua, Italy

Helen Doran, FRCPath Department of Histopathology, University Hospitals of South Manchester NHS Foundation Trust, Manchester, UK

Jean-Paul Duong Van Huyen, MD, PhD Department of Pathology, University Paris-Descartes, Hôpital Necker-Enfants Malades, Paris, France

Volkmar Falk, MD, PhD Department of Cardiothoracic and Vascular Surgery, German Heart Institute Berlin, Berlin, Germany

Marny Fedrigo, MD, PhD Cardiovascular Pathology Unit, Department of Cardiac, Thoracic and Vascular Sciences, Azienda Ospedaliera Padua, Padua, Italy

Giuseppe Feltrin, MD, PhD Operative Unit of the Regional Center for Transplant Coordination, University of Padua, Padua, Italy

Gerasimos Filippatos, MD, FESC, FACC Heart Failure Unit, Departement of Cardiology, Athens University Hospital, Athens, Greece

Alberto Foà, MD Department of Cardiology, Sant'Orsola-Malpighi University Hospital, Bologna, Italy

Gino Gerosa, MD Division of Cardiac Surgery, Department of Cardiac, Thoracic and Vascular Sciences, University of Padua, Padua, Italy

Martin Goddard, FRCS, MRCPath Department of Pathology, Papworth Hospital NHS Trust, Cambridge, UK

Heike Goebel, MD Institute of Pathology, University of Cologne, Köln, Germany

Francesco Grigioni, MD, PhD Heart Failure and Heart Transplant Program, Cardiology Unit, S.Orsola-Malpighi University Hospital, Bologna, Italy

Franck Iserin, MD Department of Pediatric Cardiology, Hôpital Necker-Enfants Malades, Paris, France

Spyridon Katsanos, MD Department of Cardiology, Leiden University Medical Center, Leiden, The Netherlands

Abdallah G. Kfoury, MD Division of Cardiovascular Disease, Intermountain Medical Center, Utah Transplant Affiliated Hospitals (U.T.A.H.) Cardiac Transplant Program, Murray, UT, USA

Kiran K. Khush, MD, MAS Division of Cardiovascular Medicine, Stanford University School of Medicine, Stanford, CA, USA

Thomas Krabatsch, MD, PhD Department of Cardiothoracic and Vascular Surgery, German Heart Center Berlin, DZHK (German Center for Cardiovascular Research), Partner Site Berlin, Berlin, Germany

David Lebeaux, MD Université Paris Descartes, Sorbonne Paris Cité, AP-HP, Hôpital Necker Enfants Malades, Centre d'Infectiologie Necker-Pasteur and Institut Imagine, Paris, France

Ornella Leone, MD Cardiovascular and Cardiac Transplant Pathology Program, Department of Pathology, Sant'Orsola-Malpighi University Hospital, Bologna, Italy

Olivier Lortholary, MD, PhD Université Paris Descartes, Sorbonne Paris Cité, AP-HP, Hôpital Necker Enfants Malades, Centre d'Infectiologie Necker-Pasteur and Institut Imagine, Paris, France

Gaia Magnani, MD, PhD Heart Failure and Heart Transplant Program, Cardiology Unit, S.Orsola-Malpighi University Hospital, Bologna, Italy

Valentina Manfredini, MD Heart Failure and Heart Transplant Program, Cardiology Unit, S.Orsola-Malpighi University Hospita, Bologna, Italy

Francesco Marchini, MD II Nephrology Unit, Azienda Ospedaliera-Universitaria Padova, Padua, Italy

Marco Masetti, PhD Heart Failure and Heart Transplant Program, Cardiology Unit, S.Orsola-Malpighi University Hospita, Bologna, Italy

Dylan V. Miller, MD Intermountain Central Lab, University of Utah, Salt Lake City, UT, USA

Desley A.H. Neil, MD Department of Histopathology, Medical School University Hospitals Birmingham NHS Foundation Trust, Birmingham, UK

Marie-Claude Parent, MD, MSc, FRCPC Division of Cardiology, Hôpital du Sacré-Coeur de Montréal, Université de Montréal, Montréal, Québec, Canada

John T. Parissis, MD, FESC Heart Failure Unit, Cardiology Department, Attikon University Hospital, Athens, Greece

Sergei Pepoyan, MD Department of Cardiology, YSMU Hospital Complex N1, Yerevan, Armenia

Sylvain Poiree, MD Service de Radiologie Adulte, Hôpital Necker-Enfants Malades, Assistance Publique-Hôpitaux de Paris, Paris, France

Jorge Pombo-Otero, MD Cardiac Pathology Department, Complejo Hospitalario Universitario A Coruña, A Coruña, Spain

Evgenij Potapov, MD, PhD Department of Cardiothoracic and Vascular Surgery, German Heart Institute Berlin, Berlin, Germany

Luciano Potena, MD, PhD Heart Failure and Heart Transplant Program, Cardiology Unit, S.Orsola-Malpighi University Hospital, Bologna, Italy

Alexandra J. Rice, BA, MB, BChir, MRCPath Department of Histopathology, Royal Brompton Hospital, Royal Brompton and Harefield NHS Trust, London, UK

Marlene L. Rose, BSc, MSc, PhD National Heart and Lung Institute, Imperial College, Heart Science Centre, Harefield Hospital, Middlesex, UK

Samuel Rotman, MD Institute of Pathology, University Hospital of Lausanne, Lausanne-CHUV, Switzerland

John D. Smith, FRCPath Tissue Tying Laboratory, Harefield Hospital, Harefield, Middlesex, UK

Alexander Stepanenko, MD Department of Cardiothoracic and Vascular Surgery, German Heart Institute Berlin, Berlin, Germany

Francesco Tona, MD, PhD Cardiology Unit, Department of Cardiac, Thoracic and Vascular Sciences, University of Padua, Padua, Italy

Claire Toquet, MD, PhD Department of Pathology, Hôpital Hôtel-Dieu, Nantes, France

Allard van der Wal, MD, PhD Department of Pathology, Academic Medical Center, University of Amsterdam, Amsterdam, The Netherlands

Marialuisa Valente, MD Pathological Anatomy, Department of Cardiac, Thoracic and Vascular Sciences, University of Padua, Padua, Italy

John P. Veinot, MD, FRCPC Department of Pathology and Laboratory Medicine, The Ottawa Hospital, Ottawa, ON, Canada

Aryan Vink, MD, PhD Department of Pathology, University Medical Center Utrecht, Utrecht, The Netherlands

Katarina Wassilew, MD, DScmed Department of Pathology, Rigshospitalet, University of Copenhagen, Copenhagen, Denmark

Andreas Zuckermann, MD Cardiac Transplantation Program, Department of Cardiac Surgery, Medical University of Vienna, Vienna, Austria

Part I

Introduction

Cardiac Transplantation and the Contribution of Pathology

1

Margaret Burke and Luciano Potena

Contents

M. Burke, MB, FRCPath (✉)
Department of Histopathology, Harefield Hospital, Royal Brompton and Harefield NHS Trust, London, UK
e-mail: mm.burke@doctors.org.uk

L. Potena, MD, PhD
Heart Failure and Heart Transplant Program, Cardiology Unit, S.Orsola-Malpighi University Hospital, Bologna, Italy
e-mail: luciano.potena2@unibo.it

1.1 Background

Heart transplantation is the one procedure providing the most durable improvement in prognosis for the treatment of patients with advanced heart failure (Lund et al. 2014). However, this has not always been the case.

Surgical techniques for heart transplantation were developed in the late 1950s to 1960s from animal experiments performed by Norman Shumway at Stanford University Medical School, CA. In the late 1960s, four surgical teams in the United States and South Africa each strove to become the first to perform a heart transplant in humans and thus write their names in history. Christian Barnard won the race in 1967 using Shumway's technique and became a global celebrity, holding heart transplantation as the shiniest trophy in the hall of fame of surgical divinity. However, the surgical miracle soon turned sour with most patients dying from rejection or infection, with a 1-year survival not exceeding 35 % (John et al. 2001). The picture started to change when therapeutic and diagnostic advances enabled effective targeting of cellular rejection. The major improvement in therapy was driven by the introduction of calcineurin inhibitors—cyclosporine in the mid-1980s, and later, tacrolimus—which reduced the incidence of rejection and improved survival up to 85 % at year 1 (John et al. 2001). The major advance in diagnosis was achieved by Caves and

O. Leone et al. (eds.), *The Pathology of Cardiac Transplantation*,
DOI 10.1007/978-3-319-46386-5_1

colleagues in Stanford who, in the 1970s, used a specially modified percutaneous transvenous catheter to obtain endomyocardial biopsies (EMBs) in which the myocardial infiltrates of rejection were identified (Caves et al. 1974). This prompted an important development of cardiovascular pathology not only in the microscopic description of allograft rejection, but also for myocarditis, cardiomyopathies, and other myocardial disorders (Leone et al. 2012). Thus was born a close collaboration between clinicians and pathologists, which was unusual in the cardiovascular setting. In those early times, the surface electrocardiogram was the "cornerstone" for rejection diagnosis, with more complex imaging techniques still at an early stage of development and cardiac biomarkers still unknown to cardiovascular clinical practice.

Forty years later, heart transplantation is no longer just an exercise of high-level surgery, but a complex therapeutic strategy involving specific knowledge and skills from several healthcare professionals, including surgeons, cardiologists, anesthesiologists, immunologists, infectious diseases specialists, psychologists, nurses, and pathologists. This active and complex professional collaboration, focused on patients' needs, represents a high-quality networking model for patient management that can be regarded as a marker of quality of global healthcare organization in a transplant hospital. The results of this model are depicted in Fig. 1.1, showing a progressive and steadily improvement in the overall survival of heart transplant recipients from the 1980s until today.

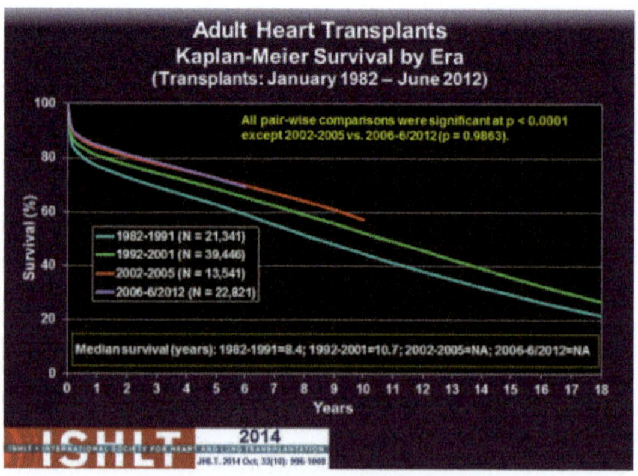

Fig. 1.1 Actuarial survival in heart transplantation by era. January 1982–June 2012 (Lund et al. 2014)

An important tool providing insights on improvements and unmet needs in heart transplantation is the registry of the International Society for Heart Transplantation, established in 1981 by a small group of clinicians to facilitate data collection on heart transplant recipients, with the publication of annual reports. From this small beginning evolved the International Society for Heart and Lung Transplantation (ISHLT) (www.ishlt.org)—*a multidisciplinary, professional organization dedicated to improving the care of patients with advanced heart or lung disease through transplantation, mechanical support, and innovative therapies via research, education, and advocacy.* Today, it has a global reach, representing over 14 different disciplines involved in the management and treatment of end-state heart and lung disease.

The latest registry report from ISHLT covers the years 1982 to June 2013 and was compiled from data on 116,104 heart transplants in recipients of all ages reported from 416 transplant centers in 34 countries worldwide. This is estimated to reflect about 66 % of global transplant activity with an 81 % survival at 1 year and 69 % survival at 5 years. A median survival of 11 years was given for all heart transplants, increasing to 14 years for those surviving the first year after transplantation (Fig. 1.1) (Lund et al. 2014).

Good though the results are, all that glitters is not gold. Several unmet needs currently limit further improvements in outcome. Late graft failure and malignancies are the most frequent causes of death after the first post-transplant year, and their incidence has only slightly reduced over the last four decades (Fig. 1.2). In addition, the fine-tuning of the perioperative management that allowed major survival improvements in the 1990s and early 2000s seems no longer adequate to support optimal results in the current era of recipients, often with multiple morbidities, frequently receiving grafts from suboptimal donors. In this setting, primary graft failure is still a threat, being responsible for up to 70 % of early deaths (Kobashigawa et al. 2014).

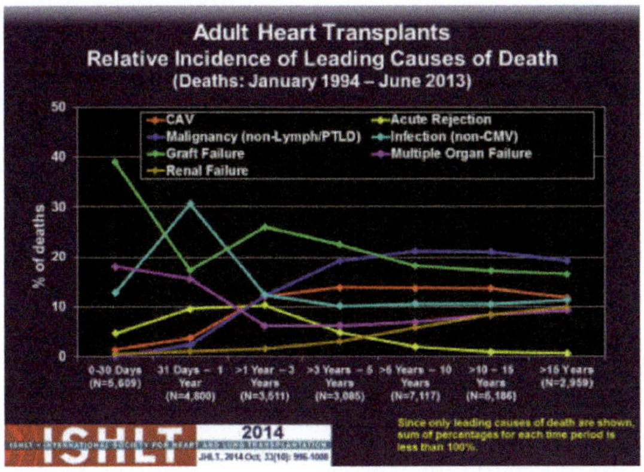

Fig. 1.2 Relative incidence of leading causes of death, January 1994–June 2013 (Lund et al. 2014). https://www.elsevier.com/journal-authors/obtaining-permission-to-re-use-elsevier-materia

1.2 Prior to Cardiac Transplantation

The journey toward a successful long-term outcome after heart transplantation begins with selection and management of suitable candidates. This is not only a matter of appropriate therapy by drug fine-tuning and device implantation—although heart failure drugs, implantable defibrillators, biventricular pacing, and ventricular assist devices have revolutionized heart failure outcomes in the last 20 years—but also a matter of appropriate diagnosis. The first part of this book provides an overview of the clinical management of heart failure, including the findings pathologists may encounter in biopsies and explanted native hearts from these patients. While standard cardiovascular imaging allows a diagnosis in the majority of patients needing heart transplantation, specific myocardial and inflammatory diseases require a pathological diagnosis. In these cases, the pathological diagnosis contributes to decision-making about heart transplantation as the preferred treatment (e.g. a myocardial infiltrative/storage disease). Of note, the pathologist's job in the diagnostic workup often needs to be completed after the transplant, when up to 30 % of clinical diagnoses of nonischemic cardiomyopathy may be proved wrong after pathological examination of the explanted heart (Luk et al. 2009).

1.3 Heart Donation and Peritransplant Pathologies

The choice of the appropriate donor is a crucial step in the process of any solid organ transplantation. In heart transplantation, this is even more important, given the falling donation rates in many countries worldwide, the high mortality rate associated with primary graft failure, and the difficulty in reliably assessing heart disease in donors. According to data from the Council of Europe, 70–85 % of hearts from multiorgan donors are currently rejected for transplantation (http://www.esot.org/news/latest-news/council-europes-newsletter-transplant-2014-now-available). In most cases, the unsuitability is the result of multiple risk factors affecting the donor, such as a high-risk profile for cardiovascular disease, a high donor age, an abnormal electrocardiogram and risk factors related to donor management such as use of inotropes in high doses, reduced ejection fraction, low sodium levels and hemodynamic instability. Pathological analysis of unused hearts provides important information to help our understanding of the mechanisms and extent of injury influencing organ suitability for transplantation.

Donor-related abnormalities may also be found in organs failing immediately after surgery (Kobashigawa et al. 2014), as well as injuries related to graft harvesting and transportation, and immediate immune-related injuries. Recognition of these aspects, as discussed in Part II of this book, is critical in the diagnostic workout of primary graft failure.

1.4 The Multiple Faces of Rejection

Following pivotal reports in the 1970s, the endomyocardial biopsy (EMB) became and has remained to this day the "gold standard" in the diagnosis and management of acute cardiac allograft rejection. Recently, its role has evolved in response to advances in the fields of immunology and molecular pathology which continue to increase our understanding of the rejection process and contribute to our current understanding of heart allograft rejection, not as a single pathological and clinical entity, but as a complex immune-mediated spectrum of changes that can lead to graft injury by several pathological mechanisms, so that often different patterns of rejection may coexist in the one biopsy. This important subject is dealt with in Part III of the book

1.4.1 Acute Cellular Rejection

In Caves et al.'s landmark publication their pathologist, Margaret Billingham, described the pathological features of acute cellular rejection (ACR) as a myocardial infiltrate of lymphocytes and devised a 4-point grading system based on its extent and intensity (Caves et al. 1974).

During the 1980s, more centers developed cardiac transplant programs, some using the Stanford biopsy rejection grading scheme. However, some centers devised their own grading schemes, and it became clear that an internationally standardized grading system was needed for multicenter clinical trials and for publication purposes to enable proper comparison of different centers' results (Billingham 1990). Thus, in 1990, the first internationally agreed Working Formulation for the pathological diagnosis of cardiac rejection, sponsored by ISHLT, was published (Billingham et al. 1990). It was based on the Stanford scheme with some modifications, and, for the first time, set standards for biopsy handling in the laboratory, and listed pathological changes in the biopsy not to be confused with rejection.

During the 1990s, the Working Formulation became the worldwide standard for diagnosis and management of ACR. Improved immunosuppression and treatment of acute rejection episodes resulted in a fall in the incidence of significant ACR ($\geq$ grade 3A) to the extent that the frequency of routine biopsies could be safely reduced. Re-evaluation of the 1990 Working Formulation led to some streamlining and updating. The revision was published by ISHLT in 2005 (Stewart et al. 2005) and is the grading system for ACR in use today, although some centers still prefer to use it alongside the 1990 Working Formulation.

1.4.2 Antibody-Mediated Rejection

The clinical observation of acute and chronic graft failure in the absence of biopsy-defined rejection, and parallel developments in immunology and immunopathology in the 1990s and 2000s, led to the recognition of antibody-mediated rejection (AMR) as a clinical, immunological and pathological entity, often coexisting with ACR. As its name suggests, AMR affects the graft by deposition of donorspecific antibodies (DSAs) with and without complement activation on capillary endothelium which becomes activated. Its clinical manifestations range from acute and severe allograft dysfunction to more indolent subclinical forms which may progress to cardiac allograft vasculopathy (CAV) (chronic rejection). Attaining a reliable, reproducible diagnosis continues to challenge clinicians, pathologists, and immunologists.

The morphological feature of endothelial activation in the early stages of AMR is "subtle," and it is likely that instances of AMR were overlooked, especially if ACR was present. The endothelial deposits of DSA and complement were initially detected in 1989 using immunofluorescence (IF) on frozen sections of myocardium, but this procedure was not easily reproducible or widely available at the time. The emergence of two further key diagnostic features identified in the 1990s—intravascular macrophages and capillary deposition of complement degradation product C4d—and the development in the 2000s of reliable paraffin tissue markers of complement C4d with sensitivity and specificity comparable to IF marked a significant advance in pathological diagnosis. A pathological grading system was proposed as part of the 2005 ISHLT Working Formulation (Stewart et al. 2005). Serological evidence of DSAs and the presence of allograft dysfunction were required to confirm the diagnosis.

Correlation of serology and the clinical findings with the EMB findings has revealed several diagnostic challenges, and it is a current unmet need in the optimization of the management of heart transplant recipients. Since 2005, we know that not everyone with biopsy-diagnosed AMR has circulating DSAs, and that C4d-negative

DSA-positive AMR and C4d-positive DSA-negative AMR may occur. Asymptomatic AMR has also been reported in association with a reduction in freedom from later CAV (Loupy et al. 2016). However, whether pathological evidence of AMR (pAMR) in the absence of circulating DSA, or vice versa, is sufficient to initiate treatment is debated. Such dilemmas require close collaboration between clinician, pathologist, and immunologist to put the pathological and serological findings into the appropriate clinical context, and thus avoid overdiagnosis and, perhaps, overtreatment. In this setting, it should be noted that while a Working Formulation for pathological diagnosis of AMR (the pAMR system) was endorsed by an international ISHLT-sponsored Task Force in 2013, (Berry et al. 2013)—which also cross-validated its reproducibility—standardization of DSA intensity assays and their interpretation is still awaited.

1.4.3 The Biopsy and Noninvasive Markers of Acute Rejection

For many years, the search has been on for sensitive and specific noninvasive markers of rejection to equal, if not surpass the EMB as the "gold standard" for diagnosis of allograft rejection. Recent understanding of the molecular basis for the inflammatory response has led to trials of molecular profiling of peripheral blood using a panel of genetic markers of inflammation and gene expression profiling (Deng et al. 2006; Mehra et al. 2008). However, it has yet to find its rightful place in the management of allograft recipients. The topic is discussed further in Part III of this book.

1.4.4 Chronic Rejection

Despite improvements in recipient management in the postoperative period and in reducing the incidence and severity of acute rejection over the last 40 years, the barriers to long-term survival remain cardiac allograft vasculopathy (CAV), primary graft failure, malignancy, and renal failure (Fig. 1.2).

The progressive, diffuse disease of CAV affects the entire coronary vascular tree and eventually leads to allograft ischemia. CAV involving the larger epicardial coronary arteries often exists alongside atheromatous plaques inadvertently "donated" as part of the allograft. There are a variety of imaging methods used to diagnose and assess the severity of CAV and correlation, where possible, with the pathology in the explanted or autopsied heart is often helpful in assessing the relative merits of the different imaging techniques. These have been reviewed and an international Working Formulation established to grade the extent and severity of epicardial CAV (Mehra et al. 2010). The heterogeneity of the clinical lesions is matched by heterogeneity of the pathological changes in CAV. However, it might be possible to identify the culprit lesion leading to the death or retransplantation of the recipient (Castellani et al. 2014; Vecchiati et al. 2014).

A current challenge to the pathologist is biopsy diagnosis of the other face of CAV—allograft microvasculopathy. Involvement of the microvasculature of the myocardium by chronic rejection may cause "late" primary graft failure and death, the process starting as early as 1 year after transplantation. It leads to diffuse myocardial ischemia through pruning of the microvascular tree by an increase in vessel wall thickness and a reduction in the number of capillaries. A number of studies have detailed the pathology (Hiemann et al. 2007) and correlated it with the coronary flow reserve (Vecchiati et al. 2014). The pathologist should carefully examine the interstitial vessels in EMBs for evidence of stenotic and inflammatory endothelial and medial disease, and, in the event of retransplantation or death, map the process in the allograft. Unlike acute rejection, universally accepted diagnostic criteria have yet to be agreed.

1.5 Nonrejection Pathology

The role of the pathologist in cardiac transplantation is wide, extending well beyond the identification of rejection and of the underlying heart disease as discussed above. Noncardiac complications, such as infections, tumors, lymphoproliferative disorders, and drug-related pathologies, especially nephrotoxicity, are commonly encountered, and their diagnosis may need involvement of pathologists expert in these areas. These may also necessitate consultation with other pathology specialties such as the microbiology or hematopathology service.

1.6 Scope of the Pathology Service

The challenge of "supply and demand" always tests the pathologist and laboratory manager who must ensure provision of a service for a broad range of clinical specialties. There is often little appreciation, especially among younger members of the clinical multiprofessional team, that pathology is not machine-driven with quick test turnaround times but a "hands-on" service where the mutual interdependency of pathologist and biomedical scientist must be effective if a responsive service tailored to the requirements of the Transplant Unit is to be provided. Regular liaison with clinical staff about the practicalities of providing this service is advised, especially at times of new clinical staff intake.

The service should include routine diagnostic histopathology, a rapid turnaround and on-call biopsy service, and access to specialist areas such as immunopathology, molecular pathology, and electron microscopy. Ideally, there should be access to a networked digital communication system to facilitate remote reporting, clinical conferencing, case consultation, teaching, and audit. This is especially helpful if the pathology service is provided remotely from the clinical service. Facilities for macrophotography and microphotography should be available. Adequate transport services both within and between hospitals are essential as is good communication between the requesting clinical team and the laboratory.

The role of the autopsy is not to be underestimated in investigating the deaths of recipients at any stage after transplantation. Reviewing the clinical course of our recipients from the perspective of the autopsy findings is important, even if only to confirm that there were no unexpected pathologies that escaped detection. However, the autopsy is also an important teaching, research, and audit tool for pathologists and clinicians alike, and if approached constructively can do much to "draw the line" under the case. It can reassure the family and the transplant team that all possible was done to help the recipient benefit from the second chance at life through the altruism of another bereaved family seeking a worthwhile legacy in memory of their loved one.

The participation of the pathologist in collaborative transplant research projects both within the institution and as multicenter projects often yield results which progress our understanding of the myriad of issues surrounding cardiac transplantation. The use of human tissues for ethically approved research must conform to national and, increasingly, international legislative requirements as well as institutional rules governing recipients'/families' consent, research, and management of tissue archives. Tissue banking is becoming more widely used to store cryopreserved and formalin-fixed tissue samples, and will ensure provision of suitable research material for future ethically approved projects.

1.7 Ensuring High Standards of Practice in Pathology

Laboratories who provide a service for Transplant Units must have achieved national accreditation standards specific to each country and comparable to international standards. Working to protocol is important in achieving this and includes using technical protocols for EMB processing based on international guidelines in the Working Formulations as well as the access to the formulations themselves for pathologists who report transplant biopsies.

Likewise, pathologists reporting transplant specimens must ensure up-to-date knowledge and experience and should subject themselves to audit and reproducibility testing by their

Table 1.1 Some useful resources for cardiac transplant pathologists

International transplant societies	Link	Main features
International Society for Heart and Lung Transplantation	http://www.ishlt.org/	Established in 1981. Annual scientific meetings, international registry for heart and lung transplants, and mechanical assist devices. Pathology representation via Pathology Council. Publishes *Journal of Heart and Lung Transplantation.* Impact factor 7.509 (2015)
European Cardiothoracic Transplant Association	http://www.esot.org/ECTTA/home	New section of the European Society for Organ Transplantation. Held its first meeting in Budapest in October 2014.
Banff Foundation for Allograft Pathology	http://www.banfffoundation.org/	Established in 1990, meets biennially. Collaborative multidisciplinary translational research in allograft pathology. Small heart transplantation working group.
Association for European Cardiovascular Pathologists	http://www.aecvp.org http://www.aecvp.org/index.php/aecvp-working-group	A cardiac transplant steering committee and network was established in 2008. It leads a Europe-wide network of pathologists involved in transplant pathology.
Society for Cardiovascular Pathology	http://www.scvp.net/acr/index.html http://www.scvp.net/amr/index.html	Links to tutorials on acute cellular rejection and antibody-mediated rejection. Publishes *Cardiovascular Pathology.* Impact factor 2.190 (2015).

peers—as indeed for any subspecialty of our discipline. Relative to other subspecialties in pathology, cardiac transplant pathology is very small—a "niche" specialty—with rarely more than one cardiac pathologist in each major center. In addition, very few pathologists are members of ISHLT; therefore, networking to draw in general pathologists who report small numbers of cardiac biopsies as part of a large general workload is very important. Using digital platforms to generate educational tools is part of this process. A new initiative by the Society for Cardiovascular Pathology and the Association for European Cardiovascular Pathology (AECVP) is the production of two online tutorials, one on ACR and the other on AMR. They have the potential to benefit all members of the transplant clinical team and not just pathologists, and their use is to be encouraged. They and other resources are listed in Table 1.1.

Falling numbers of donor organs and optimization of medical resources in many countries has led inevitably to a reduction in the number of transplant centers; therefore, local networks in each country and membership of international networks such as the AECVP Transplant Network can facilitate individual secondments to established centers by pathologists new to the field to gain experience. Networks may also facilitate reproducibility studies to ensure consistency of laboratory methodology and biopsy interpretation of the features of both forms of acute rejection. Recent developments in digital technology are suited for such studies as well as for collaborative research and consultation on challenging cases, all of which can now take place at international level from one's desktop in the workplace. This was exemplified during the 4-year evolution of the Working Formulation for pathological diagnosis of AMR, during which international multicenter questionnaires and reproducibility and validation studies by the AECVP Transplant Network and ISHLT Task Force charged with drawing up the Working Formulation contributed significantly to ironing out problems of methodology and interpretation of biopsies with AMR (Berry et al. 2013).

Conclusion

This book has been conceived to offer the reader a comprehensive review of the major pathologies encountered in heart transplant programs, viewed through the framework of the clinical problems faced during surgical and medical management of heart recipients. The aim of the authors is to underscore the importance of a continuous dialog between the pathologist and the clinician in order to put the pathological findings in the context of the clinical presentation, and thus gain as much information as possible from the description in the pathology report. This book, however, will not only provide the sound basis to chaperone the reader across the few certainties in heart transplant management, but also the shadows of the many unmet needs and uncertainties masking the path through this fascinating field of clinical practice.

References

Berry GJ, Burke MM, Andersen C, Bruneval P, Fedrigo M, Fishbein MC, et al. The 2013 International Society for Heart and Lung Transplantation Working Formulation for the standardization of nomenclature in the pathologic diagnosis of antibody-mediated rejection in heart transplantation. J Heart Lung Transplant. 2013;32(12):1147–62.

Billingham ME. Dilemma of variety of histopathologic grading systems for acute cardiac allograft rejection by endomyocardial biopsy. J Heart Transplant. 1990;9(3 Pt 2):272–6.

Billingham ME, Cary NR, Hammond ME, Kemnitz J, Marboe C, McCallister HA, et al. A working formulation for the standardization of nomenclature in the diagnosis of heart and lung rejection: Heart Rejection Study Group. The International Society for Heart Transplantation. J Heart Transplant. 1990;9(6): 587–93.

Castellani C, Angelini A, de Boer OJ, van der Loos CM, Fedrigo M, Frigo AC, et al. Intraplaque hemorrhage in cardiac allograft vasculopathy. Am J Transplant. 2014;14(1):184–92.

Caves PK, Stinson EB, Billingham ME, Shumway NE. Serial transvenous biopsy of the transplanted human heart. Improved management of acute rejection episodes. Lancet. 1974;1(7862):821–6.

Deng MC, Eisen HJ, Mehra MR, Billingham M, Marboe CC, Berry G, et al. Noninvasive discrimination of rejection in cardiac allograft recipients using gene expression profiling. Am J Transplant. 2006;6(1): 150–60.

Hiemann NE, Wellnhofer E, Knosalla C, Lehmkuhl HB, Stein J, Hetzer R, et al. Prognostic impact of microvasculopathy on survival after heart transplantation: evidence from 9713 endomyocardial biopsies. Circulation. 2007;116(11):1274–82.

John R, Rajasinghe HA, Chen JM, Weinberg AD, Sinha P, Mancini DM, et al. Long-term outcomes after cardiac transplantation: an experience based on different eras of immunosuppressive therapy. Ann Thorac Surg. 2001;72(2):440–9.

Kobashigawa J, Zuckermann A, Macdonald P, Leprince P, Esmailian F, Luu M, et al. Report from a consensus conference on primary graft dysfunction after cardiac transplantation. J Heart Lung Transplant. 2014;33(4): 327–40.

Leone O, Veinot JP, Angelini A, Baandrup UT, Basso C, Berry G, et al. 2011 Consensus statement on endomyocardial biopsy from the Association for European Cardiovascular Pathology and the Society for Cardiovascular Pathology. Cardiovasc Pathol. 2012; 21(4):245–74.

Loupy A, Toquet C, Rouvier P, Beuscart T, Bories MC, Varnous S et al. Late failing heart allografts: pathology of cardiac allograft vasculopathy and association with antibody-mediated rejection. Am J Transplant. 2016: 16(1):111–20.

Luk A, Metawee M, Ahn E, Gustafsson F, Ross H, Butany J. Do clinical diagnoses correlate with pathological diagnoses in cardiac transplant patients? The importance of endomyocardial biopsy. Can J Cardiol. 2009;25(2):e48–54.

Lund LH, Edwards LB, Kucheryavaya AY, Benden C, Christie JD, Dipchand AI, et al. The registry of the International Society for Heart and Lung Transplantation: thirty-first official adult heart transplant report – 2014; focus theme: retransplantation. J Heart Lung Transplant. 2014;33(10):996–1008.

Mehra MR, Kobashigawa JA, Deng MC, Fang KC, Klingler TM, Lal PG, et al. Clinical implications and longitudinal alteration of peripheral blood transcriptional signals indicative of future cardiac allograft rejection. J Heart Lung Transplant. 2008;27(3):297–301.

Mehra MR, Crespo-Leiro MG, Dipchand A, Ensminger SM, Hiemann NE, Kobashigawa JA, et al. International Society for Heart and Lung Transplantation working formulation of a standardized nomenclature for cardiac allograft vasculopathy-2010. J Heart Lung Transplant. 2010;29(7):717–27.

Stewart S, Winters GL, Fishbein MC, Tazelaar HD, Kobashigawa J, Abrams J, et al. Revision of the 1990 working formulation for the standardization of nomenclature in the diagnosis of heart rejection. J Heart Lung Transplant. 2005;24(11):1710–20.

Vecchiati A, Tellatin S, Angelini A, Iliceto S, Tona F. Coronary microvasculopathy in heart transplantation: consequences and therapeutic implications. World J Transplant. 2014;4(2):93–101.

Part II

Prior to Cardiac Transplantation

2 Advanced End-Stage Heart Failure: Epidemiology and Management

John Parissis, Spyridon Katsanos, Sergei Pepoyan, and Gerasimos Filippatos

Contents

J. Parissis
Heart Failure Unit, Cardiology Department, Attikon University Hospital, Athens, Greece

S. Katsanos
Department of Cardiology, Leiden University Medical Center, Leiden, The Netherlands

S. Pepoyan
Department of Cardiology, YSMU Hospital Complex N1, Yerevan, Armenia

G. Filippatos (✉)
Heart Failure Unit, Department of Cardiology, Athens University Hospital, Athens, Greece
e-mail: geros@otenet.g

2.1 Definition and Epidemiology

Advanced heart failure (HF) concerns less than 10 % of the total heart failure population and is a malignant condition with very high mortality, similar to that of aggressive human cancers (Maisel and Filippatos 2014; Adams and Zannad 1998; Metra et al. 2007; Zannad et al. 2006; Kittleson et al. 2003; Nieminen et al. 2005; Swedberg et al. 2005), with annual mortality exceeding 50 % of patients. A high rate of hospital admissions (more than two per year) due to congestion and/or peripheral hypoperfusion is also compatible with this advanced stage. This condition that concerns stage D of heart failure (AHA/ACC classification) could be defined as the syndrome with persistence of signs and symptoms of heart failure despite optimal medical and device (CRT or CRT/D) therapy (Maisel and Filippatos 2014; Adams and Zannad 1998). A definition of advanced end-stage HF is summarized in Table 2.1. The clinical features of advanced end-stage HF are described in Table 2.2, and useful prognostic factors in Table 2.3 (Maisel and Filippatos 2014; Adams and Zannad 1998; Metra et al. 2007; Zannad et al. 2006).

2.2 Management

Various therapeutic strategies recommended for the optimal management of advanced end-stage HF patients are summarized in Table 2.4 (Swedberg et al. 2005; Hunt et al. 2005).

O. Leone et al. (eds.), *The Pathology of Cardiac Transplantation*,
DOI 10.1007/978-3-319-46386-5_2

Table 2.1 Definition and characteristics of advanced heart failure

1. Severe symptoms of HF with dyspnea and/or fatigue at rest or with minimal exertion (NYHA functional class III or IV)
2. Episodes of fluid retention (pulmonary and/or systemic congestion, peripheral edema), and/or of reduced cardiac output at rest (peripheral hypoperfusion)
3. Objective evidence of severe cardiac dysfunction, shown by at least one of the following:
(a) Low LVEF (<30 %)
(b) Severe abnormality of cardiac function on Doppler-echocardiography with a pseudonormal or restrictive pattern of mitral inflow
(c) High LV filling pressures (mean PCWP > 16 mmHg, and/or mean RAP > 12 mmHg by pulmonary artery catheterization)
(d) High brain natriuretic peptide (BNP) or N-terminal (NT)-ProBNP plasma levels in the absence of noncardiac causes
4. Severe impairment of functional capacity shown by one of the following:
(a) Inability to exercise
(b) 6-minute walk test <300 m or less in females and/or patients aged ≥75 years
(c) Peak VO_2 <12 or 14 mL/kg/min
5. History of ≥1 HF hospitalization in the past 6 months

NYHA New York Heart Association, *LVEF* left ventricle ejection fraction, *PCWP* pulmonary capillary wedge pressure, *RAP* right atrial press

Table 2.2 Clinical features of advanced end-stage heart failure

Symptoms	Signs
Frequent paroxysmal nocturnal dyspnea	Resting tachycardia
Severe orthopnea	Hypotension
Poor appetite	Resting tachypnea
Weight loss with edema	Cachectic status
Frequent palpitations	Anasarca, ascites
Frequent dizziness	Somnolence
Nocturnal angina	Right ventricular lift
Abdominal bloating	Marked neck vein distension, loud S3 gallop

2.2.1 Medical Treatment

Diuretics are essential for amelioration of dyspnea symptoms in chronic HF patients with advanced disease. In congested patients, intravenous as opposed to oral administration may lead to greater clinical improvement, however at the expense of more severe renal deterioration. It should be emphasized that although diuretic therapy may be essential to relieve symptoms and to treat acute congestion, it has no proven survival benefit. On the other hand, high doses of diuretics are constantly linked to impaired survival of HF patients, albeit there is uncertainty as to whether the use of diuretics has a direct effect on disease progression, or it is just a marker of HF

Table 2.3 Prognostic factors in advanced end-stage heart failure

Demographic/clinical
Advanced age
Male gender
Frequent rehospitalizations
Advanced NYHA class
Intolerance to neurohormonal antagonists
Persistent/relapsing signs of pulmonary or peripheral congestion
Hypotension
Comorbidities (diabetes, renal failure, hepatic failure, anemia, COPD, etc.)
Electrocardiography/laboratory
Resting tachycardia
Wide QRS complex
Hyponatremia
Renal insufficiency
Anemia
Hepatic insufficiency
Neurohormones (norepinephrine, endothelin)
Natriuretic peptides
Cardiac myocyte necrosis markers (troponins)
Inflammatory markers (CRP)
Echo and hemodynamic parameters
Low LV EF/increased LV ESVI
Decreased LV long-axis systolic shortening
Mitral regurgitation/increased left atrial volume
Signs of increased LV filling pressure
Low RV EF
Increased pulmonary vascular resistance/functional capacity
Inability to perform an exercise test
Low peak VO_2 (ml/kg/min, percentage of predicted age, gender, body weight adjusted values)
Increased ventilatory response to exercise (VE/VCO_2 slope)
Low 6-minute walk test distance (<300 m)

Table 2.4 Treatment goals and available strategies for management of end-stage heart failure patients

Goal	Therapy
Improvement of morbidity and mortality	ACE inhibitors ARBs (if ACE inhibitor intolerant) Beta-blockers Mineralocorticosteroid receptor antagonists Ivabradine in selected patients with sinus rhythm CRTs/ICDs in selected patients LVAD as bridge to transplant or destination therapy in selected patients Heart transplantation in selected patients
Control of symptoms	Diuretics Digitalis (very low dose) Consider infusion of inotropes Selected antiarrhythmics
Palliation	Opioids, antidepressants, anxiolytics Oxygen Consider continuous or periodic infusion of inotropes (dobutamine, levosimendan)

deterioration. The problem of diuretic resistance has also been acknowledged in advanced HF patients, and some strategies have been proposed to overcome it, such as higher doses of diuretics, continuous infusion, combination of loop diuretic with a thiazide diuretic, torsemide or bumetanide, a higher dose of mineralocorticosteroid receptor antagonists, inotropes, vasodilators, low-dose dopamine, ultrafiltration, etc (Swedberg et al. 2005; Hunt et al. 2005).

Angiotensin-converting enzyme (ACE) inhibitors are the cornerstone of HF treatment, administered to all patients with left ventricular (LV) systolic dysfunction (LVEF) ≤35–40 % independently of NYHA functional class. They have shown to improve long-term mortality alongside with symptoms, functional capacity, and HF-related hospitalizations. Angiotensin-receptor blockers (ARBs) may also be used for patients intolerant to ACE inhibitors or as an adjunctive therapy in specific subpopulations. High doses of ACE inhibitors, in line with the doses administered in large randomized clinical trials, are favored. In doing so, regular up-titration is important with close monitoring of clinical and biomarker parameters; hypotension, renal dysfunction, hyperkalemia should be avoided. These side effects are actually responsible for the intolerance to ACE inhibitors in advanced HF patients. Symptomatic hypotension and renal failure may warrant dose reduction or even discontinuation of the medication, reflecting and imposing quick clinical deterioration (Kittleson et al. 2003; Nieminen et al. 2005; Swedberg et al. 2005).

Neurohormonal blockage with beta-blockers is another key parameter to improve clinical symptoms and survival of HF patients. Beta-blockers are recommended for all HF patients and should be titrated to optimal doses. However, associated side effects of hypotension, bradyarrhythmias, and fluid detention may prohibit administration of the targeted dose. As such, in advanced HF patients, the tolerated dose of beta-blockers may be very low, or these agents may not even be tolerated at all (Nieminen et al. 2005; Swedberg et al. 2005).

Mineralocorticoid receptor antagonists (MRA) are also recommended to NYHA III–IV patients with reduced ejection fraction already receiving ACE inhibitors/ARBs and beta-blockers. Although randomized clinical trials have shown a significant increase in survival and HF hospitalizations, end-stage HF patients commonly have low glomerular filtration rate which poses a "contraindication" to their use. Moreover, since ACE inhibitors and beta-blockers may already be poorly tolerated, the addition of another agent may be difficult. Now it is clear how useful MRA are in patients who cannot tolerate ACE inhibitors and/or beta-blockers.

It is not therefore a surprise that in advanced stages of HF, there is a remarkable inability to tolerate neurohormonal blockade; in many registries, a relatively low percentage of patients with advanced HF were treated with beta-blockers and ACE inhibitors/ARBs. For a number of these high-risk patients, some therapeutic approaches may still be applied, although never tested in clinical trials. For example captopril, as a short actin agent, may ameliorate symptomatic hypotension problems while maintaining neurohormonal blockage. Alternatively, hydralazine and nitrates can also be used in patients with renal insufficiency or hypotension, although this option has not been adequately studied. In conclusion, intolerance of first-line drugs is a very bad prognostic sign for patients with advanced HF.

A potential further improvement in the medical management of advanced heart failure could be reached in the future, thanks to LCZ 696 (sacubitril-valsartan). This is a novel compound, constituted by the combination of sacubitril and valsartan, recently demonstrated to be superior to enalapril in reducing death by 20 % for cardiovascular causes and hospitalizations by 21 % for heart failure in patients with reduced ejection fraction. Sacubitril is an inhibitor of neprilysin, an enzyme which is responsible for the breakdown of vasoactive peptides that are associated with attenuation of vasoconstriction, sodium retention, and cardiac remodeling (i.e. natriuretic peptides, bradykinin, and adrenomedullin) (Swedberg et al. 2010; McMurray et al. 2014; Filippatos et al. 2015).

Glycosides may be used in HF patients with atrial fibrillation, who are already receiving optimum beta-blocker doses. In HF patients on sinus rhythm, there may be room for low doses of glycosides for individuals with NYHA III–IV functional class and severely impaired LVEF, already treated with ACE inibitors, beta-blockers, aldosterone receptor antagonists, and diuretics. Physicians, however, should be alert to symptoms of bradyarrhythmias and ventricular arrhythmias as a result of high serum concentration levels of glycosides. Renal failure and impaired serum potassium levels are not uncommon in HF patients and may enhance the possibility of potentially life-threatening complications. This is a problem for the routine use of these pharmaceutical agents in advanced stage HF patients. Given its excretion rate and shorter half-life, digitoxin may have a safer profile as compared to digoxin.

Positive inotropic agents are a common, albeit controversial, treatment option for end-stage HF patients. These agents are stratified in two major basic categories: B-adrenergic agonists (dopamine and dobutamine) and phosphodiesterase inhibitors (i.e. milrinone). Their intravenous administration may provide short-term symptom relief in patients with reduced systemic blood pressure and signs of severe peripheral hypoperfusion, however, at the expense of severe arrhythmia and death. This is why these agents have failed to show any survival benefit in large trials. Patients with end-stage HF dependent on intravenous inotropic agents have shown a disappointing 76 % mortality at 130 days of follow-up. Although there still is room for continuous inotropic circulatory support as "bridging therapy" in patients listed for heart transplantation, infection of central venous catheters is a complication that should not be overlooked. Levosimendan is a calcium sensitizer that does not induce tachycardia or increase myocardial consumption. Although documented to improve patients' symptoms, it is not clearly superior to low-cost adrenergic agents, but it can provide some benefit in selected clinical setting and in palliative care. Omecamtiv mecarbil, a novel selective cardiac myosin activator agent, has a conceptually better profile.

There are also less used pharmaceutical agents, which may be of help in various clinical scenarios. Class III antiarrhythmic drugs, including amiodarone, are used to restore and maintain sinus rhythm in HF patients; however, no survival benefit has been demonstrated, and the side effects of pulmonary fibrosis, hepatitis, photosensitivity, and thyroid dysfunction should be taken into account. Anticoagulation is recommended for patients with atrial fibrillation, LV thrombus, or thromboembolic events. Intravenous vasodilators (nitroglycerin, nitroprusside, nesiritide) may be used for symptom relief; however, borderline systemic pressures may be a major concern in end-stage HF patients. Additionally, ivabradine may be administered to patients with sinus rhythm and heart rate greater than 70 bpm, despite adequate dose of beta-blockers—an unlikely clinical scenario for end-stage HF patients. Physicians should be aware of these pharmaceutical options and their limitations. Especially, for end-stage HF patients, the benefit of each pharmaceutical agent should be carefully weighed against the risk, and the decision to treat the patient should be made on an individual basis, considering both side effects and undertreatment. Drug therapy benefit for HF patients has been confirmed in trials using relatively stable patients, and data for end-stage HF patients are scarce. Interestingly, the point when first-line HF medication is poorly tolerated marks the beginning of end-stage HF (Adams and Zannad 1998; Hunt et al. 2005).

2.2.2 Electric Therapy and Other Implantable Devices

Cardiac resynchronization therapy (CRT) is recommended for patients with LBBB, wide QRS complex, impaired LV function, and low functional class (NYHA II–IV), despite optimal medical treatment. For non-LBBB patients, a wider (>150 ms) QRS complex is required. The efficacy of this strategy is based on the concept that delayed conduction of the electric stimulus is associated to noncoordinated contraction mechanisms of the left ventricle. Restoration of electromechanical coordination leads to a clear improvement in peak oxygen uptake, walking distance, and quality of life in line with LV reverse remodeling of these patients. Atrial fibrillation reduces the effectiveness of therapy and is a common clinical problem in end-stage HF patients. In terminal stage patients unsuitable for CRT, there are also several factors limiting overall CRT benefit, such as extensive myocardial scar, pulmonary hypertension, renal failure, and RV dysfunction. CRT has in fact been criticized for a relatively high rate (33 %) of nonresponders, which may actually be higher in terminal stage HF patients. Nevertheless, proponents of this approach point out that the annual mortality of eligible non-CRT treated patients (12.6 %) may equal or exceed that of patients suffering from aggressive cancers, and less effective and more costly therapies than CRT have never been denied for them. Awareness of this option has increased in the last years among clinical cardiologists, and a gradually increasing number of HF patients are currently treated with CRT according to standard recommendations.

There are preliminary data showing that CRT nonresponders with significant mitral regurgitation may benefit from a mitraclip procedure. An implantable cardioverter–defibrillator (ICD) is also recommended for primary prevention in symptomatic (NYHA II–IV) patients with LVEF ≤35 % to reduce the incidence of sudden death and also for secondary prevention in HF patients with documented symptomatic ventricular arrythmias. Combination of CRT and ICD enhances survival (CRT/D). The option of ICD deactivation has been offered in terminal stage HF patients to improve the quality of their remaining life (Swedberg et al. 2005; Hunt et al. 2005; Friedrich and Bohm 2007).

Preliminary data show that patients with significant mitral regurgitation may benefit from a mitraclip procedure. Mitraclip is a device that, inserted percutaneously, may reduce the hemodynamic impact of mitral regurgitation. The role of this percutaneous mitral valve “repair” of functional mitral regurgitation is currently being extensively tested, and it could emerge as a potential strategy to improve symptoms and prognosis in patients deemed unsuitable for traditional mitral valve repair.

2.2.3 Mechanical Circulatory Support

LV assist device (LVAD) or biventricular assist device (BiVAD) may be considered for patients refractory to medical and CRT device treatment, given the paucity of other available prospects. This approach concerns HF patients with LVEF < 25 %, dependent on intravenous inotropic agents, progressive end-organ dysfunction, deteriorating right ventricular function requiring frequent hospitalization for HF. Long-term survival of patients treated with mechanical circulatory support is better than those treated medically only; however, the devices may not be affordable for many healthcare providers. Right ventricular function should be carefully evaluated before implantation, and BiVAD should be preferred over LVAD when there is a high chance of postoperative right ventricular failure. Bleeding, thromboembolism, hemolysis, infection, and device failure are possible complications. Early referral of end-stage patients for device implantation is crucial, since an elective rather than an emergency procedure is more successful. Mechanical circulatory support therapy may be used as a bridge to transplantation or even as a destination therapy in selected patients. With the existing evidence, BiVAD is indicated only as a bridge to cardiac transplantation. In some cases, the term "bridge to candidacy" describes the temporary use of mechanical circulatory support in order to reverse pulmonary hypertension and/or obesity in individuals not otherwise eligible for heart transplantation. Sometimes, LV function may improve to a point where mechanical support is no longer needed (bridge to recovery) (Hunt et al. 2005; Friedrich and Bohm 2007; McMurray et al. 2012; Lund et al. 2010; Feldman et al. 2013) (see also Chap. 3). (Ref 14).

2.2.4 Other Surgical Therapies

Initial enthusiasm for aggressive surgical interventions in advanced HF patients has been toned down following the disappointing results of ventricular reconstruction trials. Revascularization is indicated in cases of documented viable myocardium when coronary artery anatomy is feasible. Mitral valve repair or replacement may be indicated in specific populations. Critical aortic stenosis may also be surgically treated when indicated.

2.2.5 Palliative Treatment

As part of the holistic approach to end-stage heart failure disease, there comes a kairotic moment: deciding whether to divert the target of treatment from prolonging life to improving the quality of the remaining life only. There is no unanimous agreement as to when, but detailed informed consent of patients is essential, and their wishes concerning invasive strategies should be considered, in accordance with the laws of the countries.

2.2.6 Transplantation

Despite therapeutic advancements and novel devices, transplantation still remains the sole therapeutic strategy able to radically change the natural history of advanced heart failure. Patients with end-stage HF, despite guideline-recommended medical, device, and surgical management, are potential candidates for transplantation. This procedure is considered the gold standard treatment for terminal stage, with an impressive 71.7 % rate of 5-year survival. Compared with medical treatment alone, functional capacity and quality of life improve dramatically after the operation as do return to work rates. Potential candidates are referred to a specialized cardiac transplantation center for further evaluation. Possible contraindications for transplantation are: age > 70 years, body mass index > 30 kg/m^2, active malignancy, pulmonary hypertension, uncontrolled diabetes, severe renal dysfunction, peripheral vascular disease, HIV and hepatitis C infection, current smoking, alcohol or illicit drug abuse, psychiatric illness, dementia, mental retardation, but not all are absolute, and the final decision is always individualized. Cardiopulmonary exercise testing also plays an important role for optimal selection of candidates. Given the shortage of donors, a dedicated team should ensure high-quality screening of possible candidates and management of patients awaiting transplantation (Hunt et al. 2005; Friedrich and Bohm 2007; McMurray et al. 2012; Mehra et al. 2006). A reasonable algorithm for the treatment of advanced end-stage HF is given in Fig. 2.1 (Friedrich and Bohm 2007; McMurray et al. 2012; Lund et al. 2010; Jaarsma et al. 2009).

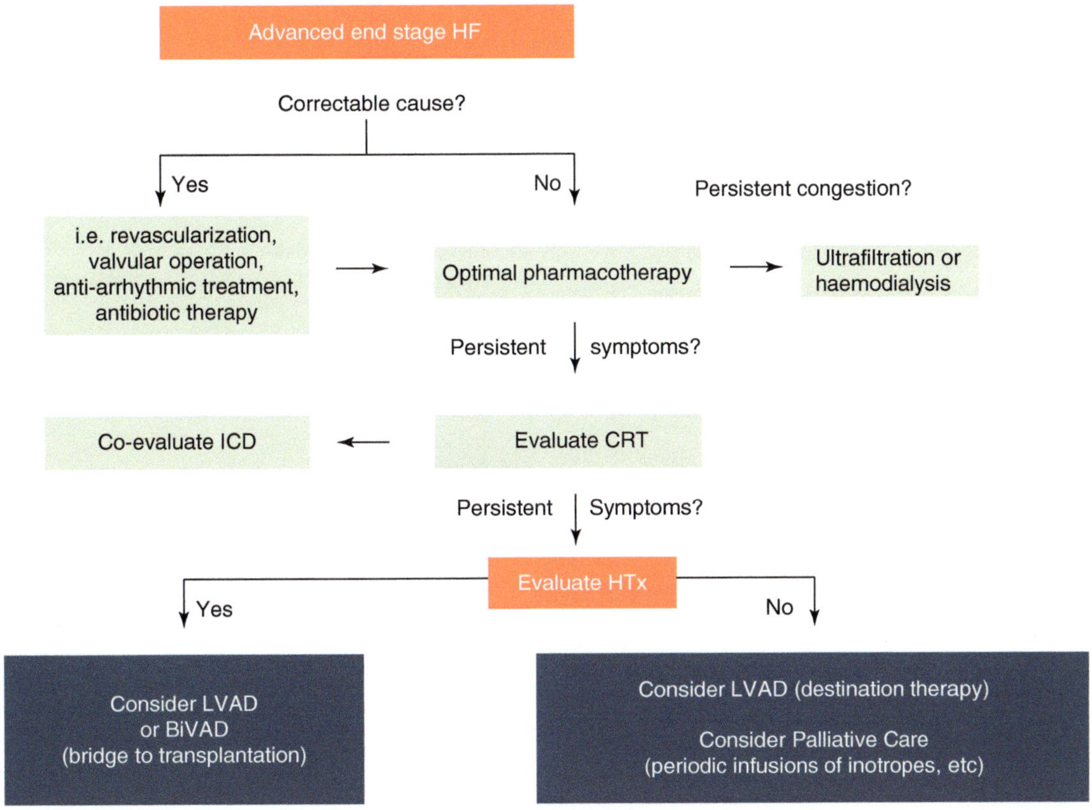

Fig. 2.1 Treatment algorithm of advanced end-stage heart failure (Modified from Friedrich and Bohm 2007). *ICD* implantable cardioverter–defibrillator, *CRT* cardiac resynchronization therapy, *HTx* heart transplantation, *VAD* ventricular assist device, *BiVAD* biventricular assist device

Key Points

- Heart failure is the clinical syndrome resulting from the acute or chronic inability of the cardiovascular system to maintain full oxygen supply and metabolic function of peripheral organs. Advanced heart failure occurs when cardiac disease progresses extensively and standard treatments are unable to relieve symptoms and prevent clinical deterioration.
- Advanced heart failure has a significant mortality rate comparable or even higher than most malignancies.
- The key to medical therapy is mainly drugs disrupting the neurohormonal mechanisms responsible for clinical syndrome progression; diuretics are necessary to control symptoms, but do not have a clear prognostic benefit; inotropic agents may be used in selected critical acute conditions, or as palliative care.
- Implantable devices including RCT/ICD may improve prognosis and symptoms in a subgroup of patients.
- Heart transplantation and ventricular assist devices are effective surgical strategies for a selected subgroup of patients with few comorbidities and severe refractory heart failure.

References

Adams Jr KF, Zannad F. Clinical definition and epidemiology of advanced heart failure. Am Heart J. 1998; 135(6 Pt 2 Suppl):S204–15.

Feldman D, Pamboukian SV, Teuteberg JJ, Birks E, Lietz K, Moore SA, Morgan JA, Arabia F, Bauman ME, Buchholz HW, Deng M, Dickstein ML, El-Banayosy A, Elliot T, Goldstein DJ, Grady KL, Jones K, Hryniewicz K, John R, Kaan A, Kusne S, Loebe M, Massicotte MP, Moazami N, Mohacsi P, Mooney M, Nelson T, Pagani F, Perry W, Potapov EV, Eduardo Rame J, Russell SD, Sorensen EN, Sun B, Strueber M, Mangi AA, Petty MG, Rogers J, International Society for Heart and Lung Transplantation. The 2013 International Society for Heart and Lung Transplantation Guidelines for mechanical circulatory support: executive summary. J Heart Lung Transplant. 2013;32(2):157–87. doi:10.1016/j.healun.2012.09.013.

Filippatos G, Farmakis D, Parissis J, Lekakis J. Drug therapy for patients with systolic heart failure after the PARADIGM-HF trial: in need of a new paradigm of LCZ696 implementation in clinical practice. BMC Med. 2015;13:35.

Friedrich EB, Bohm M. Management of end stage heart failure. Heart. 2007;93:626–31.

Hunt SA, Abraham WT, Chin MH, et al. ACC/AHA 2005 guideline update for the diagnosis and management of chronic heart failure in the adult-summary article. A report of the American College of Cardiology/American Heart Association. Task Force on Practice Guidelines (Writing Committee to Update the 2001 Guidelines for the Evaluation and Management of Heart Failure). J Am Coll Cardiol. 2005;46:1116–43.

Jaarsma T, Beattie JM, Ryder M, Rutten FH, McDonagh T, Mohacsi P, Murray SA, Grodzicki T, Bergh I, Metra M, Ekman I, Angermann C, Leventhal M, Pitsis A, Anker SD, Gavazzi A, Ponikowski P, Dickstein K, Delacretaz E, Blue L, Strasser F, McMurray J, Advanced Heart Failure Study Group of the HFA of the ESC. Palliative care in heart failure: a position statement from the palliative care workshop of the Heart Failure Association of the European Society of Cardiology. Eur J Heart Fail. 2009;11(5):433–43.

Kittleson M, Hurwitz S, Shah MR, et al. Development of circulatory-renal limitations to angiotensin-converting enzyme inhibitors identifies patients with severe heart failure and early mortality. J Am Coll Cardiol. 2003; 41:2029–35.

Lund LH, Matthews J, Aaronson K. Patient selection for left ventricular assist devices. Eur J Heart Fail. 2010;12:434–43.

Maisel A, Filippatos G. Heart failure: the expert's approach. Jaypee Brothers, New Delhi, India, 2014.

McMurray JJ, Adamopoulos S, Anker SD, et al. ESC guidelines for the diagnosis and treatment of acute and chronic heart failure 2012: The Task Force for the Diagnosis and Treatment of Acute and Chronic Heart Failure 2012 of the European Society of Cardiology. Developed in collaboration with the Heart Failure Association (HFA) of the ESC. Eur J Heart Fail. 2012;14:803–6.

McMurray JJ, Packer M, Desai AS, Gong J, Lefkowitz MP, Rizkala AR, Rouleau JL, Shi VC, Solomon SD, Swedberg K, Zile MR, PARADIGM-HF Investigators and Committees. Angiotensin-neprilysin inhibition versus enalapril in heart failure. N Engl J Med. 2014; 371:993–1004.

Mehra MR, Kobashigawa J, Starling R, Russell S, Uber PA, Parameshwar J, Mohacsi P, Augustine S, Aaronson K, Barr M. Listing criteria for heart transplantation: International Society for Heart and Lung Transplantation guidelines for the care of cardiac transplant candidates – 2006. J Heart Lung Transplant. 2006;25(9):1024–42.

Metra M, Ponikowski P, Dickstein K, et al. Advanced chronic heart failure: a position statement from the Study Group on Advanced Heart Failure of the Heart Failure Association of the European Society of Cardiology. Eur J Heart Fail. 2007;9(6–7):684–94.

Nieminen MS, Bohm M, Cowie MR, et al. Executive summary of the guidelines on the diagnosis and treatment of acute heart failure: the Task Force on Acute Heart Failure of the European Society of Cardiology. Eur Heart J. 2005;26:384–416.

Swedberg K, Cleland J, Dargie H, et al. Guidelines for the diagnosis and treatment of chronic heart failure: executive summary (update 2005): the Task Force for the Diagnosis and Treatment of Chronic Heart Failure of the European Society of Cardiology. Eur Heart J. 2005;26:1115–40.

Swedberg K, Komajda M, Böhm M, Borer JS, Ford I, Dubost-Brama A, Lerebours G, Tavazzi L, SHIFT Investigators. Ivabradine and outcomes in chronic heart failure (SHIFT): a randomised placebo-controlled study. Lancet. 2010;376(9744):875–85. doi:10.1016/S0140-6736(10)61198-1.

Zannad F, Mebazaa A, Juilliére Y, et al. Clinical profile, contemporary management and one-year mortality in patients with severe acute heart failure syndromes: the EFICA study. Eur J Heart Fail. 2006;8:697–705.

Mechanical Circulatory Support in End-Stage Heart Failure: Bridge to Transplantation and Destination Therapy

3

Alexander Stepanenko, Evgenij Potapov, Volkmar Falk, and Thomas Krabatsch

Contents

A. Stepanenko, MD (✉) • E. Potapov, MD, PhD
V. Falk, MD, PhD
Department of Cardiothoracic and Vascular Surgery, German Heart Institute Berlin, Berlin, Germany
e-mail: stepanenkoal@mail.ru

T. Krabatsch, MD, PhD
Department of Cardiothoracic and Vascular Surgery, German Heart Center Berlin, DZHK (German Center for Cardiovascular Research), Partner Site Berlin, Berlin, Germany

3.1 Background

Advances in medical treatment and the use of implantable defibrillators and cardiac resynchronization therapy have significantly improved the outcome of patients with advanced heart failure (Slaughter et al. 2009).

However, the number of patients who become refractory to these forms of treatment is constantly growing. In the case of acute deterioration and onset of cardiogenic shock, despite optimal medical and device therapy, short-term circulatory support with temporary support devices has been shown to be a valuable tool for cardiopulmonary stabilization and bridging to the next therapy step: heart transplantation or implantation of a long-term device, with the possibility of myocardial recovery.

Heart transplantation is still the gold standard for the treatment of end-stage heart failure. Hence, the acute mismatch between the number of donor organs available and the number of patients on the waiting list has increased the demand for mechanical circulatory support for bridging to heart transplantation or transplant eligibility and long-term support.

The clinical appearance of advanced heart failure varies. Most patients suffer from systolic heart failure resulting in continuously decreasing systolic function mainly of the left ventricle. A significant proportion of patients develop diastolic heart failure, which results in an increase in filling pressure and a decrease in stroke volume.

O. Leone et al. (eds.), *The Pathology of Cardiac Transplantation*,
DOI 10.1007/978-3-319-46386-5_3

In patients with isolated left ventricular dysfunction, a left ventricular assist device (LVAD) support, where blood is bypassed from the left ventricular apex to the ascending aorta or descending aorta, is usually sufficient. Prior to implantation, it must be ensured that right ventricular function is not severely impaired. In case of maintained right ventricular function, a left ventricular mechanical circulatory support device can deliver the whole volume that is reaching the left atrium to the systemic circulation. Mean blood pressure remains between 60 and 80 mmHg, with the pump producing flow of 4–7 l/min (full support pumps) or 2–4 l/min (partial support pumps). Pulsatile flow devices produce artificial ejection, mimicking the physiological heart cycle; hence, they work asynchronously with fixed stroke rate. The smallest pulsatile pump has a 10-ml blood chamber, and adult pulsatile pumps produce an artificial stroke volume of up to 80 ml.

Continuous flow VADs bypass the heart and pump blood volume independently of the heart cycle, producing a continuous flow profile in the aorta. In this case, there is no or little native ejection through the aortic valve (depending on the residual LV function), and the aortic valve leaflets may remain closed. Therefore, no pulse wave is present. Ultrasound devices or invasive methods are used for the assessment of mean arterial pressure. This kind of "unphysiological" pulseless circulation does not negatively affect end-organ function, cognitive function, or the microcirculation (Petrucci et al. 2012; Potapov et al. 2012), but may impair the structure of the aortic valve leaflets, and sometimes lead to aortic insufficiency during longer assist periods (Aggarwal et al. 2013).

Patients who present some contractility of the LV following LV unloading and/or myocardial recovery eject blood through the aortic valve. This additional cardiac output contributes little to the whole body perfusion, but it leads to an adequate blood wash-out phenomenon at the aortic root and diminishes the risk of thrombus formation in the valve area.

Early onset or late right ventricular failure in patients with an LVAD may lead to decreased pump output due to diminished transpulmonary flow and to low pump flow with subsequent hypoperfusion of the end organs and, ultimately, multiorgan failure. To avoid this dramatic complication, appropriate device selection and implanting strategy are crucial (Potapov et al. 2008a). Once the right ventricle is failing, temporary right ventricular support with short-term devices may be necessary as a bridge to RV recovery or to a permanent RVAD. If temporary RV dysfunction is expected, temporary RVAD support is started at the time of LVAD implantation and progressively weaned over weeks according to RV recovery.

When patients that present with advanced heart failure become refractory to therapy, with the involvement of both ventricles, biventricular mechanical circulatory support is required using biventricular VAD (BVAD) or a total artificial heart (TAH). BVAD support may be given with implantable pumps, using two continuous flow LVAD with one adapted for RV support, or with two extracorporeal pneumatic pumps connected to the major vessels and heart chambers by polyurethane cannulas (Berlin Heart Excor, Berlin Heart, Berlin, Germany; Thoratec, Thoratec Corporation, Pleasanton, CA, USA).

The total artificial heart is a pulsatile system containing two artificial ventricles with four valves: mechanical valves as in the temporary CardioWest total artificial heart TAH-t, Syncardia, Tucson, AZ, USA, or the Abiomed device, Abiomed Inc., Danvers, MA, USA; or biological valves as in the CARMAT TAH, CARMAT SA, France. There are some reports of the use of two adapted continuous flow LVAD connected to patients' atria and major vessels used as a continuous-flow TAH.

3.2 Devices

3.2.1 Left Ventricular Devices (Extracorporeal, Implantable)

In the current era, over 90 % of the LVADs are implantable continuous-flow pumps.

These consist of the pump body with rotor and pump housing, inflow cannula (integrated or connected), outflow graft/cannula, driveline, and driver or controller with energy source.

- *Inflow cannula*:
  (a) Material: titanium, sintered (HeartWare HVAD, M-VAD, HeartMate II, HeartMate III, Jarvik 2000), or polished (DuraHeart), complex (silicon/titanium, Incor), polyurethane cannula penetrating the skin (Berlin Heart Excor);
  (b) Insertion site: LV apex, LA in special cases (Excor, Abiomed, or Thoratec, e.g. in patients with restrictive cardiomyopathy);
  (c) Fixation to LV myocardium/sewing ring with interrupted or continuous felt-pledgeted sutures;
  (d) Optimal orientation toward the mitral valve, without contact to the LV wall.

Different devices have shown different kinds of integration into the internal surface of the LV chamber with "neo-intima" formation (Fig. 3.1).

- *Pump body*:
  (a) Material: titanium (all implantable devices), polyurethane (Excor);
  (b) Blood propulsion: volume displacement or rotary pumping using impeller;
  (c) Generated flow profile: centrifugal, axial, radial, pulsatile (pneumatic, electromechanic);
  (d) Bearings: ruby (HM II), hydrodynamic/passive magnetic (HVAD, HM III), electromechanical (Jarvik 2000), electromagnetic (INCOR, DuraHeart, HM III);
  (e) Implant position: intrapericardial (HVAD, Jarvik 2000, HM III, INCOR, HeartAssist 5), requiring pump pocket within abdominal wall (HM II, DuraHeart) or extracorporeal (Excor) (Fig. 3.2).
- *Outflow cannula*:
  (a) Dacron graft (HVAD, HM II, HM III, Jarvik 2000, HeartAssist 5, new version of Incor), silicon cannula (old version of

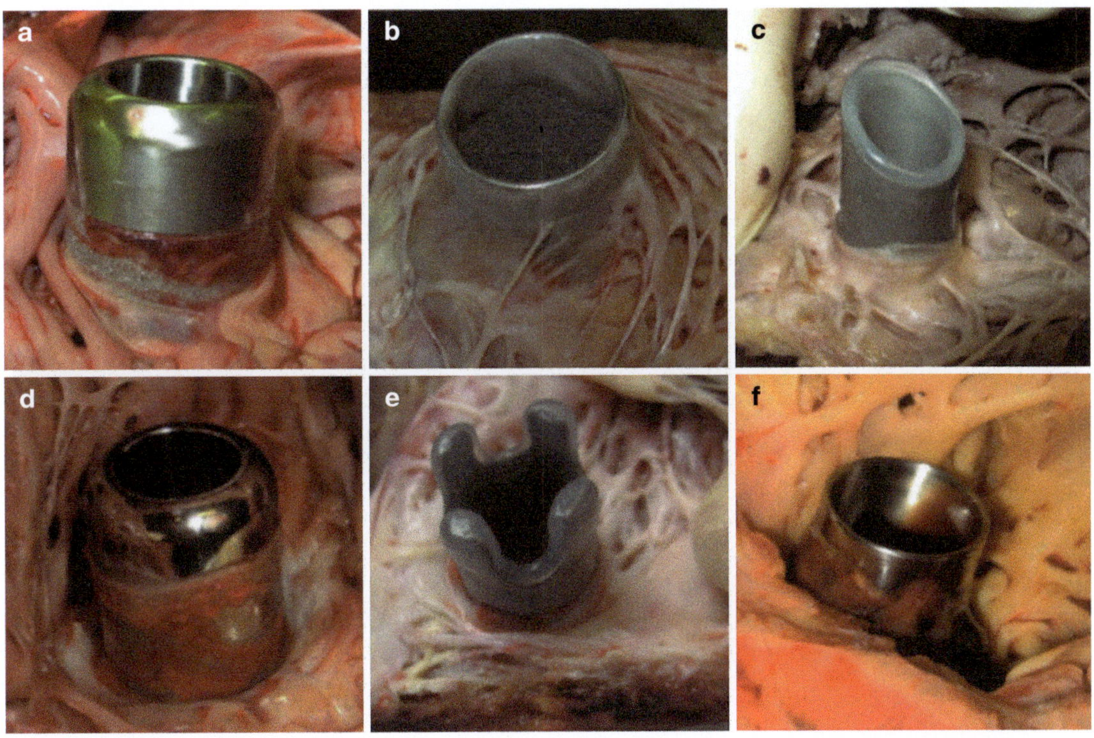

Fig. 3.1 Different types of inflow cannula present different tissue integration and "neo-intima" formation. (**a**) HeartWare cintered; (**b**) HM II; (**c**) Excor; (**d**) HeartWare noncintered; (**e**) Incor; (**f**) DuraHeart

Incor), polyurethane cannula penetrating the skin (Excor);
(b) Kinking protection/strain relief (HM II, HVAD);
(c) Anastomosis with ascending aorta or descending aorta using running or interrupted prolene sutures.

- *Driveline*:
  (a) Subcutaneous tunneling (oblique or C-shaped) with abdominal fascia perforation in the epigastral region, neck tunneling with retroauricular pedestal fixation at temporal bone (Jarvik 2000)
  (b) Exit site: Right or left lateral abdominal quadrant. It is preferable to avoid crossing the linea alba (later need for abdominal surgery, interaction with chest tubes/infection)
  (c) Tissue integration: Dacron velour covered part, silicon, titanium pedestal (Jarvik 2000) (Fig. 3.3)

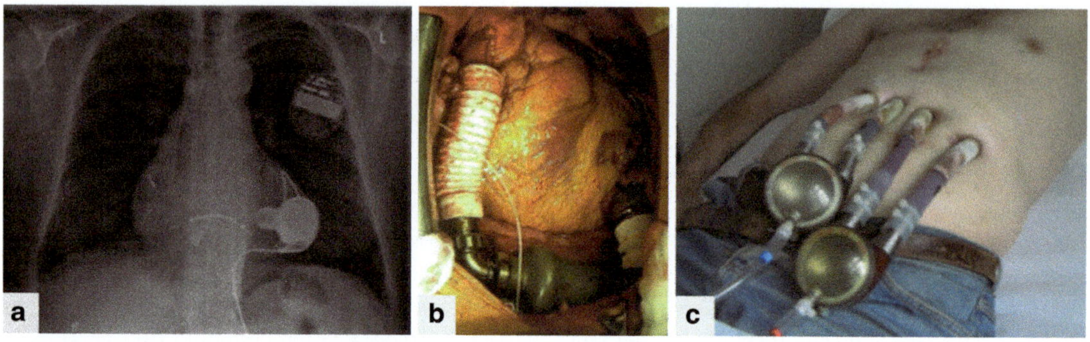

Fig. 3.2 Implant position. (**a**) HeartWare placed intrapericardially (postoperative X-ray); (**b**) HM pump body placed in created pocket (intraoperative view); (**c**) extracorporeal pump body connected to the heart chambers via long cannulas—Excor BVAD (outpatient study)

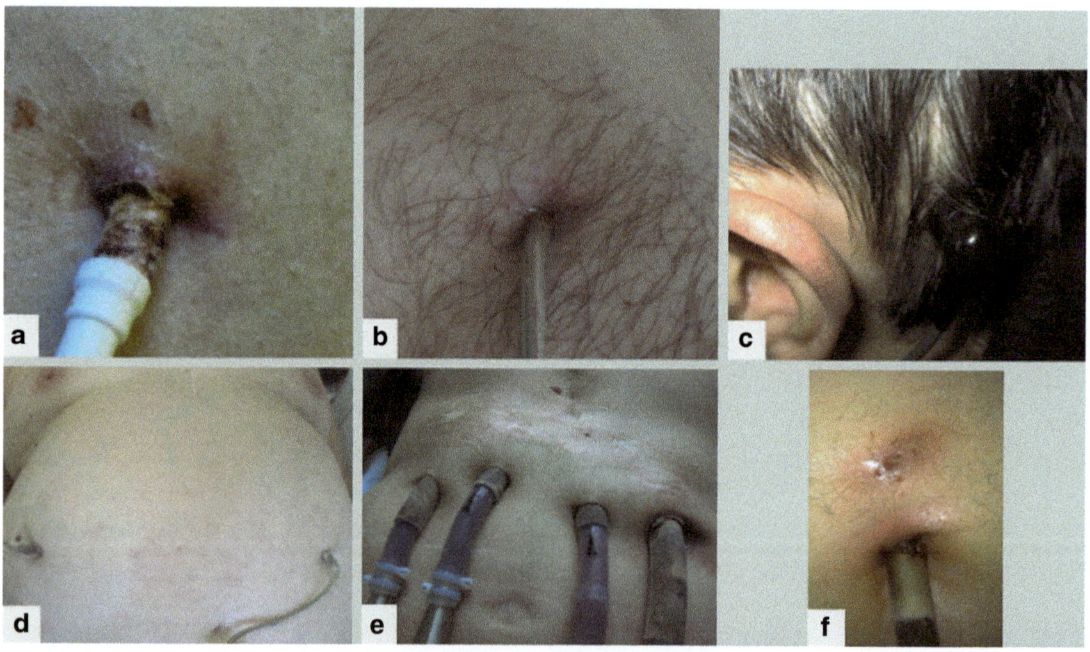

Fig. 3.3 Driveline incorporation at exit site. (**a**) HM II; (**b**) HeartWare LVAD; (**c**) Jarvik 2000 (postaurical pedestal); (**d**) HeartWare BVAD; (**e**) Excor (chronic irritation and local infection of LV-apex cannula, other three with good incorporation signs); (**f**) Incor (local infection with abscess formation along driveline)

The driveline is connected to a digital controller, lithium batteries (implantable LVADs) or to a pneumatic driver (Excor, Thoratec, CardioWest).

- *Controller and batteries*:
  (a) Air compressor (Excor, CardioWest), polyurethane tubing connecting to pump chamber, manual pump for emergencies.
  (b) The controller runs the pump and also provides text messages and audible alarms to aid system operation management.
  (c) Lithium ion batteries, cable connection of the power unit to electricity from a wall or car outlet (Fig. 3.4).
- *Implantation techniques*:
  (a) *Using cardiopulmonary bypass or extracorporeal life support through a full sternotomy (HM II, HM III, HeartWare HVAD and MVAD, DuraHeart, Incor, Jarvik 2000, HeartAssist 5).* After conventional full sternotomy and systemic heparinization, cannulation of the right atrium, using a two-stage cannula, and of the ascending aorta is performed. Cardiopulmonary bypass (CPB) with normothermia is initiated. The LV apex is exposed. The apical fixation tool is usually attached with 10–14 mattress sutures of 3–0 felt-reinforced polypropylene positioned around the apex. During a short period of induced ventricular fibrillation, a full-thickness cruciate incision inside the sewing ring is made using a special coring tool. At this time, the driveline is pulled from the pericardial space below the costal arch into the subcutaneous abdominal tissue and brought through the skin in the lower abdominal quadrant with a subcutaneous route of at least 10 cm. The aorta is partially clamped, and the distal anastomosis of the outflow graft and the ascending aorta is accomplished using a continuous polypropylene suture. Final de-airing of the outflow graft is done before the distal anastomosis is completed.
  (b) *Minimally invasive (bilateral thoracotomy/partial sternotomy), CPB standby.* The patient is placed in supine position and intubated with a double lumen tube. The first incision is made in the third right intercostal space close to the sternum, the aorta is partially clamped in its lateral portion, and anastomosis with the graft is performed. Optionally, an upper partial sternotomy may be used to approach the ascending aorta; the second incision is performed in the fifth or sixth left intercostal space, depending on the position of the LV apex. The fixation ring is attached to the apex, and the graft is passed intrapericardially under the sternum to the LV apex and connected to the pump. The driveline is tunneled out of the skin and connected to the controller. The LV apex is cored and the pump placed into the LV during continuous de-airing, fixed, and started. The procedure is done on the beating heart. If necessary, CPB can be used employing femorofemoral cannulation (Potapov and Krabatsch 2014; Hetzer et al. 2004; Cheung et al. 2011) (Fig. 3.5).

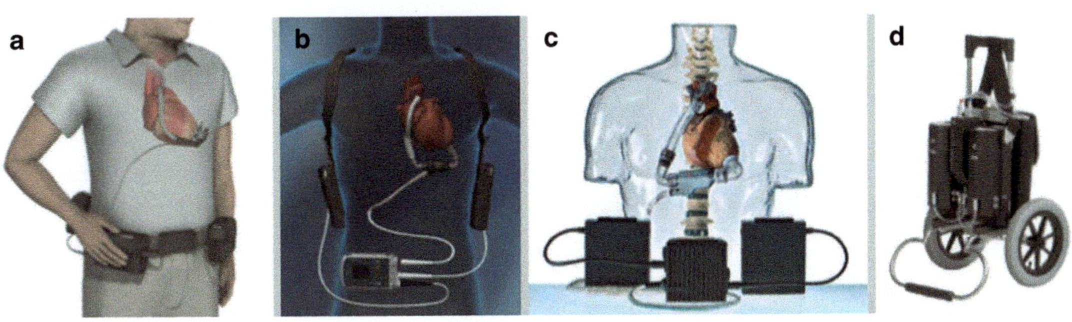

Fig. 3.4 External components. (**a**) HeartWare; (**b**) HeartMate II; (**c**) Incor; (**d**) Excor

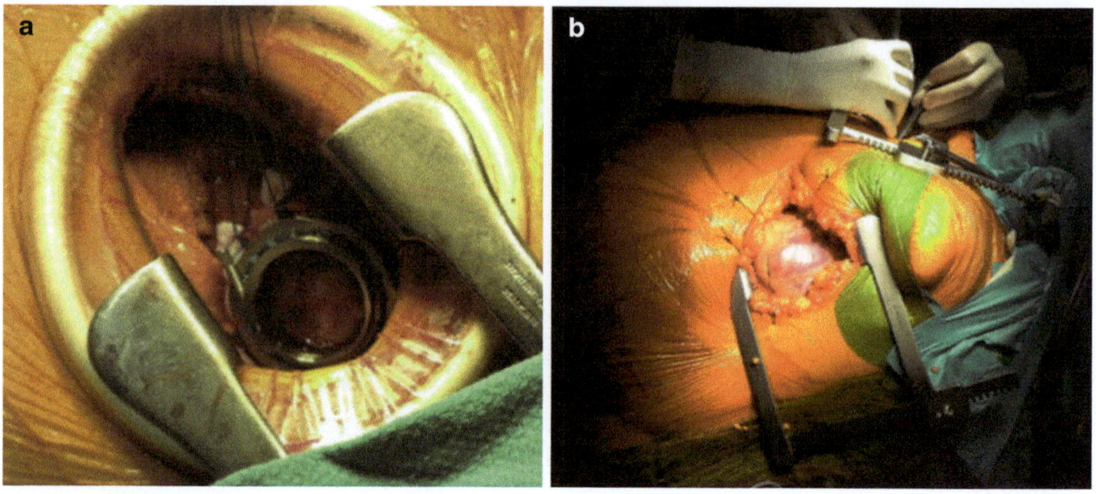

Fig. 3.5 Intraoperative view. (**a**) LV apex exposed via left-sided minithoracotomy in sixth intercostal space. (**b**) Surgeon performing outflow graft anastomosis via separate incision in the second intercostal space to the right of the sternum

(c) *Implantation technique through left lateral thoracotomy after previous cardiac operations*. In patients who have had previous cardiac operations via a median sternotomy severe adhesions may complicate intraoperative dissection. Additionally, open bypasses may cross the midline and be at increased risk for intraoperative damage. In such cases, approaching the left ventricle and descending aorta through a median sternotomy avoids these complications. In selected cases, the implantation may be performed with CPB on standby. After the patient is placed in the right lateral decubitus position with the left hip rolled back, the groin vessels are prepared and a left lateral thoracotomy is performed in the fifth intercostal space. The left lung is deflated, and the pulmonary ligament is transected up to the hilum. Placement of the sewing ring, pump insertion, and driveline tunneling are performed as described in (b). The proximal part of the descending aorta is partially excluded using a Satinsky clamp. A short longitudinal incision is made, and the distal anastomosis of the outflow graft and the descending thoracic aorta is accomplished using a continuous polypropylene suture. Tunneling of the driveline, final de-airing, and starting the LVAD are as described above (Hetzer et al. 2004) (Fig. 3.6).

3.2.2 Biventricular Devices (Extracorporeal, Implantable)

Up to 10 % of patients with end-stage heart failure experience biventricular failure that requires biventricular support. For these patients, only two long-term options are available: the total artificial heart (CardioWest, SynCardia, Tucson, AZ), which requires that the native heart be excised, and the biventricular assist device (BVAD), which uses either bulky extracorporeal or implantable displacement pumps (Krabatsch et al. 2011).

Due to improved patient selection, better understanding of right ventricular function, and early referral (preferably before RV failure), the number of individuals who require biventricular support has decreased in recent years (Kirklin et al. 2014). However, there are still patients in whom isolated LVAD support is insufficient and who are in need of biventricular support.

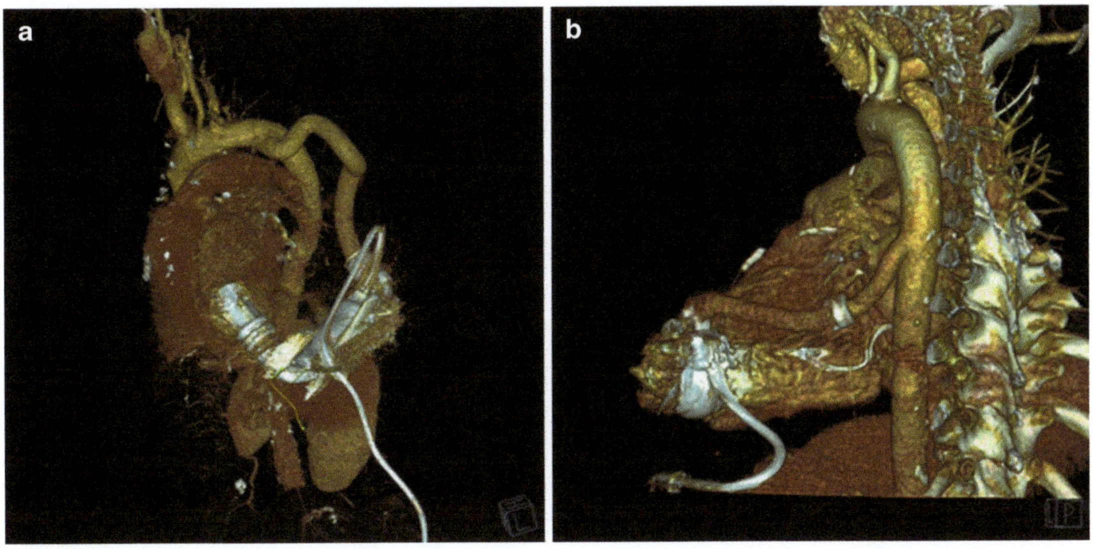

Fig. 3.6 CT scan reconstruction of LVAD implanted via left lateral thoracotomy with outflow graft connection to descending aorta: (**a**) HeartMate II; (**b**) HeartWare

3.2.2.1 Pulsatile Extracorporeal BVAD (Berlin Heart Excor)

Since the first clinical implementation of the Berlin Heart Excor device in Berlin, Germany, in the late 1980s, thousands of adults and also children have been treated with it as a bridge to heart transplantation, recovery, or destination therapy all over the world (Potapov et al. 2008b). In the recent past, this system has been most widely used in the pediatric setting.

After conventional full sternotomy and systemic heparinization, the ascending aorta and right atrium are cannulated. Cardiopulmonary bypass with normothermia is initiated. First, the left ventricular cannula is inserted. The incision is made on the left ventricular apex in the coronary-free area, and the left ventricular cannula is inserted and secured by previously placed mattress sutures supported with Teflon pledgets. Next, a side-biting clamp is placed on the ascending cannula proximal to the previously inserted aortic cannula for CPB, the aorta is incised above the clamp, and the VAD aortic cannula is fixed with continuous or mattress sutures. Afterward, the cannulas are tunneled through the skin via tight-fitting skin incisions and the pump, filled with physiological solution, is connected to the cannulas. Residual air bubbles are evacuated through a de-airing nipple that is integrated into the blood chamber, assist circulation is begun, and CPB is stopped (Hetzer et al. 2006) (Fig. 3.7).

3.2.2.2 Continuous-Flow Implantable BVAD

Since the introduction of implantable rotary blood pumps into clinical practice, there have been many attempts to adapt these pumps, once developed as left ventricular assist devices, for support of the failing right ventricle. With minor modifications of the peripheral equipment that address the lower resistance of the pulmonary circulation and anatomical issues, rotary blood-pump technology may provide an alternative in destination therapy for biventricular failure (Krabatsch et al. 2011; Kirklin et al. 2014; Strueber et al. 2010; Hetzer et al. 2010). The implantation is performed on CPB. The technique for LVAD implantation is similar to that described above; the RVAD may by connected to the diaphragmatic part or to the free wall of the right ventricle. One of the attractive sites for insertion of the inflow cannula of the implant-

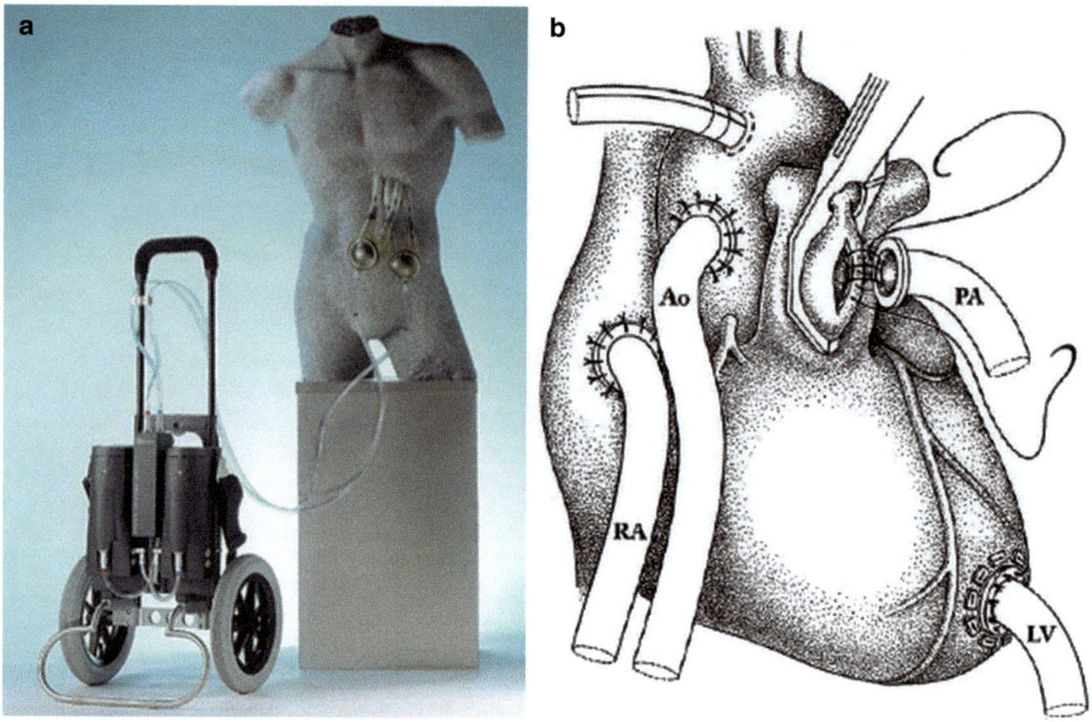

Fig. 3.7 (**a**) Berlin Heart Excor driver, connecting air tubes, pumps. (**b**) Surgical connection to the heart chambers (*RA* right atrium, *AO* aorta, *LV* LV apex, *PA* pulmonary artery)

able RVAD is the right atrium. In this case, the pump is placed outside of the pericardium into the right pleural space. The outflow graft is connected to the pulmonary artery (Fig. 3.8).

3.2.3 Total Artificial Heart

In patients who have severe biventricular failure, or if conventional connection to the heart chambers is challenging due to technical, anatomical, or pathological issues, the total artificial heart (TAH) is one of the options. Indications for its use are irreversible biventricular failure, irreversible cardiac rejection, massive myocardial infarction with or without ventricular septal defect, and massive cardiac thrombosis.

Unlike the previously described devices, a pulsatile total artificial heart is implanted into the chest in orthotopic position after the diseased heart has been explanted leaving cuffs of both atria. Both artificial ventricles are connected to patients' atria, and the major vessels produce one-way pulsatile flow (four mechanical valves). This allows the filling pressures to be kept low and the pump flow high, up to 8.4 L/min. Both drivelines are tunneled out of the skin in the epigastric region and connected to the pneumatic driver (Fig. 3.9). The only commercially available pulsatile TAH is the CardioWest-t (Copeland et al. 2004).

3.3 Survival, Long-Term Effects, and Complications

According to INTERMACS data, overall survival in patients supported with implantable rotary blood pumps is approximately 80 % at 1 year and 70 % at 2 years. Regarding biventricular support, recipients of implantable continuous flow BVAD had a better survival rate at 1 year than those with pulsatile systems: 57 % vs 45 %, respectively. Fifty-nine percent of recipients of the CardioWest-t total artificial heart survived at 1 year.

Since permanent support with ventricular assist devices has become a reality, an increasing number of patients are being supported for several years. Implantation of a VAD as destination

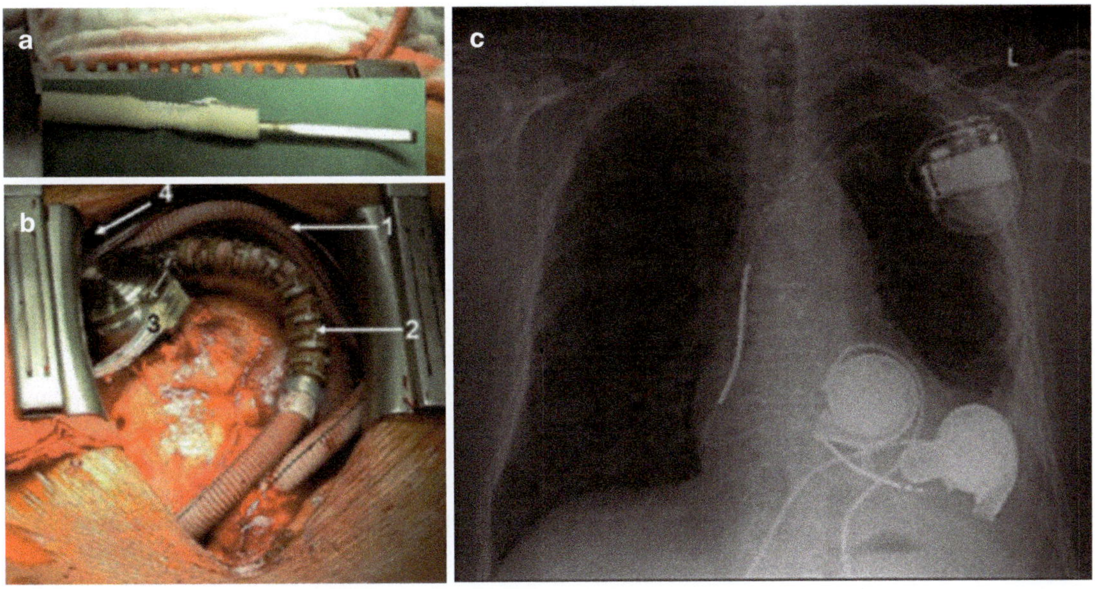

Fig. 3.8 (**a**) The narrowing of the right ventricular assist device (RVAD) outflow graft is produced before surgery by suturing 3 cm of the graft with 6-0 Prolene 2 cm from the outflow connector over a 5-mm Hegar dilator introduced into the graft. (**b**) Intraoperative view shows both pumps: *1*, outflow graft of the left ventricular assist device (LVAD) connected to the ascending artery; *2*, outflow graft of the RVAD connected to the pulmonary artery; *3*, pump of the RVAD connected to the free wall of the right ventricle; *4*, the pump of the LVAD is connected to the LV apex and is not shown (Hetzer 2010). (**c**) X-ray of two HVAD implanted as BVAD

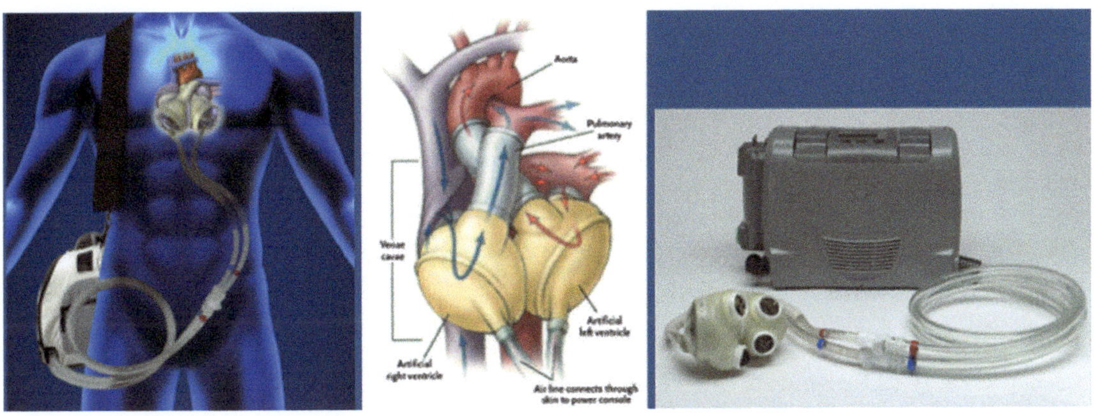

Fig. 3.9 Implantable and external components of the CardioWest-t total artificial heart

therapy or for long-term support has almost doubled during the past 6 years and now represents 43 % of all implants (Kirklin et al. 2014).

3.3.1 Thrombo-embolic and Bleeding Complications

Ventricular assist devices affect the coagulation system. All pumps come into contact with blood, and through surface activation of the clotting cascade promote thrombosis and thromboembolic events. Freedom from any thrombembolic event at 1 year is currently 85–92 % (Slaughter et al. 2009; Najjar et al. 2014). Strict anticoagulation is therefore necessary, and may in turn cause bleeding complications.

Flow stagnation around the VAD cannula or diseased myocardium, exposure to foreign surfaces (VAD cannulas and pump body), and changes in coagulation balance (over-anticoagulation, onset of acquired von Willebrand factor disease, platelet deficiency, heparin-induced thrombocytopenia (HIT), and hypercoagulable blood status) are the most important factors that disturb coagulation, with the clinical consequence of bleeding or thromboembolism (Stepanenko et al. 2014).

The incidence of bleeding of any cause (requiring red blood cell transfusion or necessitating surgery) with different types of VAD ranges between 0.16 and 2.45 events per patient per year, while the incidence of thromboembolic events is 0.05–0.28 events per patient per year (Potapov et al. 2011).

3.3.2 Pump Malfunction

Pump malfunctions due to driveline damage or thrombosis are the most important pump-related complications and, if not treated immediately, are potentially fatal. Pump exchange is a valuable option, although patients with multiple pump exchanges carry a progressive increase in mid-term mortality. Some patients with pump thrombosis may be treated with fibrinolysis if pump exchange is not possible (Najjar et al. 2014). Exceptions are extracorporeal devices, where the exchange procedure is simple by clamping of the outflow cannulas, exchange of blood chambers, de-airing, and pump restart. This is performed without a general anesthetic and at the bedside.

3.3.3 Effects of Pulseless Continuous-Flow Circulation (Aortic Valve, End-Organs, Blood Components)

Several studies have shown that during long-term support with continuous-flow blood pumps, structural alterations of the aortic valve occur. The exact mechanisms and histopathological findings have been described elsewhere (Aggarwal et al. 2013). Briefly, new onset or late progression of preexisting aortic valve regurgitation with or without a commissural fusion phenomenon significantly diminishes the clinical success of VAD therapy. Some VAD recipients require surgical treatment (conventional replacement or AV closure, transcathether valve replacement, etc.) in the later follow-up (Dranishnikov et al. 2012; Robertson et al. 2015).

Under physiological conditions, the blood flow is pulsatile from the arterial tree up to the capillary bed. The role of pulsatility in the proper function of the human body is still unclear. The discussion started with the implementation of cardiopulmonary bypass, which was nonpulsatile and came into clinical practice 60 years ago and still continues. On the basis of experience with more than 5000 patients supported with long-term CF devices in the past 13 years, it is clear that continuous blood flow seems not to have disadvantages regarding neurocognitive function, end-organ recovery, and long-term function (Potapov et al. 2012; Slaughter 2010).

Severe hemolysis is a rare complication following VAD implantation. Postoperative hemolysis may be caused by the pump design (high rotor speed operation in continuous flow pumps, artificial surface properties, mechanical bearings, high shear stress, use of mechanical valves in pulsatile devices) or by postoperative complications (hypercoagulability status, onset of heparin-induced thrombocytopenia (HIT) II, malpositioning of the apical cannula, kinking of outflow grafts, pump thrombosis).

3.3.4 Exit Site Driveline or Cannula-Related Infection

Infection is a common problem of LVAD therapy. Drivelines or device infections are reported with incidence of 0.25–0.33 events per patient per year (John et al. 2014). The driveline tunneling procedure during implantation (C-shaped, subcutaneous, intra-abdominal), externalization techniques, and exit site driveline or cannula incorporation later play a large role as a source for postoperative morbidity and mortality in the case of the onset of local infection with potential generalization and sepsis (Stepanenko et al. 2010).

Excor cannulas are covered with Dacron velour and present acceptable incorporation if the cannula position is relatively stable, without chronic moving-related irritation (Fig. 3.3e)

Drivelines of modern implantable LVADs allow good incorporation and provide long-term exit site infection-free support (Fig. 3.3a–d).

During long-term support in some cases, there is an onset of local infection at the exit site that can ascend to the mediastinum along the driveline tunnel (Fig. 3.3f). Antibiotics and local antiseptics, together with driveline or cannula immobilization, are of great value in avoiding this complication. In the case of uncontrolled ascending infection, local vacuum-assisted closure treatment, driveline relocation, or listing for heart transplantation are possible solutions.

Conclusion

VADs with their variety (univentricular of biventricular support; extracorporeal or implantable; rotary or pulsatile) have become established surgical therapy for end-stage heart failure over the last decade.

With enormous progress made in VAD technology, the incidence of complications has decreased over the years. However, with longer time on support, many forms of interaction between the implanted pump and the body have been recognized. The management of these interactions and complications during support remains challenging, but it is feasible, giving patients supported with a VAD the opportunity to return home and resume their normal lives.

Key Points

- VADs with their variety (univentricular of biventricular support; extracorporeal or implantable; rotary or pulsatile) have become established surgical therapy for end-stage heart failure.
- All devices are connected to the heart and great vessels with the aid to bypass or replace failed pumping ventricle and provide antegrade blood flow with adequate body perfusion.
- End-organ function is preserved and mild dysfunction is reversed in a large number of patients who have been supported for many years.
- Device- and treatment-related effects (driveline exit site, altered blood flow patterns, and need for anticoagulation) together with patient factors (right ventricular function, age, sex, comorbidities) may be major drivers of adverse outcomes.
- The rapid progress in VAD technology in recent years has improved survival and quality of life for patients with advanced heart failure.

Acknowledgments The authors thank Anne Gale, Editor in Life Sciences, for editorial assistance, and Ewald Hennig, PhD, and Friedrich Kaufmann, Dipl. Eng. for their technical support.

References

Aggarwal A, Raghuvir R, Eryazici P, Macaluso G, Sharma P, Blair C, et al. The development of aortic insufficiency in continuous-flow left ventricular assist device-supported patients. Ann Thorac Surg. 2013;95(2):493–8.

Cheung A, Lamarche Y, Kaan A, Munt B, Doyle A, Bashir J, et al. Off-pump implantation of the HeartWare HVAD left ventricular assist device through minimally invasive incisions. Ann Thorac Surg. 2011;91(4):1294–6.

Copeland JG, Smith RG, Arabia FA, Nolan PE, Sethi GK, Tsau PH, et al. Cardiac replacement with a total artificial heart as a bridge to transplantation. N Engl J Med. 2004;351(9):859–67.

Dranishnikov N, Stepanenko A, Potapov EV, Dandel M, Siniawski H, Mladenow A, et al. Simultaneous aortic valve replacement in left ventricular assist device recipients: single-center experience. Int J Artif Organs. 2012;35(7):489–94.

Hetzer R, Potapov EV, Weng Y, Sinawski H, Knollmann F, Komoda T, et al. Implantation of MicroMed DeBakey VAD through left thoracotomy after previous median sternotomy operations. Ann Thorac Surg. 2004;77(1):347–50.

Hetzer R, Alexi-Meskishvili V, Weng Y, Hubler M, Potapov E, Drews T, et al. Mechanical cardiac support in the young with the Berlin Heart EXCOR pulsatile ventricular assist device: 15 years' experience. Semin Thorac Cardiovasc Surg Pediatr Card Surg Annu. 2006:99–108.

Hetzer R, Krabatsch T, Stepanenko A, Hennig E, Potapov EV. Long-term biventricular support with the heartware implantable continuous flow pump. J Heart Lung Transplant. 2010;29(7):822–4.

John R, Aaronson KD, Pae WE, Acker MA, Hathaway DR, Najarian KB, et al. Drive-line infections and sepsis in patients receiving the HVAD system as a left ventricular assist device. J Heart Lung Transplant. 2014;33(10):1066–73.

Kirklin JK, Naftel DC, Pagani FD, Kormos RL, Stevenson LW, Blume ED, et al. Sixth INTERMACS annual report: a 10,000-patient database. J Heart Lung Transplant. 2014;33(6):555–64.

Krabatsch T, Potapov E, Stepanenko A, Schweiger M, Kukucka M, Huebler M, et al. Biventricular circulatory support with two miniaturized implantable assist devices. Circulation. 2011;124(11 Suppl):S179–86.

Najjar SS, Slaughter MS, Pagani FD, Starling RC, McGee EC, Eckman P, et al. An analysis of pump thrombus events in patients in the HeartWare ADVANCE bridge to transplant and continued access protocol trial. J Heart Lung Transplant. 2014;33(1):23–34.

Petrucci RJ, Rogers JG, Blue L, Gallagher C, Russell SD, Dordunoo D, et al. Neurocognitive function in destination therapy patients receiving continuous-flow vs pulsatile-flow left ventricular assist device support. J Heart Lung Transplant. 2012;31(1):27–36.

Potapov EV, Krabatsch T. Minimally invasive continuous-flow left ventricular assist device implantation: Avoiding a median sternotomy. J Heart Lung Transplant. 2014;33(11):1199–200.

Potapov EV, Stepanenko A, Dandel M, Kukucka M, Lehmkuhl HB, Weng Y, et al. Tricuspid incompetence and geometry of the right ventricle as predictors of right ventricular function after implantation of a left ventricular assist device. J Heart Lung Transplant. 2008a;27(12):1275–81.

Potapov EV, Loforte A, Weng Y, Jurmann M, Pasic M, Drews T, et al. Experience with over 1000 implanted ventricular assist devices. J Card Surg. 2008b;23(3):185–94.

Potapov EV, Stepanenko A, Krabatsch T, Hetzer R. Managing long-term complications of left ventricular assist device therapy. Curr Opin Cardiol. 2011;26(3):237–44.

Potapov EV, Dranishnikov N, Morawietz L, Stepanenko A, Rezai S, Blechschmidt C, et al. Arterial wall histology in chronic pulsatile-flow and continuous-flow device circulatory support. J Heart Lung Transplant. 2012;31(11):1171–6.

Robertson JO, Naftel DC, Myers SL, Prasad S, Mertz GD, Itoh A, et al. Concomitant aortic valve procedures in patients undergoing implantation of continuous-flow left ventricular assist devices: an INTERMACS database analysis. J Heart Lung Transplant. 2015;34(6):797–805.

Slaughter MS. Long-term continuous flow left ventricular assist device support and end-organ function: prospects for destination therapy. J Card Surg. 2010;25(4):490–4.

Slaughter MS, Rogers JG, Milano CA, Russell SD, Conte JV, Feldman D, et al. Advanced heart failure treated with continuous-flow left ventricular assist device. N Engl J Med. 2009;361(23):2241–51.

Stepanenko A, Pasic M, Potapov EV, Weng Y, Krabatsch T, Hetzer R. Accidental intraperitoneal tunneling of driveline of left ventricular assist device. Ann Thorac Surg. 2010;90(5):1690–1.

Stepanenko A, Potapov EV, Weng Y, Pasic M, Krabatsch T, Hetzer R. Anticoagulation assessment. Ann Cardiothorac Surg. 2014;3(5):538–40.

Strueber M, Meyer AL, Malehsa D, Haverich A. Successful use of the HeartWare HVAD rotary blood pump for biventricular support. J Thorac Cardiovasc Surg. 2010;140(4):936–7.

4 Clinical Indications for Heart Transplantation

Francesco Tona and Carlo Dal Lin

Contents

4.1 Background

Following the groundbreaking experience in the late 1960s and 1970s of some few centers worldwide, the improvement of immunosuppression by the introduction of cyclosporine made heart transplantation (HTx) the most successful strategy to treat *selected* patients with advanced heart failure (HF) (Shiba et al. 2004). This success is however counterbalanced by the lack of organs available for transplantation and by the early and long-term complications, often the result of immunosuppression therapies. Thus, the selection of patients who can most benefit from transplant remains a crucial issue.

According to the International Registry, worldwide HTx figures show that survival rates vary from more than 90 % at 3 months, 85 % at 1 year, 78 % at 3 years to 70 % at 5 years (Scientific Registry of Transplant Recipients: www.ustransplant.org; Lund et al. 2014). Transplanted patients' quality of life significantly improves and most are able to return to work or study (Grady et al. 1996). In the USA, more than 3000 (The Organ Procurement and Transplantation: www.optn.org) people are awaiting HTx, and about two-thirds undergo the operation each year, and worldwide, more than 4000 patients per year undergo HTx (Zaroff et al. 2002). From the early 1990s to the 2000s, the waiting time doubled and is still rising. About 16 % of patients awaiting

F. Tona, MD, PhD (✉) • C. Dal Lin, MD
Cardiology Unit, Department of Cardiac, Thoracic and Vascular Sciences, University of Padova, Padova, Italy
e-mail: francesco.tona@unipd.it

O. Leone et al. (eds.), *The Pathology of Cardiac Transplantation*,
DOI 10.1007/978-3-319-46386-5_4

transplantation die (Scientific Registry of Transplant Recipients: www.ustransplant.org; Lund et al. 2014).

4.2 Prognostic Assessment

A large array of variables and scores have been studied to assess the prognosis of HF patients, including age, heart failure etiology, widened QRS on 12-lead electrocardiogram, NYHA class, ejection fraction, decrease of peak exercise oxygen uptake, chronic hypotension, resting tachycardia, intolerance to conventional therapy, refractory volume overload, the presence of key comorbidities (such as renal dysfunction, diabetes, anemia, hyperuricemia), the degree of hyponatremia, and plasma natriuretic peptide concentration (McMurray et al. 2012). These variables may change over time, as does prognosis. The high number of prognostic markers underscores the complexity and heterogeneity of clinical course and presentation of HF. Thus, optimal prognostic evaluation needs to be based not only on evaluating multiple parameters, but also on their change over time.

Prognostic scoring systems provide an example of the interplay of multiple variables in influencing prognosis: among the many proposed, the Heart Failure Scoring System or Seattle Heart Failure Model (Alraies and Eckman 2014) have been extensively validated and are publicly available (http://www.heartfailurerisk.org/# and http://depts.washington.edu/shfm/) (Fig. 4.1).

4.3 Recipient Selection Criteria

The two main heart diseases that lead to adult end-stage heart failure requiring transplantation are ischemic heart disease and cardiomyopathies, each of which make up 45–50 % of cases

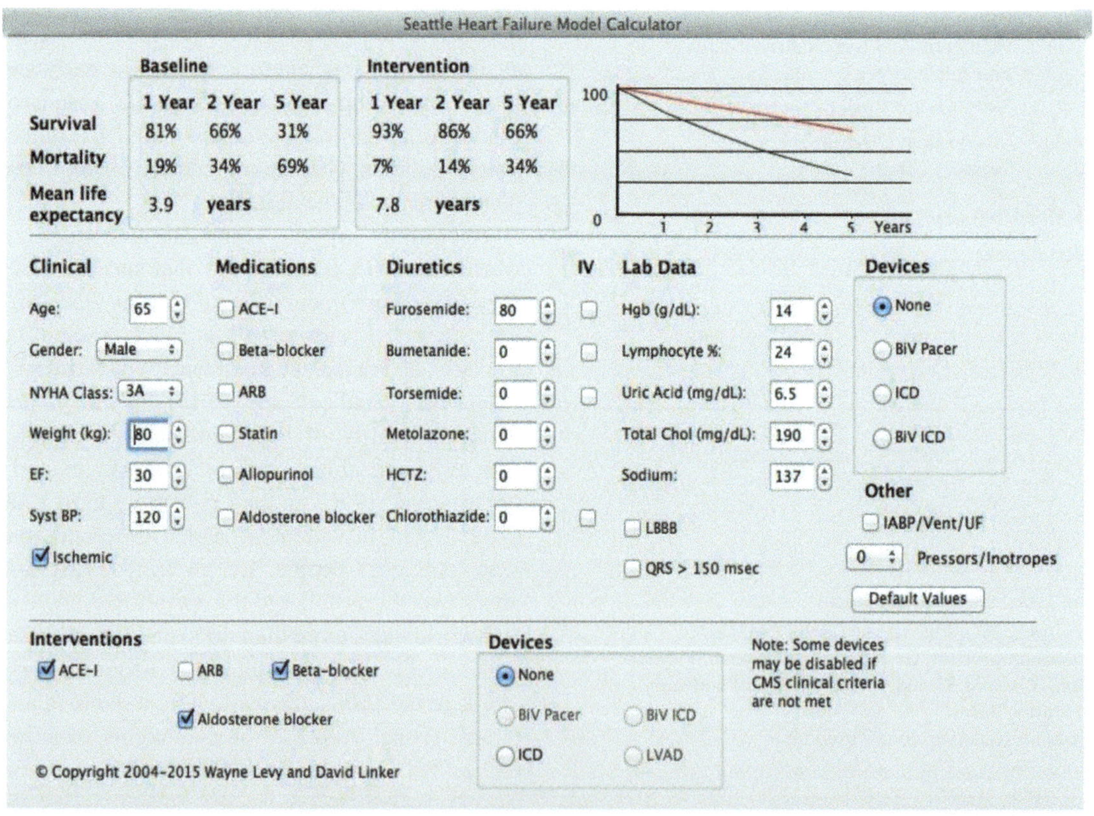

Fig. 4.1 The Seattle Heart Failure Model calculator, modified from http://depts.washington.edu/shfm/macosx.php

(Scientific Registry of Transplant Recipients: www.ustransplant.org; Lund et al. 2014). Figure 4.2 shows the details of transplanted diseases by recipient age group.

Patients with an estimated survival of <80 % at 6–12 months should be evaluated for HTx (Hunt et al. 2009; Mehra et al. 2006), after all other therapeutic approaches have failed (optimization of medical treatment, coronary or mitral valve surgery, resynchronization therapy, and ICD implantation) (Bank et al. 2000).

Most patients will have an established diagnosis of chronic heart failure due to left or biventricular systolic dysfunction not attributable to correctable structural, valvular or coronary artery disease and will fulfil the following criteria (Banner et al. 2011):

- Impaired left ventricle systolic function
- NYHA class III (e.g., marked limitation of physical activity, comfortable at rest; less than ordinary activity causes fatigue, palpitation, or dyspnea) or IV symptoms
- Already receiving optimal medical treatment (including target or maximum tolerated doses of beta-adrenergic antagonists, ACE inhibitors, and aldosterone antagonists)
- Cardiac resynchronization treatment (CRT), implantable cardioverter defibrillator (ICD), or cardiac resynchronization treatment—defibrillator (CRT-D) device implanted (if indicated)
- Evidence of a poor prognosis:
  1. Cardiorespiratory exercise testing (VO_2 max < 12 ml/kg/min if on beta-blockade, <14 ml/kg/min if not on beta-blockade, ensuring respiratory quotient ≥ 1.05)
  2. Markedly elevated B-type natriuretic peptide (or N-terminal pro-B-type natriuretic peptide) serum levels despite full medical treatment
  3. Established composite prognostic scoring system, such as the Heart Failure Scoring System or Seattle Heart Failure Model
  4. Low cardiac output at right heart catheterization (often associated with postcapillary pulmonary hypertension)

While the main indication is HF due to systolic ventricular dysfunction, transplantation may also be considered on a case-by-case basis

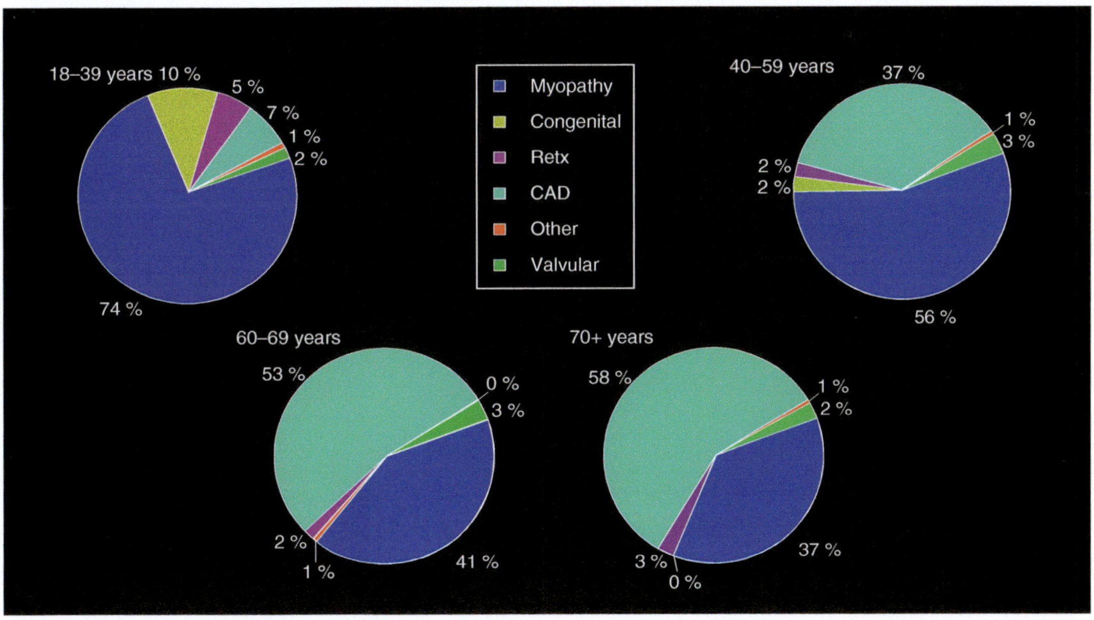

Fig. 4.2 Diagnosis by recipient age group in adult heart transplants (2006–June 2013). *CAD* coronary artery disease, *Retx* retransplants (Modified from Lund et al. 2014)

in other situations, such as persistent hemodynamically compromising ventricular arrhythmias, refractory to all conventional therapies (including antiarrhythmic drugs, catheter ablation, electrical device treatment, revascularization); refractory angina, where there is clear objective evidence of recurrent significant/debilitating myocardial ischemia that is not amenable to conventional treatment (including all forms of revascularization and full antiangina treatment); restrictive and hypertrophic cardiomyopathies with persisting NYHA III or IV symptoms refractory to conventional treatment and/or recurrent admissions with decompensated HF; congenital heart disease with NYHA functional class III–IV HF not amenable to palliative or corrective surgery (McMurray et al. 2012; Mehra et al. 2006).

In case of heart failure not associated with the dilated hypokinetic phenotype, clear echocardiographic evidence of restrictive filling pattern needs to be obtained, confirmed by hemodynamic studies. In addition, a complete and often histological diagnostic workout is needed in patients with restrictive cardiomyopathy to ascertain the presence of a possible systemic disease, amenable to other therapeutic strategies, and to assess the risk of post-transplantation recurrence (e.g. amyloidosis or glycogen storage disease) (Hunt et al. 2009; Alraies and Eckman 2014; Bank et al. 2000; Banner et al. 2011; De Jonge et al. 2008; Sidebotham et al. 2007; Camm et al. 2009; Mehra et al. 2006).

It is essential that patients be referred to the transplant center before systemic complications develop.

Clinical conditions for referral are summarized in Fig. 4.3 (McMurray et al. 2012; Hunt et al. 2009).

Heart Transplantation:
Indications and Contraindications
according to American and European Guidelines

American Guidelines

Absolute Indications in Appropriate Patients	For hemodynamic compromise due to HF • Refractory cardiogenic shock • Documented dependence on IV inotropic support to maintain adequate organ perfusion • Peak VO_2 less than 10 mL per kg per minute with achievement of anaerobic metabolism
	Severe symptoms of ischemia that consistently limit routine activity and are not amenable to coronary artery bypass surgery or percutaneous coronary intervention
	Recurrent symptomatic ventricular arrhythmias refractory to all therapeutic modalities
Relative Indications	Peak VO_2 11 to 14 mL per kg per minute (or 55 % perdicted) and major limitation of the patient's daily activities
	Recurrent unstable ischemia not amenable to other intervention
	Recurrent instability of fluid balance/renal function not due to patient noncompliance with medical regimen
Insufficient Indications	Low left ventricular ejection fraction
	History of functional class III or IV symptoms of HF
	Peak VO_2 greater then 15 mL per kg per minute (and greater than 55% predicted) without other indications

HF indicates heart failure; IV, intravenous; VO_2, oxygan consumption per unit time

European Guidelines

Patients to consider	End-stage heart failure with severe symptoms, a poor, prognosis, and no remaining alternative treatment optoons
	Motivated, well informed, and emotionallly stable
	Capable of complying with the intensive treatment required post-operatively
Contraindications	Active infection
	Severe peripheral arterial or verebrovascular disease
	Current alcohol or drug abuse
	Treated cancer in previous 5 years
	Unhealed peptic ulcer
	Recent thrombo-embolism
	Significant renal failure (e.g. creatinine clearance <50 mL/min)
	Significant liver disease
	Systemic disease with multiorgan involvement
	Other serious co-morbidity with poor prognosis
	Emotional instability or untreated mental illness
	High, fixed pulmonary vascular resistance (>4–5 wood Units and mean transpulmonary gradient >15 mmHg)

Fig. 4.3 Indications for heart trasplantation: comparison between American and European guidelines

4.4 Risk Factors and Contraindications to Heart Transplantation

Advanced HF can lead to dysfunction in other organs, which will increase the risk associated with transplantation and may eventually become irreversible; referral should be considered before these complications become established. Whenever possible, intrinsic organ damage should be differentiated from potentially reversible abnormalities secondary to heart failure (such as cardiorenal syndrome, hyponatremia, liver dysfunction, anemia, cardiac cachexia, and pulmonary hypertension) (De Jonge et al. 2008).

4.4.1 Pulmonary Hypertension and Vasoreactivity Test

Right heart failure is a common occurrence and a cause of morbidity and mortality after cardiac transplantation (Camm et al. 2009). Contemporary registry data from ISHLT indicate that approximately 20% of early deaths after cardiac transplantation are attributable to RV failure (Mehra et al. 2006).

Therefore, according to ISHLT guidelines (Mehra et al. 2006), right heart catheterization (RHC) should be performed on all candidates in preparation for listing for HTx and annually until transplantation. RHC should be perfomed at 3- to 6-month intervals in listed patients, especially in the presence of reversible pulmonary hypertension or worsening of heart failure symptoms. A vasodilator challenge should be administered when the pulmonary artery systolic pressure is ≥50 mmHg and either the transpulmonary gradient is ≥15 mmHg or the pulmonary vascular resistance (PVR) is >3 Wood units (>240 dynes·s·cm^{-5}), (De Jonge et al. 2008) while maintaining a systolic arterial blood pressure ≥ 85 mmHg.

Patients whose PVR can be acutely reduced (usually in the cardiac catheterization lab or at the bedside) are usually considered acceptable candidates for transplantation.

Although criteria have been proposed that contraindicate cardiac transplantation, increasingly, it has been recognized that absolute cutoffs do not exist, and large cohort analyses have demonstrated that elevated PVR is an incremental risk factor from low to high values (Mehra et al. 2006). Pulmonary artery hypertension and elevated PVR should be considered as a relative contraindication to cardiac transplantation when the PVR is >5 Wood units or the pulmonary vascular resistance index (PVRI) is >6 or the transpulmonary gradient (TPG) exceeds 16–20 mmHg. If the pulmonary artery pressure exceeds 60 mmHg in conjunction with any one of the preceding three variables, the risk of right heart failure and early death is increased. If the PVR can be reduced to <2.5 with a vasodilator but the systolic blood pressure falls <85 mmHg, the patient remains at high risk of right heart failure and mortality after HTx.

Vasoreactivity testing involves the administration of a short-acting vasodilator with or without inotropic properties followed by measurement of the hemodynamic response using a Swan-Ganz catheter. The drugs usually used for this acute challenge are prostacyclin, nitroglycerin, and nitroprusside. Other drugs, such as nitric oxide, dobutamine, and milrinone, can also be used (De Jonge et al. 2008).

Contraindications to vasoreactivity testing include low systemic blood pressure, low cardiac index, or the presence of severe (functional class IV) symptoms because hypotension and occasionally cardiovascular collapse can occur with the administration of the vasodilator (Banner et al. 2011). Thus, most clinicians agree that acute vasoreactivity testing should only be performed by those expert in the performance and interpretation of this procedure.

4.4.2 Potential Contraindications and Risk Factors of Poor Survival for Heart Transplantation

In light of the paucity of available organs, the selection process needs to exclude from transplant those patients presenting one or multiple conditions that will significantly reduce post-transplant survival.

Some comorbidities constitute an absolute contraindication, and others are incremental risk factors. Relative contraindications, when present in combination, may become absolute barriers to surgery.

- Age is not a contraindication to transplantation per se, but increasing age is an incremental risk factor, and it is often associated with other comorbidities: 65 years is the standard upper age limit for being considered in the waiting list for heart trasplantation for most centers, However, acceptable results have been reported in small selected series of patients older that 70.
- Multiple prior sternotomies are an incremental risk factor.
- Diabetes is not a contraindication but is a risk factor; it may become a contraindication in case of organ damage and poor glycemic control (e.g. glycosylated hemoglobin < 7.5 %).
- Symptomatic peripheral or cerebrovascular diseases are relative contraindications, given their impact on patient prognosis.
- More recently, the concept of frailty has been evaluated as an indicator of poor prognosis in heart failure patients, both after mechanical circulatory support and after transplantation (Jha et al. 2016).
- Alcohol or recreational substance abuse and dependence is a contraindication, irrespective of the legal conditions related to it.
- Obesity is a risk factor for postoperative complications and may limit the pool of organ availability: heart donors weighing more than 100 kg are unlikely, for example. In addition, a body mass index greater that 35 kg/m^2 is in any case to be considered a contraindication (Hunt et al. 2009).

4.4.3 Special Considerations

4.4.3.1 Renal Dysfunction

Renal dysfunction is often present in heart transplant candidates, often secondary to heart failure itself or to the associated cardiovascular metabolic risk factors (mainly hypertension, diabetes). It is not only a marker of heart failure severity, but also a significant marker of morbidity and mortality after transplantation (Lund et al. 2014). Therefore, patients with renal insufficiency should undergo thorough examination in order to discern a possible primary kidney-related disease from a pre-renal kidney dysfunction.

Appropriate screening requires the calculation of the estimated glomerular filtration rate (Mehra et al. 2006). However, the upper limit for acceptability is controversial and may depend on local experiences and clinical scenario. The Bethesda Conference considered irreversible renal dysfunction with serum creatinine above 2 mg/dl or creatinine clearance below 50 ml/min as a secondary exclusion criterion (Mehra et al. 2006). However, when serum creatinine was evaluated as a continuous variable, no specific level was identified beyond which the risk of heart transplant was unacceptable.

The serum creatinine value is considered an absolute contraindication at above 3 mg/dl in two-thirds of US centers and at over above 5 mg/dl in 43 % of German centers (Mehra et al. 2006), while other 43 % of centers consider above 5 mg/dl level as a relative contraindication (Mehra et al. 2006).

4.4.3.2 Malignancies and Infections

In the presence of malignancies, a patient should not be placed on the waiting list because of the risks connected to the immunosuppressive therapy that follows transplantation. However, patients who have achieved a sustained remission following cancer treatment may become transplant candidates (McMurray et al. 2012). Decision-making should include advice from an oncologist, and the outcome will be influenced by the nature of the malignancy and the patient's expected prognosis for survival free of relapse (Camm et al. 2009).

Clinically important chronic viral infections, such as HCV, HIV, and HBV, remain a subject of active debate. Chronic viral infections are relative contraindications, given the potential for organ injury, disease exacerbation by pharmacological immunosuppression, and drug interactions between antiviral and immunosuppressive drug treatment (Sidebotham et al. 2007). However, the availability of new antiviral drugs for HCV and HIV, which can lead to recovery or prolonged stabilization of the viral infection, may make it possible to consider these patients too for transplantation, in the context of a multidisciplinary environment and close collaboration with infectious disease specialists.

4.4.3.3 Comorbidities

"Contraindications" and "comorbidities" are concepts that overlap. The benefit of transplantation must be weighed against the risks associated with the recipient's comorbidities and the possible aggravation that may result from the necessary immunosuppressive therapy. It is not easy and perhaps not even possible to demarcate a clear threshold over which comorbidity can really contraindicate transplant. Therefore, from the ethical point of view, we should consider the patient's lifestyle and life expectation. It might be useful to consider the patient's "life project," that is, what he still wants to achieve in order to consider his existence satisfactory. This may help caregivers in patient care, in terms of medical and/or surgical treatment.

4.4.3.4 Psychosocial Evaluation

All cardiac transplant candidates should undergo complete psychosocial evaluation during the initial screening process. This may identify social and behavioral factors that cause difficulty during the waiting period, post-surgery recovery, and long-term postoperative management. In particular, it is important to identify risk factors that could lead to nonadherence and rule out subclinical psychiatric disorders that may jeopardize the efficacy of transplant. The patient must understand that full cooperation and adherence are critical to the safe and effective use of immunosuppressive agents (McMurray et al. 2012).

4.5 Mechanical Circulatory Support (MCS)

Transplant-eligible patients may be considered for implantation of a MCS if their clinical condition is deteriorating and if they are unlikely to receive a donor heart soon (Bank et al. 2000). These devices may be for short-term or long-term support. The latter are implantable and have been developed to assist the left ventricle (LVAD). LVAD support may also be used to reverse potential contraindications such as renal dysfunction and pulmonary hypertension secondary to heart dysfunction, thereby making the patient a better candidate for transplantation (bridge to candidacy). Permanent LVAD implant as a destination therapy is currently reccommended only for patients with an absolute contraindication for transplant (usually advanced age). In emergency situations, support with a low-cost, short-term device may be used as a "bridge to decision" to allow full assessment of the patient (Hunt et al. 2009).

Conclusion

Assessing eligibility for heart transplantation is a complex task requiring comprehensive evaluation of the patient from many aspects, with more than a single diagnostic procedure. The guiding principle is accurate prognostic evaluation weighing the benefits of transplantations against the risks linked to the procedure itself, the toxicity of the immunosuppressive drugs, and the noncardiac comorbidities that have to be carefully ruled out. In this context, the multidisciplinary work of the transplant team, including cardiologists, cardiac surgeons, pathologists, transplant coordinators, psychologists, social workers, dieticians, and physiotherapists is crucial (Banner et al. 2011).

Key points

- Assessment of eligibility for heart transplantation is a complex task, where the guiding principle is accurate prognostic evaluation while weighing the benefits of transplantation against the risks.
- Prognosis assessment systems of heart failure patients include many variables and scoring methods. The most com-

monly used and best validated are the Heart Failure Scoring System and Seattle Heart Failure Mode (http://www.heartfailurerisk.org/# and http://depts.washington.edu/shfm/).

- The majority of patients referred for transplantation have established diagnosis of chronic heart failure due to left or biventricular dysfunction not attributable to correctable structural, valvular, or coronary artery diseases.
- The main indication is HF due to systolic ventricular dysfunction. Other situations where transplantation may be considered case-by-case are as follows:
  - Persistent hemodynamically compromising ventricular arrhythmias refractory to all conventional therapies
  - Refractory angina
  - Myocardial ischemia not amenable to conventional treatment
  - Restrictive and hypertrophic cardiomyopathies with persisting NYHA III or IV symptoms
  - Congenital heart disease with NYHA functional class III–IV HF not amenable to palliative or corrective surgery
- As donor hearts are limited in number, the selection process should also consider the presence of comorbidities (one or multiple conditions) which can significantly reduce post-transplant survival.
- Some comorbidities are absolute contraindications; others, in isolation, may be relative contraindications, but absolute in combination.
- Renal dysfunction, malignancies, infections, and psychosocial factors need separate consideration.

References

Alraies MC, Eckman P. Adult heart transplant: indications and outcomes. J Thorac Dis. 2014;6:1120–8.

Bank AJ, et al. Effects of left ventricular assist devices on outcomes in patients undergoing heart transplantation. Ann Thorac Surg. 2000;69:1369–74; discussion 1375.

Banner NR, et al. UK guidelines for referral and assessment of adults for heart transplantation. Heart. 2011; 97:1520–7.

Camm AJ, Luscher TF, Serruis P W. ESC textbook of cardiovascular medicine. 2nd ed. Oxford (UK): Oxford Med; 2009. p. 1–1398.

De Jonge N, et al. Guidelines for heart transplantation. Netherlands Heart J. 2008;16:79–87.

Grady KL, Jalowiec A, White-Williams C. Improvement in quality of life in patients with heart failure who undergo transplantation. J Heart Lung Transplant. 1996;15:749–57.

Hunt SA, et al. ACCF / AHA Practice Guideline : Full Text Practice Guideline : Full Text 2009 Focused Update Incorporated Into the ACC / AHA 2005 Guidelines for the Diagnosis and Management of Heart Failure in Adults A Report of the American College of Cardiology Foundat. Circulation. 2009;119: e391–479.

Lund LH, et al. The registry of the International Society for Heart and Lung Transplantation: thirty-first official adult heart transplant report – 2014; focus theme: retransplantation. J Heart Lung Transplant. 2014;33: 996–1008.

McMurray JJV, et al. ESC Guidelines for the diagnosis and treatment of acute and chronic heart failure 2012: The Task Force for the Diagnosis and Treatment of Acute and Chronic Heart Failure 2012 of the European Society of Cardiology. Developed in collaboration with the Heart. Eur Heart J. 2012;33:1787–847.

Mehra MR, et al. Listing Criteria for Heart Transplantation: International Society for Heart and Lung Transplantation Guidelines for the Care of Cardiac Transplant Candidates. J Heart Lung Transplant. 2006;25: 1024–42.

Scientific Registry of Transplant Recipients. www.ustrasplant.org.

Shiba N, et al. Analysis of survivors more than 10 years after heart transplantation in the cyclosporine era: Stanford experience. J Heart Lung Transplant. 2004;23:155–64.

Sidebotham D, McKee A, Gillham M, Levy J. Cardiothoracic critical care. Philadelphia (USA): Elsevier; 2007. p. 1–651.

The Organ Procurement and Transplantation Network. www.optn.org.

Jha SR, Hannu MK, Chang S, Montgomery E, Harkess M, Wilhelm K, Hayward CS, Jabbour A, Spratt PM, Newton P, Davidson PM, Macdonald PS. The prevalence and prognostic significance of frailty in patients with advanced heart failure referred for heart transplantation. Transplantation. 2016;100(2):429–36.

Zaroff JG, et al. Maximizing use of organs recovered from the cadaver donor: cardiac recommendations. J Heart Lung Transplant. 2002;21:1153–60.

Pathologies Encountered in Explanted Native Hearts

5

Ornella Leone, Annalisa Angelini, Marny Fedrigo, Aryan Vink, and Allard van der Wal

Contents

O. Leone (✉)
Cardiovascular and Cardiac Transplant Pathology Program, Department of Pathology, Sant'Orsola-Malpighi University Hospital, Bologna, Italy
e-mail: ornella.leone@aosp.bo.it

A. Angelini • M. Fedrigo
Pathology of Cardiac Transplantation and Regenerative Medicine Unit, Department of Cardiac, Thoracic and Vascular Sciences, University of Padua, Padua, Italy

A. Vink
Department of Pathology, University Medical Center Utrecht, Utrecht, The Netherlands

A. van der Wal
Department of Pathology, Academic Medical Center, University of Amsterdam, Amsterdam, The Netherlands

5.1 Introduction

The primary aim of pathologic examination of hearts explanted during transplantation is the detailed study of the cardiac disease that led to heart failure and to compare the pretransplantation clinical diagnosis or the clinical–pathologic diagnosis when endomyocardial biopsy (EMB) is performed.

But this examination also offers much more.

Cardiac transplantation and availability of native hearts from live patients completely changed the anatomo-pathologic approach to cardiac diseases and gave two extraordinary opportunities:

1. It opened the way to "surgical pathology" of the entire heart, previously restricted only to autopsy.
2. It made EMB an essential routine tool in the diagnosis of cardiac diseases, given its wide use in monitoring post-transplantation rejection.

O. Leone et al. (eds.), *The Pathology of Cardiac Transplantation*,
DOI 10.1007/978-3-319-46386-5_5

Thus, today cardiovascular pathologists are no longer only mere autopsy pathologists but real surgical pathologists.

All this implies many important points. First of all, it premises having good quality tissue from live patients to examine (as with other surgical specimens) and being able to collect fresh tissue. It also encourages pathologists to follow more detailed protocols in heart examination thus opening the way to standardizing procedures and collecting large-scale data. Detailed and systematic examination of pathologic substrates of many cardiac diseases, including rare diseases, is now possible, and important diagnostic and research information is newly available. This is not yet a resource for all surgical pathologists, but it is for specialized cardiovascular pathologists and it is slowly spreading to the whole pathology community.

Another essential result is that pathologists and clinicians collaborate more closely and become used to sharing information and correlating more exhaustively clinical history and imaging findings with pathologic substrates. As a consequence all specialists involved in managing cardiac diseases should learn to give greater weight to the etiology of diseases underlying heart failure. Although the patient is of course extensively assessed prior to transplant, clinical indications for cardiac transplant are not always really etiology driven, as some unexpected diagnoses found at the pathologic examination of the explanted heart demonstrate.

This multidisciplinary work-up model in heart transplantation, where pathologists, clinicians, and surgeons usually work closely together throughout the entire transplant process should also be extended to autopsy, where pathologists all too often work in isolation, as clinician participation is limited and depends on local practice, or details of clinical history are not always available.

Examination of native hearts illuminates major aspects of heart failure, such as extending knowledge of the complex pathologic substrates of cardiomyopathies that enrich the clinical and genetic phenotypes, describing pathologic findings in the metamorphosis and evolution of diseases as a consequence of interventional procedures (e.g. coronary stents) and knowing the varied aspects of myocardial remodeling after traditional surgery (e.g. valvular heart disease, congenital heart defects).

In this chapter we want to address the pathologic examination of native hearts in this different light and to describe the pathologist's work, often underrated but essential.

Our aim is to stimulate cardiac transplant pathologists to fully explore explanted hearts and to build up a collection, as this is valuable material for increasing knowledge of cardiac disease. General surgical pathologists, who do not usually deal with cardiovascular specimens, especially explanted hearts, should also use this knowledge at autopsy examination of hearts.

5.2 Ischemic Heart Disease

5.2.1 Background and Incidence in Explanted Hearts

Ischemic heart disease (IHD) may be the first manifestation of coronary artery disease (CAD) or be the consequence of cumulative effects of coronary atherosclerosis, a chronic disease with its multifaced pathophysiology and clinically stable and unstable periods. Although not all IHD is necessarily CAD and vice versa, in clinical practice IHD and CAD have become synonymous and the incidence in the population of myocardial infarction (MI) is used to roughly define prevalence of CAD. IHD may be a limited event of a chronic disease or a major condition leading to sudden death or congestive heart failure and chronic/end-stage IHD requiring heart transplantation (HTx).

Together with cardiomyopathy, IHD is the leading underlying heart disease diagnosis for adult HTx. The percentage of heart transplantation patients with IHD has decreased over recent decades from 46 % in the 1990s to 36 % nowadays (Lund et al. 2014). As might be expected, IHD as underlying cause of HTx is related to age of the recipient: cardiomyopathy is the major diagnosis for HTx up to age 59 years, but IHD predominates thereafter (Lund et al. 2013). The decreased proportion of IHD as underlying heart disease for HTx is in line with observations of substantially decreased morbidity and mortality of CAD over the last three decades due to better medical treatment, e.g. statins, and reduction of risk factors such as smoking. Moreover, current standard treatment of CAD with balloon angioplasty and stenting, either as primary therapy or revascularization therapy in acute myocardial infarction, has modified the clinical-pathologic expression of ischemic heart disease and the need for transplant arises at a later age (>65 years).

Clinical presentation of CAD includes a wide spectrum ranging from silent ischemia, stable and unstable angina pectoris, MI, heart failure, and sudden death. These clinical events can be attributed to various pathologic lesions which, through complex cellular and molecular pathobiologic mechanisms, lead to the different patterns of myocardial muscle ischemic injury and finally to the development of chronic ischemic heart disease. This ranges from the reversible alterations of myocardial stunning to early ischemic lesions, fully developed coagulative necrosis, different stages of the reparative processes and to the development of progressive chronic disease, both chronic atherosclerosis and chronic myocardial damage with myocardial fibrosis and impaired contractile performance of the heart. Another essential factor of developing myocardial damage is ischemia–reperfusion injury, which independently contributes to cardiomyocyte death. This is particularly important today because the most effective therapy to limit the extent of MI is reperfusion of the stenosis or obstruction of the artery using primary percutaneous intervention or revascularization surgery. So, pathologists must therefore be familiar with examination of coronary stents or coronary bypass grafts. Apart from the lesions of main coronary epicardial branches, coronary microvascular dysfunction also occurs and contributes to myocardial lesions (Burke and Virmani 2007).

In explanted hearts, coronary atherosclerosis and myocardial disease are at advanced chronic stage, for which various terms are used in daily practice: ischemic cardiomyopathy vs. ischemic cardiopathy vs. chronic ischemic heart disease. The term "ischemic cardiomyopathy" was introduced in the 1995 World Heart Organization classification of cardiomyopathy referring to "a dilated cardiomyopathy with impaired contractile performance not explained by the extent of coronary artery disease or ischemic damage". Although still widely used among clinicians and pathologists, it is not currently part of either the official European Society of Cardiology or the American Heart Association clinical cardiomyopathy classification schemes (Elliott et al. 2008; Maron et al. 2006): so, due to its ambiguity and the fact that it probably refers to a more limited clinical–pathologic condition, the terms "ischemic cardiopathy" and "chronic ischemic heart disease" are preferable for a condition referring to weakness and remodeling of the heart muscle due to inadequate oxygen delivery to the myocardium consequent to CAD.

5.2.2 Specific Technical Pathology Points

5.2.2.1 Examination of Coronary Arteries

- Start with examination of the coronary origins: determine the number, position, size, and patency of the coronary ostia (Stone et al. 2012).
- Assess the size, course, and dominance of the major coronary arteries.
- Make a series of transverse cuts at 3 mm intervals in the main epicardial branches (left anterior descending, left circumflex artery, diagonal and obtuse marginal branches, right coronary artery) in order to determine patency and the degree of stenosis and presence of thrombus.
- As most cases of CAD explanted hearts have severely calcified advanced atherosclerotic lesions in the coronary arteries, in some cases it could be advisable to dissect the entire main epicardial arteries and branches including the diag-

onal and obtuse marginal for decalcification before sectioning. For decalcification, we recommend the use of ethylene-diamine-tetraacetic acid to preserve cell morphology.

- Representative sections, such as stenotic lesions and complicated thrombosed lesions, are sampled for histology.

5.2.2.2 Evaluation of Stents

Evaluation of reocclusion/restenosis of coronary arteries with implanted metallic scaffolding devices, known as stents, and subsequent histologic study cannot be done with conventional methods, which result in disruption of tissue and cellular morphology at stent–tissue interface. Although a careful study of stented coronary arteries is not needed in routine examination for diagnostic purposes, this is an important field for clinical and pathology research. Detailed methodology is described by Bradshaw and Rippstein (Bradshaw et al. 2009; Rippstein et al. 2006).

The main points to keep in mind are the following:

- Avoid sectioning the vessel through stents with scissors and scalpel or pulling out the stent from the coronary artery lumen.
- Remove the stented vessel by cutting it proximally and distally to the device.
- Before sectioning, a radiograph of the specimen is useful to identify the total length of the stent and other characteristics such as expansion, compression, or distortion.
- Fix the removed specimen in formalin before special handling.

The two main processing methods are the following:

- Processing and embedding specimens in methyl methacrylate resin (Bradshaw et al. 2009).
- Electrolytic dissolution of the stent with paraffin embedding (Rippstein et al. 2006).

Paraffin embedding method is preferred for immunohistochemical study.

5.2.2.3 Coronary Artery Bypass Grafts

Coronary artery bypass grafts (internal mammary arteries, saphenous veins, radial arteries, etc.) should be carefully dissected from the pericardial adhesions and the removed specimen also examined with transverse cuts.

For histologic study of the anastomosis, three cross sections should be obtained: one proximally, one at the anastomotic level, and one distally.

5.2.2.4 Examination of Myocardium

- Start with a transversal slice of the heart at mid-ventricular level and then parallel slices of the ventricles, working toward the apex, at 1 cm intervals (Stone et al. 2012).
- Determine the luminal diameter of both ventricles at mid-ventricular level and measure mitral valve annulus diameter.
- Document scars as subendocardial or transmural and describe their radial (anterior, lateral, posterior, and septal) and longitudinal (base, mid-ventricle, and apex) location. Document scars in papillary muscles.
- Describe wall thinning and aneurysm formation (bulge at transmural scar) and then measure wall thickness of the compact myocardium excluding the trabeculae of both ventricles in non-infarcted areas.
- Take representative sections for histology.

5.2.3 Pathologic Substrates

The pathologic study of a native heart with IHD includes morphology of atherosclerotic plaques, their stages, progression and remodeling, coronary artery stents, and bypass grafts and the multiple aspects of myocardial damage.

Systematic examination of the explanted hearts can make an important contribution to pathologically defining the chronic stage of the disease, whose spectrum varies from severe coronary atherosclerosis (obstructing or narrowing >75 % cross-sectional area of one or more major coronary arteries) and large areas of the myocardium replaced by scar tissue to less evident and not yet fully defined alterations in presence of CAD but in the absence of a recognized MI.

5.2.3.1 Coronary Atherosclerosis

Histopathological Classification

Atherosclerotic plaques develop over time. The most commonly used anatomo-clinical classification scheme of atherosclerotic lesions is that of the American Heart Association. Virmani and colleagues (2000) have produced a modified version that includes more detailed histopathologic content. The latter is the most commonly used by pathologists and divides lesions into non-atherosclerotic intimal lesions and progressive atherosclerotic lesions (Table 5.1): the scheme includes seven categories classified on the basis of accretion of lipid in relation to the formation of a fibrous cap; modifications in the lipid to form a necrotic core; thickening or thinning of the fibrous cap and thrombosis formation.

Pathologic Assessing of Stenosis Degree in Coronary Atherosclerosis

Assessment of coronary atherosclerotic lesion severity varies according to technique: angiography, intravascular ultrasound, and pathological examination. The main limiting factors for pathologic assessment are nonphysiological conditions of nonpressure-distended arteries; usually nonpressure-fixed vessels; and tissue shrinkage after fixation and processing. Although in end-stage ischemic native hearts a precise evaluation of stenosis degree is not routinely required, it should be remembered that medial collapse of the uninvolved coronary segments by an eccentric plaque can result in great overestimation of stenosis percentage. Thus, when a detailed evaluation is needed, it is advisable to allow for the collapse-related artifact by planimetry measurements as suggested by Burke et al. (2001).

Coronary Luminal Thrombus Formation

Autopsy studies have shown that occlusion of the coronary lumen due to thrombus formation is the mechanism underlying most cases of myocardial infarction. Three distinct processes are described underlying thrombus formation: plaque rupture, erosion, and, less frequently (<5 % of cases), a protruding calcified nodule (Table 5.1).

Table 5.1 Modified American Heart Association histological classification scheme of atherosclerotic lesions (Virmani et al. 2000)

Non-atherosclerotic intimal lesions	**Description**
Intimal thickening	Accumulation of smooth muscle cells (SMCs) in the intima
Intimal xanthoma or fatty streak	Accumulation of foam cells in the intima without a necrotic core or fibrous cap
Progressive atherosclerotic lesions	**Description**
Pathological intimal thickening	SMCs in a proteoglycan-rich matrix with areas of extracellular lipid accumulation without necrosis
Fibrous cap atheroma	Well-formed necrotic core with an overlying fibrous cap
Thin fibrous cap atheroma	A thin fibrous cap (<65 μm) infiltrated by macrophages and lymphocytes and an underlying necrotic core
Fibro-calcified plaque	Collagen-rich plaque with significant stenosis usually contains large areas of calcification with few inflammatory cells; a small necrotic core may be present
Lesions with thrombi	**Description**
Plaque rupture	Fibroatheroma with cap disruption; luminal thrombus communicates with the underlying necrotic core; intraplaque hemorrhage may play a role
Erosion	Luminal thrombus, no communication of thrombus with necrotic core; damaged endothelium; usually younger patients
Calcified nodule	Thrombus due to eruptive nodular calcification with underlying fibro-calcified plaque

Healed Plaque Rupture and Total Occlusion

If the patient survives myocardial infarction, the thrombus will become organized with ingrowth of microvessels and collagen formation from myofibroblasts. Eventually a new layer of connective tissue will form over the ruptured plaque, which "seals off" and stabilizes the site of rupture. In plaques complicated by total occlusion of the vessel lumen, this process of organization will increase the amount of collagen over time and remodeling of the microvessels may lead to recanalization of the artery. Since CAD HTx patients have a history of myocardial infarctions, healed plaque ruptures and total occlusions can frequently be observed in the coronary arteries of the explanted hearts (Fig. 5.1).

5.2.3.2 Coronary Stents

As stenting is the most widely performed treatment of symptomatic coronary disease today, CAD heart explants frequently contain coronary stents.

In Stent Neo-Intima Formation

Directly after stent implantation the endothelium is stripped to encourage a healing response consisting of neo-intima formation with re-endothelialization of the intimal layer. First platelets and fibrin thrombus containing neutrophils will form (Nakano and Virmani 2015). The amount of platelets in this thrombus depends on antiplatelet therapy, whereas fibrin is always present. Chronic inflammation (lymphocytes and macrophages) can also be observed, related to severity of media/plaque injury or necrotic core disruption during the procedure. The thrombus organizes with migration and proliferation of smooth muscle cells. These smooth muscle cells produce the extracellular matrix in this repair process. At first the neo-intima is rich in proteoglycans and then becomes more collagen-rich, leading to more compact scar tissue. This change in neo-intimal composition from loose to compact is thought to be responsible for the late neo-intimal regression observed in angiography studies. Neo-intima formation causes re-stenosis within the stent, defined angiographically as 50 % diameter luminal narrowing.

Late Stent Thrombosis

In recent years, drug-eluting stents have minimized the limitations of bare-metal stents. Drug-eluting stents are coated with antiproliferative drugs such as sirolimus and paclitaxel. Late stent thrombosis, defined as any platelet-rich thrombus

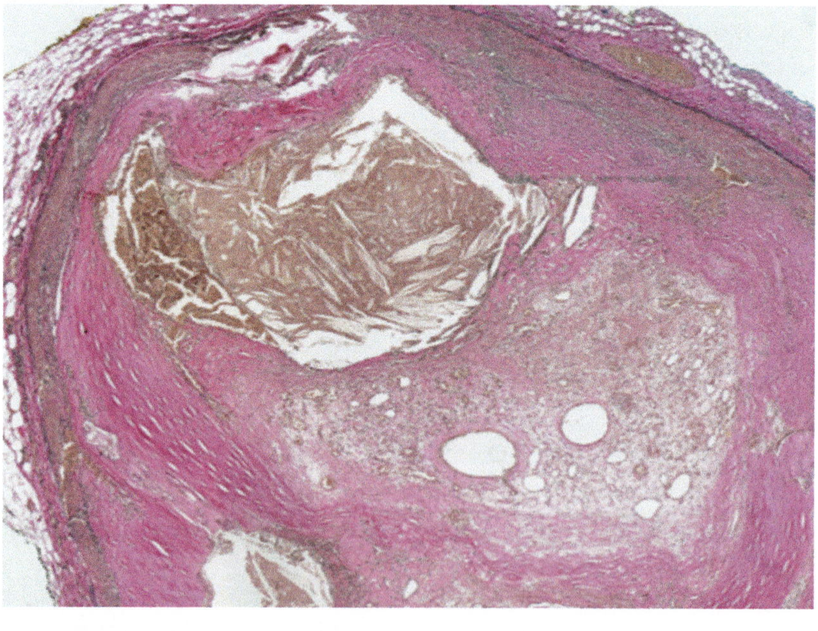

Fig. 5.1 Coronary artery with total occlusion due to previous plaque rupture. The atherosclerotic plaque shows a large necrotic core with a thin fibrous cap. In the lumen an older organized thrombus with loose connective tissue with signs of recanalization. Weigert–van Gieson elastic stain, original magnification 25×

occupying >25 % of lumen >30 days after implantation, has also been recognized as a serious long-term complication of drug-eluting stents (Fig. 5.2), where there is suppression of neo-intimal growth with poor re-endothelialization. The absence of re-endotheliaziation of the stent struts is assumed to be partly responsible for the development of late thrombosis of the stent. Additional factors that seem to be related to late stent thrombosis are incomplete apposition of the stent, penetration of necrotic core during stenting with plaque prolapse, stenting across ostia of branches, and interruption of long-term antiplatelet therapy.

In Stent Neo-atherosclerosis

Consistent with the development of native atherosclerosis, the first neo-atherosclerotic change observed in the stent area is accumulation of lipid-containing foamy macrophages around stent struts (Nakano and Virmani 2015). This can develop into the formation of unstable plaques of neo-atherosclerosis such as in-stent thin-cap fibroatheroma and plaque rupture (Fig. 5.3). These lesions can develop in both drug-eluting and bare-metal stents. In bare-metal stents neo-atherosclerosis mostly appears to develop after 5 years, whereas in drug-eluting stents these advanced neo-atherosclerotic lesions can be observed within 2 years after stent placement (Nakano and Virmani 2015). Overall neo-atherosclerosis can be observed more frequently and sooner in drug-eluting stents as compared to bare-metal stents. Probably incomplete re-endothelialization and impaired endothelial function in drug-eluting stents can partly explain the faster development of in-stent neo-atherosclerosis.

Embolization of Hydrophilic Coating

The number of interventional cardiovascular procedures has increased dramatically in recent decades and, in CAD especially, intravascular

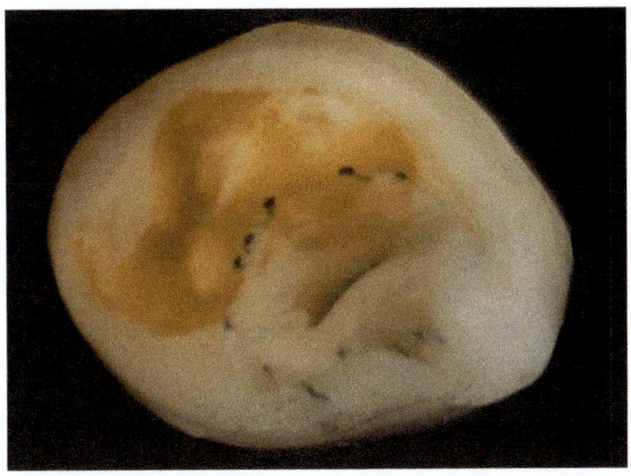

Fig. 5.3 Macroscopic picture of stented coronary artery with an in-stent atherosclerotic plaque. Note that in this case the in-stent part of the lipid-rich necrotic core is connected to the necrotic core of the original plaque outside the stent

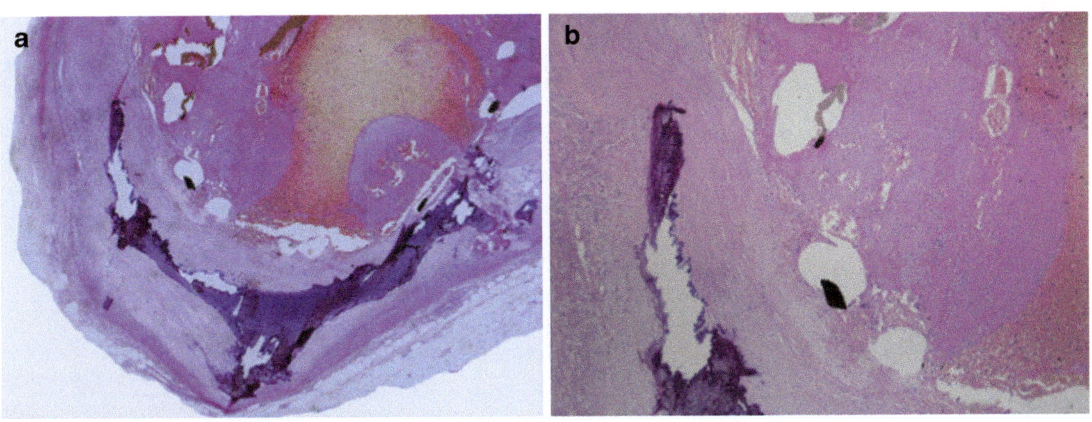

Fig. 5.2 Late stent thrombosis. (**a**) Stented coronary artery with a fibrocalcified plaque with occlusion of the lumen due to thrombus formation (Hematoxylin–eosin, original magnification 25×). (**b**) Higher magnification of late stent thrombosis (Hematoxylin–eosin, original magnification 200×). The stent struts are not covered by an endothelial layer. On top of the struts a platelet-rich thrombus has formed

angioplasty and stenting are frequently performed. The guiding catheters used in these procedures are coated with hydrophilic polymers to prevent thrombotic complications and vascular spasm. Embolization of parts of this hydrophilic coating to intramyocardial branches of coronary arteries can sometimes be observed in explanted hearts with a history of intracoronary procedures (Fig. 5.4).

5.2.3.3 Coronary Artery Bypass Grafts

In IHD native hearts, the pathologist may find segments of surgical bypass grafts, usually mammary grafts anastomosed to the left anterior descending or vein grafts sequentially anastomosed to coronary artery branches.

Chronic graft disease with significant stenosis or obstruction of the lumen is principally due to the following:

- Fibro-intimal proliferation with diffuse concentric intimal thickening by smooth muscle cells or myofibroblasts intermixed with extracellular matrix components.
- The usual atherosclerotic plaques, generally with large necrotic core and calcifications.

Organized thrombi occluding the lumen and, rarely, graft atherosclerotic aneurysms may be found (Tavora et al. 2007).

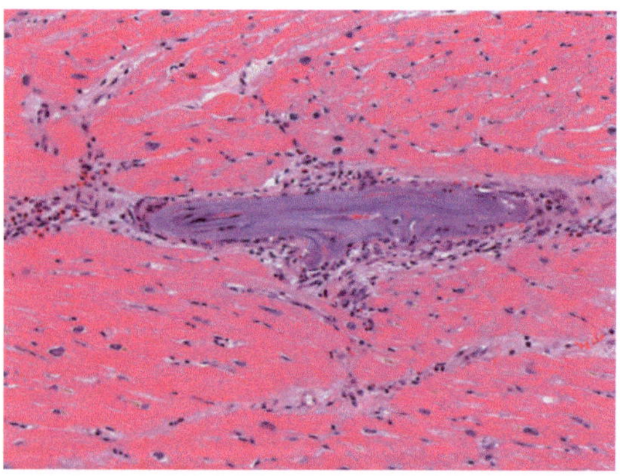

Fig. 5.4 Embolized hydrophilic coating from guide wire with blue–gray appearance in a small intramyocardial artery. The embolized material is surrounded by an inflammatory reaction with macrophages and eosinophilic granulocytes. Hematoxylin–eosin, original magnification 200×

5.2.3.4 Pathology of Myocardium

The morbidity and mortality of IHD are related to the remodeling of the myocardium that occurs in the postinfarction period. After a myocardial infarction the necrotic myocardium is replaced by scar tissue with numerous fibroblasts that produce collagen fibers. In time these areas of replacement cellular fibrosis become less cellular and dense collagenous fibrosis. Within the scars there can be fatty tissue (Fig. 5.5) or foci of calcification.

Grossly native hearts show left ventricular enlargement or biventricular dilatation, extensive and often multiple scars, either subendocardial or transmural or both (with mixed pattern), or segmental (localized) healed myocardial infarction and various degrees of hypertrophy indicative of myocardial remodeling in segments unaffected by old fibrous infarcts (Fig. 5.6). Left ventricular aneurysms or traces of aneurismectomy surgery are frequently found (Fig. 5.7).

The striking histologic finding in native hearts is the replacement fibrosis of healed infarction: it may be subendocardial or transmural, but always involves the subendocardium since this is a less well-vascularized area of the myocardium with less pO_2 as it is distant from the epicardial coronary arteries (Fig. 5.8). This distribution pattern of fibrosis is typical of IHD and is increasingly seen as an essential parameter in discriminating IHD from cardiomyopathies, especially in end-

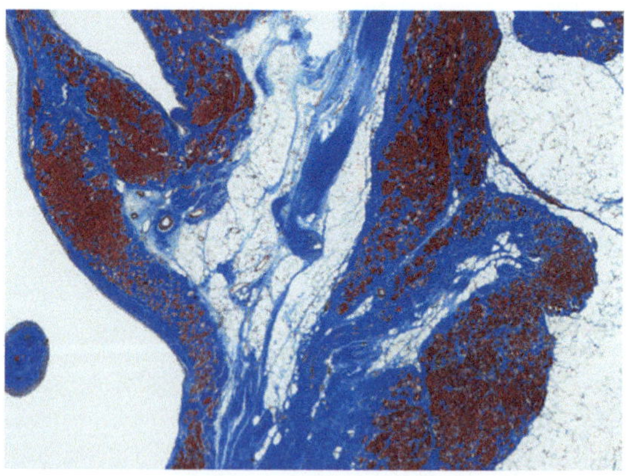

Fig. 5.5 Scar in the myocardium of the left ventricle with metaplasia of adipose tissue in the scar. Azan Mallory's trichrome stain, original magnification 25×

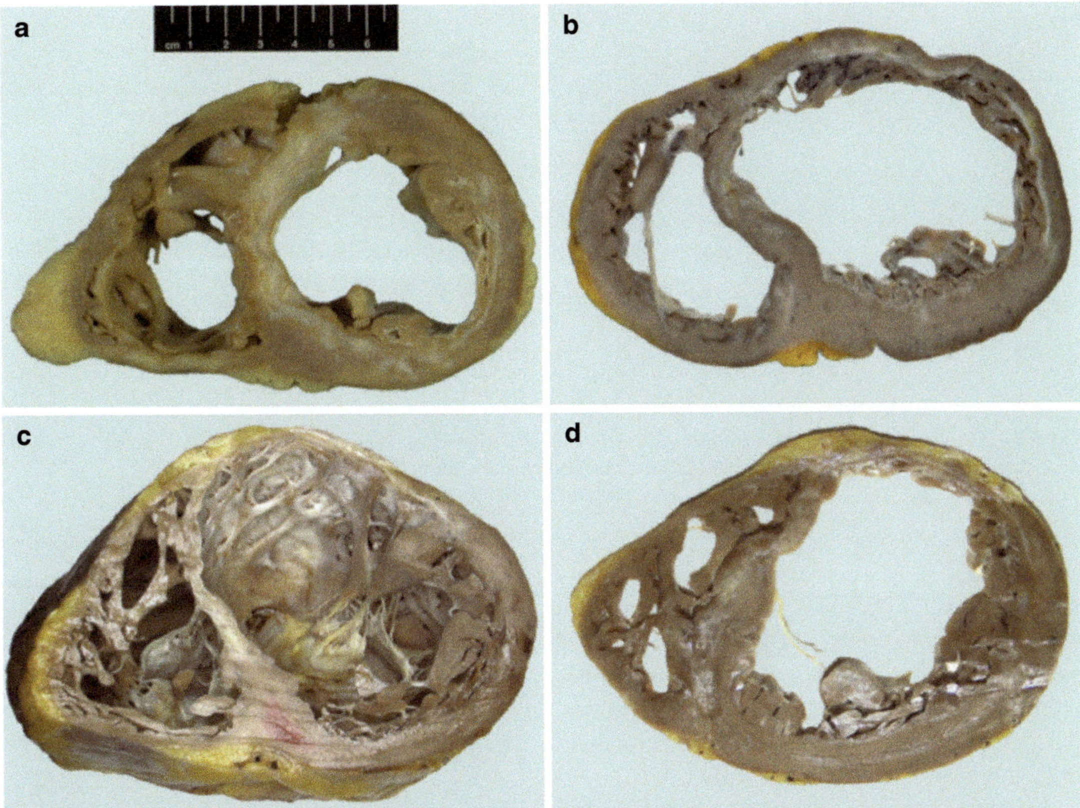

Fig. 5.6 Native explanted hearts showing variable gross appearance in IHD. (**a**) The cross section shows healed infarctions in the septum, anterior, posterior and lateral wall of the LV. Part of the scars are transmural, whereas in the LV lateral wall a subendocardial scar is present. The LAD has been removed for decalcification before sectioning. (**b**) Both ventricles are noticeably dilated. An extensive subendocardial scar is evident in the anterior-lateral LV wall and the septum. The LV inferior wall is hypertrophic as expression of myocardial remodeling. (**c**) The heart is generally enlarged. The fibrous transmural healed infarction involves the LV anterior wall and a large part of the septum, resulting in marked thinning of heart wall and initial parietal aneurysm formation. (**d**) A transmural scar is more localized in this heart (LV anterior wall), and dilatation involves only the LV. The posterior septum is hypertrophied. *LV* left ventricle, *LAD* left anterior descending coronary artery

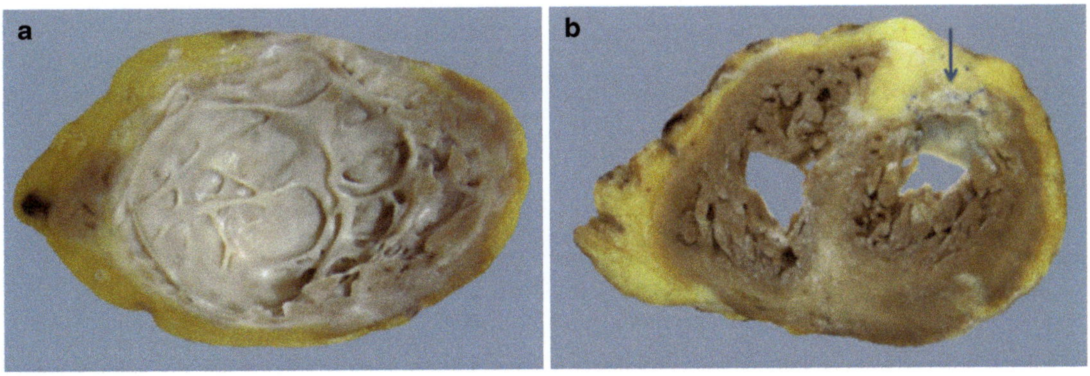

Fig. 5.7 Explanted hearts with apical aneurysms of left ventricle (**a**) or previous surgical aneurismectomy (*arrow*) (**b**)

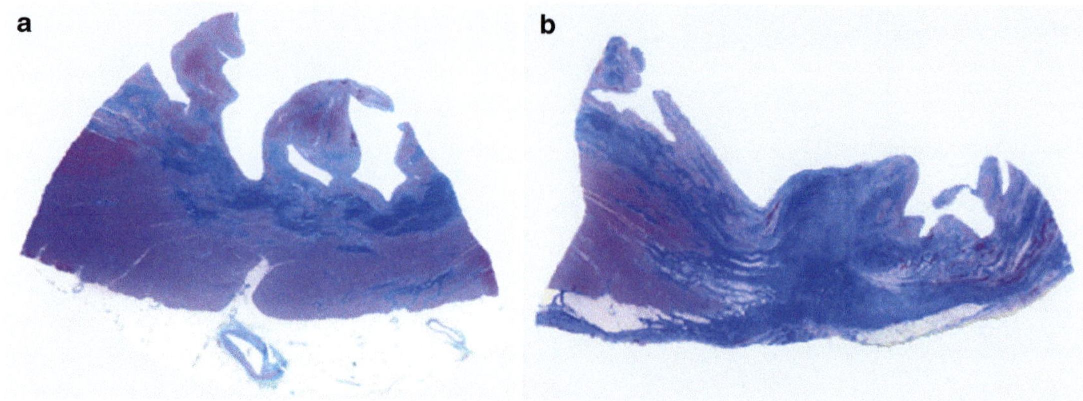

Fig. 5.8 Histologic sample of left ventricle with typical distribution of fibrosis in healed infarction: exclusively subendocardial in **a** and transmural in **b**. Azan Mallory's trichrome stain, digitalized slides

stage hearts (see Sect. 5.3). In general, in cardiomyopathies a more diffuse and differently distributed pattern of fibrosis can be seen. Recent observations suggest that the pattern of fibrosis is associated with pathogenic mutation in cardiomyopathies. In some dilated cardiomyopathies, the fibrosis is mostly located in the epicardial part of the myocardium (Gho et al. 2014).

In the myocardium surrounding the scar, reactive hypertrophy of cardiomyocytes in combination with interstitial fibrosis can be observed. In areas distant from the healed infarction replacement fibrosis of varying size may be present, caused by either prior local ischemia or embolization of parts of epicardial thrombi into small intramural arteries with subsequent microinfarctions, and nonspecific alterations of myocytes (myocytolisis, dysmetria, and vacuolization).

Another common finding in most CAD explanted hearts is cardiomyocytes with cytoplasmic vacuolization throughout the subendocardial and trabecular region of the ventricle wall: this phenomenon is due to loss of myofibrils resulting in vacuolization of myocardial cells, thereby creating a histologic pattern of empty cells (Fig. 5.9). The loss of these individual myofibrils is a cellular response to chronic nonlethal ischemia, which results in local myocardial dysfunction, and is the histological substrate of "myocardial hibernation." It has been suggested that the vacuolar changes are reversible with possible regeneration of lost myofibrils.

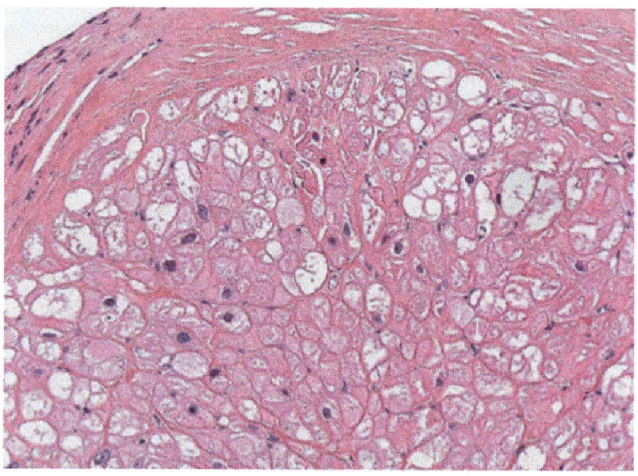

Fig. 5.9 Vacuolization of cardiomyocytes due to chronic ischemia resulting from progressive loss of individual myofibrils. Hematoxylin–eosin stain, original magnification ×200

Small vessel disease consisting of medial hypertrophy and intimal thickening/proliferation may also be found, diffusely or in multifocal areas, as histologic finding of dysfunction of the coronary microvasculature.

In some cases, there is obstructive atherosclerosis in one main coronary artery or multivessel disease with stenosis < 75 %, but no evident scar. In this case, the histology shows multifocal replacement fibrosis, decrease of myocytes, and myocell changes indicative of chronic ischemia.

5.2.4 Rare Conditions

Although coronary atherosclerosis is the main cause of IHD, it is occasionally possible to encounter non-atherosclerotic coronary artery disease, such as coronary dissection. This mainly affects young women and causes MI developing into chronic heart disease. In the native heart, the peculiar aspect is the histology of the coronary lesion, which presents the typical double lumen with neo-intima formation in the false lumen.

Another rare condition in the explanted heart is an acute myocardial infarction in cases of emergency transplantation following interventional procedures.

Illustrative Case 1 (Fig. 5.10)

A 65-year-old man suffered an anterolateral myocardial infarction 7 years ago. He was found to have severe atherosclerotic coronary artery disease of the main three coronary arteries and underwent elective coronary artery bypass graft (CABG) surgery. The left internal mammary artery (LIMA) was placed on the left anterior descending coronary artery (LAD) and a venous graft on the circumflex coronary artery and the posterior descending artery. Four years ago he again developed an acute coronary syndrome. On angiography the

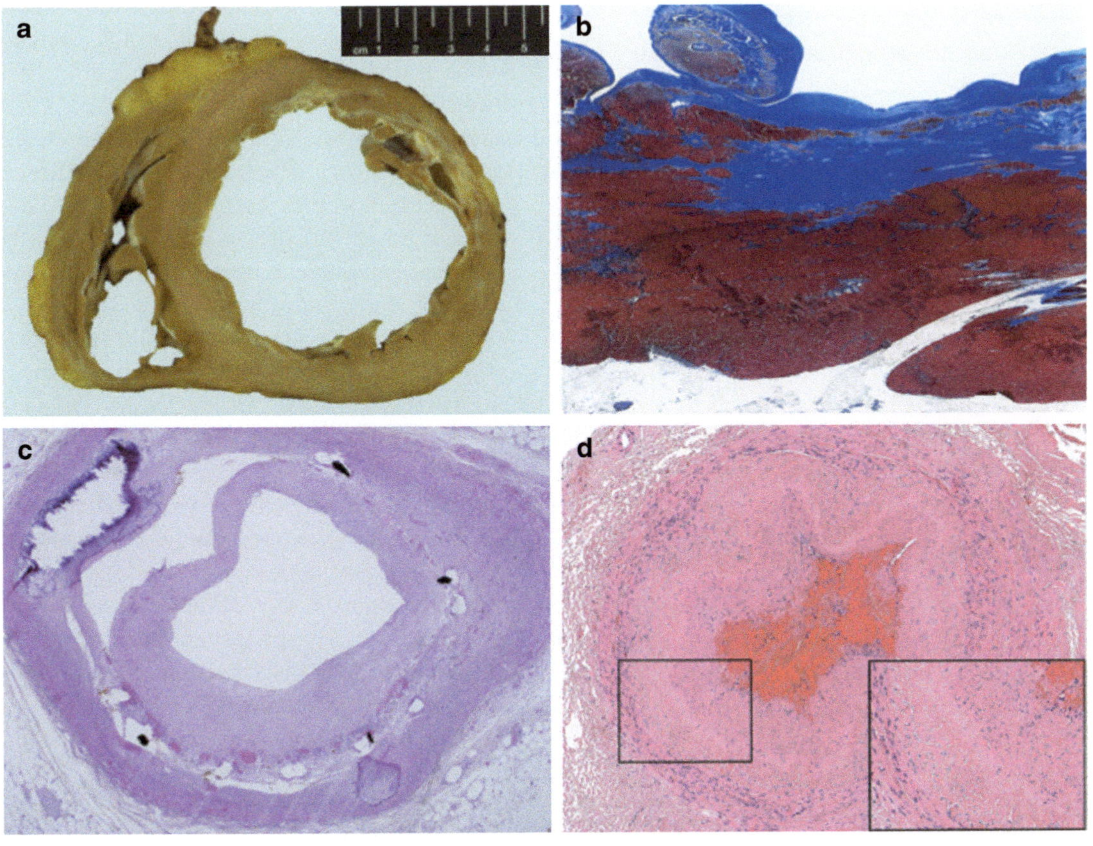

Fig. 5.10 Case 1. (**a**) Explanted heart with a large scar in the antero-lateral wall. Parts of the scar are transmural; the part in the anterior wall is mainly located in the subendocardial region. Note the LIMA graft on the LAD. (**b**) Histology of the subendocardial scar with remodeling of the surrounding myocardium (Azan Mallory's trichrome stain, original magnification ×25). (**c**) Stent in the LAD with in-stent neointima formation (Hematoxylin–eosin stain, original magnification ×25). (**d**) Distal part of the vein graft with intimal thickening and a thrombus in the lumen (Hematoxylin–eosin stain, original magnification ×25)

proximal part of the left anterior descending revealed 100 % stenosis, whereas the circumflex showed a subtotal stenosis. In addition the proximal part of the vein graft also showed 100 % stenosis with retrograde filling from the anterolateral branch. He underwent successful percutaneous transluminal coronary angioplasty (PTCA) with stenting of the proximal part of the LAD and circumflex coronary arteries. In the following years he developed severe heart failure with mitral valve insufficiency and underwent heart transplantation. The weight of the explanted heart was 460 g.

Dimensions of the heart:

- Left ventricle diameter: 7 cm
- Right ventricle diameter: 4 cm
- Left ventricle wall thickness: anterior 1.2 cm, lateral 0.9 cm, posterior 1.4 cm
- Septum thickness: 1.2 cm
- Right ventricle thickness: anterior 0.5 cm, posterior 0.3 cm

Key Points

Coronary arteries:

- Describe atherosclerotic plaques according to modified American Heart classification (Virmani et al. 2000), including the presence of lumen occlusion or degree of stenosis.
- Carefully evaluate stents and coronary by-pass.
- Identify rarer disease.

Myocardium:

- Describe presence, extent, sites, and types of myocardial scars.
- Note ventricular remodeling.
- Evaluate type, extent, and sites of myocyte and interstitial alterations.

5.3 Myocardial Disease

5.3.1 Background and Incidence in Explanted Hearts

Myocardial diseases (MDs), i.e., cardiomyopathies (CMPs), are the major reason for heart transplantation (HTx) in adults.

The International Society for Heart and Lung Transplantation (ISHLT) Registry shows that between 1982 and 2013, there were slightly more cases of CMPs than of coronary artery disease (CAD) (49 % vs. 43 %); the difference widens markedly if we consider only more recent years (2006–2013), when myocardial disease was clearly the most frequent (55 % vs. 36 %) of diseases requiring transplant (Lund et al. 2014). This difference is even more marked if we consider the geographical distribution of heart transplanted patients: in recent years in Europe and other areas, apart from the United States, CMP transplants number 57 % and 60 %, respectively (Lund et al. 2014), which could reflect different genetic and environmental factors that have a role in the origins of the diseases. In addition to the lower epidemiological frequency of CAD (see Sect. 5.2), this century has witnessed a sizeable increase in the spectrum of CMPs leading to transplant. While in the 1990s some specific CMPs – such as giant cell myocarditis, amyloidosis (AL), dystrophinopathies – represented a contraindication or controversial indication to transplant, greater knowledge, from both research and day-to-day practice, of these pathologies now makes transplant possible.

The situation is very different in pediatrics: from birth to 1-year, congenital heart disease is the main indication for transplant; for older children, CMPs rapidly increase as pathologies for transplant and, for ages 11–17 years, they account for as much as 66 % (Dipchand et al. 2014).

The term cardiomyopathy includes a broad and heterogeneous spectrum of myocardial disease, primary and secondary, familial/genetic and nonfamilial/nongenetic, idiopathic and acquired, so distinguishing among all these requires experience in the field. There have been many definitions and classification schemes of

CMPs over the years and the literature and textbooks often offer contradictory definitions, terms, and nosography. Only recently classifications that try to systemize this complex topics reflecting the impressive advances in knowledge and diagnosis of these diseases have been produced, although with different approaches (Elliott et al. 2008; Maron et al. 2006). According to the Position Statement from the European Society of Cardiology (ESC) (Elliott et al. 2008) we define CMP as "a myocardial disorder in which the heart muscle is structurally and functionally abnormal, in the absence of coronary artery disease, hypertension, valvular disease and congenital heart disease sufficient to cause the observed myocardial abnormality." CMPs are grouped into specific morphological and functional phenotypes: dilated cardiomyopathy (DCM), hypertrophic cardiomyopathy (HCM), arrhythmogenic right ventricular cardiomyopathy (ARVC), restrictive cardiomyopathy (RCM), and unclassified cardiomyopathy (UC) (Elliott et al. 2008). The aim of ESC classification scheme for CMPs is "*to help clinicians look beyond generic diagnostic labels in order to reach more specific diagnoses that may be useful for tailored clinical management of patients and their families*" (Elliott et al. 2008).

It is difficult to have general data on different types of transplanted CMPs, mainly because pre-transplant clinical diagnoses are listed in broad categories and MDs are often simply mentioned as non-ischemic cardiomyopathy. The really few pathologic studies comparing clinical and histological diagnosis of explanted hearts in a meaningful number of cases demonstrate that CMPs are the group most prone to pretransplant misdiagnoses, especially in CMPs secondary to a specific disease (e.g. various types of myocarditis, cardiac sarcoidosis) (Waller et al. 1998; Roberts et al. 2014a; Luk et al. 2009). This is partly the result of the habit of using pretransplant EMB (see Chap. 6).

DCM, the most common CMP and the leading cause of end-stage heart failure, is the most frequent clinical indication for orthotopic heart transplantation (c.a. 65 %) (Roberts et al. 2014b; Zhang et al. 2012). CMPs other than DCM leading to transplant are selected forms of HCM, arrhythmogenic cardiomyopathy (ACM), idiopathic RCM, left ventricular noncompaction (LVNC), myocarditis, and amyloidosis. For some of these, the data are limited to short series or single-center experiences. Single cases or limited case series of rarer CMPs or of CMPs restricted to endemic areas are also reported: sarcoidosis, storage disease, distrophinopathies, laminopathies, rheumatic heart disease, eosinophilic endomyocardial disease, eosinophilic granulomatosis with polyangitiis, Chagas disease, etc.

First-year and long-term survival in adult patients with CMPs is higher compared to patients transplanted for CAD (Lund et al. 2014). Recent data indicate that ACM has excellent posttransplant survival and HCM better survival than ischemic heart disease; for RCM patients, the worse outcomes are in the post-chemotherapy/ radiotherapy form group (DePasquale et al. 2014).

5.3.2 Specific Technical Pathology Points

5.3.2.1 Gross Examination

The approach to heart examination and especially sectioning and sampling should be guided by clinical history and diagnosis. Examination must be standardized and as detailed as possible.

Although the heart is quite frequently sent formalin-fixed, when it is available fresh, small pieces from the left ventricle (LV) should be frozen for possible molecular studies or be fixed in glutaraldehyde for ultrastructural examination (this last especially for suspected or previously diagnosed storage or mitochondrial diseases).

Apart from general details of native heart examination (see Appendix) and the more general recommendations for processing surgically resected hearts laid down in guidelines of the Association for European Cardiovascular Pathology and the Society for Cardiovascular Pathology (Stone et al. 2012), the essential points for CMP specimens are the following:

- Weight, dimensions (longitudinal and transverse), shape ("normal", globular, conical, altered volumetric ratio between the ventricles, possible aneurysms), amount, and distribution of epicardial fat.
- Chamber sizes (normal, small, dilated).
- Thickness of free wall of both ventricles and the interventricular septum (IVS) (parietal myocardium, excluding trabeculae) at basal, mid, and apical levels. When significant differences are present, thickness of various ventricular walls should be measured.
- Gross appearance of the myocardium with detailed description of recent lesions, scars, or fibrosis, fatty or fibro-fatty replacement, specifying their extent (transmural, subendocardial, mediomural, subepicardial) and location (anterior, lateral, posterior at basal, medium, and apical levels).

It should be noted that pathology examination of ventricle volumes and of myocardial thickness is conditioned by the non-physiological state of the heart, which is stiffened by formalin fixation or flattened when unfixed.

5.3.2.2 Sectioning

There are two main approaches for sectioning a heart affected by CMPs, using the echocardiographic short axis or four-chamber cuts. In the short axis cut, serial transverse sections (i.e., perpendicular to the long axis of the heart) are obtained from the apex to the mid-ventricular level (or to the base as far as the apex of papillary muscles) at 1 cm intervals (Fig. 5.11a, b); the cardiac basal segment can then be sectioned along its longitudinal axis. The second option is to perform an entire four-chamber section from the base to the apex along the acute and obtuse edges and the atrio-ventricular valves (Fig. 5.11c, d). The former method is better because the volume of ventricles and wall alterations can be assessed on different multiple planes; with the latter these alterations can only be assessed in a single cut.

Although significant coronary atherosclerosis is not usually present in native hearts with CMPs, careful examination of the coronary tree with serial sections is still good practice, at least in the proximal sites, especially in idiopathic DCM, where an occult CAD might be the underlying cause of the disease.

5.3.2.3 Sampling

Sampling for histological examination should be wide ranging and any minimalist approach should be avoided: currently histology is key to the study of CMPs in order to detect the various pathological aspects both in different types and within the same group of diseases and also to detail pathologic features of rare forms.

Standard sampling for CMPs should include the following:

- A complete section of the heart at mid-ventricular level (Fig. 5.12).
- One sample from the right ventricle (RV), two from the LV (anterior and inferior walls), and one from the IVS, all from both basal and apical segments.

All the samples must be taken from the most altered areas and further significant specimens should be obtained from areas with clear-cut macroscopic alterations.

It is also recommended that representative specimens of the myocardium of the atrial cap, of any valve lesions and of coronary arteries be obtained.

5.3.2.4 Staining

Apart from the usual hematoxylin–eosin, stains for collagen and elastic fibers (Masson or Mallory trichrome, Movat pentachrome, Weigert–Van Gieson, etc.) should also be requested in representative sections.

When warranted by hematoxylin-eosin, further additional stains and immunohistochemistry should be performed.

5.3.3 Pathologic Substrates

Of all cardiac diseases, CMPs, both common and rare forms, have probably benefited the most from the information obtained from pathologic study of native hearts.

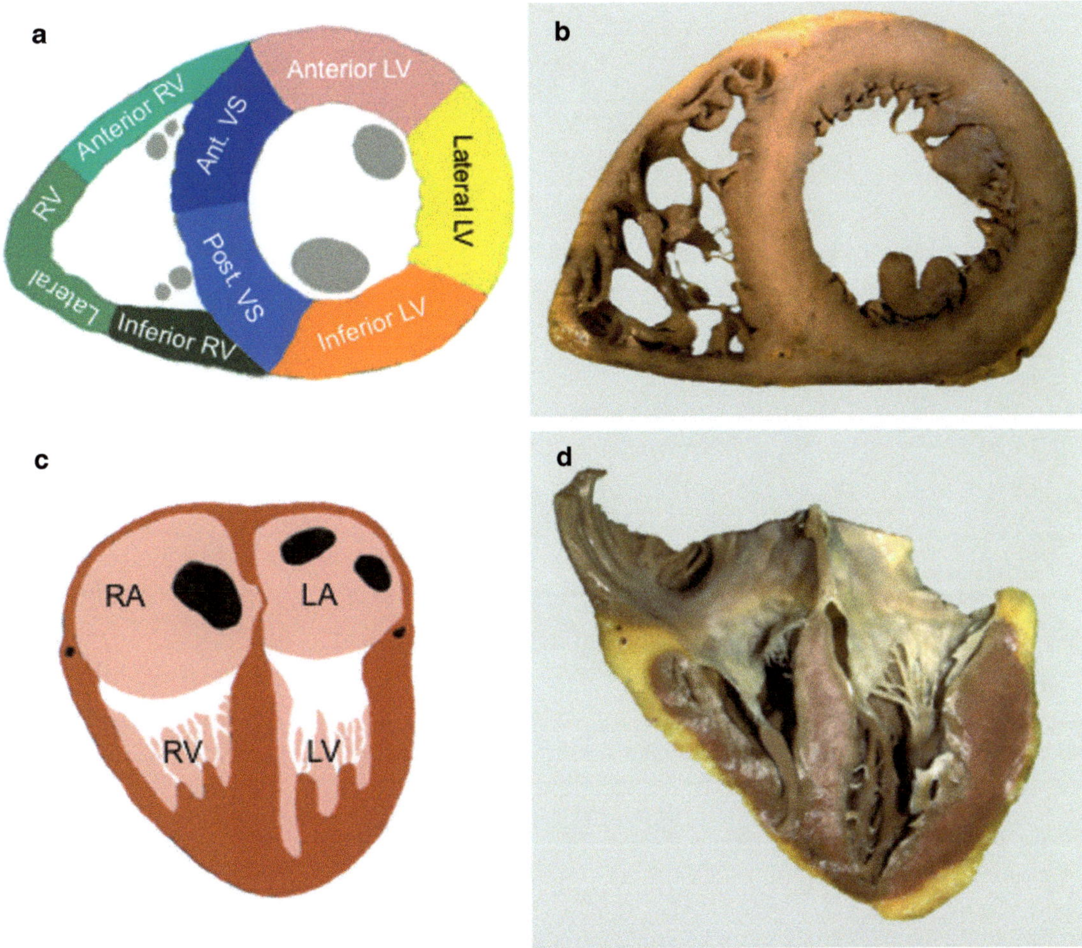

Fig. 5.11 On the left diagram (**a**) an echocardiographic mid-short axis cut, and in diagram (**c**) an echocardiographic four-chamber cut. On the right (**b**) and (**d**), the corresponding sections of native hearts. *LA* left atrium, *LV* left ventricle, *RA* right atrium, *RV* right ventricle, *VS* interventricular septum. Modified from Galati et al. 2016

Today identifying etiology is the main goal in CMPs and detailed pathologic examination of native hearts is a major step, both to confirm clinical diagnosis and to identify specific forms, which were not clear enough before transplantation (Rapezzi et al. 2013).

As these are usually end-stage heart failure cases, the pathologic examination too may have significant limits in tracing back the etiology, especially in the most frequent group, DCMs, which cover various diseases and where pathologic findings too are usually non-specific.

In CMPs transplanted at earlier phases of the disease, the pathologic substrate can really identify the etiology (e.g. myocarditis) and so give detailed confirmation of the pretransplant clinical diagnosis or even modify it.

In other CMP groups, such as dilated end-stage HCM, ARCV, or specific CMPs, the role of pathologic examination is also to provide additional information on the pathologic substrates underlying the diseases, so increasing knowledge of the pathogenesis and the phenomenology.

It should be emphasized that pathologic findings in chronic diseases differ from those of the active stage, so the pathologist must be aware of this and interpret subtle features in order to provide the fullest description of the disease.

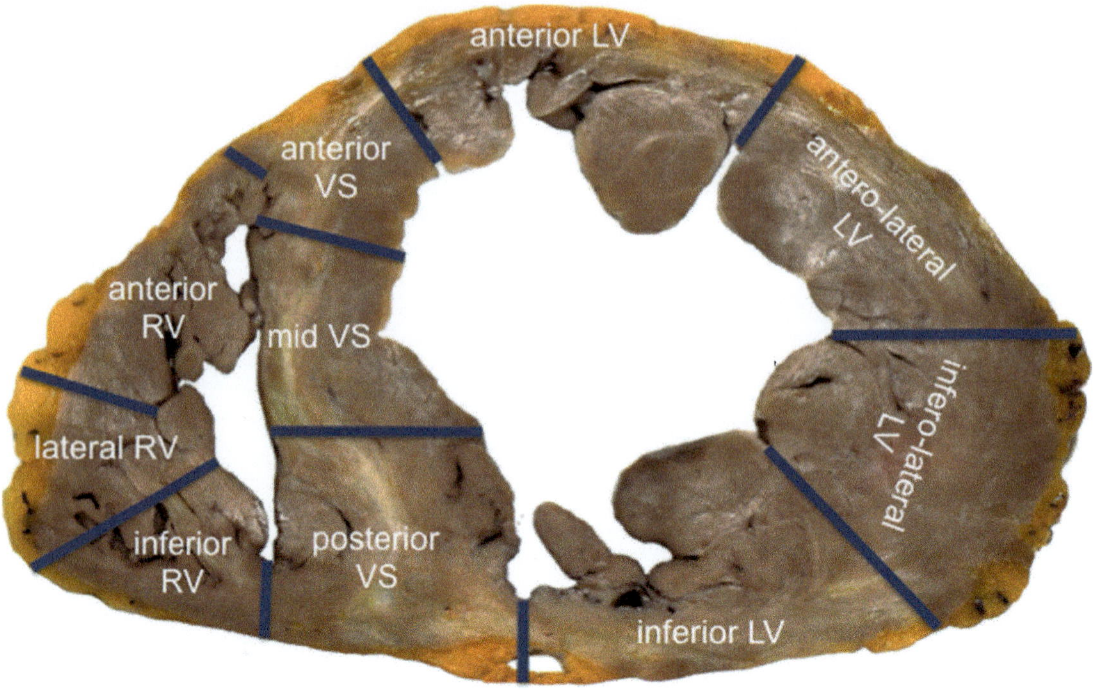

Fig. 5.12 Sampling of ventricles and septum should be taken from the segments shown in the photo in order to enable correlation with echocardiographic or magnetic resonance images. *LV* left ventricle, *RV* right ventricle, *VS* interventricular septum. Modified from Galati et al. 2016.

We will examine the pathological substrates of major groups/phenotypes of CMPs and of some specific forms.

5.3.3.1 Dilated Cardiomyopathy

Dilated cardiomyopathy is a melting-pot of a number of diseases including familial and acquired diseases. Familial forms (up to 35 % of patients) include variable pattern of inheritance, predominantly autosomal dominant and X-linked, autosomal recessive, or mitochondrial inheritance. Secondary causes include nutritional deficiency, endocrinopathies, systemic disease, cardiotoxic drugs, cardiac infective or immune inflammation at late stage, peripartum cardiomyopathy, and alcohol.

The majority of patients with dilated hearts are transplanted with the generic diagnosis of idiopathic DCM (c.a. 85 %), a diagnosis of exclusion. The pathologic features of this group are not usually indicative of any specific disease: they are able to confirm the generic diagnosis of DCM but the only real way to reach a specific diagnosis is to carefully correlate pathological findings with clinical data. Moreover a considerable proportion of cases are probably genetic and the final diagnosis must combine clinical and genetic data, which entails a long and expensive diagnostic process, not yet always standard procedure, even in specialized centers.

In *idiopathic DCM*, the heart is increased in weight, enlarged, and globular with markedly dilated left ventricle or biventricular dilatation (Fig. 5.13a, b). The ventricular mural myocardium is usually thinned, although it may be normal or thickened in some areas (Fig. 5.13b, c). Except for the typical thinning, the ventricular myocardium may be grossly normal in appearance or show whitish fibrotic areas, variable in extent and irregularly distributed (Fig. 5.13d); the endocardium is thickened diffusely or irregularly. Minor changes or atherosclerotic plaques narrowing the lumen for ≤50 % in cross-sectional area can be found in the major coronary arteries. When significant (≥75 %) atherosclerosis in one or more major epicardial branch is present, the

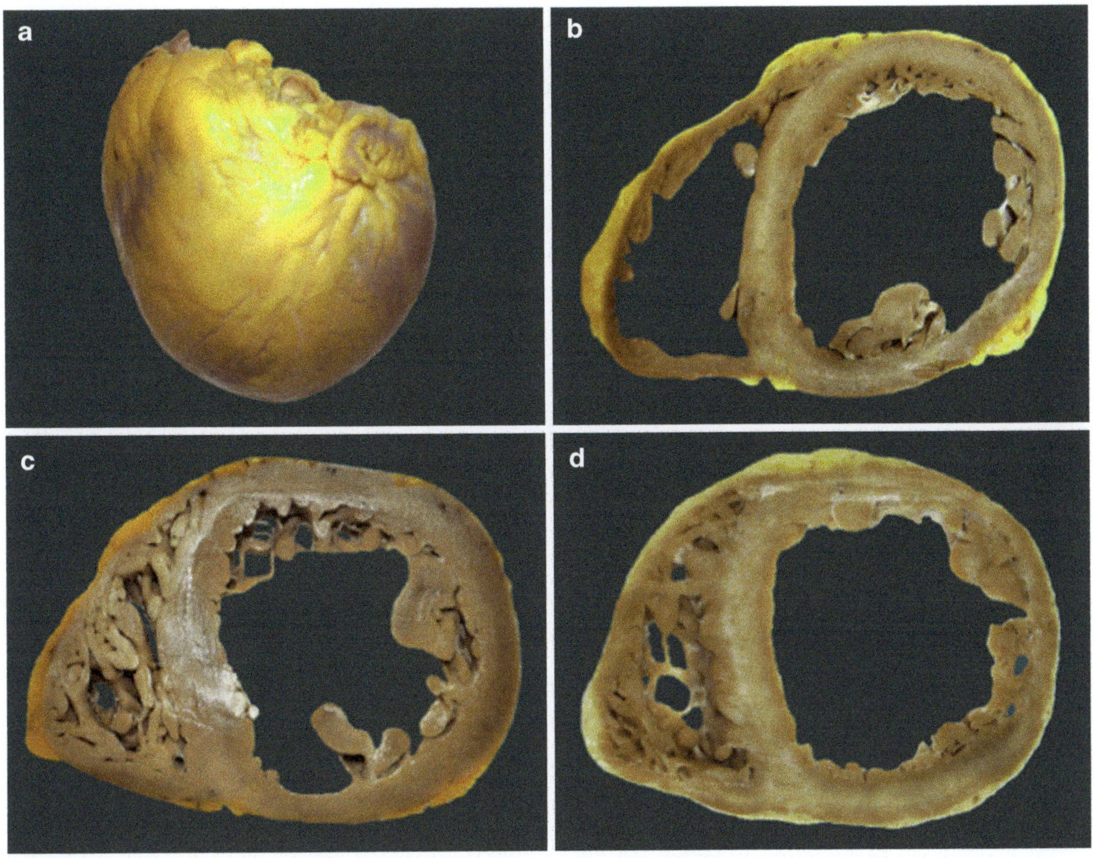

Fig. 5.13 Macroscopy of idiopathic DCM. In typical idiopathic DCM the heart is very enlarged and shows a rounded apex (**a**). Biventricular dilatation is evident in **b** as well as marked thinning of LV mural myocardium. In **c**, the myocardium of LV is very thin in the inferior wall, less thinned in the antero-lateral and almost normal in the infero-lateral wall. LV myocardium may show focal subendocardial and mural whitish areas (**b**) or be grossly normal (**c**); extensive whitish fibrotic areas mainly involving the mid LV and the IVS may be seen in post-inflammatory cases (**d**) (see section "Myocardites/Inflammatory CMPs/Postmyocarditis DCM"). *DCM* dilated cardiomyopathy, *LV* left ventricle, *IVS* interventricular septum

diagnosis of ischemic cardiomyopathy should be considered, both as first etiology of the disease and as a concurrent cause:

Histologic features are non-specific and mainly consist of fibrosis and myocyte chronic damage: their extent varies considerably and the severity does not usually correlate with clinical dysfunction. Interstitial (perivascular or perimyocyte) and replacement fibrosis is seen in variable degrees, diffuse or irregularly distributed (Fig. 5.14a, b); irregular fibrotic thickening of the subendocardium is also common. The most frequent myocyte alterations are variations in dimension, from true hypertrophy or simple increased size to attenuation; sarcoplasmic vacuolization/myofibril loss; foci of subendocardial colliquative myocytolisis (Fig. 5.14c–f). Minor inflammatory cell infiltrates can be found in the myocardial interstitium. It is noteworthy that interstitial myocardial fibrosis is increasingly recognized as central to the pathogenesis of CMPs and there is research ongoing into identification of specific patterns of fibrosis. For idiopathic DCM little data are available and there are various descriptions of fibrosis patterns; diffuse reactive (interstitial and/or perivascular) rather than reparative (replacement); increasing in the left ventricular free wall from epicardium to endocardium; intramyocardial band-like with septal involvement (Fig. 5.14a).

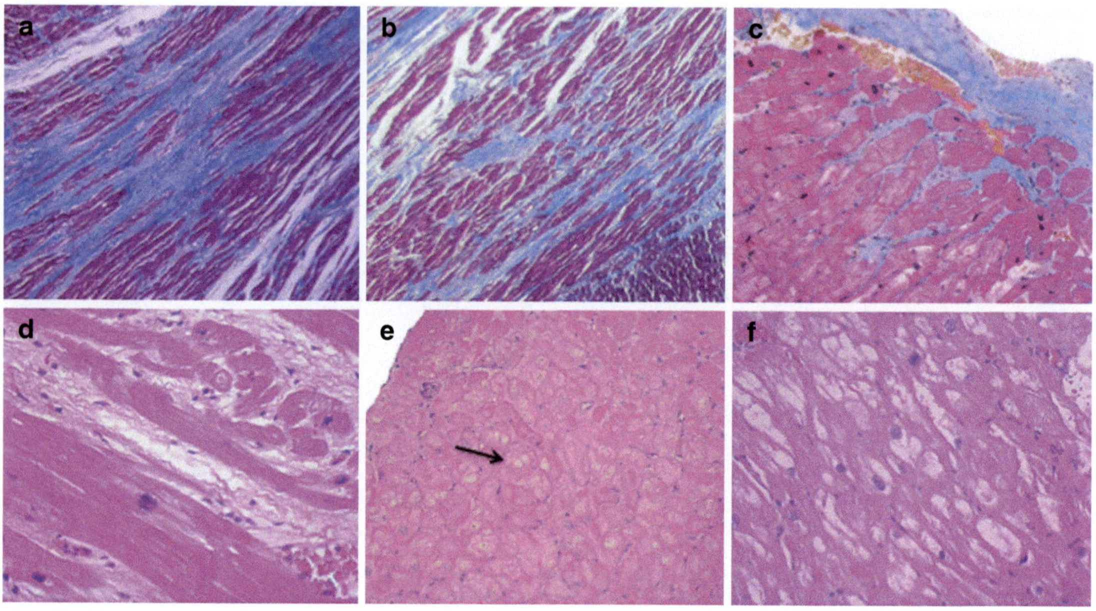

Fig. 5.14 The most frequent histologic alterations in idiopathic DCM are replacement intramyocardial band-like fibrosis of the septum (**a**: Azan Mallory trichrome; 100×) or interstitial perimyocyte fibrosis (**b**: in blue with Azan Mallory trichrome stain; 100×); variation in dimension of myocytes with hyperchromic and irregular nuclei (**c**, **d**: Hematoxylin–eosin 200×); progressive myofibril loss in myocells with sarcoplasmic vacuolization (**e**, *arrow*; hematoxylin–eosin 200×) or foci of colliquative myocytolisis (**f**: Hematoxylin–eosin 200×). *DCM* dilated cardiomyopathy

As mentioned, in a number of cases, etiology can be recognized by combining pathologic features and clinical history (see below "Specific cardiomyopathies") as well as pretransplant EMB findings.

5.3.3.2 Hypertrophic Cardiomyopathy

Historically, the term HCM identifies "sarcomere protein disease" and is defined as unexplained left ventricular hypertrophy in the absence of hypertension and valve disease. But the clinical phenotypic spectrum of an increased ventricular wall thickness (i.e. the *hypertrophic cardiomyopathies*) may be caused by an increase of left ventricular mass due to interstitial infiltration (amyloid) or intracellular accumulation of metabolic substrates (storage disease) as well as to some mitochondrial disease. These possibilities must be excluded through appropriate diagnostic work-up.

HCM/sarcomeric protein disease is the most common genetically transmitted heart disease (≥13 genes encoding proteins of cardiac sarcomere) with tremendous phenotypic heterogeneity in its clinical expression, genetics, and pathologic substrates. Heart transplantation is required in selected patients, prevalently those who have developed refractory end-stage heart failure with a hypokinetic and dilated left ventricle. Less frequently do those with life-threatening arrhythmias unresponsive to medical therapy need transplantation (Biagini et al. 2008).

The end-stage phase is a well-recognized part of HCM and its clinical profile is turning out to be more heterogeneous than expected: the prevalence, although varying in the literature, can be set around 5 % (Harris et al. 2006; Biagini et al. 2005), while a paper using a large population of patients gives the incidence as 5.3 per 1000 patient/years (Biagini et al. 2005).

The pathology of end-stage evolution is very interesting and differs from that of common HCM: its macroscopic spectrum shows three main patterns:

- Variable LV dilatation, depending on the distribution of myocardial hypertrophy, which may persist markedly in the IVS and the LV lateral

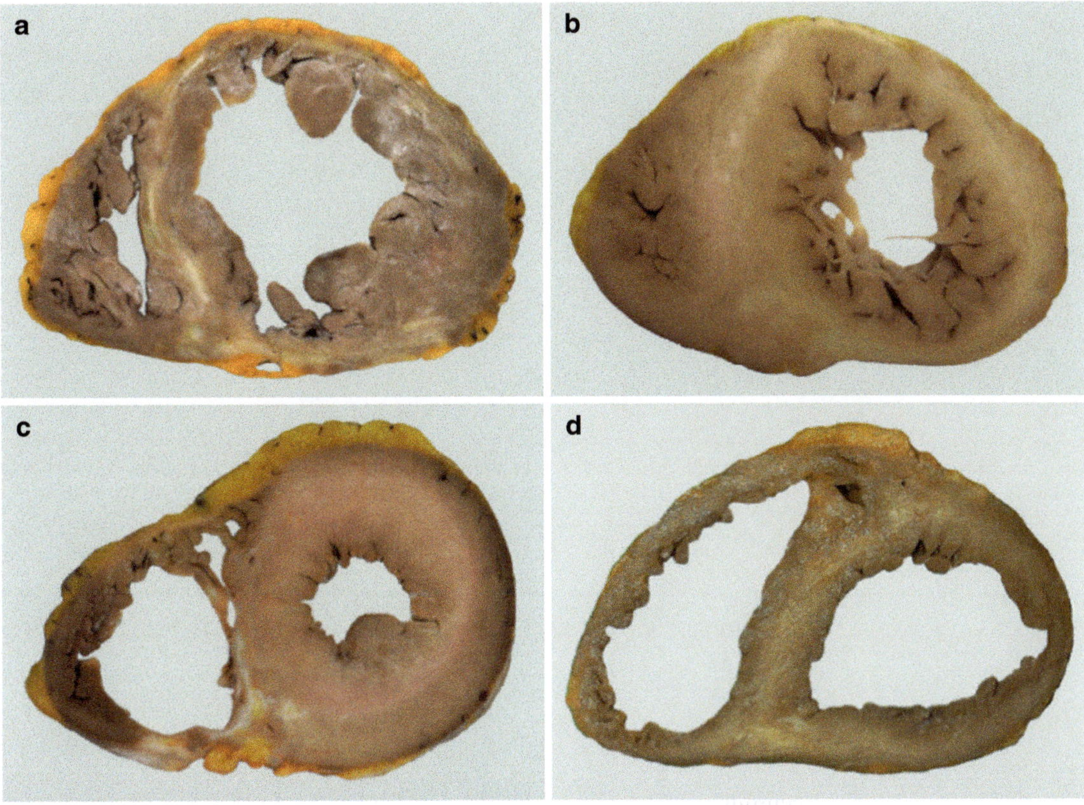

Fig. 5.15 Macroscopic spectrum of end-stage heart failure HCM. (**a**) Male transplanted at 47 years of age with LV dilatation, severe thinning of the anterior and posterior LV walls and hypertrophy of the lateral wall. The posterior septum is hypertrophic and in lesser degree the anterior. Fibrosis is extensive in midmural septum and in the posterior and anterior walls of LV with subepicardial–mediomural distribution or transmural focal areas. (**b**) Heart of a young female transplanted at 23 years. Marked hypertrophy of the IVS, RV, and the lateral wall of the LV is evident together with thinning of the anterior and inferior LV walls. LV cavity is mildly and irregularly dilated and extensive whitish areas of fibrosis are evident in the IVS and LV. (**c**) In the native heart of this 39-year-old male marked concentric hypertrophy of LV and IVS is present, associated with striking fibrosis, prevalently mediomural and irregularly subendocardial. The RV cavity is dilated. (**d**) Explanted heart of a 41-year-old female with marked biventricular dilatation and irregularly alternating myocardial hypertrophy or thinning. *LV* left ventricle, *RV* right ventricle, *IVS* interventricular septum

wall and be associated with severe thinning of the anterior and posterior LV walls or of the anterior septum. White areas of scarring, sometimes transmural, are evident and mostly involve the IVS and the LV. RV may also be hypertrophic and show fibrotic areas (Fig. 5.15a).

- Persistent more diffusely distributed marked hypertrophy of IVS and LV with mild ventricular dilatation. Wide areas of fibrosis are also seen in this pattern (Fig. 5.15b, c).
- Marked biventricular dilatation, irregularly alternating myocardial hypertrophy or thinning (Fig. 5.15d).

The main histologic features are the following:

- Myocyte hypertrophy with bizarre enlarged nuclei.
- Multifocal myocyte disarray as in typical sarcomeric HCM (Fig. 5.16a).
- Extensive areas of marked sarcoplasmic vacuolization at times resembling storage disease (Fig. 5.16b).
- Extensive interstitial fibrosis showing two main patterns:
  - Striking replacement fibrosis with a typical distribution (see below).
  - Interstitial perimyocytic fibrosis.

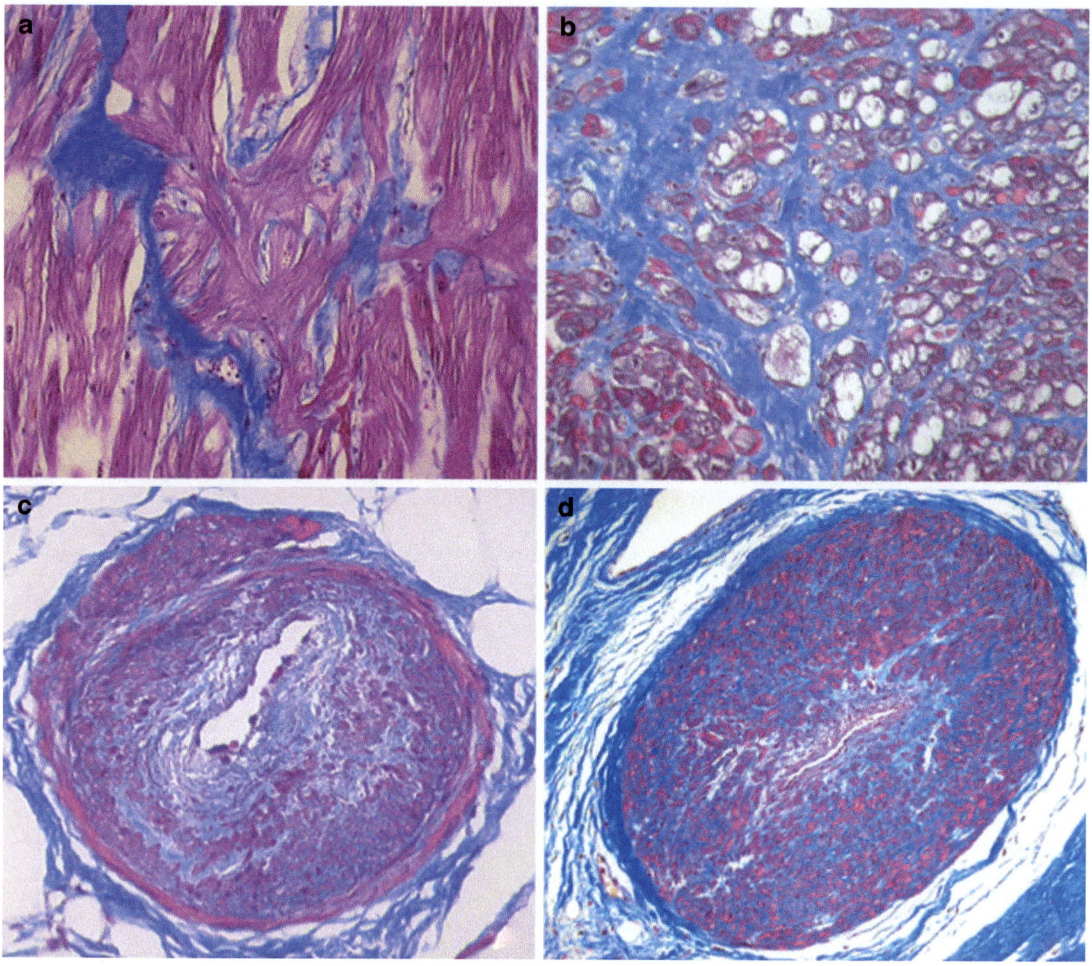

Fig. 5.16 Histology of end-stage HCM. A Multifocal typical myocyte disarray (**a**) is associated with large areas of sarcoplasmic vacuolization (**b**). Small vessel disease is always present, moderate to severe at this stage: image **c** shows combined intimal–medial disease with fibrous intimal hyperplasia and hypertrophy of medial smooth muscle cells; in image **d**, almost complete obstruction of the lumen is caused by marked medial hypertrophy and fibrosis. Mallory trichrome stain: **a** (400×); **b** (200×); **c** (400×); **d** (400×). Modified from Galati et al. 2016

- Small vessel disease made up of several abnormal intramural coronary arteries with thickened walls and narrowed/obstructed lumen due to intimal disease (eccentric or concentric hyperplasia of loose or mature fibrous tissue) or medial disease (hypertrophy with or without fibrosis of medial layer) or both, sometimes with hamartomatous appearance (Fig. 5.16c, d).

Pathogenetic mechanisms of dilated-hypokinetic evolution have been widely discussed in the literature and there is general agreement that small vessel disease is to be considered as one of the keys to myocardial ischemia-mediated myocyte death and ultimately to replacement fibrosis (Harris et al. 2006; Biagini et al. 2005; Maron et al. 2009).

Histologic examination of the hearts of 31 patients transplanted for end-stage HCM at the Bologna center between 1991 and 2014 (19 males and 12 females; median age at transplant 46.5 ± 11.9 years; 6.4 % of total heart transplanted patients) showed very marked intramyocardial fibrosis, interstitial perimyocytic or replacement or mixed, with certain prevalent patterns of distribution in the ventricular and septal walls (Fig. 5.17):

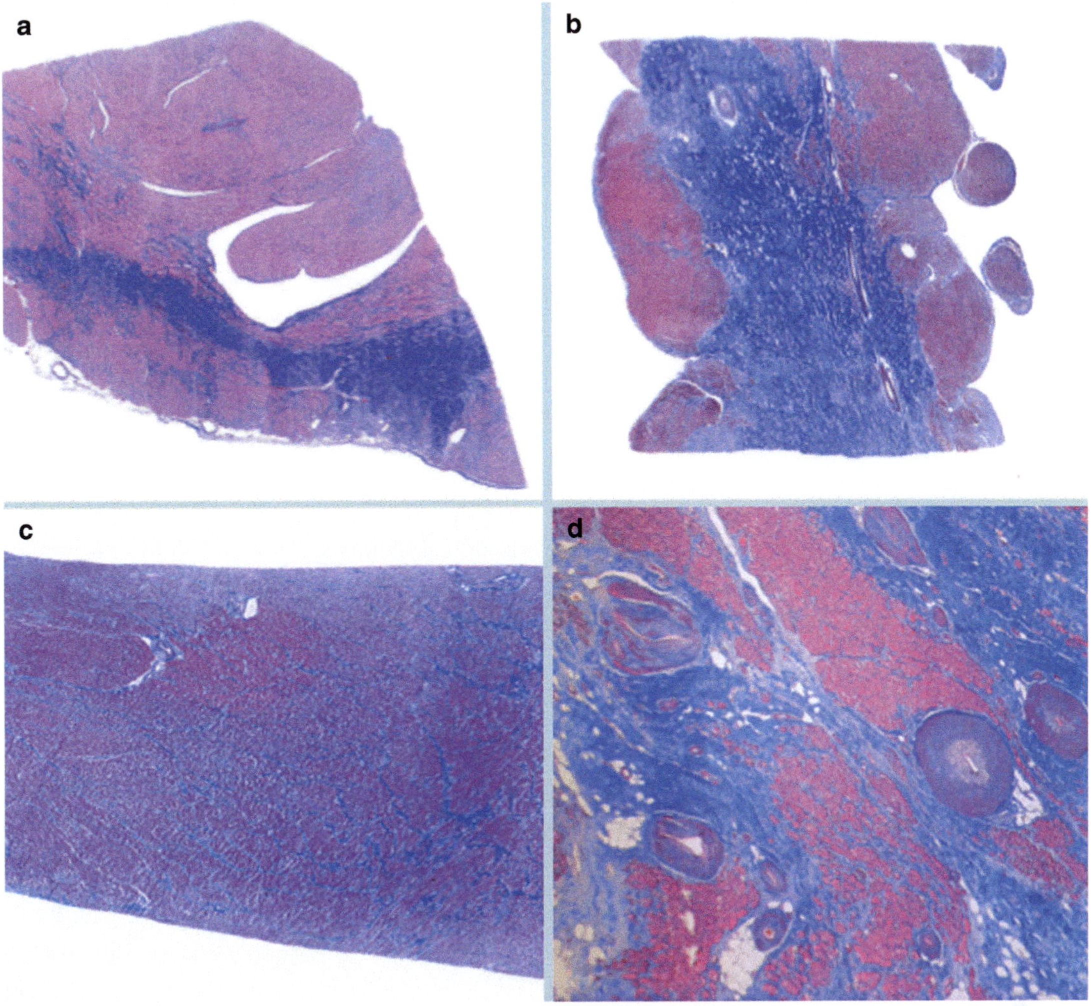

Fig. 5.17 Types of fibrosis in specimens from LV (**a**, **c**) and IVS (**b**, **d**) in end-stage HCM cases. (**a**, **b**) Replacement fibrosis with mediomural/subepicardial distribution in LV wall (**a**) and mostly localized in the IVS midwall (**b**). Interstitial perimyocyte fibrosis with plexiform distribution around myocardial fibers (**c**). Severe small vessel disease in close relation with scar-like fibrosis: small arteries on the left show hamartomatous disorganization of the wall (**d**). Mallory trichrome stains. *LV* left ventricle, *IVS* interventricular septum. Modified from Galati et al. 2016

1. Highest midmural distribution (33.4 %), with possible involvement of subepicardial (20.3 %) and subendocardial (20.2 %) layers, but never in isolation.
2. Radial/circumferential distribution at midventricular short-axis level with mostly affected LV inferior (24.3 % of total fibrosis) and antero-lateral (15.8 %) and anterior walls (11.9 %), and relatively spared infero-lateral wall (7 %). The septum is more homogeneously involved by fibrosis.
3. Longitudinal distribution with evident base/apex gradient pattern resulting in fibrosis notably increasing toward the apex (31.9 % ± 14.5 %, at base to 46.2 % ± 14.9 % at apex).

Pattern 1 sharply differentiates end-stage HCM from post-ischemic cardiopathy, where fibrosis is mainly subendocardial; pattern 3 differentiates end-stage HCM from other CMPs (e.g. amyloidosis where amyloid deposits typically spare the apex).

Fibrosis is also present in RV, with an increasing gradient toward the inferior wall (Galati et al. 2016).

The most striking small vessel disease is typically seen in association with the most extensive areas of replacement fibrosis.

5.3.3.3 Restrictive Cardiomyopathy

Restrictive cardiomyopathy is a primary abnormality of diastolic function characterized by elevated ventricular filling pressures and relatively preserved systolic function. Restrictive ventricular physiology may occur in a wide range of different pathologies, so the term RCM includes idiopathic and familial forms or may result from various disorders.

Idiopathic RCM is a rare disease and should be considered only after carefully ruling out restrictive forms secondary to amyloidosis, sarcoidosis, endomyocardial fibrosis, radiation/chemotherapy, late stage of hypertrophic dilated, valvular, hypertensive and ischemic heart diseases, carcinoid heart disease, scleroderma. Endomyocardial biopsy should be performed when diagnosing a patient with RCM because specific causes may need specific treatment or may change the indication to transplant (see paragraph 5.3.3.6).

The prevalence of heart transplantation for overall RCMs (idiopathic and secondary) in a large US cohort is 1.4%, similar to HCM but significantly lower than DCM (De Pasquale et al. 2012).

Gross cardiac specimens of idiopathic form demonstrate typical bi-atrial enlargement with normal-sized or small ventricles and absent or mild hypertrophy (Fig. 5.18a, b). Prominent trabeculation may be present.

Although the histology is nonspecific, commonly found alterations are fibrous subendocardial thickenings; marked interstitial fibrosis, increased myocyte dimension alternating with normal sized myocells; and areas of sarcoplasmic vacuolization (Fig. 5.18c). Myocyte disarray is not uncommon but unlike HCM involves bundles of myocytes rather than single fibers.

The patterns of fibrosis are little known: diffuse perimyocytic fibrosis is most frequent, but replacement or band-like fibrosis has been described in the mediomural LV myocardium.

5.3.3.4 Arrhythmogenic Right Ventricular Cardiomyopathy/ Arrhythmogenic Cardiomyopathy

Arrhythmogenic right ventricular cardiomyopathy is a progressive disorder of the cardiac muscle, whose pathologic hallmark is fibro-fatty replacement of myocardium. Unlike the other wider phenotypic categories of DCM, HCM, and RCM, this histologic definition makes possible to confine the term ARCV to a specific form of CMP, although these pathologic abnormalities had also be found in some neuromuscular diseases.

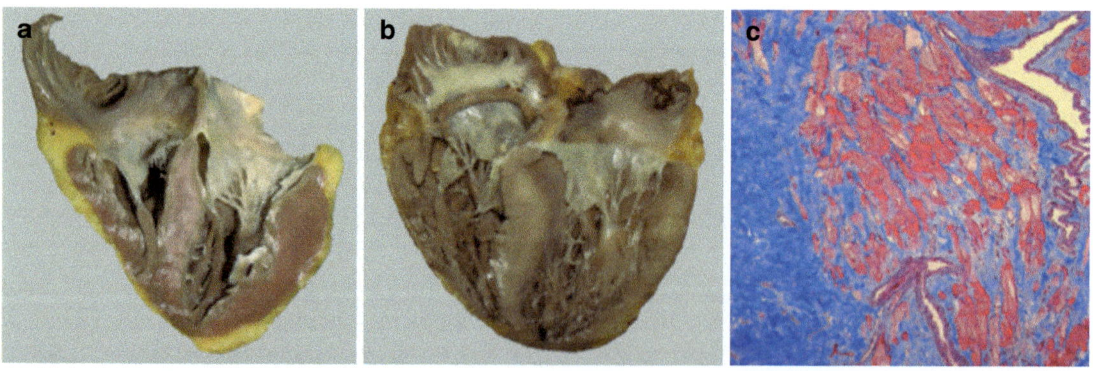

Fig. 5.18 (**a**, **b**) Explanted hearts with idiopathic restrictive cardiomyopathy of two female patients (41 and 19 years old). In both hearts bi-atrial enlargement is evident; ventricles are small in **a** and mildly dilated in **b**, where a Carpentier ring is placed in the tricuspid annulus. (**c**) The histologic picture shows marked interstitial fibrosis, varying myocyte size and sarcoplasmic vacuolization

We think it is more correct to call this CMP "arrhythmogenic cardiomyopathy (ACM)" rather than ARVC because, although it came to light as a disease exclusively of the right ventricle, recently three different patterns have been recognized: RV dominant disease, biventricular CMP, and LV dominant form (Sen-Chowdhry et al. 2007). There are still numerous questions as to the etiopathogenesis of this interesting CMP and in spite of excellent research into its genetic origin, how defects in genes codifying for desmosomal proteins can cause massive and progressive fibro-fatty replacement of ventricular myocardium is still underrecognized.

As in HCM the phenotype in native hearts differs from the clinical–pathologic profile of the disease in sudden death cases. The main indication for heart transplantation is end-stage heart failure and refractory ventricular arrhythmias account for a small number of patients.

Thanks to successful transplantation in 17 patients in Bologna Transplant Centre, we have been able to analyze the pathology features of this end-stage subgroup, consisting in nine males, eight females, median age of 45.7 years (range 24–64 years), representing 2.7 % of heart transplanted patients (Graziosi et al. 2013).

All the hearts had biventricular disease and were heavily dilated. RV involvement was always diffuse with transmural fibro-fatty replacement and typical inflow and outflow aneurysms in almost all cases; LV showed various degrees of involvement, mainly in the posterolateral wall; the IVS was almost always affected by the disease, predominantly in the posterior portion. Apical segments were involved in all cases. It should be noted that in some cases careful examination of LV is required, as findings may be attenuated. At histology, diffuse fibro-fatty replacement involved RV throughout the wall; LV was affected in multifocal areas with a prevalent pattern of fibrous replacement, mainly subepicardial/mediomural and more focally transmural. Typical myocyte damage (hypertrophy, dysmetria, sarcoplasmic vacuolization) was present in both ventricles, multifocally in the LV (96 %) and diffusely in the RV (100 %). Lymphocytic infiltrates in both ventricles and IVS, with both active myocarditis and quiescent patterns, were frequently seen (Fig. 5.19). It should be noted that four of these patients had previously been clinically diagnosed as suffering from idiopathic DCM.

5.3.3.5 Left Ventricular Noncompaction

Left ventricular noncompaction cardiomyopathy (LVNC), a disease characterized by prominent LV trabeculation and deep intertrabecular recesses (Jenni et al. 2007), is included in the ESC Position Statement under unclassified CMPs and is considered by the American Heart Association classification as primary genetic CMP. Its nosography is debated as it is unclear whether it is a separate, distinct CMP or a morphologic trait common to various CMPs, most frequently DCM and sporadic in hypertrophic and restrictive phenotypes (Biagini et al. 2006).

Examination of explanted hearts mostly supports the second hypothesis of morphologic findings common to a spectrum of CMPs: in some cases, often pediatric, the hypertrabeculation is very striking and remembers the structure of the embryonic heart; in other cases attenuated, partly due to the degree of ventricular cavity dilation.

In addition it should be noted that the anatomic definition and parameters of this disease have never really been agreed on, so pathologists have continued with the echocardiographic criteria (noncompacted portion of LV myocardium ≥ 2 times as thick as the compacted portion) which are probably inadequate for pathologic analysis.

Further research is needed into this heterogeneous condition in order to define diagnostic criteria and genetic substrates.

5.3.3.6 Specific Forms of Cardiomyopathies

Myocardites/Inflammatory CMPs/Post-myocarditis DCM

In dilated hearts, several kinds of inflammatory process may be observed, occurring in various phases. In general, the incidence of myocarditis in the native hearts of transplant recipients has been reported to range from 1 to 8 %, with lymphocytic myocarditis as the most frequent form. Other rare

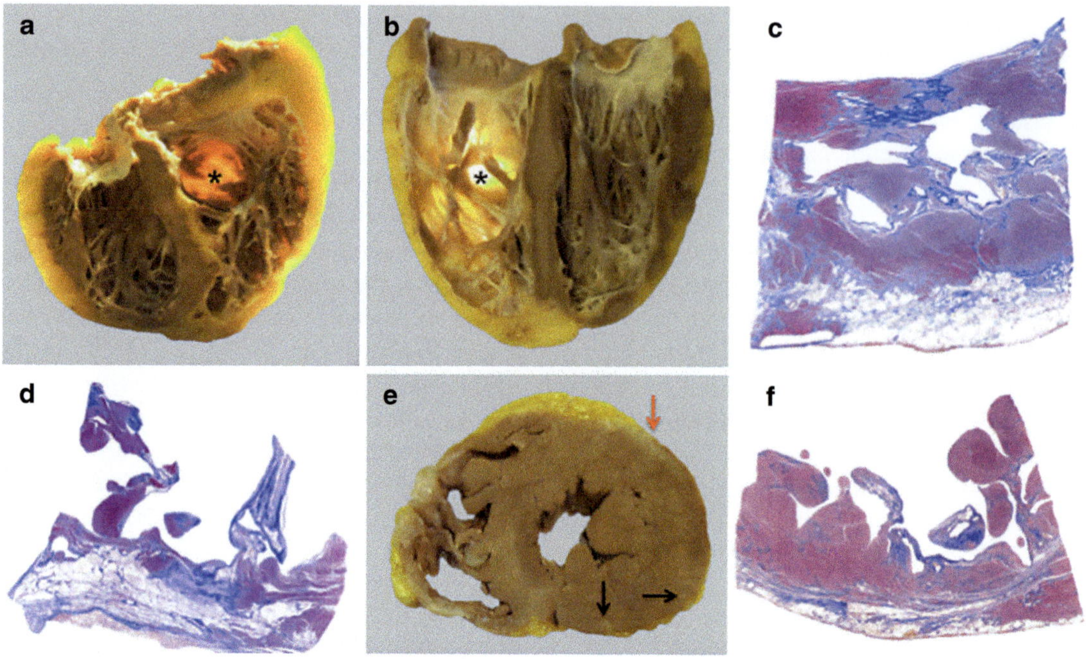

Fig. 5.19 Explanted hearts of patients with end-stage biventricular arrhythmogenic cardiomyopathy. (**a**) Longitudinal cut of the heart of a 64-year-old male with massive involvement of the RV, where a significant aneurysm of the RV outflow is emphasized by transillumination (*asterisk*). (**b**) Posterior view of a longitudinal cut of the native heart of a 27-year-old female, showing an aneurysm of the RV posterior wall, typically localized below the tricuspid valve (*asterisk*); the LV lateral wall is multifocally involved by the disease with typical scalloped contour of the myocardial wall. Histology reveals typical fibro-fatty replacement, originating from the subepicardium and involving the LV midwall (**c**: LV specimen; Azan Mallory trichrome) and entire RV wall (**d**: Azan Mallory trichrome). (**e**) In this other case (34-year-old male) the LV is focally involved: in the anterior wall a subepicardial whitish fibrotic area is evident (*red arrow*) and in the infero-lateral wall subepicardial yellow foci (*black arrows*). (**f**) Histology of this case confirms that the LV involvement is limited but with the same distribution as in other cases. *LV* left ventricle, *RV* right ventricle

forms such as giant cell myocarditis (GCM), cardiac sarcoidosis, or cardiac involvement in systemic inflammatory disorders may be present, although in limited cases. There was at one time some concern about cardiac transplantation for myocarditis, but today this is largely accepted and current data on patients transplanted with lymphocytic myocarditis are promising in terms of rejection or death risk; for rare forms the data are still very limited (Moloney et al. 2005).

In *post-lymphocytic myocarditis DCM*, abnormalities vary depending on the stage of the disease, from nonextensive dilatation of ventricles in the subacute phase, sometimes with marbled aspect of the myocardium, to significant enlargement of the heart with irregularly distributed focal fibrotic areas, or very evident and extensive scars in the subepicardial-mediomural areas or transmural, with infarction-like distribution or not (Fig. 5.20).

Similarly, the histology can show a still active disease with multiple interstitial lymphocytic inflammatory infiltrates associated with myocyte damage or healing/healed myocarditis, where mild interstitial inflammation is associated with reparative changes ranging from loose granulation tissue to replacement by collagenous scar tissue and associated chronic myocyte damage (post-myocarditis DCM) (Fig. 5.21).

GCM is a particularly malignant form of myocarditis, which leads to more pronounced pathological abnormalities in the heart, and both ventricles are often uniformly involved. In explanted hearts, the disease is commonly

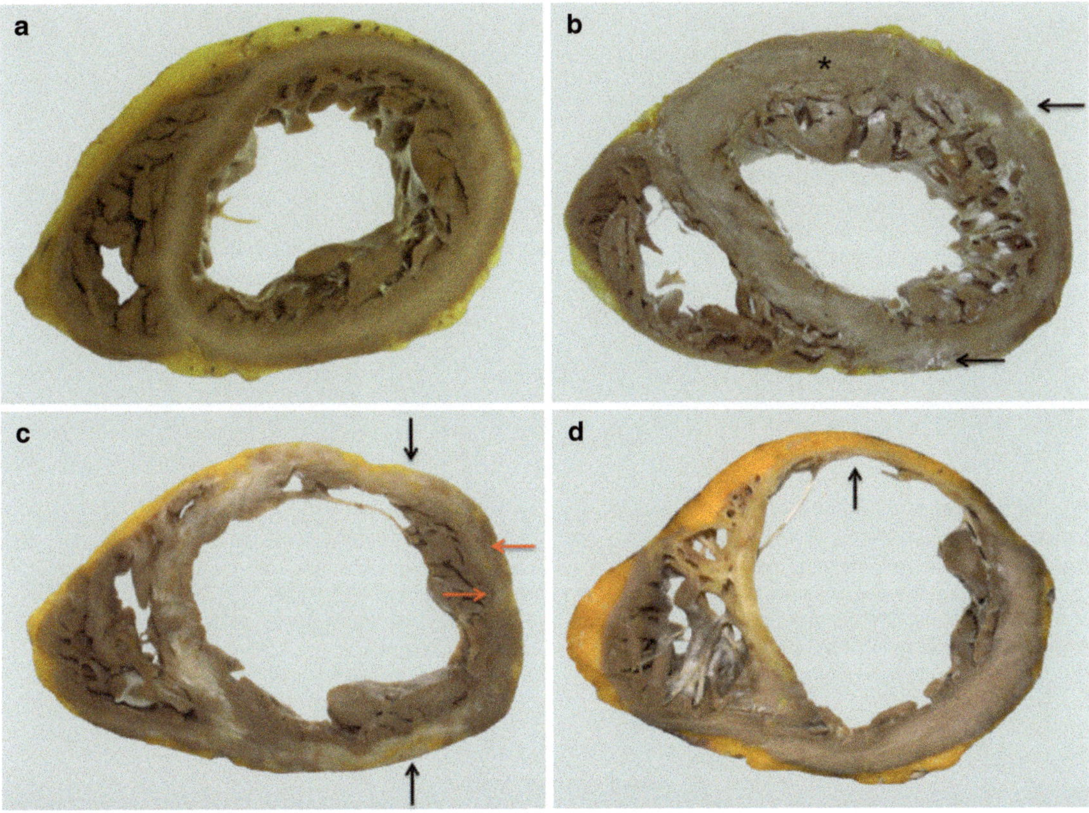

Fig. 5.20 Explanted hearts of patients with post-lymphocytic myocarditis DCM. (**a**) Macroscopic spectrum is evident: different degrees of ventricle dilatation, irregular thinning of myocardial walls with possible reactive hypertrophied myocardium areas (**b**: *asterisk*), irregularly distributed focal fibrotic areas (**b**: *arrows*), extensive subepicardial-mediomural replacement fibrosis (**c**: *red arrows*) or transmural scars (**c**: *black arrows*); infarction-like scar with parietal aneurysm (**d**: *arrow*)

found in the late healing or healed stage (still active on-going GCM has a significant chance of relapse in the transplanted heart) (Maleszewski et al. 2015; Cooper et al. 1997).

The ventricular walls are thin due to diffuse fibrous scarring, prevalently of the outer half of the myocardium, or even with a pseudo-infarction distribution; the typical polymorphous inflammation (numerous giant cells, lymphocytes or mononuclear cells, eosinophils and plasma cells) and the extensive myocardial damage of the acute phase are not seen and only a few giant cells or small areas of mild inflammation are scattered within wide areas of granulation tissue or of immature vs. mature replacement fibrosis (Fig. 5.22 a–d). On occasion aspects of granulomatous inflammation may appear in the native heart probably as a result of immunosuppressive therapy.

Within inflammatory diseases, *cardiac sarcoidosis* is probably the most frequently missed pre-transplant diagnosis and although there have been few cases, these could have benefit from more appropriate management in order to delay progression and timing of transplant. The heart shows marked ventricular cavity dilatation and focal but extensive scars, mainly subepicardial, in the free walls of both ventricles and in the IVS with thinning of the basal septum or the anterior LV wall. The septum is extensively involved from the base to the apex with scars limited to the mid-wall or sparing the mid portions at various points (Strauss et al. 2011). At histology the typical non-caseating granulomas with giant cells showing

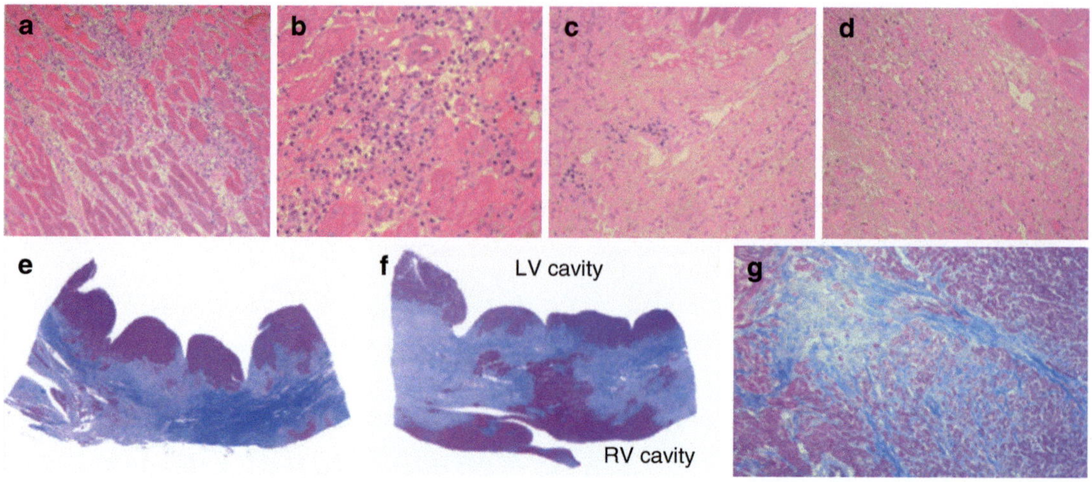

Fig. 5.21 Histology of post-lymphocytic myocarditis DCM. Histology reflects the varied macroscopic aspects: multiple foci of active interstitial lymphocytic inflammatory infiltrates associated with myocyte damage (**a**, **b**: Hematoxilyn–eosin, 200×); foci of healing myocarditis with scant inflammation within reparative/granulation tissue (**c**, **d**: Hematoxilyn–eosin, 200×); LV replacement transmural scar (**e**, Azan Mallory trichrome) and IVS mediomural replacement fibrosis (**f**, Azan Mallory trichrome). The remaining myocardium shows chronic myocell damage (**g**: Azan Mallory trichrome, 100×). *DCM* dilated cardiomyopathy, *LV* left ventricle, *IVS* interventricular septum

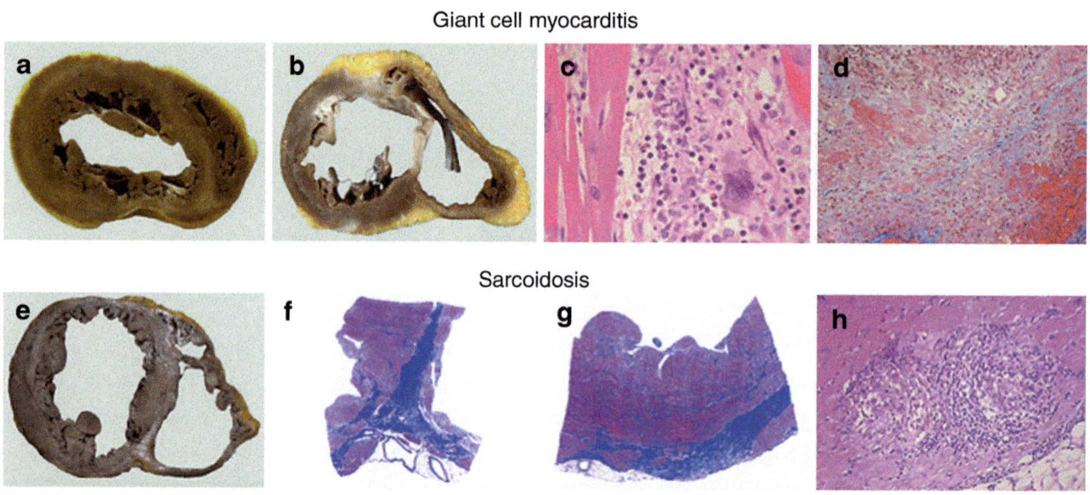

Fig. 5.22 (**a**–**d**) Giant cell myocarditis. (**a**) Heart of a 47-year-old male with LV dilatation, irregular myocardium thickness and fibrous scars in the anterior and posterior LV walls and in the mediomural IVS. (**b**) Native heart from a 40-year-old female with biventricular dilatation and antero-septal pseudo-infarction scar. Foci of inflammation with few giant cells are present at histology in myocardial interstitium (**c**: Hematoxylin–eosin, 250×) or within interstitial fibrosis (**d**: Hematoxylin–eosin, 250×) or areas of granulation tissue and immature fibrosis (**d**: Azan Mallory trichrome, 200×). (**e**–**h**) Sarcoidosis. (**e**) Heart of a 35-year-old male with marked biventricular dilatation and thinning of RV and anterior and posterior LV walls as well as of anterior IVS; extensive whitish replacement fibrosis is evident. Histologic sections of IVS (**f**) and LV (**g**) specimens reveal large mediomural or subepicardial areas of replacement fibrosis, highlighted in *blue* with Azan Mallory trichrome. In **h** a typical compact noncaseating granuloma with giant cells is shown (Hematoxylin–eosin, 400×). *LV* left ventricle, *IVS* interventricular septum

asteroid bodies are localized within mature fibrous tissue along with viable myocytes and lymphocytic inflammatory infiltrates (Fig. 5.22e–h) (Roberts et al. 2014b).

Although today the ISHLT does not consider sarcoidosis or other inflammatory CMPs associated with systemic diseases to be contraindications for heart transplantation, these patients require closer post-transplant follow-up due to the risk of disease recurrence and more frequent episodes of rejections.

Apart from other rarer forms of inflammatory CMPs, it should be remembered that histologic examination of explanted hearts can reveal *hypersensitivity myocarditis* (HSM), usually not clinically diagnosed before transplantation. First recognized by Gravanis et al. in 1991 (Gravanis et al. 1991), this disease affects some 3–7 % of transplanted patients and although it does not seem to influence post-transplant survival, it is associated with an increased frequency of acute cellular rejection (Kanai-Yoshizawa et al. 2013). Pathologists should be aware that HSM is consequent on multiple drug therapy and is not usually the original disease of the native heart but a superimposed picture due to heart failure therapy. The most common histologic pattern is interstitial or perivascular eosinophilic inflammatory infiltrates, associated to variable numbers of lymphocytes, macrophages, giant cells, neutrophils and small epithelioid granulomas, and the absence of significant myocardial necrosis or fibrosis.

CMPs Resulting from Chemotherapy or Radiotherapy

CMPs resulting from chemotherapy or radiotherapy involve an important group of explanted hearts that share dilated or restrictive phenotypes, although numbers are limited as underestimated at initial diagnosis. At the Bologna Centre ten patients (seven women and three men; median age: 43.5 ± 14.4) underwent heart transplantation following chemotherapy or mediastinum irradiation for lymphomas, acute lymphoblastic leukemia, Ewing sarcomas, and breast cancer.

In *actinic CMPs*, pathologic findings are very clear and the hearts significantly altered: ventricles may be dilated or show restrictive features, with various degrees of myocardium thinning or hypertrophy and marked subendocardial fibrosis. Organizing mural thrombi are frequently present. Fibrosis is extensive, mainly subendocardial, but also interstitial or replacement, and more prominent in LV lateral and anterior walls. Myocyte degenerative alterations, especially myofibril loss, are usually very marked; coronary involvement concurs, both in subepicardial main branches, which can show fibrocalcified plaques severely narrowing the lumen, and microvessel loss, narrowing, and obstruction (Fig. 5.23).

In *post-chemotherapy CMPs*, pathologic findings are more attenuated and less specific: fibrosis is less extensive and degenerative myocyte alterations more variable in degree.

In both types sparse lymphocytic infiltrates may be present and alterations of intramyocardial small vessels concur.

Apart from transplanted cases, this is a major group of CMPs caused by the toxic effects of many other drugs or agents. Cardiovascular pathologists should further research these diseases, as they are frequently an unrecognized cause of sudden death.

Cardiac Amyloidosis

Cardiac amyloidosis is the prototype of infiltrative cardiomyopathies. The general term amyloidosis covers a protein metabolic disorder and includes a number of heterogeneous diseases, characterized by extracellular deposition of anomalous and insoluble fibrillary proteins, which alter the structure of tissues and organs involved and impair their function (Falk and Dubrey 2010). The term *cardiac amyloidosis* refers to the specific presence of amyloid deposits in the heart, both in systemic forms and in rarer localized ones. The presence and extent of cardiac involvement is highly variable: in some cases, cardiac localization is the main cause of patient morbidity and mortality; in others it is only an incidental finding without any functional consequences (Garcıa-Pavıa et al. 2011; Rapezzi et al. 2009, 2010).

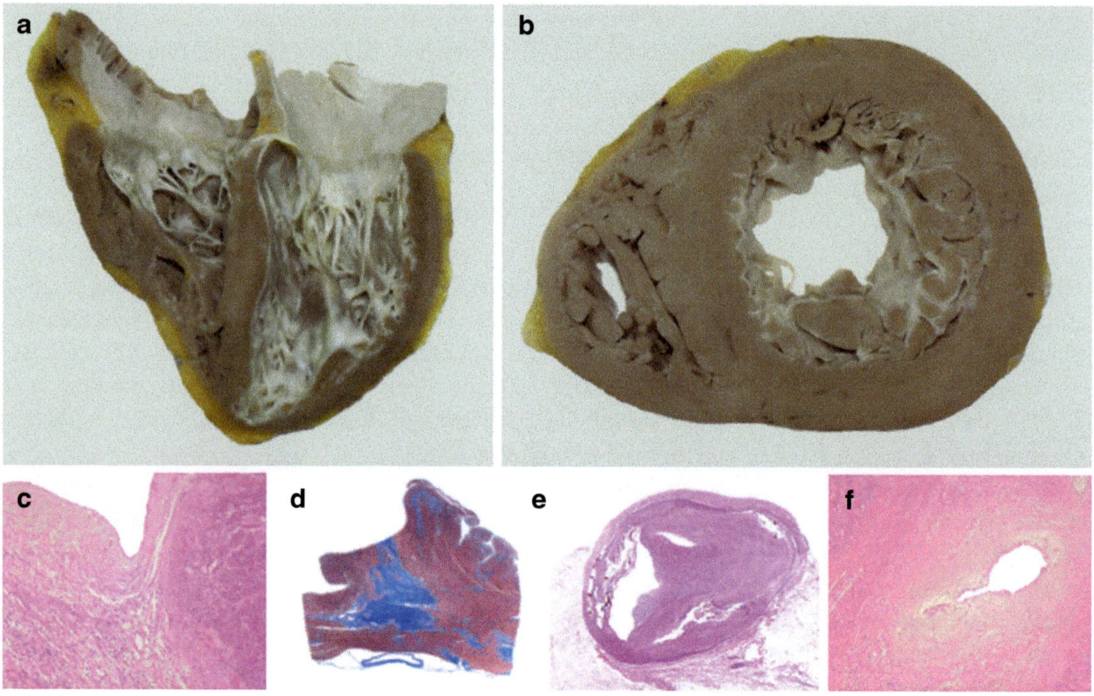

Fig. 5.23 Actinic CMP. (**a**) Explanted heart of a 56-year-old female treated with radiotherapy following breast cancer: LV shows diffused and marked subendocardial fibrosis causing restrictive physiology. (**b**) Actinic CMP of a 31-year-old female who underwent radiotherapy after lymphoblastic leukemia when she was a child of 4. The heart is dilated and marked biventricular trabeculations are evident, along with diffuse LV subendocardial fibrosis. Some histologic findings in these CMPs: extensive subendocardial fibrosis, sometimes with scarce lymphocytes. (**c**) Hematoxylin–eosin, 250×); interstitial or replacement fibrosis evident in the cardiac specimen of (**d**) (Azan Mallory trichrome) in the RV and LV anterior walls and in the septum; fibro-calcified plaque severely narrowing the lumen of a descending anterior coronary artery. (**e**) Hematoxylin–eosin); loose concentric intimal hyperplasia with severe stenosis of the lumen in an intramural artery. (**f**) Hematoxylin–eosin, 400×). *CMP* cardiomyopathy, *LV* left ventricle, *RV* right ventricle

Pathologists usually encounter native explanted hearts with cardiac amyloidosis within combined organ transplantations: most frequently heart–liver transplantation for hereditary transthyretin-related amyloidosis (ATTR) or heart transplantation combined with autologous peripheral blood stem cell transplantation in primary immunoglobulin light chain amyloidosis (AL) (see Chap. 23).

Macroscopically the heart is usually enlarged and stiffened: both atria are dilated, the RV is regular or slightly dilated, and the LV cavity may be normal or reduced. On the cut surface, the myocardium has a homogeneous waxy appearance; more rarely large accumulations of amyloid are visible at macroscopy (Falk and Dubrey 2010) (Fig. 5.24).

At histology amyloid appears as deposits of homogeneous and amorphous pink substance, which, when stained with Congo Red, is red-orange in color under ordinary light and has a typical green birefringence under polarized light, whose brightness may considerably vary depending on whether amyloid fibrils are formed from full-length proteins or from fragments (Fig. 5.25a–c).

In the heart, deposits are localized in the myocardial interstitium with two main patterns:

- Variably thin intercellular deposits around the myocytes (perimyocytic pattern) separating and compressing myocells (Fig. 5.25d, e).
- Nodular substitutive aggregates of varying size (nodular pattern) (Fig. 5.25f, g).

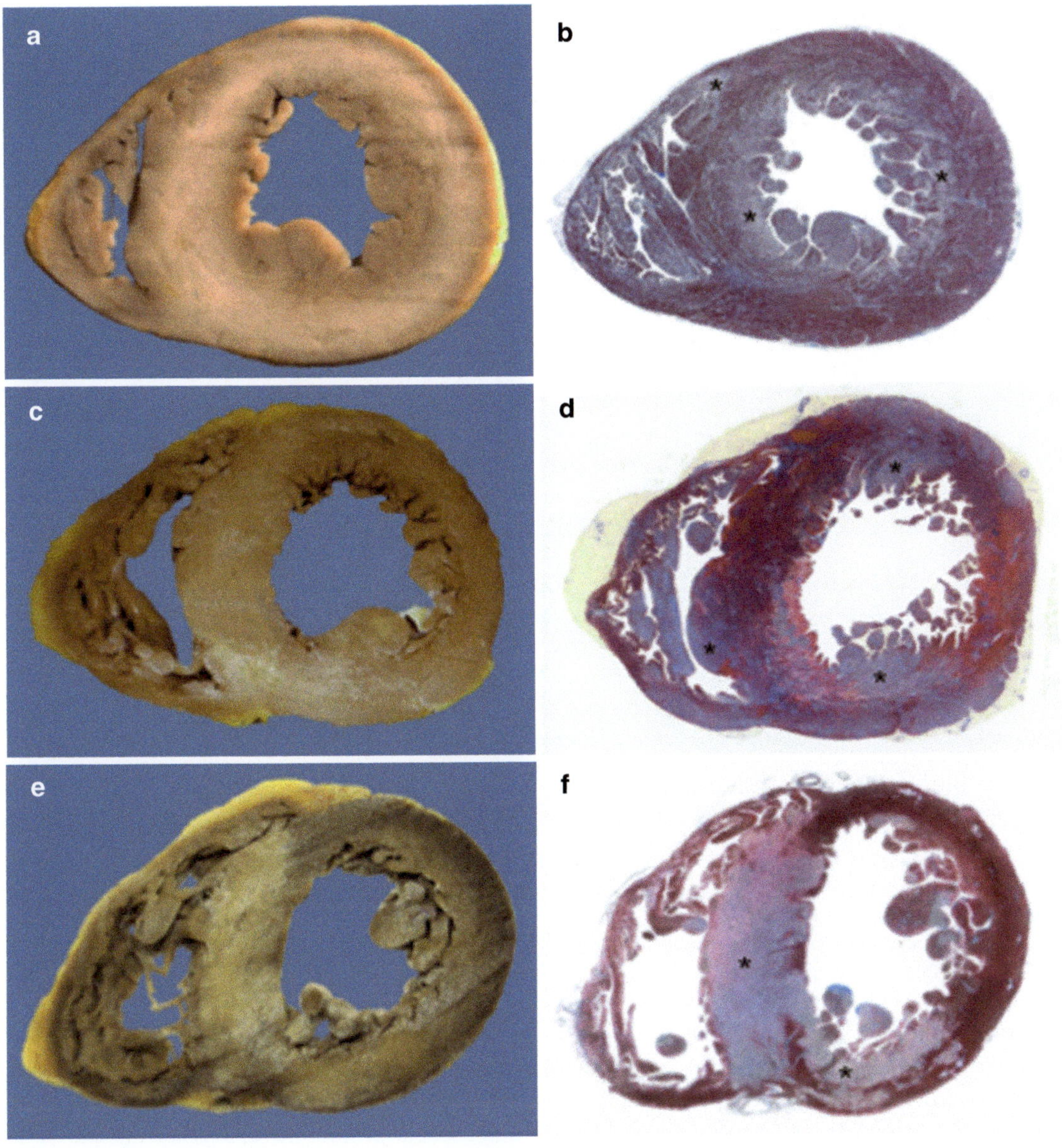

Fig. 5.24 (**a**, **c**) Amyloidotic cardiomyopathy in native hearts of two patients who underwent combined heart-liver transplantation for familial transthyretin-related systemic amyloidosis. (**a**) Heart of a 60-year-old man with Gln89 mutation in transthyretin gene; (**c**) heart of a 46-year-old man with Asn23 mutation in transthyretin gene. (**e**) Autoptic heart of a 56-year-old woman with monoclonal immunoglobulin lambda chain systemic amyloidosis. The three macroscopic transverse slices are compared with the same histologic macrosections stained with Azan Mallory trichrome, which highlights amyloid as bluish-gray deposits (*asterisks*). In the first heart (**a**, **b**), amyloid is diffusely distributed giving the waxy appearance to the myocardium; in the other two (**c**, **d** and **e**, **f**), amyloid is aggregated in larger nodules and masses, already evident at macroscopic examination

The subendocardium is frequently involved with nodular deposits; small intramyocardial vessels may be involved (Fig. 5.25h, i) to varying degrees causing microinfarcts or resulting in a condition of chronic myocardial ischemia, even in the absence of significant interstitial involvement. Surprisingly, subepicardial coronary arteries are spared or only occasionally involved. Atrio-ventricular valve tissue is usually thickened due to nodular deposits of amyloid.

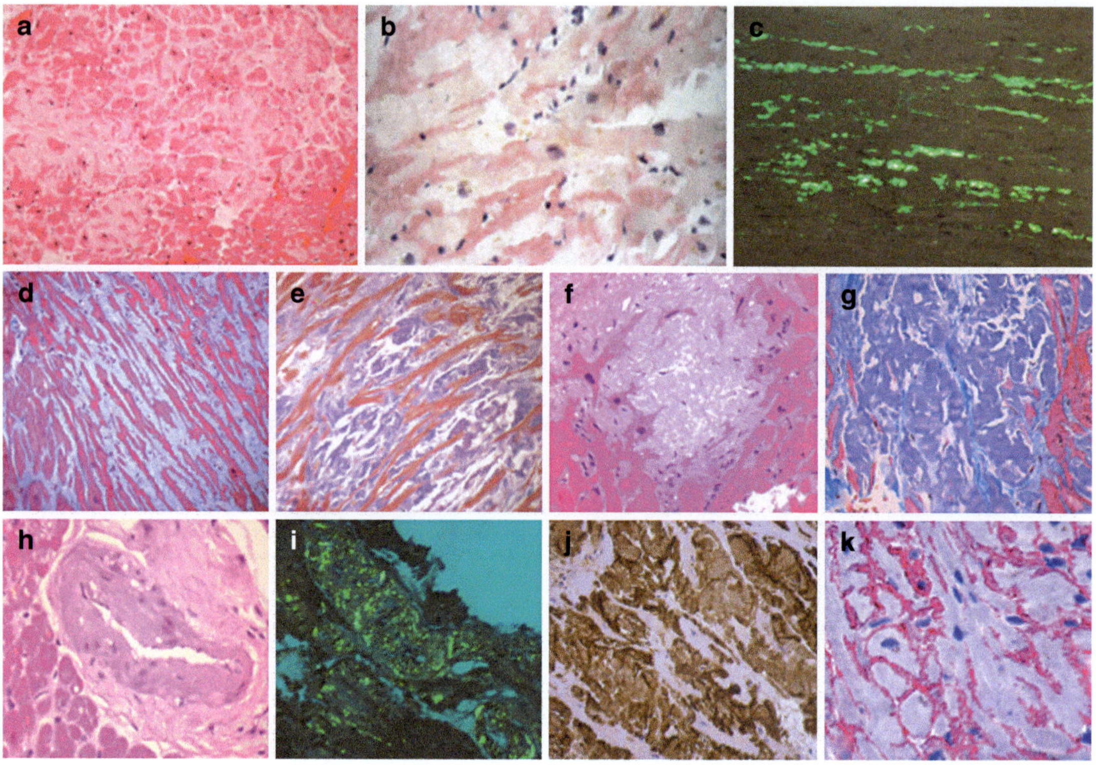

Fig. 5.25 Histology and immunohistochemistry of amyloid. The interstitial amorphous amyloid deposits (**a**: Hematoxylin–eosin, 200×) acquire a typical green birefringence when Congo Red (**b**: 400×) is observed under polarized light (**c**: 200×). (**d**–**e**) Perimyocytic pattern of amyloid distribution with varying degrees of intercellular deposits (Azan Mallory trichrome, 200×). (**f**–**g**) Nodular pattern of amyloid deposition (**f**: Hematoxylin-eosin 200×; **g**: Azan Mallory trichrome, 400×). (**h**, **i**): Vascular deposits of amyloid narrowing the lumen of the small intramyocardial arteries (**h**: Hematoxylin-eosin, 400×; **i**: Congo Red under polarized light, 100×). (**j**, **k**) Immunoperoxidase for amyloid showing transthyretin-positive deposits in **j** (200×), and immunoglobulin lambda chain positive deposits in **k** (200×)

A crucial point in the long and complex process of diagnosis of cardiac amyloidosis, which lies beyond the aims of this chapter, is defining the type of amyloidosis, which conditions prognosis and appropriate treatment, including the option of transplantation (Garcıa-Pavıa et al. 2011). To help identify amyloid fibril types, pathologists can use antibodies directed against amyloid proteins with both immunohistochemical (both immunoperoxidase and immunofluorescence) (Fig. 5.25j, k) and immunoelectron microscopic techniques. The results need to be carefully interpreted within the clinical–instrumental context; but due to sensitivity and specificity problems and technical and interpretative difficulties, referral centers are turning to highly sensitive methods, which combine laser microdissection of amyloid deposits from formalin-fixed paraffin-embedded samples and the analytical power of tandem mass spectrometry–based proteomic analysis (Larsen et al. 2015; Vrana et al. 2009).

Today native hearts with amyloid are increasingly available and it is important to analyze these to obtain detailed information on distribution and patterns of amyloid deposition, to be correlated with clinical and imaging data (Leone et al. 2012).

Native Hearts and Genetic CMPs Associated with Systemic Muscle Disorders

Several inherited skeletal myopathies may be associated with cardiac myopathies leading to

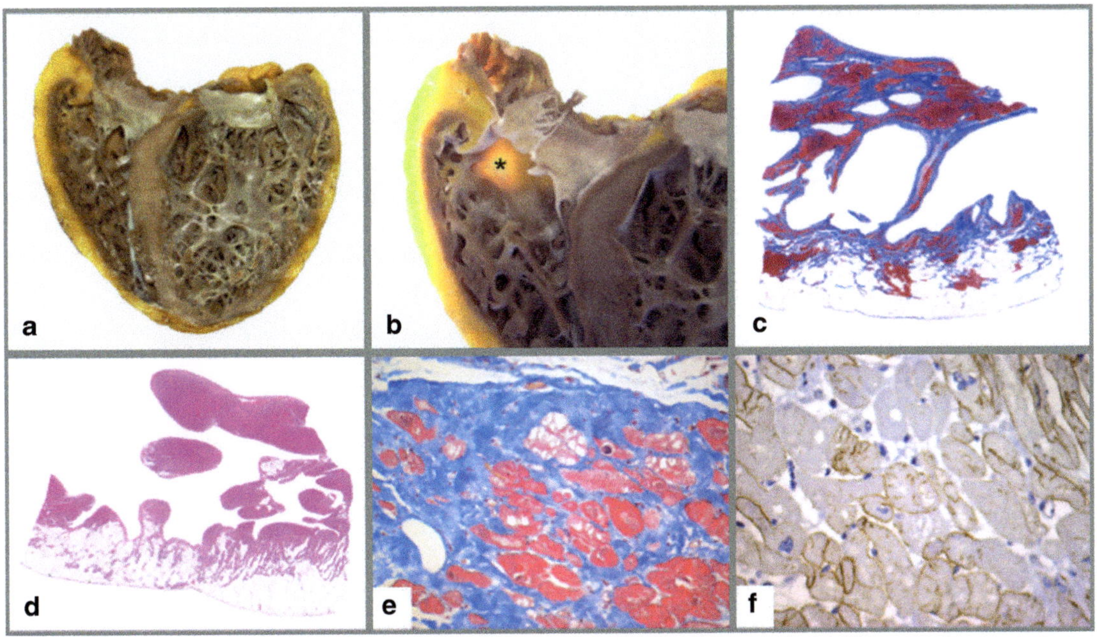

Fig. 5.26 Explanted heart of a 40-year-old male affected by Becker disease. (**a**) Left ventricle is very enlarged and shows marked trabeculations and subendocardial fibrosis. Ventricle walls are thinned and areas of fibro-fatty replacement starting from the subepicardium and progressing towards the endocardium are evident in both ventricles. (**b**) A detail of the posterior view of the right ventricle highlights a localized area below the tricuspid valve where myocardium is totally absent and replaced by fatty tissue (*asterisk*) like the aneurysms described in ACM. (**c, d**) Histology shows extensive fatty and/or fibro-fatty replacement of myocardium in both ventricles and marked trabeculations (**c**, specimen from LV, Azan Mallory trichrome; **d**: specimen from RV, Hematoxylin–eosin). (**e**) High power reveals interstitial fibrosis, and hypertrophy, attenuation, sarcoplasmic vacuolization and myofibril loss of myocytes (Azan-Mallory trichrome, 250×). (**f**) Immunohistochemistry for dystrophin shows the altered labeling of myocyte sarcolemma ranging from irregular and fragmented to diminished to absent (250×). *ACM* arrhythmogenic cardiomyopathy, *LV* left ventricle, *RV* right ventricle

end-stage heart failure. Some of these CMPs are suitable for transplant.

The majority of available reports concern Becker's muscular dystrophy (Komanapalli et al. 2006), where mutations in the dystrophin gene can result in mild functional skeletal involvement and more profound myocardial involvement. Other sporadically transplanted cases concern Emery–Dreifuss muscular dystrophy, or also desmin-related cardiomyopathy (DRM) a clinically heterogeneous group of diseases due to mutations in the intermediate filament desmin (DES) gene, characterized by progressive skeletal and/or cardiac myopathy with dilated, restrictive, and occasionally ACM-like phenotypes.

Hearts with Becker and Emery–Dreifuss muscular dystrophy share the DCM phenotype with wall thinning: histology shows profound alterations alternating extensive replacement fibrosis with fibro-fatty replacement of myocardium of both ventricles, mimicking ACM. Myocytes are diffusely altered and show hypertrophy, attenuation, irregular nuclei, sarcoplasmic vacuolization, and myofibril loss (Fig. 5.26).

In Fig. 5.27, the heart of a 31-year-old female transplanted for DCM as a consequence of a mutation (Leu183Pro) in lamin A/C proteins is shown. The heart is enlarged, LV dilated and ventricular wall thinned. Histology is non-specific and shows interstitial perimyocytic fibrosis, prevalently in the subendocardium, to various degrees associated to fibrous thickening of the endocardium and to areas of replacement fibrosis. Myocytes are increased in size and show marked nuclear contour irregularity. Mutations

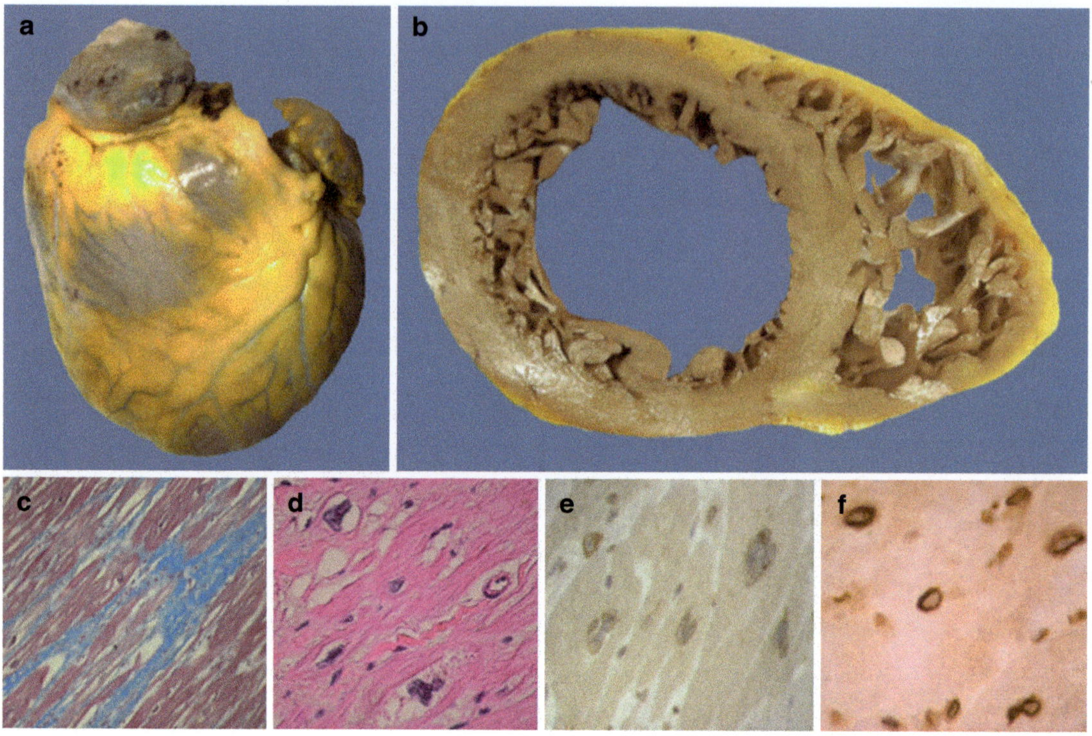

Fig. 5.27 Heart of a 31-year-old female transplanted for cardio-laminopathy (Leu183Pro mutation in lamin A/C proteins). On the anterior view the heart is markedly enlarged (**a**) and the short-axis cut shows a severe dilation of LV; marked trabeculation of RV and mild thinning of both ventricular walls (**b**). Histology shows a specific findings: interstitial perimyocytic fibrosis (**c**, Azan Mallory trichrome, ×400), increased size of myocells and marked nuclear contour irregularity (**d**, Hematoxylin–eosin, ×400). Immunohistochemical staining with anti-lamin A/C antibody shows absent or irregular perinuclear labeling (**e**, ×400) compared to a normal control (**f**, ×400). *LV* left ventricle, *RV* right ventricle

in the LMNA gene produce several distinct syndromes (Charcot–Marie–Tooth disease type 2, mandibuloacral dysplasia, familial partial lipodystrophy-Dunnigan type, restrictive dermopathy, and premature aging syndromes) as well as CMPs.

In this group, a potential role for immunohistochemistry (IHC) is emerging although standardization is still to come. The most documented use of immunohistochemical tests is for dystrophin, where antibodies are commercially available for both paraffin and frozen tissues recognizing three epitopes of the molecule (COOH-terminal; NH_2-terminal, rod-domain). In Becker MD, labeling of myocyte sarcolemma with dystrophin antibodies is markedly altered and ranges from irregular and fragmented to diminished to absent (Fig. 5.26f). Similar results are evident with anti-lamin A/C antibody, which show absent or irregular perinuclear labeling (Fig. 5.27e). MD myocardia disease.

Anti-emerin antibody is also available for routine use, whose normal continuous labeling around nuclei is completely lacking in affected cases. The desmin antibody can show positive aggregates of the protein in the myocyte sarcoplasm of affected cases.

Native hearts should ideally be used for detailed study and validation of the diagnostic use of IHC in EMB.

Other Cardiomyopathies

Other CMPs are more rarely transplanted, such as non-tropical eosinophilic endomyocardial fibrosis (Loeffler disease) (Fig. 5.28a, b) or peripartum cardiomyopathy (PP-CMP) (Fig. 5.28c, d).

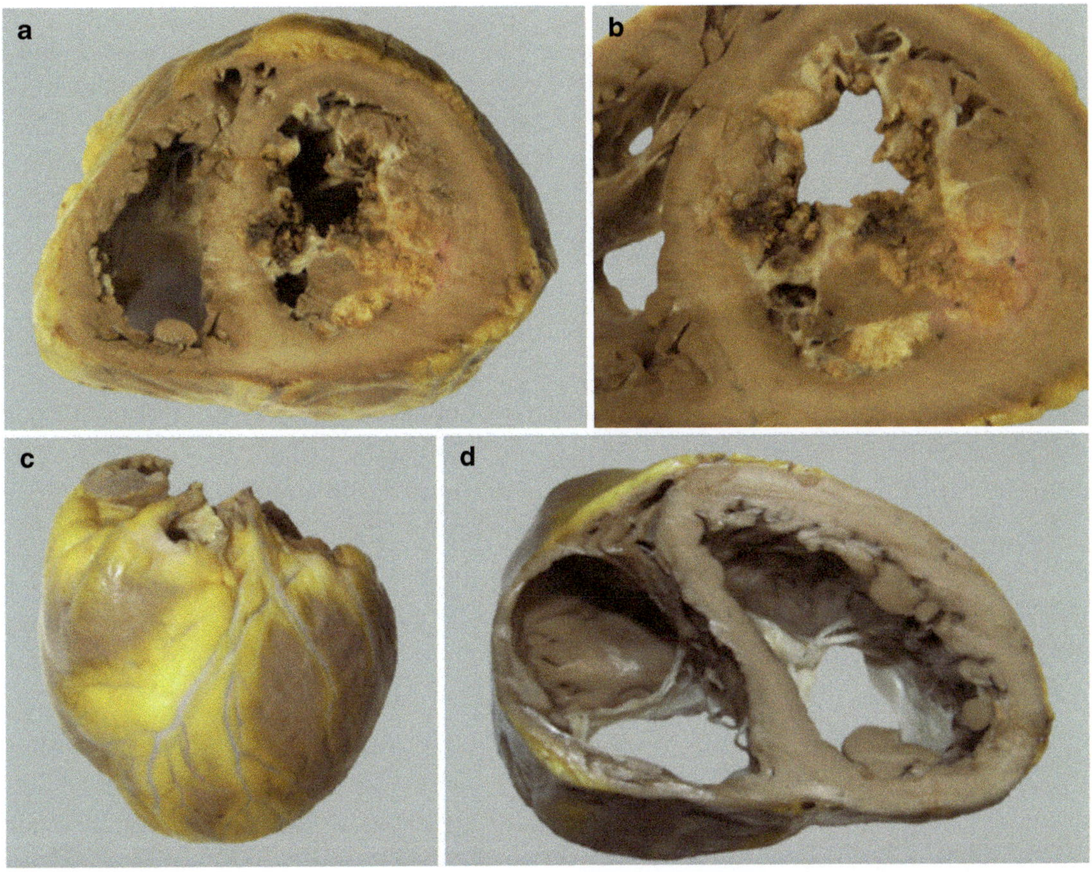

Fig. 5.28 (**a**, **b**) Heart of a 43-year-old male with non-tropical eosinophilic endomyocardial fibrosis (Loeffler disease) in chronic stage. On transverse mid-section the left ventricular cavity is almost occluded by an organized thrombus, with many calcified areas. Histology showed diffuse and marked subendocardial fibrous thickening due to the organization of the thrombotic material. The myocardium was characterized by nonspecific alterations such as mild interstitial fibrosis and myocytes of various sizes. (**c**, **d**) Heart of a 37-year-old female who developed peripartum cardiomyopathy 1 month after the birth. The heart weighted 290 g. and was dilated: transverse cut shows marked biventricular dilatation with severe thinning of ventricular walls

PP-CMP is idiopathic heart failure occurring during the last month of pregnancy or the first 5 months postpartum, whose incidence is high in developing nations: nearly 25% of patients require heart transplantation (Rasmusson et al. 2012). Macroscopic findings may vary considerably from significant DCM with marked biventricular dilatation and ventricular myocardial thinning to less dilatation and irregular ventricular wall thickness. In this CMP, histology is non-specific: fibrotic subendocardial thickening and irregularly distributed interstitial fibrosis – sometimes very extensive – may be seen. Myocytes reveal various non-specific alterations indicative of remodeling (hypertrophy or attenuation) or myofibril loss. Scant interstitial lymphocytic infiltrates are frequently seen, focally associated with myocell damage. Graft failure and death are more frequent in this type of patient because of higher allosensitization, higher pretransplant acuity and increased rate of rejection.

It should be noted that Chagas' cardiomyopathy is the third leading indication for heart transplantation in Brazil; given the severe prognosis of the disease, transplantation is really the only therapeutic option for these patients (Bocchi and Fiorelli 2001).

Pediatric Cardiomyopathies

In pediatric cardiomyopathy morbidity and mortality are high and these diseases are the most common cause of a heart transplant in children older than 1 year (Lipshultz et al. 2013).

The North American Pediatric Cardiomyopathy Registry (PCMR), one of the largest cohorts, recognized various types of cardiomyopathies in several thousand children over the past two decades (Lipshultz et al. 2003). Cardiac transplantation remains the only definitive treatment for children with DCM progressing to end-stage heart failure and, in this group, PCMR identified a specific cause in 34% of cases.: postmyocarditis, neuromuscular disorders, familial cardiomyopathies, and inborn metabolism errors (Harmon et al. 2009). RCM is the least common pediatric cardiomyopathy phenotype (around 4.5 %) and has the poorest prognosis. The majority of patients die or undergo cardiac transplantation within a few years of diagnosis, although criteria for listing these children for heart transplantation are not generally agreed.

In Fig. 5.29, the explanted heart of a 3-year-old female transplanted with clinical diagnosis of "Concentric hypertrophic cardiomyopathy with restrictive ventricular filling pattern". Metabolic study protocol identifies only a partial reduction of complex III enzymes of mitochondrial respiratory chain. The heart was enlarged, weight 90 g and was 5.3 cm along the longitudinal diameter and 5.7 cm along the transverse one. On the anterior view, we see the removal of semilunar valves for the valve tissue bank and on the posterior face, LV is larger than the right, whose apex reaches the mid-portion of the heart. On the longitudinal cut this discrepancy is very clear: the RV is small, its cavity is almost inexistent, and it appears to be an accessory chamber. The IVS is

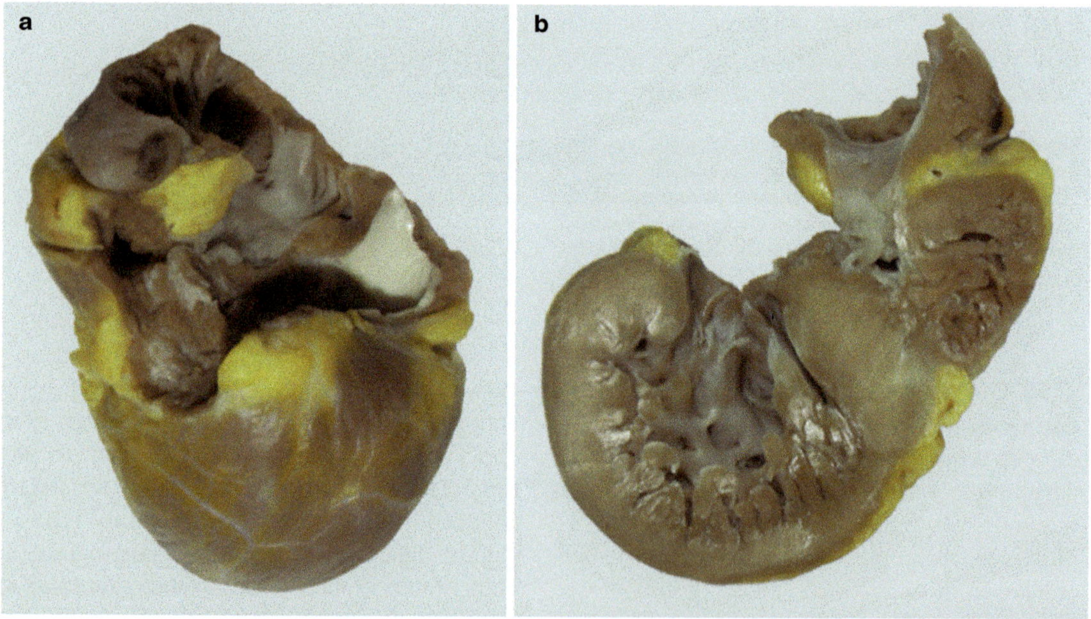

Fig. 5.29 Native heart of a 3-year-old female transplanted with clinical diagnosis of "Concentric hypertrophic cardiomyopathy with restrictive ventricular filling pattern" and the final pathologic diagnosis of unclassifiable cardiomyopathy with mixed pattern: biventricular hypertrophy, restrictive characteristic and marked trabeculation of the left ventricle. (**a**) Anterior view of the heart. (**b**) Entire longitudinal cut clearly showing different sized ventricular cavities

markedly hypertrophic (maximum thickness of 1.5 cm at the medium third) and extensive fibrosis is present; the LV shows dilated cavity with marked trabeculations in the mid-apical portion and irregular thickness of the parietal myocardium, hypertrophied in the basal segments (1.4 cm) and thinned out in the inferior third. The right ventricular myocardium has irregular thickness and shows diffuse trabeculation. Histology revealed diffuse endocardial and interstitial fibrosis, this last pericellular, perivascular, and substitutive. Myocardial disarray was evident and myocells showed focal hypertrophy, various degrees of sarcoplasmic vacuolization, and subendocardial myocytolisis. Pathology diagnosis was of unclassifiable CMP with mixed pattern: biventricular hypertrophy, restrictive characteristic and marked trabeculation of the left ventricle.

5.3.4 Pre- and Post-transplant Diagnosis

In conclusion it should be emphasized that the congruity or discrepancy between clinical pre-transplant diagnosis and pathologic diagnosis at post-transplant examination of CMPs depends on many factors:

- The period of transplant (pre-2000 or post-2000): in recent years there has been a greater clinical interest in the etiology of cardiac disease.
- Whether the transplant center has a referral center for CMPs in general or for some specific forms.
- Whether the center usually includes EMB in the work-up for CMPs, according to the recent guidelines (Rapezzi et al. 2013) which suggest tissue evaluation and genetic tests in selected cases, in order to reach a comprehensive diagnosis.
- Availability of specialized cardiovascular pathologists able to give detailed diagnosis in this complex field.

Illustrative Case 2 (Figs. 5.30–5.31)

Two very interesting complex cases involving two first-degree female family members are described to exemplify the approach to cardiomyopathies. The main diagnostic hypotheses to consider in such cases include sarcomeric HCM, Anderson–Fabry disease, glycogen storage diseases, and mitochondrial disease.

A woman and her daughter with similar HCM phenotypes progressed to LV systolic dysfunction and underwent heart transplantation at the age of 47 and 23, respectively, with the diagnosis of "sarcomeric" HCM with end-stage evolution.

The mother's medical history started at age 35 years and the daughter's at 7 years, when she was completely asymptomatic but underwent familiar screening.

The main clinical findings of both cases are shown here.

Clinical findings	Mother, 35 years of age	Daughter
Echocardiography findings	LV hypertrophy (14 mm); LV enlargement (end-diastolic diameter: 56 mm); LVEF: 30 %; relative wall thinning at the basal segment of the IVS with marked akinesia	*At 7 years of age* extreme LV hypertrophy (maximal wall thickness: 16 mm); normal ventricular cavity (end-diastolic diameter of 35 mm); LVEF: 78 %; relative wall thinning at the basal IVS with hypoakinesia *At 23 years of age* thinned LV walls and LV enlargement (end-stage evolution); thinning of the basal IVS still evident

Clinical findings	Mother, 35 years of age	Daughter
Extracardiac/multisystemic manifestations (renal insufficiency, acroparesthesias, angiokeratomas, neurological-musculoskeletal or ocular involvement)	Absent	Absent
Mode of transmission	Autosomal dominant. Autosomal recessive form and matrilinear/mitochondrial inheritance unlikely X-linked inheritance excluded	
Most likely clinical diagnosis	Sarcomeric HCM in end stage	

Pathology of the explanted hearts. Mother's heart weighted 510 g and was enlarged and rounded (Fig. 5.30a). The short axis slice at mid-ventricular level showed LV dilatation and LV hypertrophy pattern characterized by hypertrophy of the septum, mildly hypertrophied areas in the antero-lateral wall, and thinned areas in the posterior wall. The anterior right ventricular wall was also hypertrophic (Fig. 5.30c).

Daughter's heart weighted 490 g and was less enlarged and less rounded at the apex (Fig. 5.30b). At the transverse mid-ventricular cut marked LV hypertrophy (maximum wall thickness of 25 mm at the level of the septum), mildly hypertrophied areas in the antero-lateral wall, thinned inferior wall, and diffuse hypertrophy of the right ventricular myocardium were evident (Fig. 5.30d).

At histology, extensive fibrosis throughout the septum and the LV was present in both hearts (Fig. 5.31a, b). In the mother, fibrosis was prominent in the anterior LV wall (with transmural areas of replacement fibrosis) and in the LV inferior wall with subepicardial/mediomural distribution; in the septum it was discontinuous and mediomural. In the daughter, fibrosis was more extensive and circumferentially distributed throughout the LV, mainly with subepicardial–mediomural distribution and transmural replacement fibrosis in a very thinned inferior area; in the hypertrophied septum, fibrosis was significant, continuous, and mediomural. The extent and distribution of fibrosis are also evident in the macroscopic transverse sections (Fig. 5.30c, d) as whitish areas.

Other histologic findings common to both hearts were myocyte hypertrophy and multiple myocardial disarray (Fig. 5.31c, d), extensive and marked myocyte sarcoplasmic vacuolization (Fig. 5.31e), and mild to moderate small mural vessel disease (Fig. 5.31f).

Although hypertrophic vacuolated myocytes are usual in end-stage HCM, the widespread vacuolization present in these cases could suggest a diagnosis of glycogen storage disease: periodic acid Schiff (PAS) and PAS-diastase stainings revealed no glycogen storage; ultrastructural examination showed no intracellular accumulation substances, electron dense concentric lamellar bodies (as in Anderson–Fabry disease) or significant mitochondrial proliferation or inclusions and giant mitochondria typically seen in mitochondrial CMPs. All these findings are largely consistent with the diagnosis of sarcomeric end-stage HCM.

Genetic analysis was performed on samples of both blood and explanted hearts with the same results, testing eight sarcomeric genes (MYH7-myosin heavy chain 7; MYBPC3-myosin binding protein 3; TNNT2-Troponin T type 2; TNNI3-Troponin I type 3; TPM1-tropomyosin alfa1; ACTC1-actin alpha cardiac muscle 1; MYL3-myosin essential light chain; MYL2-myosin regulatory light chain), and three metabolic genes (GLA-alpha-galactosidase A; LAMP2-lysosome associated membrane glycoprotein 2; PRKAG2-AMP activated protein kinase).

In the mother two new mutations of uncertain significance were found: p. Thr106Ile in MYL3 gene and p. Gly80Val in LAMP2 gene; in the daughter none.

These mutations are of uncertain pathogenetic significance as they have not been previously described in literature: the mutation in MYL3 gene could be related to a sarcomeric HCM with an autosomal dominant inheritance, while the mutation in the LAMP2 gene may correlate with a lyso-

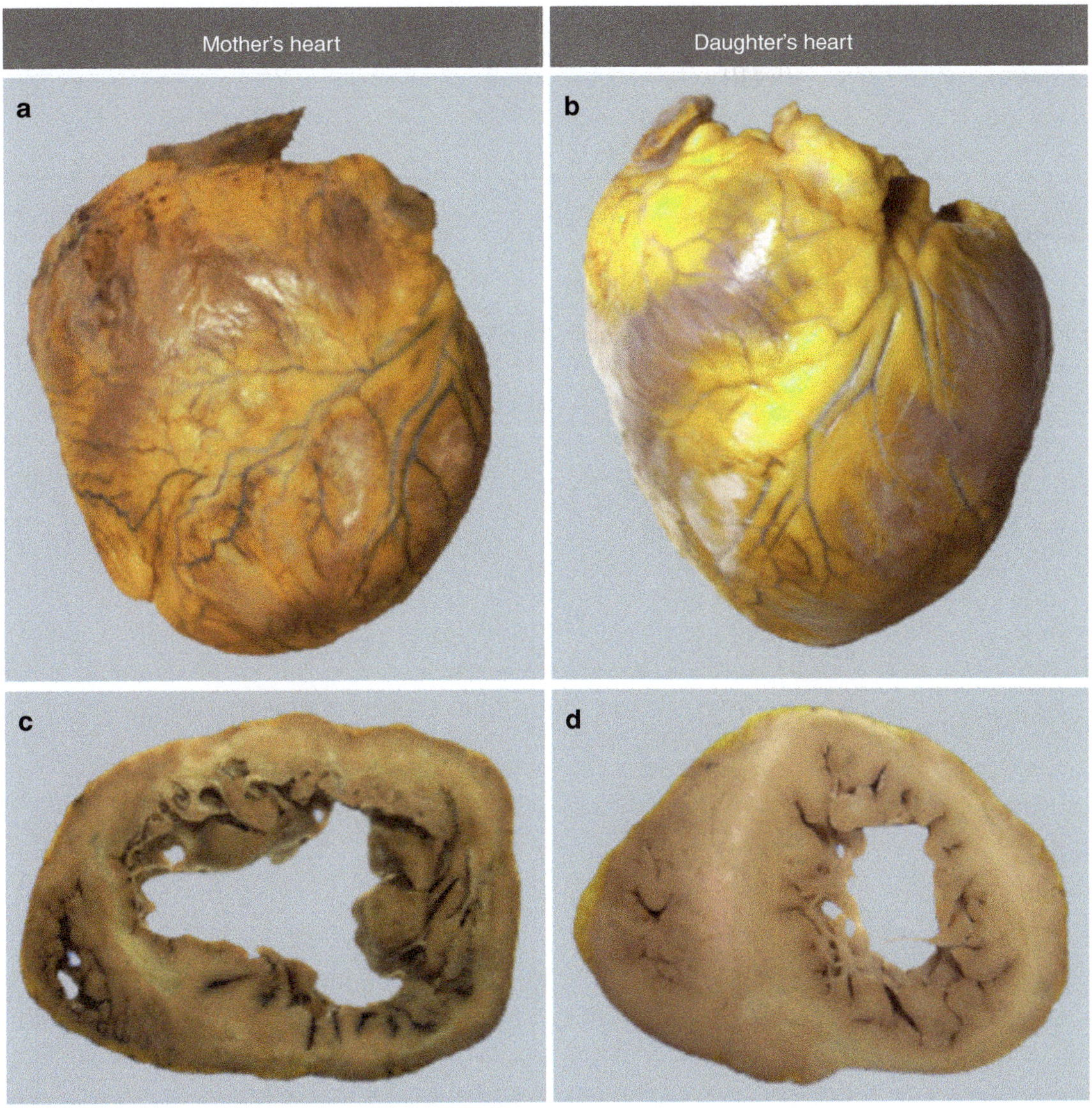

Fig. 5.30 Illustrative case 2. Macroscopic aspects of the explanted hearts. (**a**, **b**) Anterior view of the hearts. (**c**, **d**) Transverse short axis slices

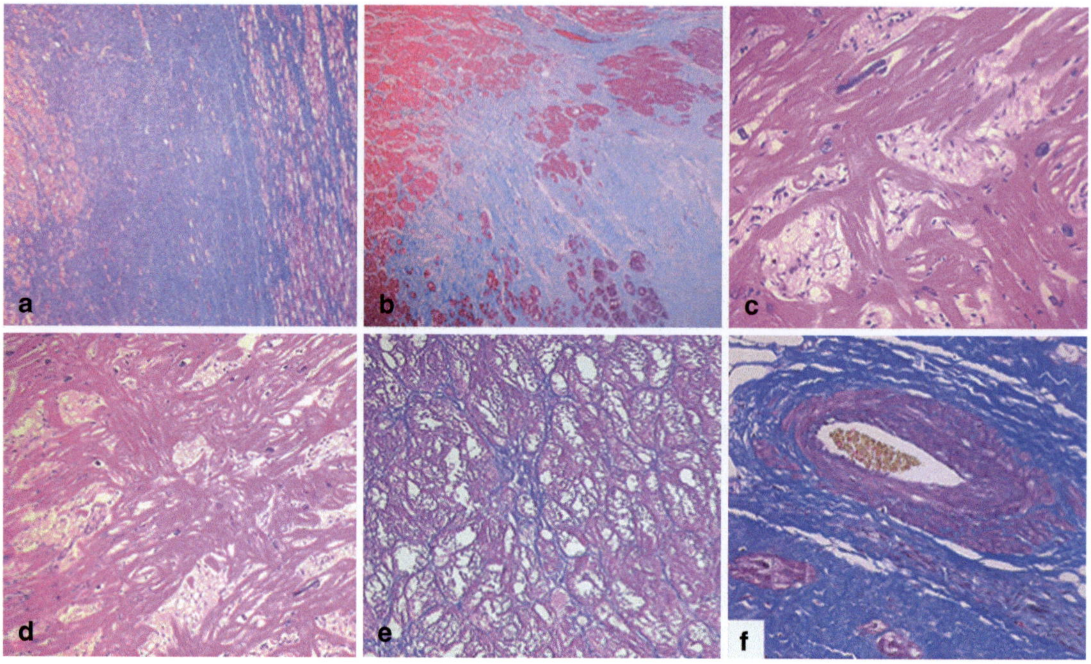

Fig. 5.31 Illustrative case 2. Histologic findings. (**a**, **b**) Marked extensive fibrosis (Azan Mallory trichrome, 100×); (**c**, **d**) myocyte Hypertrophy and myocardial disarray (Hematoxilyn–eosin, 400×); (**e**) myocyte sarcoplasmic vacuolization (Azan Mallory trichrome, 200×); (**f**) moderate parietal thickening of small mural artery due to intimal hyperplasia and medial hypertrophy (Azan Mallory trichrome, 200×)

somal glycogen storage diseases (Danon disease) with an X-linked inheritance.

Conclusion: These two cases well illustrate the complexity of some CMPs and the importance of a complete diagnostic work-up.

The similar HCM phenotypes with progression to LV systolic dysfunction with superimposable pathologic findings in these two first-degree female family members associated with a probable autosomal dominant inheritance could support a final diagnosis of "sarcomeric HCM" with end-stage evolution, although genetic analysis failed to confirm this diagnosis.

It should be noted that genetic screening is an essential tool in CMPs, especially in HCM, but diagnosis cannot rely on it alone.

Key Points

- Familiarity with the disease, epidemiology, and clinics.
- Familiarity with indications to transplant various forms of CMPs.
- Accurate macroscopic examination: try to recognize the macroscopic phenotype of the disease through examination of relative volumes of cardiac chambers, thickness of myocardium, and macroscopic lesions.
- Sectioning the heart appropriately to the disease (short-axis vs. four chamber cuts).
- Careful examination of coronary arteries in order to exclude unrecognized primary or concurrent ischemic cardiopathy.
- Adequate and standardized sampling.
- Histology:

- Check for a specific etiology by studying myocardium alterations, extent, and distribution of fibrosis (usually chronic and not active diseases), intracellular or interstitial deposits, presence and type of inflammatory infiltrates.
- Detailed knowledge required of subtle histological features, which can help in distinguishing various CMPs.

• Fully describe all features in order to collect data and correlate pathologic findings with clinical data.

5.4 Heart Valve Disease

5.4.1 Background and Incidence in Explanted Hearts

Heart valve disease (HVD) is a large chapter of cardiac disease, and although less frequent than coronary artery disease or hypertension, it is still quite common and continues to be a major cause of morbidity. It includes many and different forms (Fig. 5.32):

- Congenital disorders: ranging from very rare diseases (e.g. unicommissural aortic valve or congenital pulmonary stenosis) to less rare forms (Ebstein anomaly of the tricuspid valve –1 % of congenital heart disease overall) and to the common bicuspid aortic valve, whose prevalence is 1–2 % of the general population (see also Sect. 5.5).
- Disease associated to genetic disorders (e.g. Marfan or Ehlers–Danlos disease).
- Primary and secondary acquired disease. In primary forms intrinsic anatomic alterations affect the valves themselves or the "valve complex" (annulus, leaflets and commissures, subvalvular apparatus) (Fig. 5.33): the most frequent etiologies are myxomatous degeneration, rheumatic valve disease, infective endocarditis, degenerative age related process – such as mitral valve calcification or senile calcific aortic stenosis – non-bacterial thrombotic endocarditis. Secondary forms are associated to other cardiac diseases, mainly ischemic heart disease or dilated cardiomyopathy: valve tissue and valvular apparatus are not significantly altered and valve dysfunction is related to modified geometrical relationships between the myocardial disease and the valve apparatus.

Due to valve anatomy or structure, each is designed to ensure optimal function, and/or to hemodynamic reasons, some etiologies are more common in left-sided valves (degenerative, rheumatic forms), others are specific to right-sided valves (carcinoid heart disease).

In industrialized countries, the degenerative valve diseases are the most common as a result of increasing longevity, coupled with a background incidence of rheumatic and infective endocarditis, whereas in developing countries patients are mainly affected by inflammatory (principally rheumatic) diseases.

Despite the epidemiologic importance of HVD there are few registers unlike for other major heart diseases. A European prospective survey conducted around 10 years ago on 5000 adult patients with HVD found that the most frequent origin is degenerative, especially causing aortic stenosis and that patients are mostly elderly and with a number of risk factors and comorbidities (Iung et al. 2003).

HVD is an infrequent indication for HTx and accounts for only a minor percentage of heart transplanted patients. The ISHLT Registry data show that between 1982 and 1999 the percentage of patients transplanted because of HVD was 4 %; in more recent years (2000–2015) it has fluctuated between 2 and 3 % (Fig. 5.34).

This low percentage is also due to progressive improvements in surgical replacement and repair and to the new percutaneous techniques for treating cardiac valve disease (catheter-deployed bioprosthetic valve inserted percutaneously in the aortic position; coated metallic clip devices applied to mitral leaflets).

When HTx is considered in patients with severe HVD, the outcome of valve surgery and

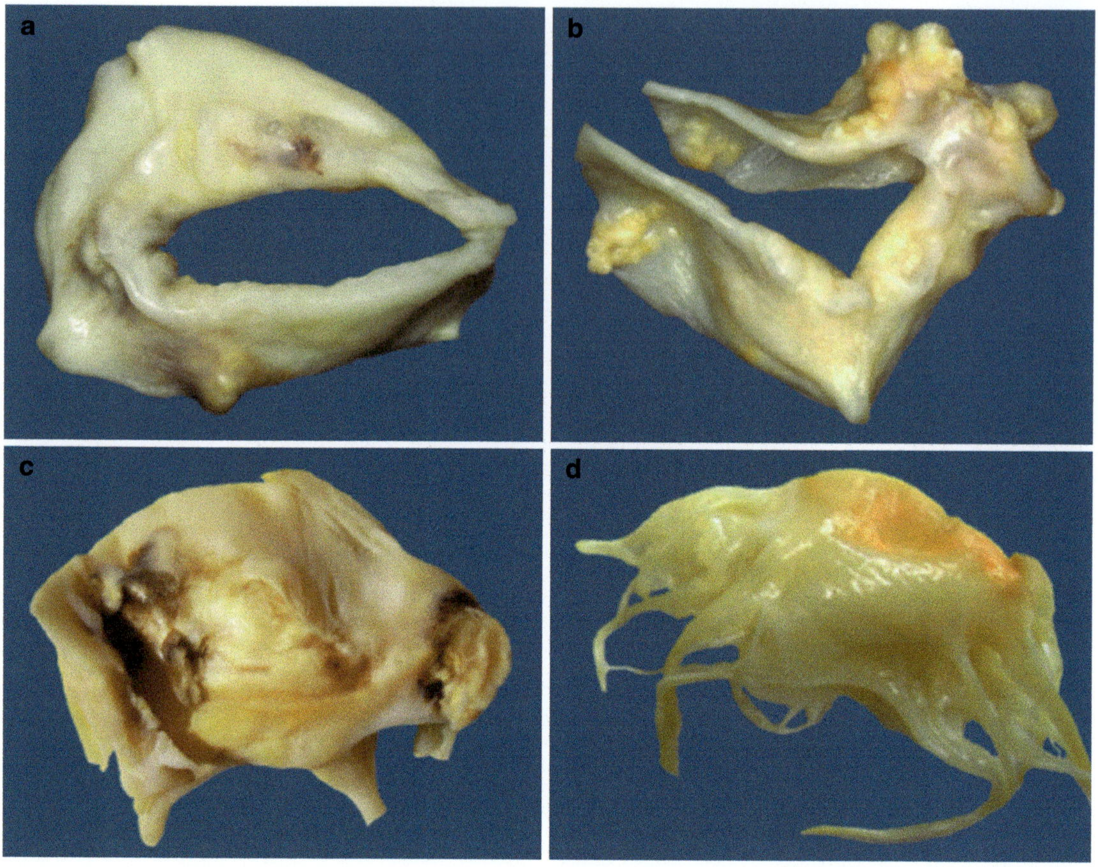

Fig. 5.32 Surgical valve specimens. (**a**) Unicommissural aortic valve with whitish thickened tissue and focal erosion in the leaflet (ventricular view). (**b**) Bicuspid aortic valve. The two leaflets are markedly thickened and show multiple calcific nodules; median rafe is present in the greatest cusp. (**c**) Chronic rheumatic mitral valve disease with leaflet fibrosis, commissure fusion, calcification and chordal thickening. (**d**) Floppy mitral valve with significant myxomatous degeneration of the anterior leaflet

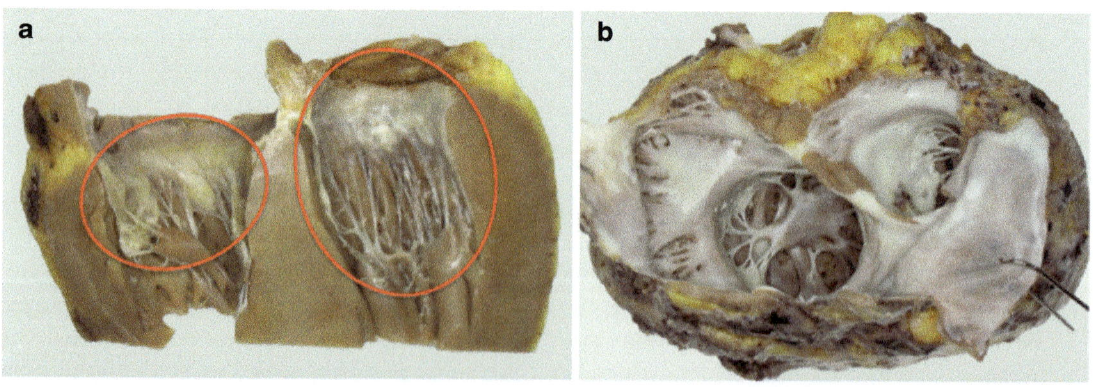

Fig. 5.33 The "valvular complex" of atrioventricular valves includes the annulus, the leaflets and commissures, the subvalvular apparatus, chordae tendineae and papillary muscles, and atrial and ventricular myocardium. (**a**) Posterior view of a longitudinal cut of the heart. (**b**) Atrioventricular valvular complex viewed from the atria

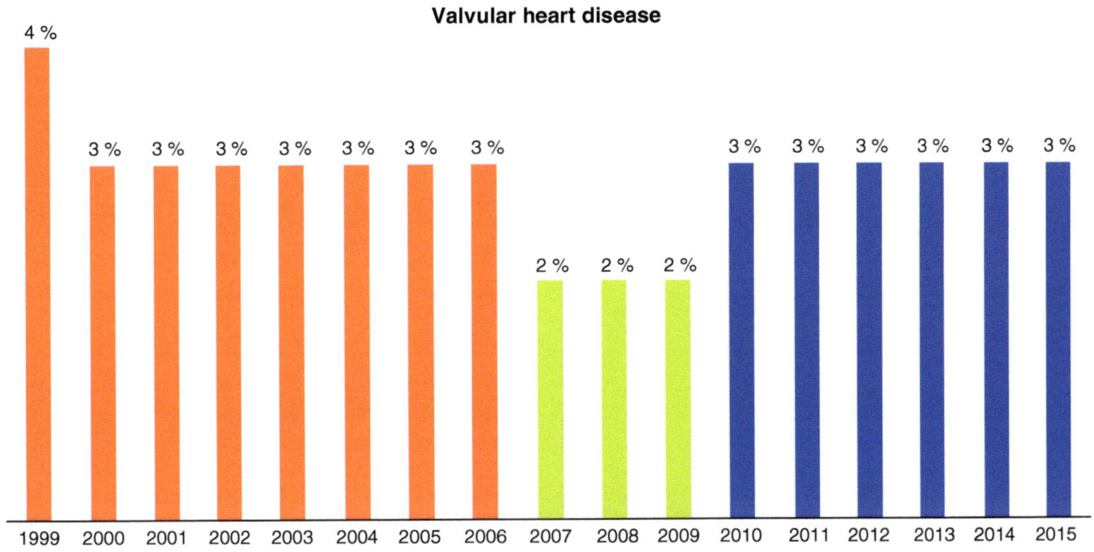

Fig. 5.34 Percentages of valvular heart disease in native hearts 1999–2015 (Data from the ISHLT Registry)

interventional techniques should be weighed against that of heart transplantation (Costanzo et al. 1995).

However, HTx must be considered when the disease progresses beyond the point where other therapies are effective and patients develop end-stage valvular cardiomyopathy with a life expectancy of a few months (Pellegrini et al. 2012).

5.4.2 Specific Technical Pathology Points

Native hearts with end-stage valvular cardiomyopathy usually include prosthetic valves or, in the mitral and tricuspid positions, annuloplasty rings: when encountered these should be evaluated in situ in order to recognize type and note any complication.

Pathology examination of hearts with valvular disease is the same as for hearts with myocardial diseases and has been treated in depth in Sect. 5.3.

In our case, the best approach for sectioning the heart is to perform the echocardiographic short axis cut, i.e. to obtain serial transverse sections (i.e. perpendicular to the long axis of the heart) from the apex to the mid-ventricular level at 1 cm intervals (for details and figures see Sect. 5.3). In this way prosthetic atrioventricular valves can be examined from the atrial view and, after the heart has been sectioned, from the ventricular view (Fig. 5.35).

When an aortic valve prosthesis is present, it can be easily examined from the aortic view and, if necessary, from the ventricular side by opening the outflow tract of the left ventricle basal segment along the anterior surface (Fig. 5.36).

Sampling and staining follow the scheme for cardiomyopathy; when biological prosthesis are present valve leaflets can also be sampled.

5.4.3 Pathologic Substrates in Native Hearts and in Surgical Valve Specimens

Owing to significant improvements in valvular surgery, new technology for treating cardiac valve disease and advances in pre-operative and post-operative care, an increasing number of patients – many of them elderly – undergo valve replacement or repair procedures. Consequently, today, at autopsy the pathologist rarely encounters

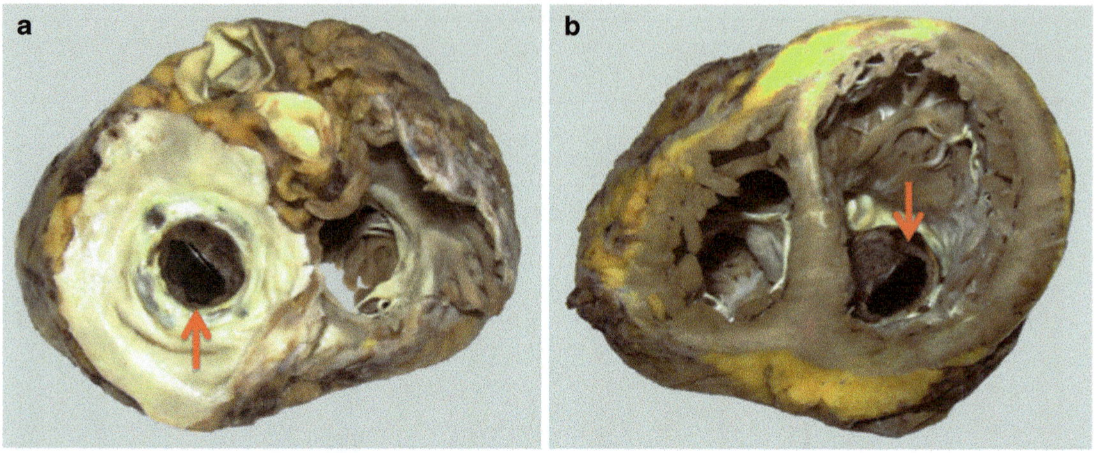

Fig. 5.35 Mitral mechanical prosthesis from the atrial view (**a**) and the ventricular view (**b**) (*arrows*)

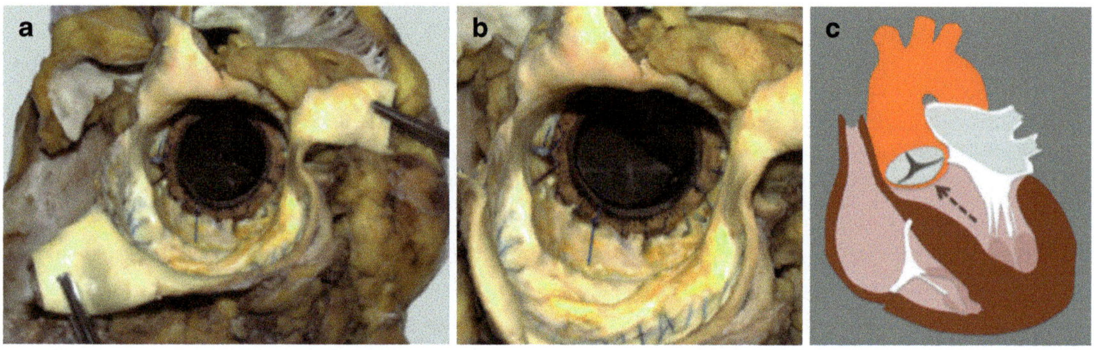

Fig. 5.36 (**a**, **b**) Aortic view of mechanical bileaflet prosthesis in aortic position. (**c**) Scheme showing the outflow tract of the left ventricle (*arrow*) to be opened to evaluate the inferior side of aortic prosthesis

valvular heart disease that has followed its natural course, but ever more frequently examines surgical specimens of diseased valves. Those native hearts with end-stage valvular cardiomyopathy allow the pathologist to study structural alterations of ventricles due to myocardial remodeling consequent on the underlying valve disease before valve surgery, late degenerative alterations in leaflets of bioprosthetic valves, as well as tissue reaction around sutures of ring prosthesis.

Thus, as in other fields of cardiovascular pathology, pathologic valve examination has progressed from autopsy to surgical pathology, and enriched the pathological perspective with detailed histological study. This passage from macrostructure to microstructure has led to an even better understanding: the relationship between valvular tissue framework and function, how valvular tissue components react to damage, the pathological substrates and the mechanisms of valvular dysfunction and the relationships between molecular, cellular, and morphological aspects. All in all the fullest understanding so far of heart valve biology and pathobiology. All valve diseases place a hemodynamic burden on the left and right ventricles: the general changes in myocardial structure and function in response to stimuli that accompany valvular dysfunction are known as remodeling. At tissue level, the process of myocardial remodeling includes molecular and cellular changes and alterations in gene expression leading to hypertrophy of individual myocytes, death of some myocytes by apoptosis, hyperplasia of interstitial cellular components, and changes in both the quantity and quality of the extracellular matrix (Yacoub and Cohn 2004a, b).

Valve prostheses encountered in native hearts can be mechanical or biological tissue valves. The most frequent mechanical valves are bileaflet tilting disc type. Bioprosthetic valves are either xenografts or homografts. Xenografts are made from animal tissue (usually porcine) or bovine parietal pericardium; homografts are human tissue grafts harvested from cadavers or from live donors. Bioprosthesis can be mounted on a frame or stent or without these (stentless) (Butany et al. 2003; Butany and Collins 2005).

In tricuspid position annuloplasty rings may be found (a full ring or a C-shaped flexible prosthesis); in mitral position, valve repair with annuloplasty is usually associated with a partial resection of the leaflet. These devices are mainly found in patients with severe end-stage dilated or ischemic cardiomyopathy, where functional mitral regurgitation in particular is one of the most challenging problems, with negative impact on survival (Szalaya et al. 2003).

Recently a percutaneous mitral valve repair using MitraClip devices has been developed as a catheter-based option for correction of functional and degenerative mitral regurgitation instead of the traditional surgical repair or replacement. The histopathological healing response to this catheter-based mitral valve repair device has been documented in a recent paper by Ladich et al., the first large pathologic study in humans (Ladich et al. 2011). In patients with functional mitral regurgitation following advanced heart failure in dilated cardiomyopathy, MitraClip implantation has also been successfully used as a bridge therapy to heart transplantation (Garatti et al. 2015).

In native hearts acute/early complications of valve prosthesis, such as thrombosis, endocarditis, dehiscence of commissural insertion or significant paravalvular leak, are usually not seen. In bioprosthetic valves, structural valve tissue degeneration, mainly leaflet degeneration with thickening of cuspal tissue with or without calcifications, may be found (Khan et al. 2010; Siddiqui et al. 2009). Pannus or fibrous reaction to the device can occur at the host fabric or host tissue interface and can sometimes be found as overgrown tissue in the sewing cuff or within the biological components, causing stiffening and progressive stenosis and dysfunction.

The experience of explanted native hearts with end-stage valvular cardiomyopathy from the Heart Transplant Centre of Sant'Orsola Hospital of Bologna reflects the data in the international registries.

From October 1991 to December 2014, 28 patients (4.4 %) out of 631 underwent heart transplantation for end-stage "valvular" cardiomyopathy, subdivided as follows:

- Trivalvular disease with mitral and aortic mechanical prosthesis and tricuspid valvuloplasty: 9 %.
- Trivalvular rheumatic disease with mitral and aortic mechanical prosthesis and tricuspid porcine bioprosthesis: 4.5 %.
- Mitro-aortic disease with mechanical prosthesis: 23 % (40 % with tricuspid annuloplastic).
- Mitral disease with mechanical prosthesis: 18 % (75 % with tricuspid annuloplasty).
- Aortic disease with aortic mechanical prosthesis: 36.5 % (12.5 % with mitral valvuloplasty, 12.5 % with tricuspid valvuloplasty, and one Marfan patient with mitral and tricuspid valvuloplasty).
- Mitral valve disease with mitral valvuloplasty: 4.5 %.
- Previous Ross surgery (pulmonary homograft in aortic position and second homograft in pulmonary valve position): 4.5 %.

All the hearts had significantly increased in weight (medium 696 g, range 380–1040 g) and were enlarged with prevalent increase in transverse diameter, typically larger than those usually observed in DCM.

In a majority of cases ventricular cavities were dilated: there was irregularly distributed hypertrophy of the left ventricle and the septum, more markedly so in the isolated aortic disease group. Even at gross examination, some hearts showed significant fibrotic whitish areas. The main histological findings were extensive fibrosis (subendocardial, interstitial, and replacement) and marked nonspecific myocyte alterations (hypertrophy, sarcoplasmic vacuolization, myocytolysis, and dysmetry close to fibrosis areas).

Case 1. A 45-year-old woman transplanted for cardiopathy following trivalvular rheumatic heart disease. The heart was rounded and weighted 380 g. The epicardial surface was diffusely opaque due to marked fibrotic reaction of chronic pericarditis. The tricuspid valve had been replaced by a porcine bioprosthesis and the aortic and mitral ones by bileaflet mechanical valves. The porcine leaflets were thickened, swollen, and bulging due to tissue degeneration; pannus with fibrous reaction was evident in the sewing cuff and starting to extend to the cusps. Mild hypertrophy of the left ventricle lateral wall and of the septum were evident; the left ventricle inferior wall showed fibrous replacement areas (Fig. 5.37).

Case 2. A 52-year-old man who underwent heart transplantation for end-stage rheumatic car-

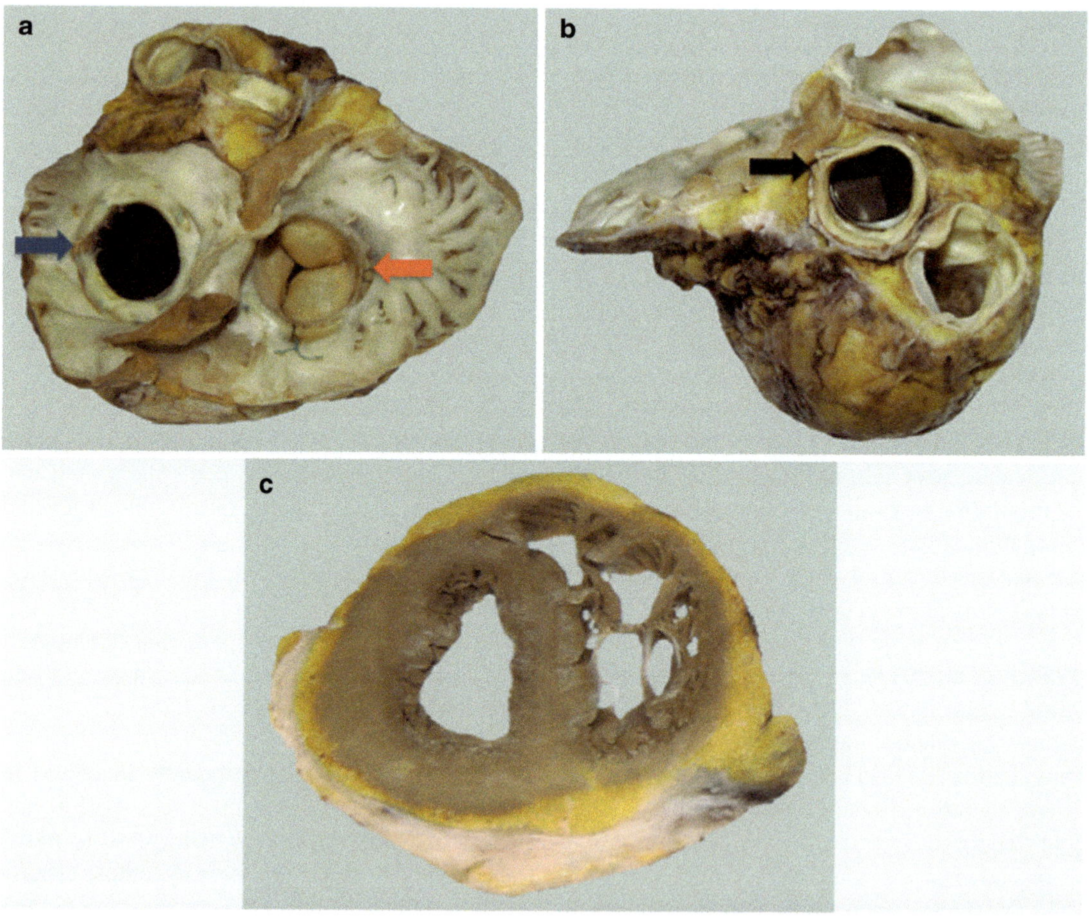

Fig. 5.37 Native heart with end-stage valvular cardiomyopathy due to rheumatic heart disease. (**a**) Atrial view showing mechanical bileaflet prosthesis in mitral position (*blue arrow*) and porcine bioprosthesis in tricuspid one (*red arrow*). Porcine leaflets are thickened, swollen and bulging due to tissue degeneration; fibrous reaction is evident in the sewing cuff of both prostheses, starting to extend into the cusps in the tricuspid bioprosthesis. (**b**) Superior view of great artery orifices showing a mechanical prosthesis in aortic position (*black arrow*). (**c**) In the transverse midventricular cut of the heart fibrous chronic pericarditis and mild left ventricle and septum hypertrophy are present

diomyopathy. The heart weighed 760 g and was severely enlarged. The epicardium was diffusely thickened and whitish with a wrinkled surface due to previous surgery. The left ventricle was considerably dilated and the mid-apical septum showed an extensive scar-like fibrous area. The coronary arteries revealed no significant atherosclerotic stenosis. The mechanical prostheses were evident in the mitral and aortic positions; the tricuspid valve, whose leaflets were thickened and swollen, had a Carpentier ring around the annulus (Fig. 5.38).

Apart from extensive subendocardial and replacement fibrosis and nonspecific alterations of myocells, the noteworthy finding at histology was a number of lymphocytic inflammatory infiltrates within the fibrous tissue or in the interstitium associated with focal myocyte damage, witness to the previous autoimmune inflammatory myocardial disease.

Today, the relative incidence of postinflammatory rheumatic disease varies from 30 to 50 % in surgically excised valves. Pathologic findings of the chronic phase of rheumatic valve disease are leaflet fibrosis, commissure fusion, calcification, and chordal thickening or fusion. Histologically, these thickened leaflets show dense fibrosis, which obliterates the layered architecture of the cusps, neovascularization, and mild chronic inflammation (Fig. 5.39). The chronic aspect is the result of healing and remodeling of recurrent acute valvulitis, characterized by small flat vegetation (verrucae) histologically made of platelets and fibrin and areas of fibrinoid necrosis and lympho-histiocytic inflammation with occasional giant cells.

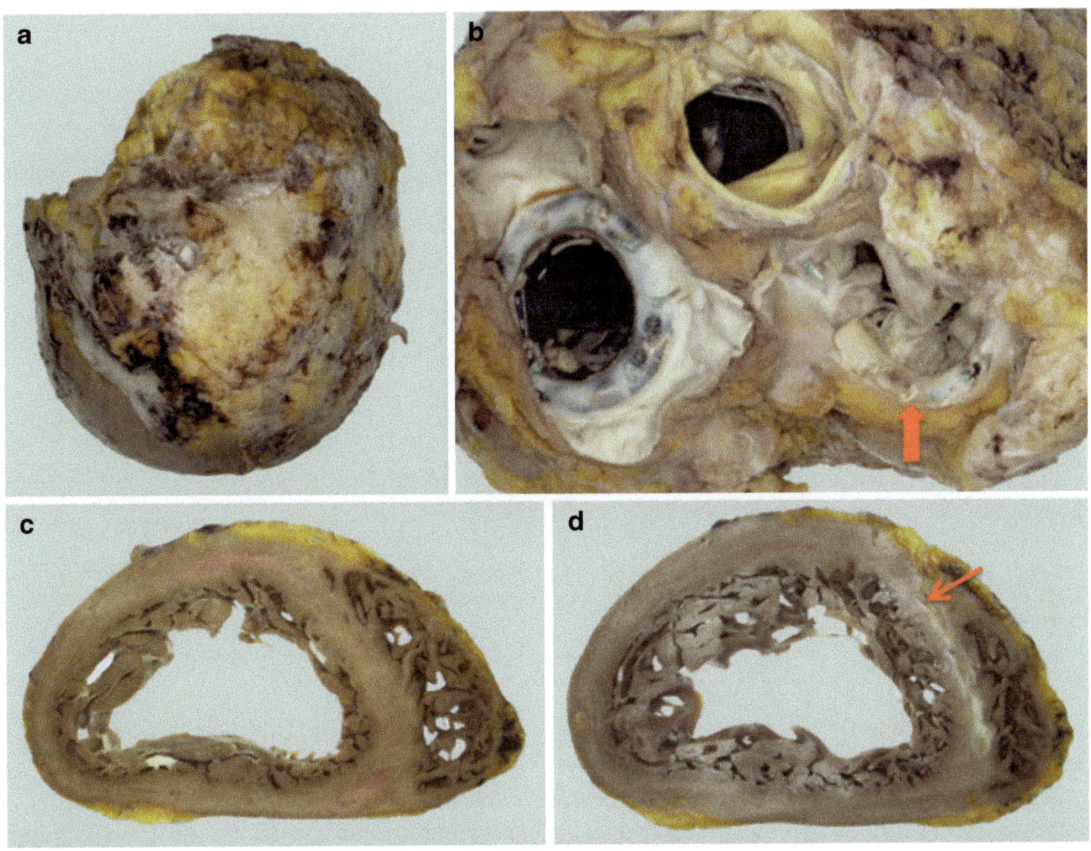

Fig. 5.38 (**a**) Native heart with end-stage rheumatic cardiomyopathy. (**b**) Atrial view showing mechanical prosthesis in mitral and aortic position and Carpentier ring around tricuspid annulus (*arrow*). (**c**, **d**) Short-axis cuts of the heart showing marked dilatation of left ventricle and extensive septal fibrous scar (*arrow*)

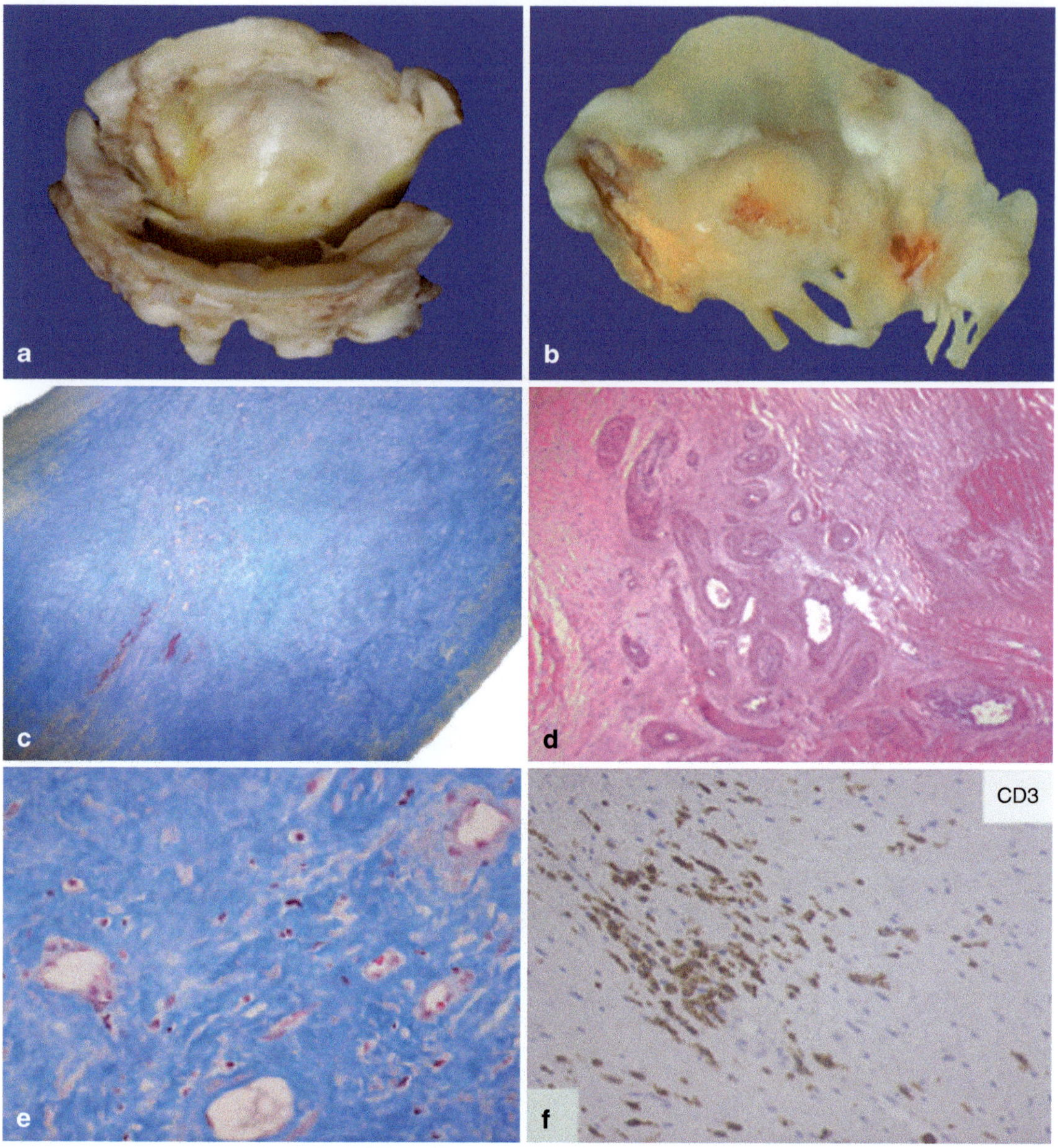

Fig. 5.39 Chronic phase of rheumatic valve disease. (**a**, **b**) Macroscopy of surgical specimens of mitral valve with marked leaflet fibrosis, commissure fusion and calcification. Histology shows dense fibrosis (**c**, Azan Mallory trichrome, 25×), neovascularization with thickened (**d**, Hematoxylin–eosin, 200×) and thinned (**e**, Azan Mallory trichrome, 400×) vessel walls and mild chronic inflammation (**f**, CD3 immunohistochemistry, 400×)

Granulomatous Aschoff bodies are very rare in valve tissue.

The involvement of the tricuspid valve is not uncommon in patients with rheumatic heart disease and is virtually always associated with mitral disease. The pathological pictures are similar, but commissural fusion and calcification are less common in the former than in mitral and aortic rheumatic valves.

Case 3. A 43-year-old man transplanted for ischemic heart disease. The explanted heart showed severe dilatation of the left ventricle, an extensive fibrous scar in the left ventricle anterior wall and in the septum, and apical aneurysmatic dilatation with thrombus stratification. The patient underwent MitraClip implantation in the central position of mitral valve leaflets (Fig. 5.40).

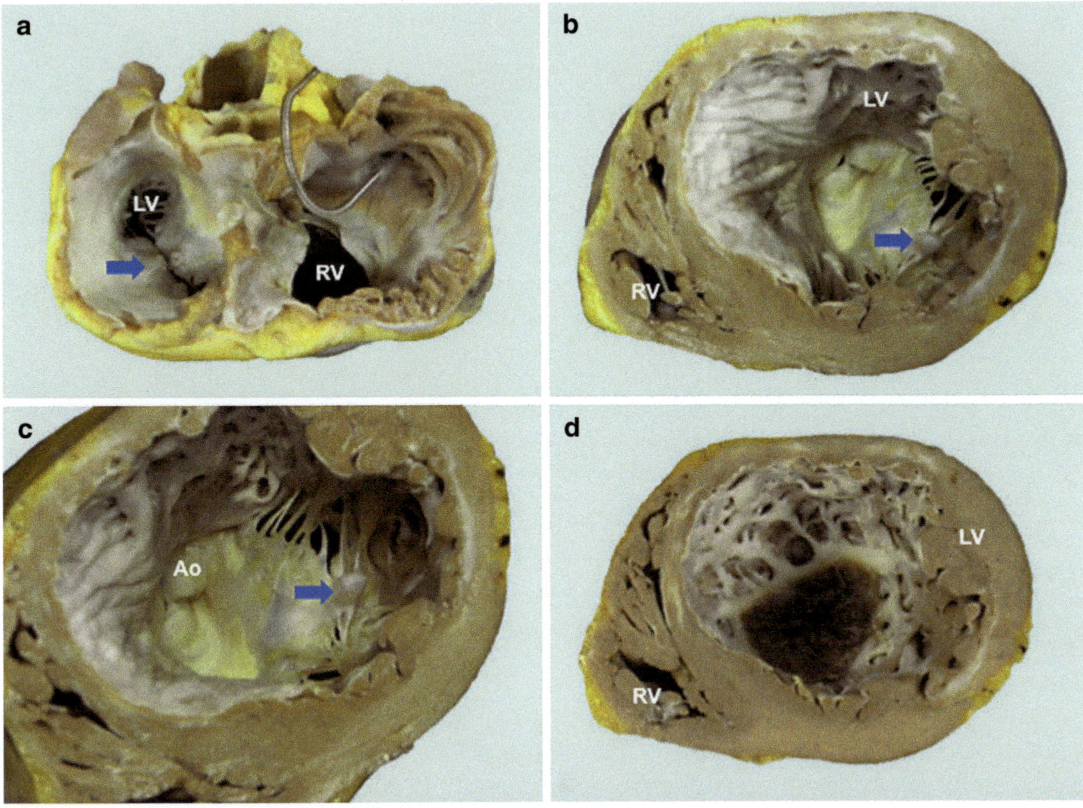

Fig. 5.40 Macroscopic view of the native heart. (**a**) View from above showing the atrio-ventricular junction. Both atria appear dilated and a catheter has been placed into the right atrial appendage. Note the mitral valve with two ostia due to a mitral clip. (**b**) View from below after a cross section at mid-ventricular level, showing the dilated left ventricle with postischemic antero-septal myocardial scar. Note the mitral clip covered by fibrous tissue (*arrow*). (**c**) High-power view of **b** with the mitral clip anchoring the anterior and posterior leaflets of the mitral valve in the central position. (**d**) View from above of the apical part of the heart with apical aneurysm and mural thrombosis. *Ao* aortic valve, *LV* left ventricle, *RV* right ventricle

Prosthesis in mitral position or mitral repair aspects and annuloplasty may be found in native hearts with end-stage dilated cardiomyopathy or ischemic heart disease (Fig. 5.41). The mechanism of mitral valve dysfunction is functional and due to alterations in heart geometry, although organic/structural alterations of valve tissue probably concur (Grande-Allen et al. 2005).

Heart valve disease is a paradigm of the changing etiology of human disease, which today separates developing countries, where patients are mainly affected by inflammatory disease (especially rheumatic disease) and industrialized countries, where the highest incidence is due to degenerative valve disease as a result of increasing longevity (Soler-Soler and Galve 2000).

Degenerative valve disease increases with age but aging is probably not the only factor (Fig. 5.42a). Its histopathological changes include the following (Fig. 5.42b–f):

- Fibrous and elastic thickening (due to collagen deposition and degeneration).
- Lipid deposition (ranging from a nodule to a horizontal bar-shaped deposit).
- Myxomatous degeneration.
- Dystrophic calcification at leaflet and annulus levels.

Myxomatous degeneration affects up to 5 % of the population and may represent a genetic condition or be a secondary manifestation of leaflet adaptation or repair. It is the histopathological basis of the floppy valve and the most frequent

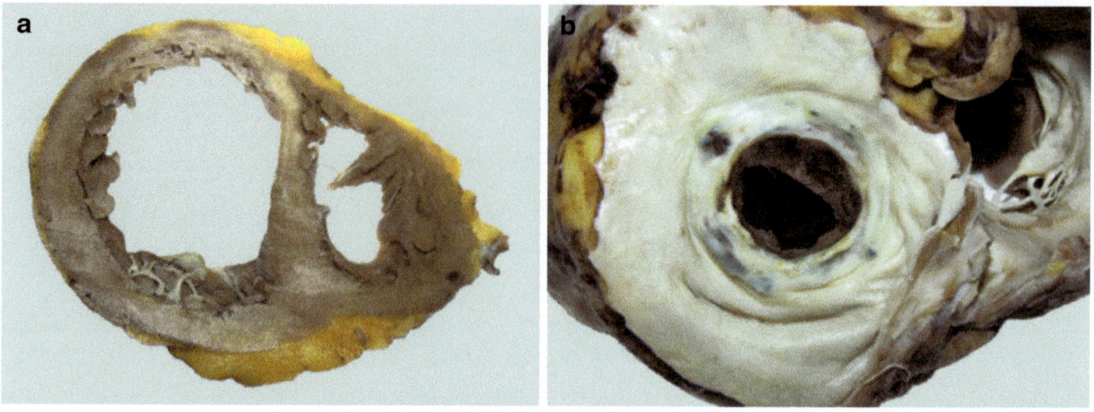

Fig. 5.41 (**a**) Transverse cut of native heart with end-stage ischemic disease showing an antero-septal fibrous scar. (**b**) Atrial view of the mechanical prosthesis in mitral position with pannus and fibrous reaction

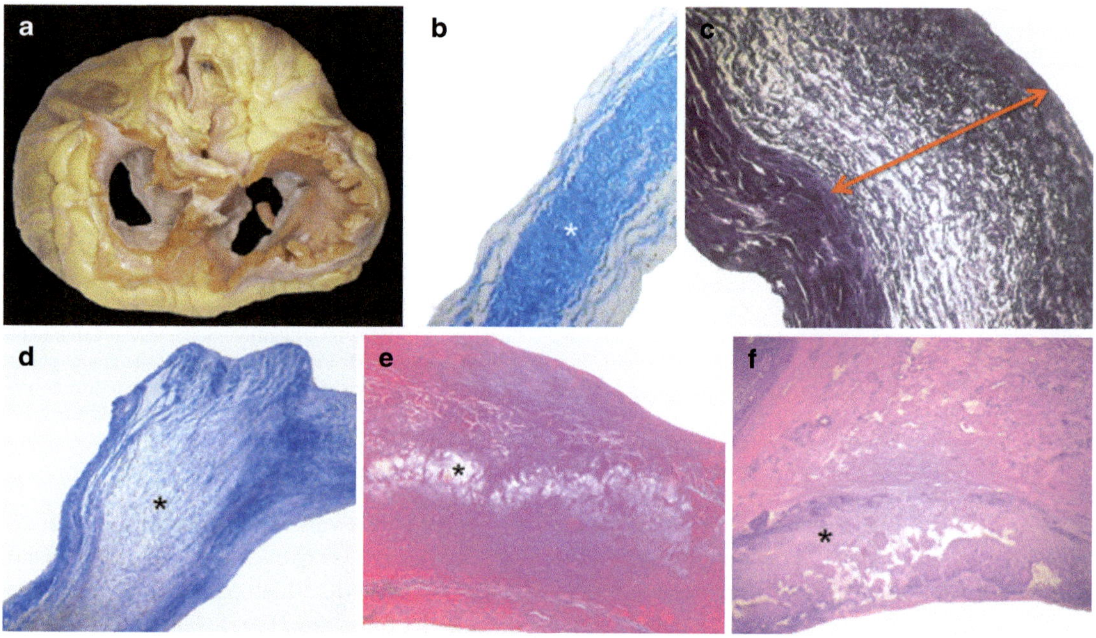

Fig. 5.42 (**a**) Native heart with degenerative valve disease associated to the primary dilated cardiomyopathy disease: atrial view of the bulging atrioventricular valves with jelly appearance. Histology of degenerative valve disease including: fibrous thickening (**b**, Azan Mallory trichrome, 25× – *asterisk*); elastic thickening (**c**, Weigert–van Gieson stain, 100× – *arrow*); myxomatous degeneration (**d**, Azan Mallory trichrome, 25× – *asterisk*); lipid deposition (**e**, hematoxylin–eosin, 100× – *asterisk*); dystrophic calcification (**f**, Hematoxylin–eosin, 200× – *asterisk*)

cause of mitral valve prolapse (Grau et al. 2007). Histologically, there is a myxomatous thickening of the leaflets due to expansion of the spongiosa and replacement of the solid fibrosa with loosely arranged myxomatous tissue rich in mucopolysaccharides and spindle-shaped fibroblastic cells (Fig. 5.43). Unlike the mitral, the tricuspid valve rarely develops degenerative changes.

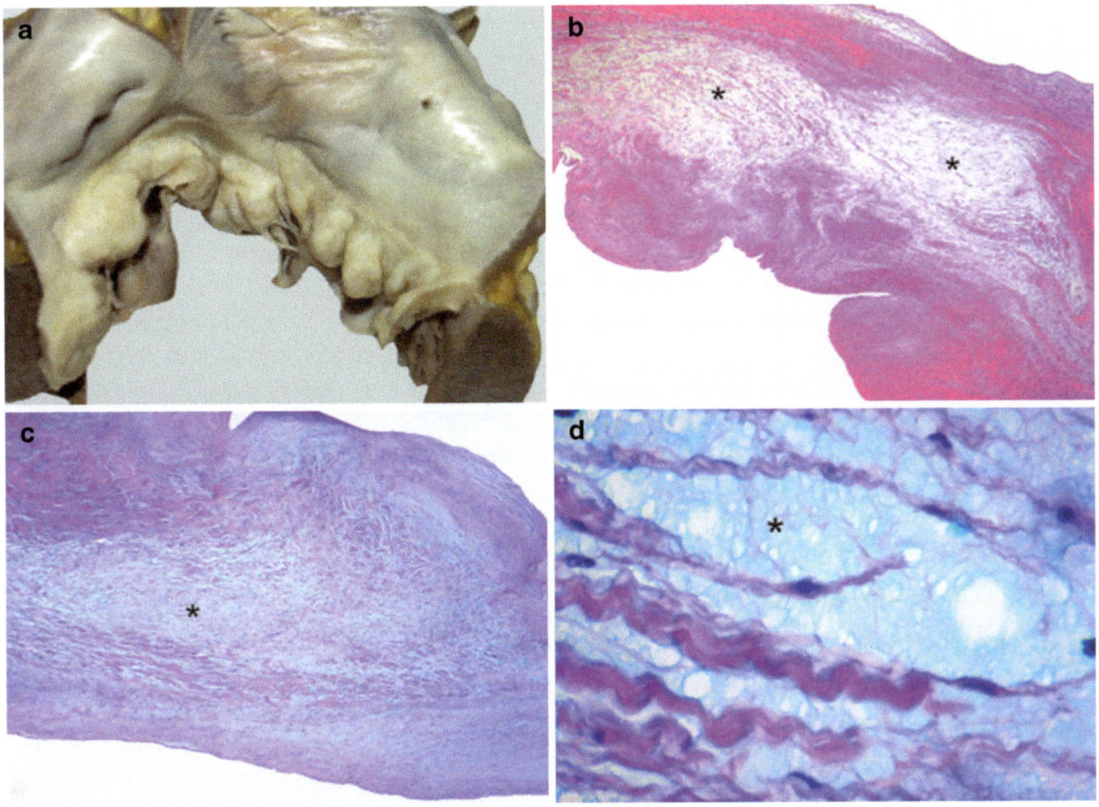

Fig. 5.43 (**a**) Autoptic heart opened along the obtuse margin of left ventricle with mitral valve prolapse. Histology of myxomatous degeneration showing loosely arranged myxomatous tissue rich in mucopolysaccharides expanding the spongiosa (**b**: Hematoxylin–eosin 25×; **c**: Alcian blue stain, 100×, **d**: Alcian blue stain, 400× – *asterisks*)

Key Points

- Heart valve disease is very frequent and includes many and different forms, of which the most frequent are degenerative and rheumatic.
- Heart valve disease is an infrequent indication for heart transplantation and accounts for only 3 % of heart transplanted patients.
- The majority of native hearts with end-stage cardiomyopathy will have had surgery or repair for primary heart valve disease.
- Native hearts with end-stage valvular cardiomyopathy usually include prosthetic valves or annuloplasty rings, which should be examined in situ.
- The pathologist should be familiar with the major types of prosthesis and main complications of surgery/repair or percutaneous implants.
- However, prosthesis or annuloplasty may also be found in native hearts with end-stage dilated cardiomyopathy or ischemic heart diseases.

5.5 The Spectrum of Congenital Heart Defects

5.5.1 Background and Incidence in Explanted Hearts

The first pediatric heart transplant was performed in 1967 in a neonate for a congenital heart disease affecting the right ventricle, an Ebstein anomaly, with a disastrous outcome of only 6 hours of life.

Only after the introduction of cyclosporine as immunosuppressive therapy 20 years later did heart transplantation become a consistent option for pediatric as well as adult patients.

In patients, younger than 18 years of age, the indications for HTx can be grouped into three main categories: cardiomyopathies (CMPs), congenital heart diseases (CHD), and other diseases/retransplantations. Relative percentages of these three groups have changed since the early experience in the 1990s, with the decreasing incidence of CHD (Dipchand et al. 2013).

Better management of CHD patients and dramatic improvements in surgical techniques and intensive care unit management have modified the indications for transplantation as primary therapeutic option for many congenital defects. Various palliative options are now offered as first treatment to neonates affected by hypoplastic left heart syndrome and/or tricuspid atresia and hypoplastic right ventricle.

However, large-volume data from the United States centers demonstrates increasing incidence of transplantation for CHD (Lamour et al. 2009; Schumacher et al. 2015).

Data from the 2013 International Society for Heart and Lung Transplantation Report showed that according to age distribution and time, CHD is the first cause of transplantation within the first year of life. In this group, a significant decrease from 1988–1999 (76 %) to the present 2003–2013 (55 %) was observed (Dipchand et al. 2013). CHD is also decreasing in 11- to 17-year-old patients, falling as low as one-fourth of all indications. In adults, CHD represents up to 3 % of all indications (Coskun et al. 2007; Boucek et al. 2014).

According to the literature on outcomes in pediatric heart transplant patients, CHD has a worse prognosis than CMP, due to the technical complexities of surgery and more complicated perioperative care (Seddioa et al. 2013; Voeller et al. 2012; Gambino et al. 2007; Chen et al. 2004; Griffiths et al. 2009).

Impressive improvements in modern surgical techniques mean that in most centers surgical palliation is now preferred to HTx for CHD, so the majority of patients reach adulthood, thus shifting the issue of childhood mortality to adult age (Attenhofer Jost et al. 2013).

As a consequence, the number of CHD adult patients is greatly increasing and only later in life do they present with congestive heart failure and end-stage disease. This is changing the scenario of transplants for CHD, as it is expected that 10–20 % of patients suffering from complex CHD will require HTx as adults (Schweiger et al. 2015).

Thus, when considering CHD in native transplanted hearts the pathologist can find a wide range of situations: previously operated and non-operated explanted hearts, both pediatric and adult, and ventricular-assisted devices implanted as a bridge to transplantation.

Examination and dissection of these hearts require great expertise and care.

In centers not specialized in pediatric transplantation, adult hearts with previous surgery are the most frequent.

5.5.2 Specific Technical Pathology Points

Methods for evaluating CHD native hearts vary depending on whether we are dealing with primary diseases transplanted or with previously palliated end-stage CHD.

What is really essential in both situations is collation of all the clinical information, notes on native heart structural diseases and also of the various surgical procedures previously performed.

5.5.2.1 Non-operated CHD

For these hearts, there is no standard sectioning method due to heterogeneity of the underlying structural abnormalities.

A transverse cut at mid-ventricle is not usually recommended; generally it is preferable to dissect the heart following blood flow.

The best classification system for these specimens is the *sequential segmental approach (SSA)*, whose main steps are as follows:

- Definition of atrial situs.
- Morphologic identification of atria, ventricles, and great arteries.
- Recognition of atrioventricular and ventriculo-arterial connections.

It is beyond the scope of this chapter to detail this approach; excellent publications (Shinebourne et al. 1976; Anderson and Wilcox 1996; Anderson and Shirali 2009) or textbooks (Anderson et al. 1991 cover this subject).

Some points to emphasize when managing non-operated CHD native heart specimens according to the SSA are as follows:

- The absence of the venous pole of the atria does not interfere with situs identification, as there are the atrial appendages, with their striking morphology.
- Examination of the ventricular cavities with careful evaluation of trabecular components and assessment of the atrio-ventricular junction and related valve apparatus viewed from above and below are major steps in identifying right and left ventricles.
- Before dissection the presence of a biventricular or univentricular condition should be checked; with univentricular physiology it is essential to identify the rudimentary ventricle.

Histology is not required in non-operated CHD except for research.

5.5.2.2 Operated CHD

In cases of previously operated hearts, the sample can be managed according to the general recommendations for surgically resected hearts in the guidelines of the Association for European Cardiovascular Pathology and the Society for Cardiovascular Pathology (Stone et al. 2012).

Any devices related to previous surgical or interventional procedures must also be assessed. Most frequently these are found at the atrial septum following closure of interatrial septal defects, or at the ventriculo-arterial junction (mechanical or biological valves).

Check also for any catheters within the cavities and any epicardial leads.

With Fontan procedures identify patches or biological grafts used for palliation.

A ventricular-assisted device should be photographed before removal from the apex, and carefully evaluated.

In dissecting the heart it is preferable to use the echocardiographic short axis cut with serial transverse sections, each of 1 cm, from the apex to the medium third of the heart, as shown in Section 5.2. As the structure and morphology of the heart can be very altered, it is advisable to have a clear idea of the original diagnosis and of the subsequent surgery steps and if possible with the surgeon or cardiologist present.

The various main branches of the coronary arteries should be cut transversally to the main longitudinal direction, as previously described in Section 5.2, in order to identify atherosclerotic plaques, which could be present in association with the congenital heart disease of an adult patient.

Histology should include sampling from both ventricles and from coronary arteries if lesions are identified.

When a ventricular-assisted device is found, a transverse section at 1 cm from the insertion point of the device can be taken for histologic study.

5.5.3 Pathologic Substrates

According to the literature on single-center experiences (Seddioa et al. 2013; Voeller et al. 2012; Gambino et al. 2007; Chen et al. 2004) or on multi-institutional studies (Lamour et al. 2009; Schumacher et al. 2015; Boucek et al. 2014), a

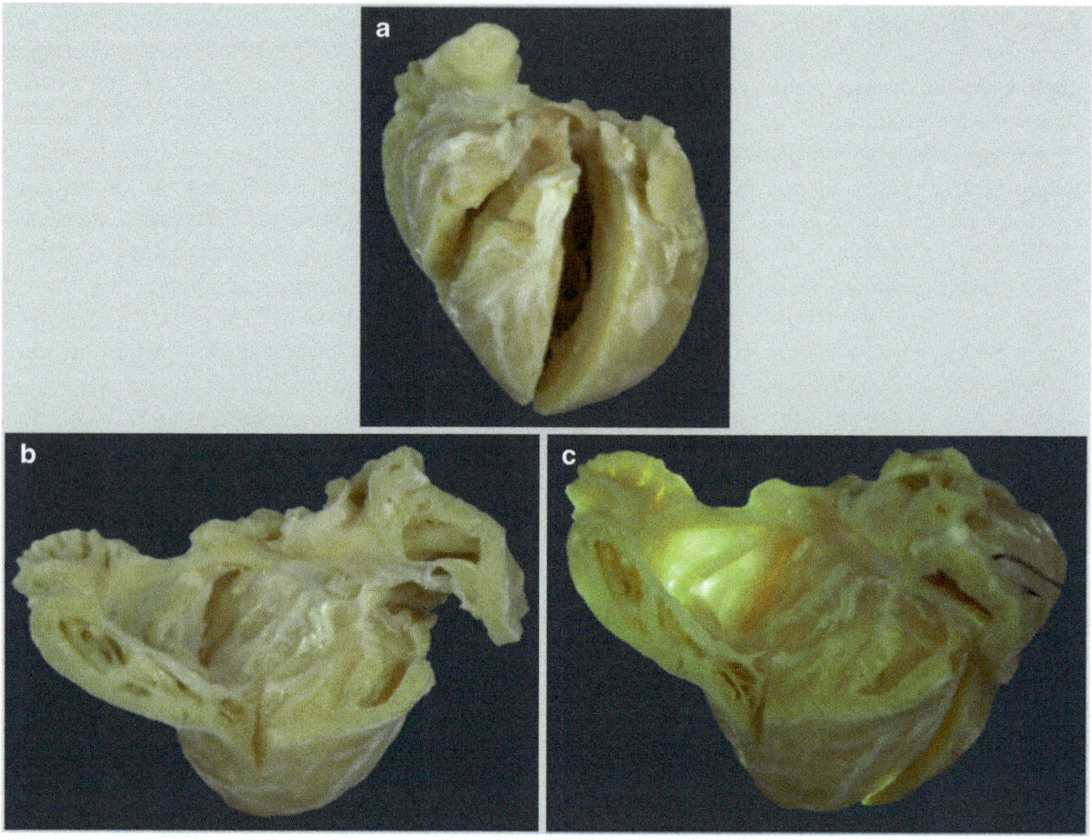

Fig. 5.44 The heart of a female infant affected by Ebstein's anomaly of the tricuspid valve and transplanted at the age of 2. (**a**) Anterior view of the native heart. (**b**) The right ventricle has been opened to show the displacement of the leaflets inside the ventricular cavity. (**c**) The heart has been transilluminated to show the papiraceous appearance of the atrialized part of the ventricular posterior wall

wide range of congenital heart defects are found among those leading to heart transplantation. The types of congenital heart defect depend on local experience and policy in managing CHDs over time. A minority of hearts removed at time of transplantation are unrepaired (7–15 %) and the main diseases in this group are hypoplastic left heart syndrome (HLHS); severe Ebstein's anomaly (Fig. 5.44); congenitally corrected transposition of the great arteries (Fig. 5.45); anomalous left coronary artery origin; severe congenital mitral valve insufficiency; and unclassified forms of severe congenital heart disease.

However, most have been previously palliated or corrected for complex congenital heart defects, both in pediatrics and in adults (90–93 %). The main pathological substrates are two-ventricle defects in more than half of cases and single ventricle in the rest (36–44 %). The most frequent two-ventricle and single-ventricle defect types are listed in Table 5.2; the most common types of reparative surgery in Table 5.3.

There is extreme pathologic variety in these operated CHDs, which need therefore to be studied case by case. Usually the hearts are very enlarged and dilated. Morphology of ventricles varies depending on the primary CHD, previous palliative or corrective surgery, and myocardial remodeling phenomena. Frequently endocardium is thickened. Histology is non-specific and shows various degrees of subendocardial or interstitial fibrosis, and reactive or degenerative alterations of myocytes (hypertrophy, dysmetria, sarcoplasmic vacuolization, myocytolisis). Foci of myocardial coagulative necrosis related to the end-stage heart failure and foci of mild lymphocytic inflammation related to remodeling may be seen.

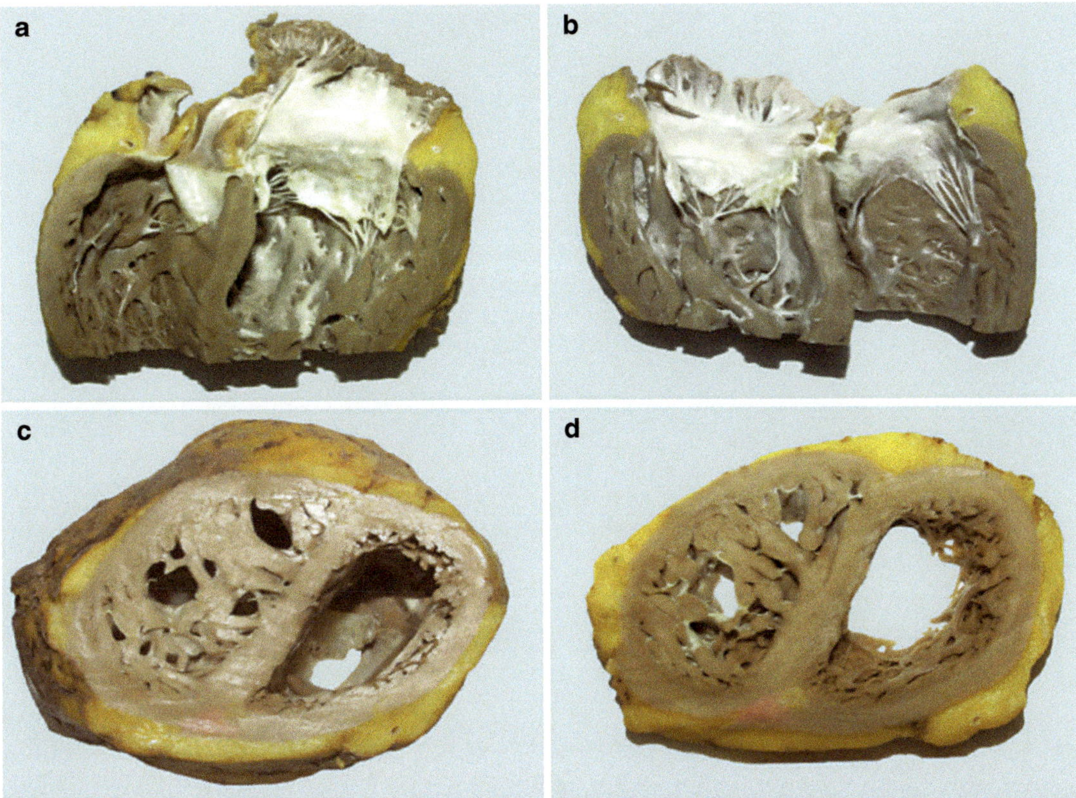

Fig. 5.45 A 25-year-old male transplanted for congenitally corrected transposition of great arteries. Heart weighed 780 g and was enlarged (12 cm along the longitudinal diameter and 11.5 along the transverse diameter). (**a**, **b**) Anterior (**a**) and posterior (**b**) views of longitudinal cuts. (**c**, **d**) Short-axis sections. RV is dilated and shows hypertrophy of the parietal myocardium (1 cm at superior third; 0.9 cm at medium third; 0.6 cm at inferior third) and a prominent trabecular myocardium. LV is relatively decreased in volume and shows regular or thinning parietal myocardium. *LV* left ventricle; *RV* right ventricle

Table 5.2 Congenital heart disease usually transplanted after previous surgery

Biventricular defects	Single ventricle defects
D-transposition of the great arteries (12 %)	Tricuspid atresia
Right ventricular outflow tract obstruction (10 %)	Hypoplastic left heart syndrome
Atrial/ventricular septal defects (8 %)	Double inlet left ventricle with left atrio-ventricular atresia
L-transposition of the great arteries (8 %)	Unbalanced artrio-ventricular canal with aortic atresia
Left ventricular outflow tract obstructions (8 %)	
Complete atrio-ventricular canal defect (8 %)	
Others (11 %)	

Table 5.3 The most common types of reparative surgery encountered in native hearts

Four-chamber repair: 29 %
Fontan procedure: 22 %
Glenn procedure: 16 %
Norwood procedure: 5 %
Pulmonary artery banding/shunting: 11 %
Mustard/Senning procedure: 10 %

Other cases of operated CHD are shown in Figs. 5.46 and 5.47.

Special attention should be given to patients who have already undergone Fontan-type palliative surgery and now present with failure requiring transplantation (failing Fontan). These patients have increased risk of death both early

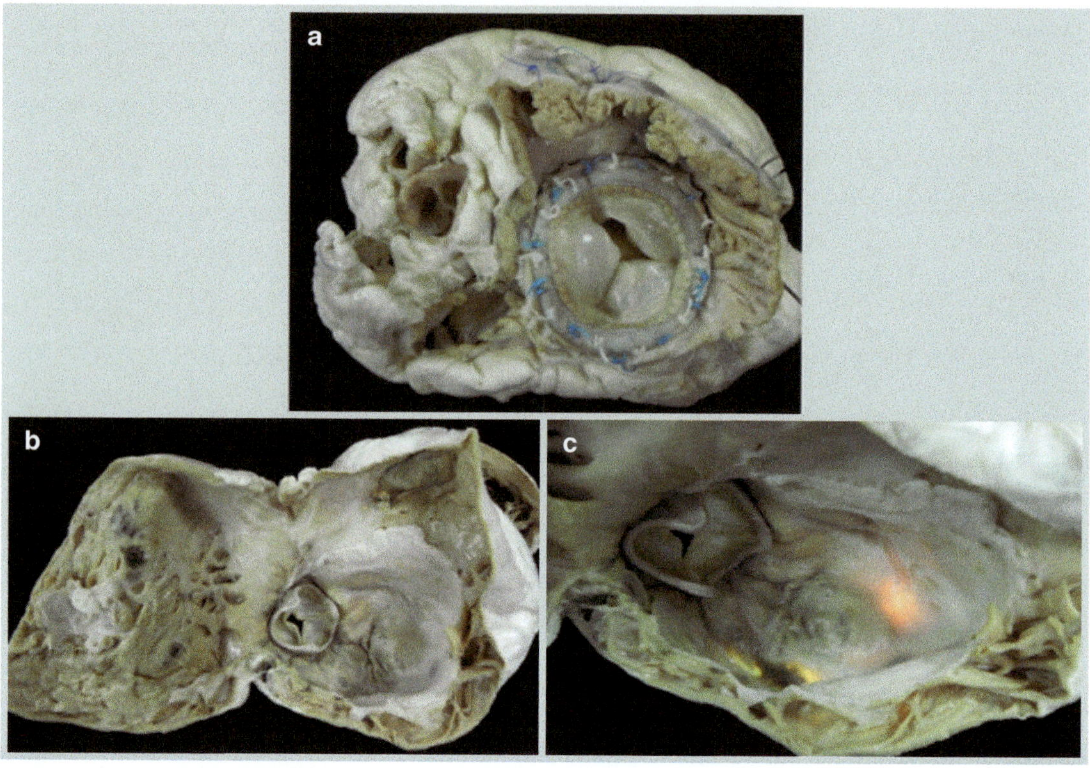

Fig. 5.46 The heart of a male infant affected by Ebstein's anomaly and previously operated for tricuspid valve replacement and ventricular cavity reduction. (**a**) Superior view of the native heart, showing the bioprosthesis in the tricuspid position. (**b**) The right ventricular cavity is opened to show the bioprosthesis located at the atrioventricular junction; the native leaflets, dysplastic and displaced toward the ventricular cavity, have been in part removed. The original tricuspid annulus is still visible. Note the posterior wall which has been folded. (**c**) A closer view with transillumination of the atrialized component

and late after HTx (Kanter et al. 2011; Michielon et al. 2011; Jayakumar et al. 2004; Davies et al. 2012). The Fontan palliative procedure is used for various univentricular circulation or single ventricle diseases, with the aim of diverting venous blood from systemic venous return to pulmonary arteries, without passing through the subpulmonary tract of the ventricle. Many variations of the original procedure have been performed, to favor systemic oxygen saturation and avoid or reduce ventricular volume overload. These variations fall into three main subcategories: internal Fontan (lateral tunnel), atrio-pulmonary connection, and extracardiac tunnel.

In internal Fontan, a lateral tunnel is constructed with a baffle inside the right atrium to direct the blood from the systemic venous circulation to the pulmonary artery.

In the second group, an atrio-pulmonary connection is created between the right atrium and the pulmonary artery, directly or by interposing the native removed pulmonary valve or by a valvular duct (the classic Fontan).

In the third category, an extracardiac duct directs the blood from the inferior vena cava to the pulmonary artery, while the superior vena cava is anastomosed to the pulmonary artery as in bidirectional Glenn anastomosis.

Transplant surgery involves removing all of these connections/anastomosis, so hearts sent for pathologic examination are no longer intact. All the parts removed at surgery must, however, be included for examination and

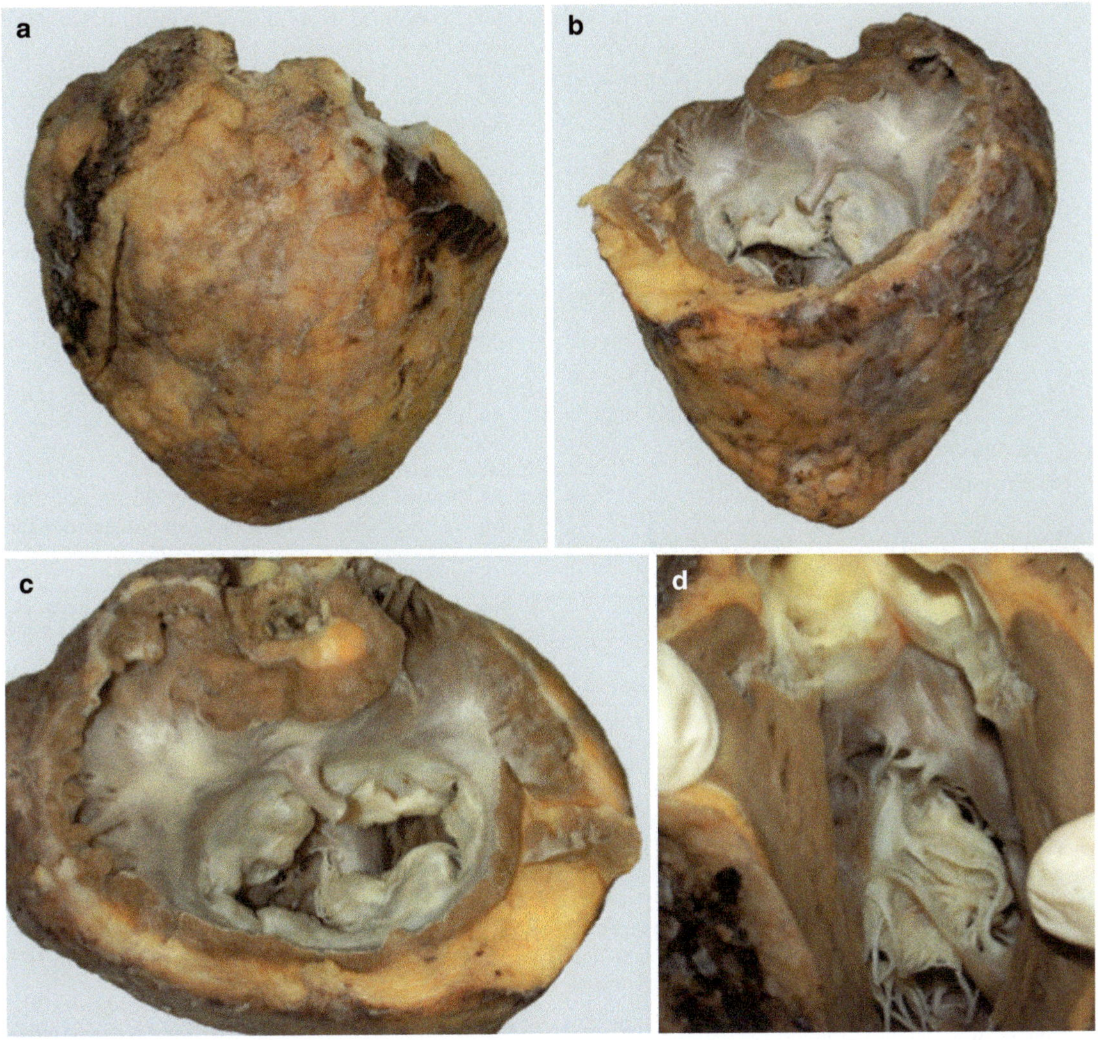

Fig. 5.47 Native heart of a 15-year-old female with complete atrio-ventricular septal defect (complete atrio-ventricular canal defect) transplanted due to arrhythmia. The heart showed concordant biventricular atrio-ventricular connection, with a common valve, concordant ventriculo-arterial connection, usual atrial arrangement, and levocardia. RV is decreased in size and shows wall hypertrophy; LV is dilated with thinned walls. (**a**) Anterior view of the heart. (**b**) Posterior view of the heart. (**c**) Superior view showing the common orifice with common atrio-ventricular valve with its four thickened leaflets (anterior, posterior, and two lateral). (**d**) RV with a large ventricular septal defect and redundant valve leaflet tissue. *LV* left ventricle; *RV* right ventricle

evaluated for stenosis, calcifications, and baffle or duct distortions. Cardiac complications of failing Fontan are systemic venous pathway obstruction, pulmonary venous obstruction, left ventricular outflow tract obstruction, valvular abnormalities, and systolic ventricular dysfunction, the last being a major indication for transplantation.

Key Points

- Transplanted CHD hearts are heterogeneous.
- Hearts can be operated or non-operated (nowadays, c.a. 10–15 % of CHD hearts are non-operated).

- Fontan-like procedures for single ventricle are the most common previous surgical techniques.
- The sequential segmental approach is the best system for classification of CHDs.
- No standardized dissection technique for explanted CHD has been established.
- Dimension and remodeling of the ventricle cavities should be noted.
- Acquired coronary lesions may coexist in adult hearts.
- Possible anastomosis or graft materials or conduits must be carefully evaluated.

References

Anderson RH, Shirali G. Sequential segmental analysis. Ann Pediatr Cardiol. 2009;2(1):24–35.

Anderson RH, Wilcox BR. How should we optimally describe complex congenitally malformed hearts? Ann Thorac Surg. 1996;62:710–6.

Anderson RH, Becker AE, Robertson WB, editors. The cardiovascular system. Part A: general considerations and congenital malformations, chap. 4. Churchill Livingstone; London (1993). p. 53–70.

Attenhofer Jost CH, Schmidt D, Huebler M, Balmer C, Noll G, Caduff R, Greutmann M. Heart transplantation in congenital heart disease: in whom to considerand when? J Transplant. 2013;2013:376027.

Biagini E, Coccolo F, Ferlito M, Perugini E, Rocchi G, Bacchi-Reggiani L, Lofiego C, Boriani G, Prandstraller D, Picchio FM, Branzi A, Rapezzi C. Dilated-hypokinetic evolution of hypertrophic cardiomyopathy. J Am Coll Cardiol. 2005;46:1543–50.

Biagini E, Ragni L, Ferlito M, Pasquale F, Lofiego C, Leone O, Rocchi G, Perugini E, Zagnoni S, Branzi A, Picchio FM, Rapezzi C. Different types of cardiomyopathy associated with isolated ventricular noncompaction. Am J Cardiol. 2006;98:821–4.

Biagini E, Spirito P, Leone O, Picchio FM, Coccolo F, Ragni L, Lofiego C, Grigioni F, Potena L, Rocchi G, Bacchi-Reggiani L, Boriani G, Prandstraller D, Arbustini E, Branzi A, Rapezzia C. Heart transplantation in hypertrophic cardiomyopathy. Am J Cardiol. 2008;101:382–92.

Bocchi EA, Fiorelli A. The Brazilian experience with heart transplantation: a multicenter report. J Heart Lung Transplant. 2001;20(6):637–45.

Boucek D, Yetman AT, Yeung E, Miyamoto SD, Stehlik J, Kfoury AG, Kaza AK, Weng C, Everitt MD. Survival based on patient selection for heart transplant in adults with congenital heart disease: a multi-institutional study. Int J Cardiol. 2014;172:e89–90.

Bradshaw SH, Kennedy L, David F, Dexter DF, Veinot JP. A practical method to rapidly dissolve metallic stents. Cardiovasc Pathol. 2009;18:127–33.

Burke AP, Virmani R. Pathophysiology of acute myocardial infarction. Med Clin North Am. 2007;91:553–72.

Burke A, Tavora F, editors. Chronic ischemic heart disease, chap. 6. In: Practical cardiovascular pathology. Philadelphia: Lippincott Williams & Wilkins; 2001. p. 73.

Butany J, Collins MJ. Analysis of prosthetic cardiac devices: a guide for the practicing pathologist. J Clin Pathol. 2005;58:113–24.

Butany J, et al. Mechanical heart valve prostheses: identification and evaluation (erratum). Cardiovasc Pathol. 2003;12(6):322–44.

Chen JM, Davies RR, Mital SR, Mercando ML, Addonizio LJ, Pinney SP, Hsu DT, Lamour JM, Quaegebeur JM, Mosca RS. Trends and outcomes in transplantation for complex congenital heart disease: 1984 to 2004. Ann Thorac Surg. 2004;78:1352–61.

Cooper Jr LT, Berry GJ, Shabetai R. Idiopathic giant-cell myocarditis - natural history and treatment. N Engl J Med. 1997;336:1860–6.

Coskun O, Coskun T, El-Arousy M, Parsa MA, Reiss N, Blanz U, Von Knyphausen E, Sandica E, Schulz U, Knobl H, Tenderich G, Bairaktaris A, Kececioglu D, Korfer R. Heart transplantation in adults with congenital heart disease. ASAIO J. 2007;53:103–6.

Costanzo MR, Augustine S, Bourge R, Bristow M, O'Connell JB, Driscoll D, Rose E. Selection and treatment of candidates for heart transplantation. A statement for health professionals from the Committee on Heart Failure and Cardiac Transplantation of the Council on Clinical Cardiology, American Heart Association. Circulation. 1995;92(12):3593–612.

Davies RR, Sorabella RA, Yang J, Ralph S, Mosca RS, Chen JM, Jan M, Quaegebeur JM. Outcomes after transplantation for "failed" Fontan: a single-institution experience. J Thorac Cardiovasc Surg. 2012;143: 1183–92.

De Pasquale EC, Nasir K, Jacoby DL. Outcomes of adults with restrictive cardiomyopathy after heart transplantation. J Heart Lung Transplant. 2012;31:1269–75.

DePasquale EC, Schweiger M, Ross HJ. A contemporary review of adult heart transplantation: 2012 to 2013. J Heart Lung Transplant. 2014;33:775–84.

Dipchand AI, Kirk R, Edwards LB, et al. The Registry of the International Society for Heart and Lung Transplantation: Sixteenth Official Pediatric Heart Transplantation Report-2013; focus theme: age. J Heart Lung Transplant. 2013;32:979–88.

Dipchand AI, Edwards LB, Kucheryavaya AY, Benden C, Dobbels F, Levvey BJ, Lund LH, Meiser B, Yusen RG, Stehlik J, for the International Society of Heart and Lung Transplantation. The Registry of the International Society for Heart and Lung Transplantation: Seventeenth Official Pediatric Heart Transplantation Report-2014; Focus Theme: Retransplantation.

J Heart Lung Transplant. 2014;33(10):985–95 (online eSlides).
Elliott P, Andersson B, Arbustini E, Bilinska Z, Cecchi F, Charron P, Dubourg O, Kuhl U, Maisch B, McKenna WJ, Monserrat L, Pankuweit S, Rapezzi C, Seferovic P, Tavazzi L, Keren A. Classification of the cardiomyopathies: a position statement from the European Society of Cardiology Working Group on myocardial and pericardial diseases. Eur Heart J. 2008;29(829): 270–6.
Falk RH, Dubrey SW. Amyloid heart disease. Prog Cardiovasc Dis. 2010;52:347–61.
Galati G, Leone O, Pasquale F, Olivotto I, Biagini E, Grigioni F, Pilato E, Lorenzini M, Corti B, Foà A, Agostini V, Cecchi F, Rapezzi C. Histologic and histometric characterization of myocardial fibrosis in end-stage hypertrophic cardiomyopathy: a clinical-pathological study of 31 explanted hearts. Circ Heart Fail. 2016;9:e003090.
Gambino A, Cerutti A, Feltrin G, Toscano G, Tarantini G, Milanesi O, Angelini A, Gerosa G. Outcome after pediatric heart transplantation: two decades of a single center experience. Eur J Cardiothorac Surg. 2007;32: 220–4.
Garatti A, Castelvecchio S, Bandera F, Medda M, Menicanti L. Mitraclip procedure as a bridge therapy in a patient with heart failure listed for hearth transplantation. Ann Thorac Surg. 2015;99(5):1796–9.
Garcıa-Pavıa P, Tomé-Esteban MT, Rapezzi C. Amyloidosis. Also a heart disease. Rev Esp Cardiol. 2011;64:797–808.
Gho JM, van Es R, Stathonikos N, Harakalova M, te Rijdt WP, Suurmeijer AJ, van der Heijden JF, de Jonge N, Chamuleau SA, de Weger RA, Asselbergs FW, Vink A. High resolution systematic digital histological quantification of cardiac fibrosis and adipose tissue in phospholamban p.Arg14del mutation associated cardiomyopathy. PLoS One. 2014;9(4), e94820.
Grande-Allen KJ, Barber JE, Klatka KM, Houghtaling PL, Vesely I, Moravec CS, McCarthy PM. Mitral valve stiffening in end-stage heart failure: evidence of an organic contribution to functional mitral regurgitation. J Thorac Cardiovasc Surg. 2005;130:783–90.
Grau JB, Pirelli L, Yu P-J, Galloway AC, Ostrer H. The genetics of mitral valve prolapse. Clin Genet. 2007;72:288–95.
Gravanis MB, Hertzler GL, Franch RH, Stacy LD, Ansari AA, Kanter KR, Tazelaar HD, Rodeheffer R, McGregor C. Hypersensitivity myocarditis in heart transplant candidates. J Heart Lung Transplant. 1991;10(5 Pt 1):688–97.
Graziosi M, Leone O, Berardini A, Lorenzini M, Rotundo MG, Biagini E, Potena L, Grigioni F, Boriani G, Rapezzi C. Arrhythmogenic right ventricular cardiomyopathy as cause of severe heart failure leading to heart transplantation. Eur Heart J. 2013. P1188 | BEDSIDE. doi:http://dx.doi.org/10.1093/eurheartj/eht308.P1188.
Griffiths ER, Kaza AK, Wyler von Ballmoos MC, Loyola H, Valente AM, Blume ED, del Nido P. Evaluating failing Fontans for heart transplantation: predictors of death. Ann Thorac Surg. 2009;88:558–64.
Harmon WG, Sleeper LA, Cuniberti L, et al. Treating children with dilated cardiomyopathy (from the North American Pediatric Cardiomyopathy Registry). Am J Cardiol. 2009;104:281–6.
Harris KM, Spirito P, Maron MS, Zenovich AG, Formisano F, Lesser JR, Mackey-Bojack S, Manning WJ, Udelson JE, Maron BJ. Prevalence, clinical profile, and significance of left ventricular remodelling in the end-stage phase of hypertrophic cardiomyopathy. Circulation. 2006;114:216–25.
Iung B, Baron G, Butchart EG, Delahaye F, Gohlke-Barwolf C, Levang OW, Tornos P, Vanoverschelde JL, Vermeer F, Boersma E, Ravaud P, Vahanian A. A prospective survey of patients with valvular heart disease in Europe: The Euro Heart Survey on Valvular Heart Disease. Eur Heart J. 2003;24:1231–43.
Jayakumar KA, Addonizio LJ, Kichuk-Chrisant MR, Galantowicz ME, Lamour JM, Quaegebeur JM, Hsu DT. Cardiac transplantation after the Fontan or Glenn procedure. J Am Coll Cardiol. 2004;44:2065–72.
Jenni R, Oechslin EN, van der Loo B. Isolated ventricular non-compaction of the myocardium in adults. Heart. 2007;93:11–5.
Kanai-Yoshizawa S, Sugiyama Kato T, Mancini D, Marboe CC. Hypersensitivity myocarditis and outcome after heart transplantation. J Heart Lung Transplant. 2013;32(5):553–9.
Kanter KR, Mahle WT, Vincent RN, Berg AM, Kogon BE, Kirshbom PM. Heart transplantation in children with a fontan procedure. Ann Thorac Surg. 2011;91: 823–30.
Khan NA, et al. Morphological changes in porcine bioprosthetic valves of a HearthMate left ventricular assist device. Can J Cardiol. 2010;26(7):e270–2.
Komanapalli CB, Sera V, Slater MS, Burdette M, Tripathy U, Brady G, Hegnell L, Ravichandran PS, Hershberger RE, Song HK. Becker's muscular dystrophy and orthotopic heart transplantation: perioperative considerations. Heart Surg Forum. 2006;9(2):E604–6.
Ladich E, Michaels MB, Jones RM, McDermott E, Coleman L, Komtebedde J, Glower D, Argenziano M, Feldman T, Nakano M, Virmani R. On behalf of the Endovascular Valve Edge-to-Edge Repair Study (EVEREST) Investigators. Pathological healing response of explanted MitraClip devices. Circulation. 2011;123:1418–27.
Lamour JM, Kanter KR, Naftel DC, Chrisant MR, Morrow WR, Clemson BS, Kirklin JK, on behalf of the CTRD (Cardiac Transplant Registry Database) and the PHTS (Pediatric Heart Transplant Study). The effect of age, diagnosis, and previous surgery in children and adults undergoing heart transplantation for congenital heart disease. J Am Coll Cardiol. 2009;54: 160–5.
Larsen BT, Mereuta OM, Dasari S, Fayyaz AU, Theis JD, Vrana JA, Grogan M, Dogan A, Dispenzieri A, Edwards WD, Kurtin PJ, Maleszewski JJ. Correlation of histomorphological pattern of cardiac amyloid

deposition with amyloid type: a histological and proteomic analysis of 108 cases. Histopathology. 2016;68:648–56.

Leone O, Longhi S, Quarta CC, Ragazzini T, De Giorgi LB, Pasquale F, Potena L, Lovato L, Milandri A, Arpesella G, Rapezzi C. New pathological insights into cardiac amyloidosis: implications for non-invasive diagnosis. Amyloid. 2012;19:99–105.

Lipshultz SE, Sleeper LA, Towbin JA, Lowe AM, Oray EJ, Cox FG, Lurie PR, McCoy KL, McDonald MA, Messere JE, Colan SD. The incidence of pediatric cardiomyopathy in two regions of the United States. N Engl J Med. 2003;348:1647–55.

Lipshultz SE, Cochran TR, Briston DA, Brown SR, Sambatakos PJ, Miller TL, Carrillo AA, Corcia L, Sanchez JE, Diamond MB, Freundlich M, Harake D, Gayle T, Harmon WG, Rusconi PG, Sandhu SK, Wilkinson JD. Pediatric cardiomyopathies: causes, epidemiology, clinical course, preventive strategies and therapies. Future Cardiol. 2013;9:817–48.

Luk A, Metawee M, Ahn E, Gustafsson F, Ross H, Butany J. Do clinical diagnoses correlate with pathological diagnoses in cardiac transplant patients? The importance of endomyocardial biopsy. Can J Cardiol. 2009;25(2):e48–54.

Lund LH, Edwards LB, Kucheryavaya AY, Dipchand AI, Benden C, Christie JD, Dobbels F, Kirk R, Rahmel AO, Yusen RD. Stehlik J; International Society for Heart and Lung Transplantation. The Registry of the International Society for Heart and Lung Transplantation: Thirtieth Official Adult Heart Transplant Report--2013; focus theme: age. J Heart Lung Transplant. 2013;32(10):951–64.

Lund LH, Edwards LB, Kucheryavaya AY, Dipchand AI, Benden C, Christie JD, Dipchand AI, Dobbels F, Goldfarb SB, Levvey BJ, Meiser B, Yusen RD, Stehlik J, for the International Society for Heart and Lung Transplantation. The Registry of the International Society for Heart and Lung Transplantation: Thirty-first Official Adult Heart Transplant Report-2014; focus theme: retransplantation. J Heart Lung Transplant. 2014;33(10):996–1008 (online eSlides).

Maleszewski JJ, Orellana VM, Hodge DO, Kuhl U, Schultheiss HP, Cooper LT. Long-term risk of recurrence, morbidity and mortality in giant cell myocarditis. Am J Cardiol. 2015;115(12):1733–8.

Maron BJ, Towbin JA, Thiene G, Antzelevitch C, Corrado D, Arnett D, Moss AJ, Seidman CE, Young JB. Contemporary Definitions and Classification of the Cardiomyopathies. An American Heart Association Scientific Statement From the Council on Clinical Cardiology, Heart Failure and Transplantation Committee; Quality of Care and Outcomes Research and Functional Genomics and Translational Biology Interdisciplinary Working Groups; and Council on Epidemiology and Prevention. Circulation. 2006;113:1807–16.

Maron MS, Olivotto I, Maron BJ, Prasad SK, Cecchi F, Udelson JE, Camici PG. The case for myocardial ischemia in hypertrophic cardiomyopathy. J Am Coll Cardiol. 2009;54:866–75.

Michielon G, Carotti A, Pongiglione G, Cogo P, Parisi F. Orthotopic heart transplantation in patients with univentricular physiology. Curr Cardiol Rev. 2011;7:85–91.

Moloney ED, Egan JJ, Kelly P, Wood AE, Cooper Jr LT. Transplantation for myocarditis: a controversy revisited. J Heart Lung Transplant. 2005;24:1103–10.

Nakano M, Virmani R. Histopathology of vascular response to drug-eluting stents: an insight from human autopsy into daily practice. Cardiovasc Interv Ther. 2015;30(11):1–11.

Pellegrini C, Nicolardi S, Di Perna D, Totaro P, Tinelli C, Pagani F, Viganò M. Heart transplantation for end-stage valvular cardiomyopathy: a 26-year single-center experience. J Heart Lung Transplant. 2012;31(4S):S58.

Rapezzi C, Merlini G, Quarta CC, et al. Systemic cardiac amyloidoses. disease profiles and clinical courses of the 3 main types. Circulation. 2009;120:203–1212.

Rapezzi C, Quarta CC, Riva L, et al. Transthyretin-related amyloidoses and the heart: a clinical overview. Nat Rev Cardiol. 2010;7:398–408.

Rapezzi C, Arbustini E, Caforio ALP, Charron P, Gimeno-Blanes J, Helio T, Linhart A, Mogensen J, Pinto Y, Ristic A, Seggewiss H, Sinagra G, Tavazzi L, Elliott PM. Diagnostic work-up in cardiomyopathies: bridging the gap between clinical phenotypes and final diagnosis. A position statement from the ESC Working Group on Myocardial and Pericardial Diseases. Eur Heart J. 2013;34:1448–58.

Rasmusson K, Brunisholz K, Budge D, Horne BD, Alharethi R, Folsom J, Connolly JJ, Stehlik J, Kfoury A. Peripartum cardiomyopathy: post-transplant outcomes from the united network for organ sharing database. J Heart Lung Transplant. 2012;31(2): 180–6.

Rippstein P, Black MK, Boivin M, Veinot JP, Ma X, Chen YX, et al. Comparison of processing and sectioning methodologies for arteries containing metallic stents. J Histochem Cytochem. 2006;54(6):673–81.

Roberts WC, Roberts CC, Ko JM, Filardo G, Capehart JE, Hall SA. Morphologic features of the recipient heart in patients having cardiac transplantation and analysis of the congruence or incongruence between the clinical and morphologic diagnoses. Medicine. 2014a;93: 211–35.

Roberts WC, Chung MS, Ko JM, Chapehart JE, Hall SA. Morphologic features of cardiac sarcoidosis in native hearts of patients having cardiac transplantation. Am J Cardiol. 2014b;113(4):706–12.

Schumacher KR, Almond C, Singh TP, Spicer R, Hoffman TM, Hsu D, Naftel DC, Pruitt E, Zamberlan M, Canter CE, Gajarski RJ, on behalf of the PHTS Study Group Investigators. Predicting graft loss by 1 year in pediatric heart transplantation candidates: an analysis of the pediatric heart transplant study database. Circulation. 2015;131:890–8.

Schweiger M, Stiasny B, Dave H, Cavigelli-Brunner A, Balmer C, Kretschmar O, Bürki C, Klauwer D, Hübler M. Pediatric heart transplantation. J Thorac Dis. 2015;7(3):552–9.

Seddioa F, Gorislavetsb N, Iacovonib A, Cugolac D, Fontanab A, Gallettia L, Terzib A, Ferrazzi P. Is heart transplantation for complex congenital heart disease a good option? A 25-year single centre experience. Eur J Cardiothorac Surg. 2013;43:605–11.

Sen-Chowdhry SS, Syrris P, Ward D, Asimaki A, Sevdalis E, McKenna WJ. Clinical and genetic characterization of families with arrythmogenic right ventricular dysplasia/cardiomyopathy provides novel insights into patterns of disease expression. Circulation. 2007;115: 1710–20.

Shinebourne EA, Macartney FJ, Anderson RH. Sequential chamber localization-logical approach to diagnosis in congenital heart disease. Br Heart J. 1976;38:327–40.

Siddiqui RF, et al. Bioprosthetic heart valves: modes of failure. Histopathology. 2009;55(2):135–44.

Soler-Soler J, Galve E. Worldwide perspective of valve disease. Heart. 2000;83:721–5.

Stone RJ, Basso C, Baandrup UT, Bruneval P, Butany J, Gallagher PJ, Halushka MK, Miller DV, Padera RF, Radio SJ, Sheppard MN, Suvarna K, Tan CD, Thiene G, van der Wal AC, Veinot JP. Recommendations for processing cardiovascular surgical pathology specimens: a consensus statement from the Standards and Definitions Committee of the Society for Cardiovascular Pathology and the Association for European Cardiovascular Pathology. Cardiovasc Pathol. 2012;21(1):2–16.

Strauss DG, Selvester RH, DiBernardo LR. Myocardial scar in sarcoidosis by 12-lead ECG and pathology. Ann Noninvasive Electrocardiol. 2011;16(2):219–22.

Szalaya ZA, Civeleka A, Hohea S, Brunner-LaRoccab HP, Klovekorna WP, Knezc I, Vogtc PR, Bauera EP. Mitral annuloplasty in patients with ischemic versus dilated cardiomyopathy. Eur J Cardiothorac Surg. 2003;23:567–72.

Tavora FR, Jeudy J, Burke AP. Multiple aneurysms of aorto-coronary saphenous vein grafts with fatal rupture. Arq Bras Cardiol. 2007;88:e107–10.

Virmani R, Kolodgie FD, Burke AP, Farb A, Schwartz SM. Lessons from sudden coronary death: a comprehensive morphological classification scheme for atherosclerotic lesions. Arterioscler Thromb Vasc Biol. 2000;20(5):1262–75.

Voeller RK, Epstein DJ, Guthrie TJ, Gandhi SK, Canter CE, Huddleston CB. Trends in the indications and survival in pediatric heart transplants: a 24-year single-center experience in 307 patients. Ann Thorac Surg. 2012;94:807–16.

Vrana JA, Gamez JD, Madden BJ, Theis JD, Bergen III HR, Dogan A. Classification of amyloidosis by laser microdissection and mass spectrometry–based proteomic analysis in clinical biopsy specimens. Blood. 2009;114:4957–9.

Waller TA, Hiser WL, Capehart JE, Roberts WC. Comparison of clinical and morphologic cardiac findings in patients having cardiac Transplantation for ischemic cardiomyopathy, idiopatic dilated cardiomyopathy, and dilated hypertrophic cardiomyopathy. Am J Cardiol. 1998;81:884–94.

Yacoub MH, Cohn LH. Novel approaches to cardiac valve repair from structure to function: part I. Circulation. 2004a;109:942–50.

Yacoub MH, Cohn LH. Novel approaches to cardiac valve repair from structure to function: part II. Circulation. 2004b;109:1064–72.

Zhang M, Tavora F, Huebner T, Heath J, Burke A. Allograft pathology in patients transplanted for idiopathic dilated cardiomyopathy. Am J Surg Pathol. 2012;36:389–95.

Pretransplant Endomyocardial Biopsy: When and Why

6

John P. Veinot

Contents

J.P. Veinot, MD, FRCPC
Department of Pathology and Laboratory Medicine, The Ottawa Hospital, Ottawa, ON, Canada
e-mail: jpveinot@toh.ca

6.1 Background

The utility of endomyocardial biopsy (EMB) has been challenged with issues of nonspecific pathological diagnoses and significant complication rates mentioned. In skilled operator hands, the complication rate is low (Veinot 2002a).

A recent scientific statement from the American Heart Association, American College of Cardiology, and the European Society of Cardiology (Cooper et al. 2007) revitalized the role of EMB on the basis of evidence-based medicine criteria. The document was written from a clinical viewpoint. Fourteen clinical scenarios when EMB should be performed included unexplained heart failure, with or without heart block or arrhythmias, eosinophilia, chemotherapy, restrictive myocardial physiology, cardiac tumors, unexplained heart failure in children, unexplained ventricular hypertrophy, arrhythmogenic right ventricular cardiomyopathy, and ventricular arrhythmias.

The Association for European Cardiovascular Pathology (AECVP) and the Society for Cardiovascular Pathology (SCVP) have prepared a consensus statement regarding when and how EMB assists in the clinical workup of patients with heart failure, arrhythmias, and cardiac masses (Leone et al. 2012). It was deemed necessary to inform clinicians of the potential of pathological analysis of the cardiac biopsy and to urge clinicians and pathologists to collaborate and

O. Leone et al. (eds.), *The Pathology of Cardiac Transplantation*,
DOI 10.1007/978-3-319-46386-5_6

share protocols for EMB indications. A preliminary version had been previously published (Leone et al. 2009).

EMB may biopsy the right or left side of the heart. This directly allows assessment of the heart tissues, including endocardium, myocardium, and interstitium. Access to the heart is most often via the venous route through the internal jugular or femoral vein. The left ventricle may be biopsied with trans-septal puncture or by direct access through a peripheral artery (Veinot 2002a). Left-sided biopsies are thought to be more risky in terms of complications, and they are seldom warranted unless there is a specific left ventricular mass, lesion, or region of interest. One of the recognized diagnostic limitations with endomyocardial biopsies is sampling error, although this issue is related to the type and extent of the disease, and it may be overestimated. For focal myocardial lesions or disorders, additional biopsy specimens might be recommended, or more targeted sampling using imaging or electrophysiology guidance could be utilized. A negative biopsy specimen may not rule out a disease. A positive biopsy specimen, no matter how few pieces were obtained, may be diagnostic. The pathological interpretation of the biopsy specimens should be approached similar to other medical biopsy specimens. These specimens are well fixed, and all the endomyocardial components can be commented upon including the endocardium, myocardium, small blood vessels, and interstitium.

6.2 Triage: Sampling and Handling

Management of a myocardial sample is no longer limited to histology, but may include immunohistochemistry for the identification of inflammatory cell type populations, polymerase chain reaction (PCR) and reverse transcriptase (RT)-PCR, either qualitative or quantitative, for the detection of DNA and RNA viruses, search for cytokine expression and apoptosis, ultrastructural investigation for extracellular or intracellular storage disease, immune markers for malignancy cell type, and other parameters. The cardiac biopsy complements new developments in cardiac imaging, electrophysiological, and molecular investigations that may increase biopsy utility.

Pathological analysis of EMB is complex and requires standard protocols (Leone et al. 2009). It is vital that the pathologist be provided with sufficient clinical information as an aid for diagnosis and to guide the most appropriate triage and technical choices. Recommendations for triage and analysis are outlined in Tables 6.1 and 6.2.

6.3 Pretransplant Versus General Indications for EMB

Pretransplant EMB is somewhat different from EMB use in nontransplant candidates, as the indications for transplantation are exclusively based on clinical criteria.

The issues supporting pretransplant biopsy are:

- *Clinical misdiagnosis* (Luk et al. 2009): In many cases, clinical misdiagnosis would be of little significance for transplant candidates, especially today when the spectrum of diseases suitable for transplantation has notably

Table 6.1 Specimen procurement and triage

At least three, preferably four, endomyocardial fragments, each 1–2 mm^3 in size, should immediately be fixed in 10 % buffered formalin at room temperature for light microscopic examination. When myocardial lesions, which may be characterized by focal distribution, are suspected, additional sampling is recommended
If indicated, one or two specimens may be snap-frozen in liquid nitrogen and stored at −80 °C for possible molecular tests or specific stains. Otherwise, fragments may be stored in RNA-later at room temperature
If indicated, one fragment fixed in 2.5 % glutaraldehyde or Karnowsky solution for ultrastructural tests
A sample of peripheral blood (5–10 ml) in EDTA or citrate from patients with suspected myocarditis allows for molecular testing for the same viral genomes sought in the myocardial tissue and from patients with genetic cardiomyopathies allows for genetic tests

Table 6.2 Pathological analysis

Light microscopic examination is routinely performed on formalin-fixed and paraffin-embedded tissue and includes, when appropriate:
Multiple and numbered hematoxylin–eosin section examination
Additional histochemical, histomorphological, and immunohistochemical stains performed on paraffin-embedded fragments or on frozen sections
Semiquantitative evaluation or morphometric analysis on sections cut for histochemical, histoenzymatic, and immunohistochemical tests
Additional stains include Masson/Mallory trichrome, Movat pentachrome, Weigert-Van Gieson stain, Congo Red, sulfated Alcian Blue, and iron stain. PAS stain, with and without diastase, is often useful to assess intramyocardial glycogen and also to assess blood vessels in the interstitium.
Molecular tests, such as polymerase chain reaction (PCR), quantitative or qualitative, and reverse transcriptase-PCR on the fragments frozen in liquid nitrogen or stored in RNA-later.
Transmission electron microscopy examination on fragments fixed in glutaraldehyde or Karnowsky solution and embedded in resin. Ultrastructural analysis is preceded by examination of semi-thin sections stained with Toluidine blue.

widened, but in some cases (e.g. sarcoidosis or myocarditis/inflammatory cardiomyopathy), a correct and detailed diagnosis can influence management—with drug therapy to delay transplantation, or mechanical circulatory support to delay or even avoid transplantation, or by giving information on post-transplant prognostic stratification. Furthermore, cardiac transplant therapy is extremely intense as patients may undergo considerable morbidity and complications due to both the procedure and immunosuppression.

- *Etiological rather than generic diagnosis* is valuable both as good medical practice and as a workup methodology, or even for familial counseling, especially in referral centers for heart disease/cardiomyopathies.
- The importance of a *systematic approach* in transplant centers in order to achieve comparable and standardized diagnostic and therapeutic pathways.
- The valuable opportunity to *correlate the bioptic diagnosis* with pathological findings of the explanted heart in order to improve diagnostic criteria with EMB.

The greatest diagnostic contribution of pretransplant EMB is when it is able to define specific forms of heart disease/cardiomyopathy. When findings are nonspecific, EMB may confirm a clinical dilated/hypertrophic/restrictive phenotype, whose etiology might fall into a genetic category or where the advanced stage of the disease does not allow the initial disease to be traced.

6.4 EMB Contribution in Specific Forms of Heart Disease

6.4.1 Myocarditis/Inflammatory Cardiomyopathies

The role of EMB in diagnosing myocarditis/inflammatory cardiomyopathies is probably the most controversial and subject of lively debate.

During the 1990s, the negative results in the Myocarditis Treatment trial reduced EMB use in myocarditis, but this is not surprising as there was no distinction between viral and nonviral myocarditis. The pathological diagnosis of myocarditis was based upon the 1987 Dallas criteria which require the presence of an inflammatory infiltrate associated to myocyte damage for the diagnosis of "active" myocarditis (Aretz 1987).

Today, the technical tools for diagnosing different forms of myocarditis are significantly improved, and the routine use of immunohistochemistry to assess the extent and composition of inflammatory infiltrates as well as the development of highly sensitive molecular biology techniques (PCR or in situ hybridization) allows a judicious use of cardiac biopsy which may become relevant for a detailed diagnosis and for deciding whether antiviral or immunosuppressive therapy is indicated (Liu et al. 1996). In order to assess immune etiology, cardiac autoantibodies in the blood might also be investigated.

Improvements in imaging techniques, especially cardiac magnetic resonance (CMR), can be usefully integrated with EMB to determine the extent of the disease and to define the best place to biopsy; this approach may reduce the main limitation of biopsy, which is sampling error due to micromultifocal distribution of the disease. However, CMR cannot replace EMB, the essential tool able to define the etiology of myocarditis. This concept is now included in the position statement from the European Society of Cardiology on the current state of knowledge on etiology, diagnosis, management, and therapy of myocarditis.

At histology, routine (hematoxylin and eosin) stained serial sections should be evaluated for the presence of the inflammatory infiltrate (immunotype and semiquantitative or qualitative analysis), myocyte damage type (myocytolysis, apoptosis, or other myocyte alteration), and fibrosis (type and semiquantitative or morphometric analysis).

The nature or type of the infiltrating cell allows the characterization of the cause of the myocarditis and may also be helpful in suggesting additional investigations. Lymphocytic, macrophagic, or plasmacytic infiltrates suggest a viral or autoimmune pathoetiology (Fig. 6.1). Eosinophilic myocarditis may be seen with Churg–Strauss, drug-related myocarditis, parasite infections, or with hypereosinophilic syndrome. Toxic myocarditis (catecholamines and pressor agents, pharmaceutical drugs, illegal drugs, pheochromocytoma) usually presents as scanty multifocal neutrophilic or mixed neutrophilic–macrophagic infiltrate associated with microfoci of myocells fragmented or with band necrosis or real necrosis. Giant cells suggest drug hypersensitivity, specific infections (fungal and protozoal), or primary giant cell myocarditis. Giant cell myocarditis can produce a severe acute clinical scenario with heart failure and ventricular arrhythmias and is important to diagnose, as it may be very responsive to immunosuppression and may reoccur in the graft after transplant (Fig. 6.2).

It has been suggested that a mean lymphocyte count of >5 lymphocytes per high power field (HPF) is necessary to diagnose myocarditis. Other authors have required >10 lymphocytes/HPF or a minimum of 14 infiltrating leukocytes/mm^2 (Maisch et al. 2000). As an adjunct to routine histopathological examination,

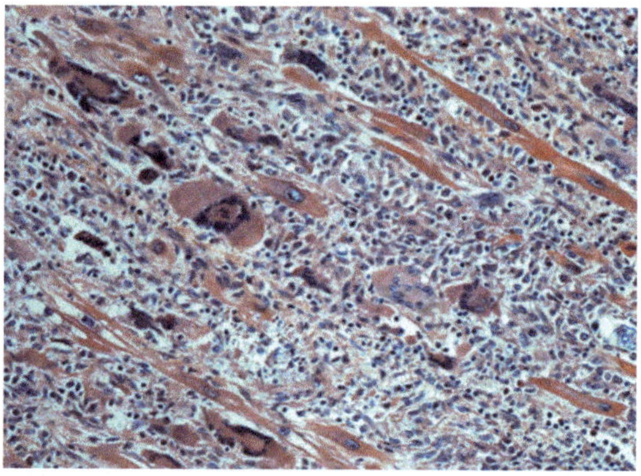

Fig. 6.2 Giant cell myocarditis—EMB specimen from a young male patient with heart failure and numerous refractory ventricular arrhythmias. Numerous giant cells are observed along with cardiomyocyte injury and fibrosis. No well-formed granulomas are seen (Hematoxylin phloxine saffron ×200)

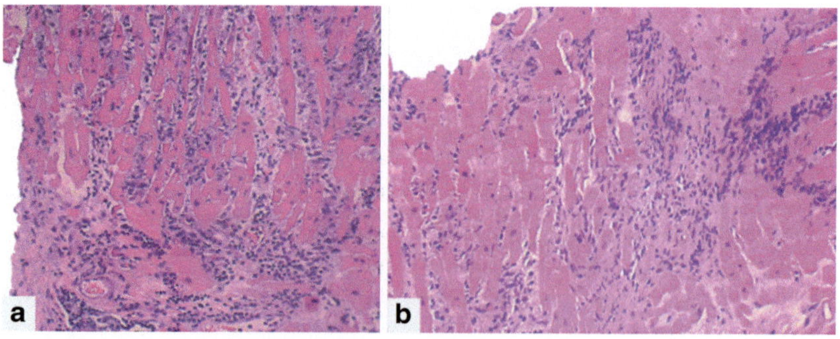

Fig. 6.1 (**a**, **b**) Lymphocytic myocarditis. EMB specimen from a young woman with recent onset heart failure. There is lymphocytic inflammation and injury to several cardiac myocytes (Hematoxylin–Eosin ×200)

immunohistochemical or immunofluorescence staining for lymphocytes (anti-CD45, CD45RO, CD3, CD20, CD4, CD8, CD79a), and macrophages (anti-CD68) may be performed. Major histocompatibility complex (MHC) antigens (MHC I and MHC II) are sometimes performed, according to local practice (Maisch et al. 2000).

Enteroviral RNA has been detected in myocardial biopsies of patients with dilated cardiomyopathy and myocarditis and has been associated with an adverse prognosis (Why et al. 1994). Detection of viral nucleic acid using PCR or RT-PCR has also been employed (Maisch et al. 2000). The controversy surrounding the routine use of molecular viral genome detection to diagnose myocarditis is mainly as to whether it is necessary to know the status of the virus and its load in the peripheral blood (in order to determine if viral detection in a myocardial sample represents blood contamination or actual myocardial pathology) and also the incidence of the virus in the general population. In situ hybridization has been proposed to circumvent this conundrum. Appropriate controls are also important. The use of viral genome detection should be performed in a molecular biology laboratory with expertise in these molecular techniques (microbiology or pathology laboratories). It should be borne in mind that molecular findings need to be interpreted along with knowledge of the myocardial histopathology and pathology expertise, rather than evaluated in isolation.

The pathological diagnosis of myocarditis should report: histological findings including the cell type, immunophenotypic characterization of the inflammatory infiltrate, and molecular viral data, if these are available.

6.4.2 Amyloid

Amyloidoses comprise a group of disorders characterized by the deposition of abnormally folded proteins. At least 11 types of amyloidosis may involve the heart (Collins et al. 2009). EMB is an important modality in the workup of patients with cardiac amyloidosis. In hematoxylin–eosin stained sections, the amyloid appears as a homogeneous, eosinophilic, amorphous substance (Fig. 6.3). When this is recognized, it is recommended that biopsies be stained with Congo Red to confirm the presence of amyloid, whose deposits appear with a characteristic green birefringence under polarized light. Modified sulfated Alcian Blue or Thioflavin T may also be used. After confirming the presence of amyloid in the heart, it must be typed. EMB has been proven useful in helping to establish the type of cardiac amyloid, using techniques such as immunohistochemistry, immunofluorescence (on frozen tissue) (Collins et al. 2009), or immune-electron microscopy (Arbustini et al. 1997). But due to the low specificity of these techniques or possible overlap of the different antibodies, referral centers are turning to molecular techniques, such as

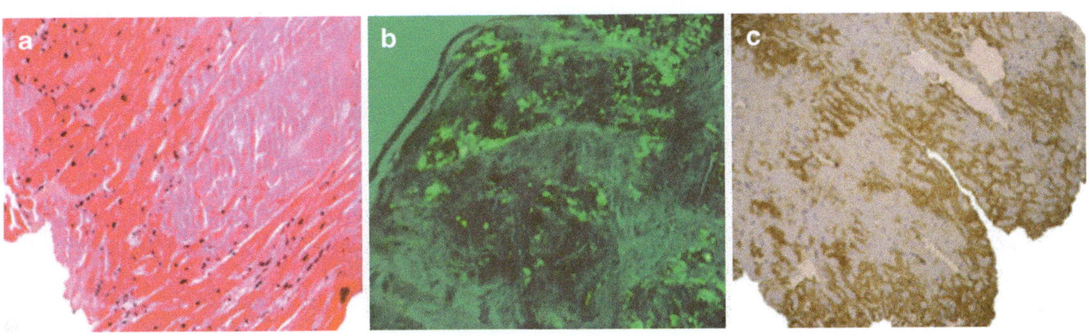

Fig. 6.3 Amyloid—EMB from a patient with diastolic heart failure. The biopsy specimen demonstrated interstitial nodular and perimyocyte homogeneous pink material (**a**, Hematoxylin–Eosin ×200). In the section stained with Congo Red (**b**), the subendocardial/interstitial nodular deposits show the typical green birefringence (Congo Red ×200). This was transthyretin protein positive by immunotyping (section **c**, ×200)

protein sequencing (Benson et al. 2009) and mass spectrometry (Vrana et al. 2009). Subclassification of amyloid deposits is not trivial, and mistyping of amyloid can have catastrophic effects, as the prognosis is very different and treatment options are specific for the type of amyloid present. Amyloid subtyping should be performed in a center with experience, using techniques that have been validated to be reliable in that center.

6.4.3 Storage Disease

EMB can play a significant role in diagnosing storage disease.

Histological findings for this group are not really specific but can be strongly suggestive and can point the direction for further investigations (other stainings, immunohistochemistry, electron microscopy), which in an appropriate clinical context, can together arrive at the definite diagnosis.

6.4.3.1 Myocardial Iron Storage

The heart normally contains no iron, and therefore, finding stainable iron in the cardiomyocyte indicates the presence of pathology (Lombardo et al. 1995). Iron tends to initially deposit subepicardially, and may not always be found in the right ventricle septal region; thus, the possibility of sampling error exists.

The histological appearance of iron storage on hematoxylin–eosin stained sections is that of intramyocytic granular brownish deposits, which are blue by Prussian Blue (Perls) staining. Moreover, biopsy may also be useful in patient monitoring to verify therapeutic results.

In some candidates, for liver transplant, EMB may sometimes be performed to evaluate an unexpected cardiac alteration with dilatation of ventricles or restrictive physiology prevailing on dilatation. In such a case, the most frequent need is to check for hemosiderosis.

6.4.3.2 Glycogen Storage Disease

Glycogenoses involving the heart are generally the result of defects in genes and enzymes involved in the glycogen metabolism; the most widely known diseases are type II (Pompe disease), type III (Cori disease), and type IV (Andersen disease) glycogen storage diseases. At the cardiac level, they have prevalently hypertrophic/restrictive features, with possible terminal evolution to a dilated hypokinetic form.

At histology, myocytes show severe vacuolization in central areas due to massive glycogen deposits, which displace myofibrils to the periphery. Glycogen may be detected with periodic acid Schiff (PAS) stain, which colors deposits in a purple/violet red (Fig. 6.4); this coloration disappears after diastase digestion (PAS-diastase). PAS staining may be carried out on paraffin sections, although a fresh sample (when available) would be more appropriate. Ultrastructural analysis is essential to confirm and typify glycogen deposits.

6.4.3.3 Anderson-Fabry Disease

It is a form of sphingolipidosis due to a deficiency of the lysosomal enzyme alpha-galactosidase A, which determines intracellular storage of trihexosylceramide. It may be difficult to differentiate this disease from other causes of ventricular hypertrophy, for example, HCM or hypertensive cardiomyopathy; in the literature, it is reported that Anderson-Fabry disease has been diagnosed using EMB in 3 % of patients with unexplained cardiac hypertrophy.

Histology is similar to glycogen storage and shows hypertrophied and vacuolated myocytes. Electron microscopy shows osmiophilic aggregates of concentric and parallel lamellae composed of variably dense alternate bands, typical of this disease, although not exclusive to it (Fig. 6.5).

6.4.3.4 Desmin-Related Cardiomyopathy

In this disease, there is excessive deposition of intermediate desmin filament in skeletal and cardiac muscle, causing progressive cardiac failure.

Histology is nonspecific and characterized by interstitial fibrosis, myocyte dysmetry, and intrasarcoplasmic small vacuoles. Electron microscopy is necessary for diagnosis, as it shows the presence of intramyocytic granule—filamentous deposits in the interfibrillar areas or at the Z band level.

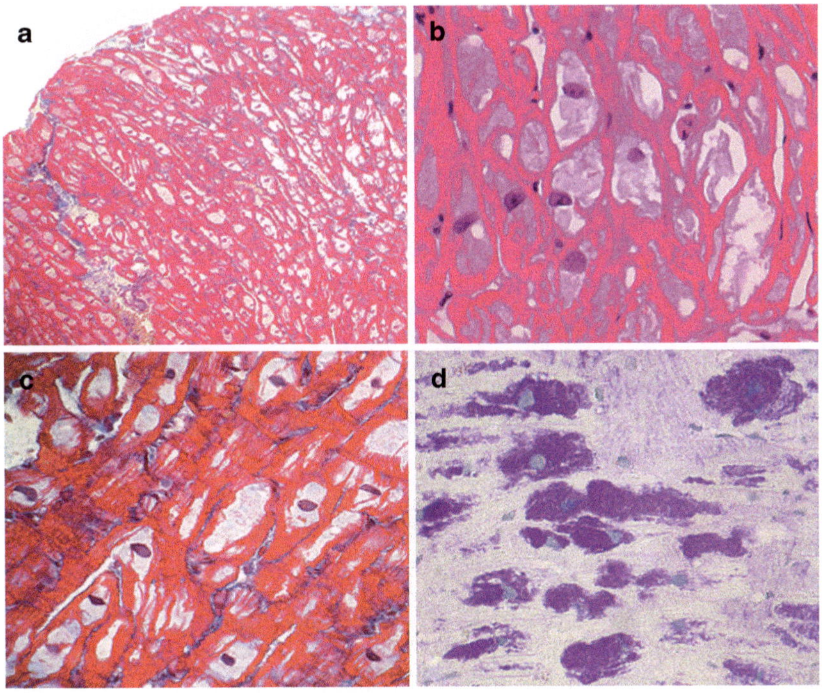

Fig. 6.4 Glycogen storage disease. EMB from a 47-year-old male with glycogen storage disease, who underwent heart transplant 3 years later. (**a**–**c**) Histology shows severe, diffuse vacuolization of myocytes containing deposits, which appear pale pink with Hematoxylin–Eosin stain (**b**, ×100) and grayish with Mallory trichrome (**c**, ×400). PAS staining demonstrates typical purple/violet red deposits corresponding to glycogen (**d**, ×400)

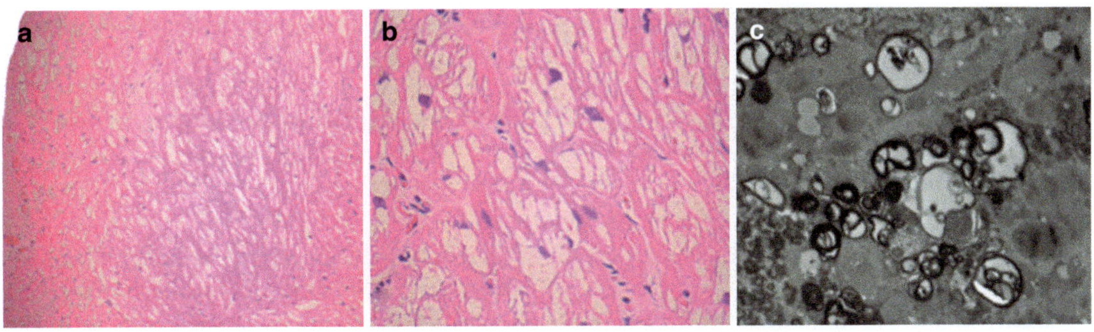

Fig. 6.5 Anderson-Fabry disease. EMB performed for clinical suspicious of infiltrative/storage disease in a 69-year-old male with hypertrophic heart. (**a**, **b**) Histology shows hypertrophied and vacuolated myocytes (Hematoxylin–Eosin: **a** ×100; **b** ×400), and electron microscopy shows the typical lamellar bodies within the cytoplasm of cardiac myocytes (**c**, Courtesy of Giovanna Cenacchi)

6.4.4 Arrhythmia Investigation: Sarcoidosis and Arrhythmogenic Cardiomyopathy

EMB may be useful in the workup of arrhythmia (d'Amati and Factor 1996). Biopsy specimen findings are often nonspecific, but abnormal, with changes suggestive of cardiomyopathy (Vignola et al. 1984). Strain and colleagues, in their study of patients with spontaneous ventricular fibrillation but no apparent structural heart disease, found 89 % of biopsies to be abnormal (50 % suggestive of cardiomyopathy, 17 %

myocarditis, 11 % abnormal intramyocardial arteries, 11 % arrhythmogenic cardiomyopathy (ARVC), and 11 % normal) (Strain et al. 1983).

Apart from myocarditis with arrhythmic presentation, as previously discussed, EMB may be of use in diagnosing sarcoidosis or arrhythmogenic cardiomyopathy.

Sarcoidosis is a systemic granulomatous disease and may involve the heart in association with other organs or, less commonly, in isolation, which is more difficult to recognize. This disease is the most frequently missed clinical diagnosis, and in some cases an unexpected diagnosis of sarcoidosis is made on biopsy of patients with ventricular tachycardia, suspected arrhythmogenic cardiomyopathy, or restrictive cardiomyopathy (Ladyjanskaia et al. 2010; Corrado and Thiene 2009).

Histological findings are pathognomonic or highly suggestive of the disease, showing the typical granulomatous inflammation with epithelioid compact granulomas.

Due to the focal nature of the infiltrates and the fact that sarcoid tends to involve the base of the heart, which is not the area usually biopsied (Veinot 2002a), EMB has been reported to have poor sensitivity in systemic sarcoidosis with presumed cardiac involvement, being positive in 19–25 % of cases (Ardehali et al. 2005). A positive biopsy guides management with corticosteroids and prophylactic use of a defibrillator. To increase the sensitivity of the procedure, electrophysiological (electro-anatomic mapping) or image-guided biopsy procedures have been utilized.

In arrhythmogenic cardiomyopathy, right ventricle EMB may serve as a diagnostic tool, especially in sporadic forms (not familial), or to exclude mimics (i.e. myocarditis, sarcoid, etc.). Histological examination shows fibrous or fibrofatty replacement and myocardial atrophy, which are not specific (e.g. also seen in muscular dystrophies). Fatty tissue alone is not considered diagnostic for ARVC, since fat is normally found in the endocardium and myocardium, particularly at the anterolateral apical right ventricular free wall. Currently, the principal findings are: myocyte alterations (hypertrophy and vacuolization) and comingling of fibrous and fatty tissue. Inflammatory infiltrates can also be present.

Histomorphometry evaluation of right ventricle EMB is supported for research to gather data concerning its utility for diagnosis. According to the updated diagnostic criteria, fibrous or fibrofatty replacement with <60 % residual myocardium in at least 1 EMB sample is a major criterion and 60–75 % residual myocardium is a minor criterion for ARVC (Basso et al. 2008; Marcus et al. 2010). EMB samples from the septum may not be particularly helpful. Biopsying the affected area, including the right ventricle free wall, may be considered.

Diagnostic accuracy increases if the EMB sampling site is guided by imaging (magnetic resonance imaging) or electrophysiological (electroanatomical mapping) techniques.

Immunohistochemistry for plakoglobin and other cellular junction proteins is promising since it may decrease the need for free wall biopsy as it works on morphologically preserved myocardium and thus on septal bioptic samples. Attention to specific antibody dilutions and technique is important. This test needs validation before entering routine practice and cannot at present replace morphological diagnosis.

6.4.5 Eosinophilic Endomyocardial Disease/Hypereosinophilic Syndrome

Hypereosinophilic syndrome, although rare, may frequently involve the heart with an eosinophilic endomyocarditis and thrombus formation. The best known diseases are tropical (Davies) endomyocardial fibrosis and Loeffler endocarditis although many synonyms have accumulated through the years.

Tropical (Davies) endomyocardial fibrosis is typical in the tropical areas, and usually occurs in children and young adults: it is commonly associated with nutritional deficiency, hypersensitivity to malaria, viral and parasitic infections, magnesium deficiency, and high cerium intake. Pathologically, there is fibrotic endocardial thickening at the apex and inflow of right or both ventricles, with atrioventricular valve apparatus entrapment; endocardial calcification and mural thrombosis, as well as variable degrees of subendocardial necrosis or degeneration of the underlying myocardium (Iglezias et al. 2008).

Loeffler endocarditis (also known as nontropical eosinophilic endomyocardial disease or fibroplastic parietal endocarditis) usually manifests in the fourth decade of life: at gross examination, there is diffuse deposition of mural thrombus over the ventricular endocardium incorporated into a whitish fibrous plaque. Three stages can be distinguished: an eosinophilic endomyocarditis/necrotic (rarely symptomatic) stage; a thrombotic stage (with risk of thromboembolism); and a fibrotic stage with cardiac and atrioventricular valvular dysfunction (Fauci et al. 1982).

EMB can allow a "definite" diagnosis only in the acute/active phase, with the demonstration of eosinophilic endomyocarditis, endocardial damage, and thrombotic deposition infiltrated by eosinophils (Fig. 6.6). A "probable/possible" diagnosis can be reached in the chronic phase of Loeffler endocarditis and in tropical endomyocardial fibrosis, with the evidence of endocardial fibrous thickening and subendocardial myocyte abnormalities.

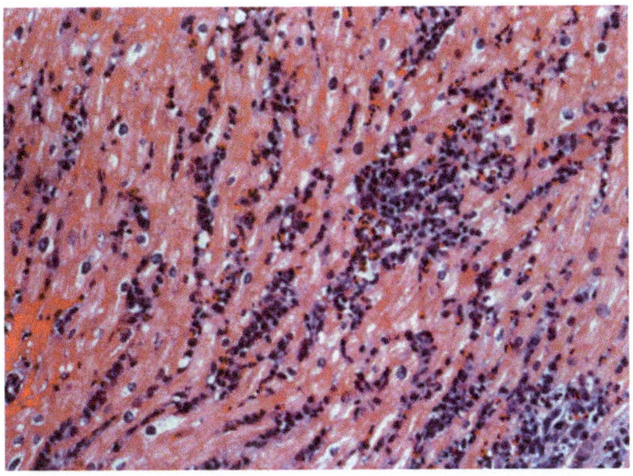

Fig. 6.6 Hypereosinophilic heart disease—EMB from a young woman with a high eosinophil blood count and restrictive heart hemodynamics. Ventricular thrombus was noted on imaging. The biopsy specimen showed eosinophilic myocarditis. Eosinophil-rich thrombus material was also obtained at the time of biopsy (Hematoxylin phloxine saffron ×200)

6.4.6 Neoplasms

In rare instances, a patient with a primary cardiac neoplasm may be considered for transplant, and EMB may be pivotal in the diagnostic workup, guide to therapy, or palliation if appropriate (Fig. 6.7). The main limit is bioptic accessibility of the tumor mass. EMB is relatively successful only for intracavitary tumors and routinely performed only for right-sided lesions easily accessible for transvenous biopsy; left-sided tumors may be biopsied with trans-septal puncture or retrograde via arterial access (Chan et al. 2001).

6.5 EMB When Histology Findings Are Nonspecific

The utility of biopsy for primary cardiomyopathies presenting as dilated, hypertrophic, or restrictive phenotypes is mixed.

In genetic cardiomyopathies or in end-stage forms of transplant candidates, where etiology has not been recognized, histological myocardial appearance on endomyocardial biopsy usually has a broadly similar aspect because of the nonspecificity of the myocardial response to injury which may impose diagnostic limitations.

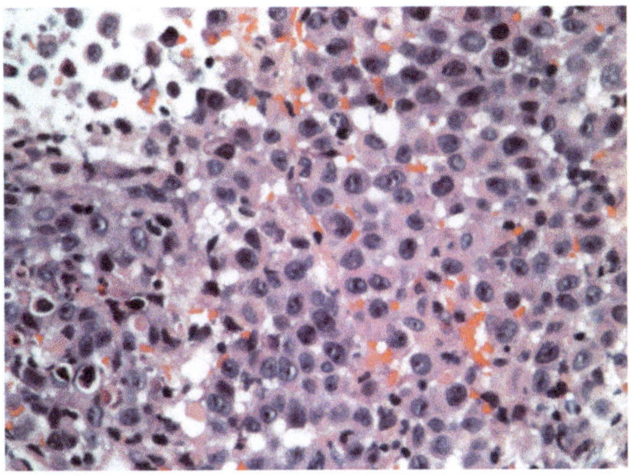

Fig. 6.7 Melanoma—EMB of a right atrial mass in a patient with suspected cardiac and lung metastases. He had a clinical history of melanoma. Biopsy was done to obtain diagnostic tissue prior to medical therapy (Hematoxylin–Eosin ×400)

The two most commonly encountered abnormalities, myocyte hypertrophy and interstitial fibrosis, are both nonspecific.

In spite of this, EMB diagnosis may be valuable in the workup of heart failure of unknown cause (active myocarditis vs. acute exacerbation of a chronic disease) to exclude specific diseases and even in the pretransplant setting.

In dilated cardiomyopathy (DCM), nonspecific histology includes fibrosis, myocyte nuclear enlargement, and often sarcoplasmic degenerative changes such as a perinuclear halo, and myocyte clearing or vacuolization (Fig. 6.8). Myofiber attenuation and stretching may be marked. Nuclei may be irregular in shape and hyperchromatic.

But EMB can reveal active myocarditis or a subacute phase where the disease is evolving into DCM, as the initial viral infection led to myocyte destruction, followed by a chronic immunological attack of the myocytes with autoantibodies and with the involvement of the cellular immune system (Kawai 1999).

Many immunostains for muscle fiber abnormality can be attempted in cardiomyopathies associated with skeletal myopathy to characterize the disease, although their use is not still standardized for routine use (see Chap. 5).

In cases of nontypically sarcomeric hypertrophic or in restrictive phenotypes, EMB may be helpful in excluding infiltrative (amyloid) or storage diseases or may demonstrate a myocardial cause for restriction such as eosinophilic and noneosinophilic primary restrictive cardiomyopathy (Veinot 2002b).

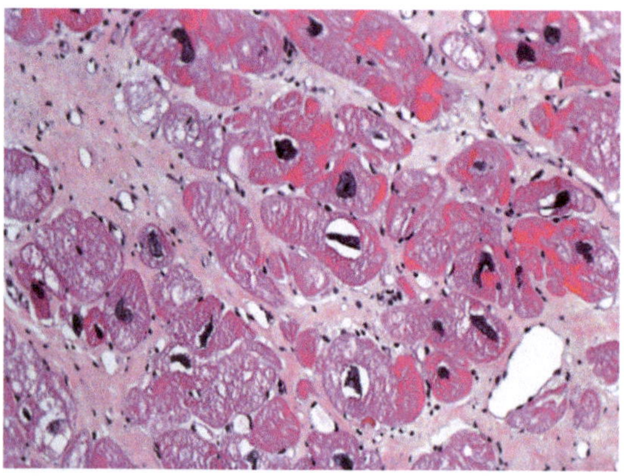

Fig. 6.8 Idiopathic-dilated cardiomyopathy: EMB specimen from a young woman with chronic congestive heart failure. Cardiomyocytes of various sizes with nuclear enlargement, irregularly shaped, sarcoplasmic vacuolization, and interstitial fibrosis are present (Hematoxylin–Eosin ×200)

Key Points

- Endomyocardial biopsy is a safe and useful diagnostic procedure.
- The utility of biopsy is variable depending upon the disease entity and its pathological characteristics, and is particularly valuable in defining specific forms of heart disease/cardiomyopathy.
- Many histological myocardial findings are diagnostically abnormal but nonspecific, while other disorders have diagnostic biopsy findings.
- In dilated cardiomyopathy phenotypes or in arrhythmia investigation, the ability of EMB to evaluate inflammatory heart disease and define its etiology might be a major step in timing of transplantation and prognostic stratification.
- In nontypically sarcomeric hypertrophic and in restrictive phenotypes, EMB may provide specific diagnosis.
- The main point is to standardize a systematic clinical–pathological approach to diagnosing pretransplant diseases in the single transplant center.

Illustrative Case (Fig. 6.9)

This 56-year-old male patient had been previously healthy but presented complaining of episodes of presyncope. Electrocardiogram showed right bundle branch block and first degree AV block. Transthoracic echocardiogram and coronary angiography were unremarkable. During a stress test, he had near-syncope, and complete heart block was noted on electrocardiogram. The patient was referred for further evaluation.

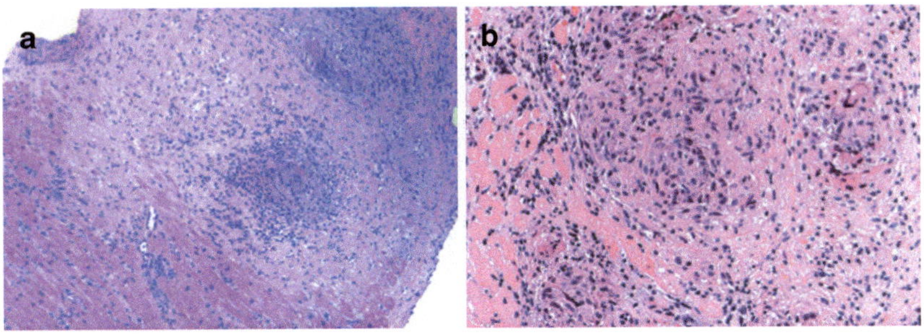

Fig. 6.9 Illustrative case: Cardiac sarcoid—Electrophysiologically guided right ventricle biopsy specimen showing several nonnecrotizing granulomas consistent with involvement of the heart by sarcoidosis (Hematoxylin–Eosin: **a** ×100; **b** ×200). Special stains for microorganisms were negative

An intravenous pacemaker (ICD) was inserted, and the patient was referred for an FDG-PET (fluorodeoxyglucose-positron emission tomography) scan which showed multifocal FDG uptake, suggestive of cardiac sarcoidosis.

Electroanatomical mapping showed numerous areas of low voltage; the right ventricular outflow region had normal mapping.

A CARTO-guided EMB was performed and was not diagnostic, so a dual chamber ICD was inserted.

A second CARTO-guided EMB was performed, and the right ventricular biopsy specimens showed nonnecrotizing granulomatous inflammation consistent with sarcoid (Fig. 6.9). Special stains for acid-fast bacilli and fungi were negative.

The patient was placed on an oral steroid and an angiotensin-converting enzyme inhibitor and did well.

References

Arbustini E, Morbini P, Verga L, Concardi M, Porcu E, Pilotto A, et al. Light and electron microscopy immunohistochemical characterization of amyloid deposits. Amyloid. 1997;4:157–70.

Ardehali H, Howard DL, Hariri A, Qasim A, Hare JM, Baughman KL, et al. A positive endomyocardial biopsy result for sarcoid is associated with poor prognosis in patients with initially unexplained cardiomyopathy. Am Heart J. 2005;150(3):459–63.

Aretz HT. Myocarditis: the Dallas criteria. Hum Pathol. 1987;18:619–24.

Basso C, Ronco F, Marcus F, Abudureheman A, Rizzo S, Frigo AC, et al. Quantitative assessment of endomyocardial biopsy in arrhythmogenic right ventricular cardiomyopathy/dysplasia: an in vitro validation of diagnostic criteria. Eur Heart J. 2008;29(22):2760–71.

Benson MD, Breall J, Cummings OW, Liepnieks JJ. Biochemical characterisation of amyloid by endomyocardial biopsy. Amyloid. 2009;16(1):9–14.

Chan KL, Veinot J, Leach A, Bedard P, Smith S, Marquis JF. Diagnosis of left atrial sarcoma by transvenous endocardial biopsy. Can J Cardiol. 2001;17(2):206–8.

Collins AB, Smith RN, Stone JR. Classification of amyloid deposits in diagnostic cardiac specimens by immunofluorescence. Cardiovasc Pathol. 2009;18(4):205–16.

Cooper LT, Baughman KL, Feldman AM, Frustaci A, Jessup M, Kuhl U, et al. The role of endomyocardial biopsy in the management of cardiovascular disease – a scientific statement from the American Heart Association, the American College of Cardiology, and the European Society of Cardiology. Circulation. 2007;116(19):2216–33.

Corrado D, Thiene G. Cardiac sarcoidosis mimicking arrhythmogenic right ventricular cardiomyopathy/dysplasia: the renaissance of endomyocardial biopsy? J Cardiovasc Electrophysiol. 2009;20(5):477–9.

d'Amati G, Factor SM. Endomyocardial biopsy findings in patients with ventricular arrythmias of unknown origin. Cardiovasc Pathol. 1996;5:139–44.

Fauci AS, Harley JB, Roberts WC, Ferrans VJ, Gralnick HR, Bjornson BH. NIH conference. The idiopathic hypereosinophilic syndrome. Clinical, pathophysiologic, and therapeutic considerations. Ann Intern Med. 1982;97(1):78–92.

Iglezias SD, Benvenuti LA, Calabrese F, Salemi VM, Silva AM, Carturan E, et al. Endomyocardial fibrosis: pathological and molecular findings of surgically

resected ventricular endomyocardium. Virchows Arch. 2008;453(3):233–41.
Kawai C. From myocarditis to cardiomyopathy: mechanisms of inflammation and cell death: learning from the past for the future. Circulation. 1999;99(8):1091–100.
Ladyjanskaia GA, Basso C, Hobbelink MG, Kirkels JH, Lahpor JR, Cramer MJ, et al. Sarcoid myocarditis with ventricular tachycardia mimicking ARVD/C. J Cardiovasc Electrophysiol. 2010;21(1):94–8.
Leone O, Rapezzi C, Sinagra G, Angelini A, Arbustini E, Bartoloni G, et al. Consensus document on endomyocardial biopsy of the Associazione per la Patologia Cardiovascolare Italiana. G Ital Cardiol (Rome). 2009;10(9 Suppl 1):3S–50.
Leone O, Veinot JP, Angelini A, Baandrup UT, Basso C, Berry G, et al. 2011 Consensus statement on endomyocardial biopsy from the Association for European Cardiovascular Pathology and the Society for Cardiovascular Pathology. Cardiovasc Pathol. 2012; 21(4):245–74.
Liu P, Martino T, Opavsky MA, Penninger J. Viral myocarditis; balance between viral infection and immune response. Can J Cardiol. 1996;12(10):935–43.
Lombardo T, Tamburino C, Bartoloni G, Morrone ML, Frontini V, Italia F, et al. Cardiac iron overload in thalassemic patients: an endomyocardial biopsy study. Ann Hematol. 1995;71:135–41.
Luk A, Metawee M, Ahn E, Gustafsson F, Ross H, Butany J. Do clinical diagnoses correlate with pathological diagnoses in cardiac transplant patients? The importance of endomyocardial biopsy. Can J Cardiol. 2009;25:e48–54.
Maisch B, Portig I, Ristic A, Hufnagel G, Pankuweit S. Definition of inflammatory cardiomyopathy (myocarditis): on the way to consensus. A status report. Herz. 2000;25(3):200–9.
Marcus FI, McKenna WJ, Sherrill D, Basso C, Bauce B, Bluemke DA, et al. Diagnosis of arrhythmogenic right ventricular cardiomyopathy/dysplasia. Proposed Modification of the Task Force Criteria. Circulation. 2010;121:1533–41.
Strain JE, Grose RM, Factor SM, Fisher JD. Results of endomyocardial biopsy in patients with spontaneous ventricular tachycardia but without apparent structural heart disease. Circulation. 1983;68(6):1171–81.
Veinot JP. Diagnostic endomyocardial biopsy pathology – general biopsy considerations, and its use for myocarditis and cardiomyopathy: a review. Can J Cardiol. 2002a;18(1):55–65.
Veinot JP. Diagnostic endomyocardial biopsy pathology: secondary myocardial diseases and other clinical indications – a review. Can J Cardiol. 2002b;18(3): 287–96.
Vignola PA, Aonuma K, Swaye PS, Rozanski JJ, Blankstein RL, Benson J, et al. Lymphocytic myocarditis presenting as unexplained ventricular arrythmias: diagnosis with endomyocardial biopsy and response to immunosuppression. JACC. 1984;4:812–9.
Vrana JA, Gamez JD, Madden BJ, Theis JD, Bergen III HR, Dogan A. Classification of amyloidosis by laser microdissection and mass spectrometry-based proteomic analysis in clinical biopsy specimens. Blood. 2009;114(24):4957–9.
Why HJF, Meany BT, Richardson PJ, Olsen EGJ, Bowles NE, Cunningham L, et al. Clinical and prognostic significance of detection of enteroviral RNA in the myocardium of patients with myocarditis or dilated cardiomyopathy. Circulation. 1994;89:2582–9.

Part III

Heart Donation and Peritransplant Pathologies

Donor Selection Criteria: Clinical and Pathological Insights

7

Ornella Leone, Luciano Potena, Alberto Foà, and Andreas Zuckermann

Contents

O. Leone (✉)
Cardiovascular and Cardiac Transplant Pathology Program, Department of Pathology, Sant'Orsola-Malpighi University Hospital, Bologna, Italy
e-mail: ornella.leone@aosp.bo.it

L. Potena
Heart Failure and Heart Transplant Program, Cardiology Unit, S.Orsola-Malpighi University Hospital, Bologna, Italy

A. Foà
Department of Cardiology, Sant'Orsola-Malpighi University Hospital, Bologna, Italy

A. Zuckermann
Department of Cardiac Surgery, Medical University of Vienna, Vienna, Austria

7.1 Background

Careful evaluation of donors and donor organs is essential for all solid organ transplantations, as their characteristics affect recipient outcome.

In heart transplantation, particularly, two additional aspects are also crucial:

- Donor age, which is closely related to age-dependent risk of transmission of donor sub-clinical diseases, most commonly coronary artery atherosclerosis.
- The effects – still poorly understood – that potentially reversible myocardial abnormalities can have in the immediate/early postoperative period for an organ with largely mechanical properties.

Currently these two aspects are particularly significant in light of the notable increase in donor mean age over the last 10 years and the more critical management of brain-dead donors, where pathophysiology of brain death can negatively affect the heart.

The clinician's final decision as to whether to accept a heart comes at the end of a complex process, starting with identification of a potential deceased donor and proceeding through various steps including referral to procurement team, local legislation, donor management and assessment of donor risk (Kransdorf and Stehlik 2014).

O. Leone et al. (eds.), *The Pathology of Cardiac Transplantation*,
DOI 10.1007/978-3-319-46386-5_7

In this chapter, we will review the main principles guiding the decision-making on donor heart suitability for transplantation and the pathological abnormalities that can be found in a discarded donor heart.

7.2 Clinical Considerations for Donor Selection

Although many studies have examined the impact of recipient characteristics on survival after heart transplantation, emerging data suggest that donor parameters are also a major factor in post-transplant mortality (Lund et al. 2014; Smits et al. 2012; Khush et al. 2013). When offered a candidate heart from a suboptimal donor, clinicians are inclined to reject it in the expectation of an unfavorable outcome.

Despite the organ shortage, only 36.9 % of donors reported to Eurotransplant Registry were considered potential candidates, and of these only 64.6 % were ultimately used for transplantation (Smits et al. 2012). Furthermore in Europe, donors are significantly older than in the USA (Lund et al. 2014): the median age for heart donors in Eurotransplant has increased from 34 years in 1996 to 45 years in 2011. There is clearly an imperative to balance increasing waiting times and the risk of mortality while awaiting a transplant versus poor post-transplant survival due to marginal donor hearts. To this end, an objective donor quality assessment tool to supplement clinical experience would be helpful for centers deciding whether or not to accept a donor heart that is suboptimal but which may be usable.

To evaluate a potential donor heart, a series of examinations and inquiry of demographic data of the donor are necessary.

These first sets of data define the primary quality of the donor heart and determine the intensive care of the donor.

7.2.1 General Donor Criteria

7.2.1.1 Donor Age

Medical literature shows contradictory evidence on the risk of donor age for early and long-term outcome after cardiac transplantation. The definition of an 'old' cardiac donor varies among centers and reports: some centers define donor old age as >40 years, whereas others give 50, 55 or 60 years. There have been reports of good transplant outcomes using donor hearts >60 years of age (Smits et al. 2012; Roig et al. 2015; Wittwer and Wahlers 2008); however, most published data, especially large registry data, show a clear association with greater donor age and worse outcome. The International Society for Heart and Lung Transplantation (ISHLT) Registry shows a steadily increasing risk with every 10 years of donor age (i.e. 1 year death risk for a 40 years donor is 1.14 times that of under 40 years donors; for a 50 years donor the risk is 1.30 and for a 60 years donor 1.48) (Lund et al. 2014). Thirty-day survival especially seems much decreased with older donors. Although some studies also suggest decreased long-term survival, most studies show little influence after the first month (Young 1999; Lietz et al. 2004).

Besides direct influence on survival, older donor hearts have a higher risk of developing graft vasculopathy (Li et al. 2006; Stehlik et al. 2010; Caforio et al. 2004). Increased age is associated with the development of cardiovascular risk factors which may affect chances of subclinical coronary artery disease: if undetected, the disease can be transmitted to the recipient through the transplant. Besides coronary lesions, arterial hypertension, diabetes mellitus and left ventricular hypertrophy may also impact donor heart quality (Kuppahally et al. 2007; Marelli et al. 2000).

Every risk factor increases the potential for intra- and perioperative complications due to graft dysfunction. Therefore, close cardiac examination is of prime importance with older donors and those with risk factors. In addition, an expected longer ischemic time might have a significant negative effect on primary graft function. Some authors report up to 40 % 1-year mortality in older donor hearts with long ischemic time (see ischemic time section) (Lund et al. 2014).

Recipient selection for older donor hearts has been discussed from more than a decade. Strategies of old-for-old allocation or older donor hearts for alternative waiting list patients have been reported with acceptable results (Roig et al. 2015; Dark 2015). Newer reports have not found any negative interaction between donor and recipient age concerning mortality or graft vasculopathy (Eskandary et al. 2014).

7.2.1.2 Donor Size and Weight

For the selection of a donor heart, donor size and weight combined or body mass index (BMI) seem to be more important than weight alone (especially in smaller donors). In general, an average size/weight donor (175 cm, 75 Kg) seems to be acceptable for most recipients. Moderate oversize, especially for recipients with elevated pulmonary vascular resistance, seems to be helpful, although controversial and little supported by evidence (Sethi et al. 1993; Hosenpud et al. 1989; Patel et al. 2008). Nevertheless, extreme oversizing might be problematic for patients with previous cardiac surgery or small normal-sized hearts and can lead to restrictive dysfunction of the graft. Moreover there have been reports of higher rates of graft vasculopathy in donors > 90 kg (Li et al. 2006).

Female donor hearts are smaller and are associated with lower cardiac output than male hearts in equal-sized persons, partially explaining the increased early mortality observed in undersized female donor hearts transplanted into male recipients (Weiss et al. 2009; Reed et al. 2014). Thus, appropriate size match between donor and recipient should be a major guiding principle for acceptance and appropriate allocation of organs.

7.2.1.3 Donor History

Information on cardiovascular risk factors (hypertension, diabetes mellitus, smoking, drinking habits and family history) as well as cardiotoxic substances (cocaine, cardiotoxic medication, previous chemotherapy, CO- or cyanid-intoxication) and indirect evidence of risk factors need to be examined (Smits et al. 2012). Many donors with intracerebral bleeding had untreated hypertension for years. Patient history might also reveal known cardiac disease (coronary artery disease, valve disease, rhythm disorders).

If donors underwent cardiopulmonary resuscitation (CPR), it is important to have information about time, duration and cause of CPR. If any cardiac disease is associated with CPR, the donor heart should not be used; if no cardiac cause can be detected and heart function was restored to normal after CPR, donor heart procurement can be performed (Ali et al. 2007).

7.2.1.4 Cause of Death

Brain death cause can negatively influence donor heart function (impaired contractility, arrhythmia and increased cardiac enzymes) and therefore impact post-operative prognosis (Mohamedali et al. 2014; Berman et al. 2010).

In non-traumatic intracranial bleeding, a catecholamine surge can develop that is associated with temporary cardiac dysfunction. Optimal donor management and postponing of organ procurement can reduce non-acceptance rates for donor hearts and the risk of primary graft dysfunction (Mohamedali et al. 2014). A potential pitfall here, however, is left ventricular hypertrophy: patients dying from cerebral hemorrhage are often hypertensive and may be carriers of unknown hypertensive cardiac disease, which can lead to a restrictive syndrome, difficult to manage in the post-operative phase (Kuppahally et al. 2007).

In traumatic brain death by gunshot, the sudden increase of intracerebral pressure can also lead to an increase of endogenous catecholamines. But in this case, in addition to the negative impact on myocardial contractility, there have been reports of increased antigen expression in donor tissue after brain death due to explosive brain injury associated with higher risk of graft rejection (Karamlou et al. 2005).

7.2.1.5 Malignancies

Most malignancies are contraindicated for transplantation: only supratentorial brain malignancies without metastasis can be used for organ donation. In donors with malignancies in remission, data on grading, staging, therapeutic history, last oncological control are mandatory for a decision on potential procurement.

When unexpected donor lesions are found, histology examination may be extremely useful (Desai et al. 2014; Warrens et al. 2012).

7.2.1.6 Infection

Information on donor infection status is important. Besides syphilis serology, antibody data on human immunodeficiency virus (HIV), Hepatitis B and C viruses (HBV and HCV) as well as Cytomegalovirus (CMV), Epstein Barr virus (EBV) and Toxoplasma are the most frequent routine analyses (Smits et al. 2012). HIV and HCV positive donors are not normally accepted (only for HIV and HCV positive recipients). However, the availability of new and effective drugs for Hepatitis C now offers an opportunity to use those organs and prophylactically treat the recipients. Donors with positive HBV serology can be used either for positive recipients or if donor is not infectious. CMV and EBV positive donors can be accepted if prophylaxis is used in negative recipients. In syphilis or toxoplasmosis positive donor organs, long-term prophylaxis in the recipient is mandatory.

7.2.2 Cardiac Specific Donor Criteria

7.2.2.1 Electrocardiogram (ECG)

ECG provides important information on cardiac pathology. Rhythm disturbances, signs of left ventricular hypertrophy and ischemic areas in the donor heart can easily be detected.

7.2.2.2 Echocardiography

Transthoracic or transesophageal echocardiography is now a routine donor examination in most hospitals.

The following parameters are used for decision-making:

1. Ventricular dimensions (left ventricular end diastolic diameter <56 mm; right ventricular end diastolic diameter <30 mm).
2. Ventricular function: with a left ventricular ejection fraction (LVEF) >45 % most donor hearts can be accepted. In hearts with LVEF <45 % one should consider temporary impairment of heart function due to catecholamine surge during brain death (or excess of catecholamine support in the intensive care unit). Therefore, after donor optimization there should be serial examinations (Mohamedali et al. 2014; Casartelli et al. 2012).

   Global, as well as regional wall motion abnormalities due to brain death can be temporary. Nevertheless, regional wall motion abnormalities may be signs of coronary artery disease and need to be examined by coronary angiography, if available. Stress echocardiography has also been found to give promising results (Bombardini et al. 2014).

   Impaired right ventricular function (tricuspid annular plain systolic excursion >1.8 - TAPSE) can be temporary and also a sign of catecholamine surge. Nevertheless, persistent right ventricular dysfunction in the donor is associated with post-operative right ventricular failure.
3. Left ventricle (LV) myocardial thickness: mild to moderate LV hypertrophy per se has no negative effect on early and long-term survival. However, septum thickness >13 mm, especially in older donor grafts with cardiovascular risk factors, is associated with higher perioperative death and worse long-term outcome (Marelli et al. 2000; Goland et al. 2008; Kuppahally et al. 2007).
4. Valve morphology: any stenosis or moderate to severe insufficiency of any valve is a contraindication for organ donation. In selected cases, a valve reconstruction or replacement strategy might be considered.
5. Congenital heart disease: non-complicated atrium-septal defect and normally functioning bicuspid aortic valve are the only congenital diseases that can be accepted for heart donation. However, close visual examination of right ventricular size by the retrieving team is essential before the heart can be accepted. Any defects are closed at a back-table before the heart is implanted.

Apart from all this however and besides clearly pathological conditions, it should be remembered that acceptance should not rely on single ultrasound measurements since repeated assessment may show improvement (Casartelli et al. 2012); the technique itself is also subject to considerable measurement variability (Khush et al. 2015).

7.2.2.3 Coronary Angiography

Donor hearts with a preexisting coronary artery disease (CAD) (stenosis >50%) have two to three times higher risk of early graft failure after transplantation. The results are even worse in hearts with two- or three-vessel disease (Grauhan et al. 2007). Mild arteriosclerotic lesions however largely without significant stenosis can be found in younger patients and the hearts may be acceptable for transplantation. Nevertheless, preexisting lesions do not tend to lead to faster or severe disease progression (Caforio et al. 2004; Li et al. 2006).

Coronary angiography should be performed whenever possible in cases with high risk of CAD or signs of potential CAD in ECG or echocardiography. In older donors (>55 years) especially coronary angiography should be scheduled more frequently in order to lower age-related organ decline rate, as donor hearts without signs of CAD can be transplanted with good short- as well as long-term outcomes (Hauptman et al. 2001). As an alternative to angiography, a coronary computed tomography (CT) scan with calcium-score can be performed to detect potential CAD.

7.2.2.4 Targets of Donor Support

Most organ donors are treated with vasopressor (norepinephrine) and/or inotropic (dobutamin, dopamine) drugs. Before brain death, medical treatment centers on protection of brain perfusion and reduction of brain edema. However, immediately after brain death, therapy should focus on organ protection and vasopressor support should be minimized to achieve organ perfusion (Smits et al. 2012). Hypovolemic donors should receive enough volume infusion to achieve normovolemia. Ideally inotropic support should not exceed 7.5 g/kg/min dopamine/dobutamine and 0.4 g/kg/min norepinephrine. Any higher dose catecholamine support above these thresholds is associated with potential organ damage and should be carefully considered in the decision-making process (Abuanzeh et al. 2015).

Absolute contraindications for donor heart acceptance are summarized in Table 7.1.

Table 7.1 Absolute contraindications for accepting donor hearts

Severe global hypokinesia after optimization of donor treatment (central venous pressure, inotropic drugs)
Severe diffuse CAD in coronary angiography
Myocardial infarction in donor history
Complex ventricular arrhythmia
Severe congenital heart disease
Extracranial or infratectorial malignancy
CO intoxication with Met-HB >20%
Systemic uncontrolled bacterial infection
Active endocarditis

7.3 Pathology in the Donor Selection Process

Despite the wide variability worldwide in the criteria and pieces of information needed to assess heart suitability, pathological assessment of heart biopsy is not part of the routine workout, as it may be for abdominal organs.

In donor renal biopsy, histologic scoring to evaluate the sum of interstitial fibrosis, tubular atrophy, glomerulosclerosis and vascular damage is used to predict delayed graft function risk, now that donor criteria have been expanded due to organ shortage (Jochmans and Pirenne 2011; Balaz et al. 2013).

In allograft liver biopsy too, the predictive value of histologic analysis of steatosis, fibrosis and necrosis is evaluated for the development of primary non-function or poor function as well as allograft dysfunction (D'Alessandro et al. 1991; Markin et al. 1993). A single liver biopsy may be sufficient for assessing the extent of macrovesicular steatosis and frozen sections permit rapid evaluation of steatosis, fibrosis, inflammation and hepatocyte necrosis, which can contraindicate transplantation. But independently of steatosis and fibrosis, the usefulness of liver biopsy for assessment of elderly donor or hemodynamically unstable allografts still remains unclear (Durand et al. 2008).

There are no conclusive data on the true predictive value of donor organ histology during assessment, and many problematic issues must be considered, especially for the heart, whose anatomic and functional features make it very different from other organs for transplant.

Although from a technical point of view a myocardial biopsy can be performed during a multiorgan donation, the need for the heart to limit ischemic time as much as possible does not allow adequate sample processing, as even the rapid process requires around 2 hours. Extemporary frozen sections are not adequate for assessing the type of histologic lesions to evaluate and definite specimens are necessary.

Moreover non-targeted bioptic sampling is not representative; even if lesions are recognized, the essential parameter is their extent throughout the whole myocardium.

In addition, clinical or instrumental data (echocardiography, angiography) frequently make it possible to obtain extensive information on the whole heart.

In this context, the substantial contribution of pathology in heart donation is the opportunity to routinely evaluate the whole discarded organ in order to recognize possible correlations between pathological alterations and clinical-instrumental data obtained before rejection. If generally adopted, this could be one relatively simple means to improve current criteria for accepting hearts and help identify a subgroup of potentially usable organs, currently discarded. Protocols shared within single transplant centers would provide additional pathologic information with little effort.

7.4 Pathology Findings in Donor Discarded Hearts

The evaluation of non-procured donor heart specimens or of the entire organ in order to obtain pathologic information is not routine procedure in transplant centers, and this is probably due to variation in local legislation and also religious aspects.

Available data, although lacking in detail, concern legislation and directives on tissue banking (e.g. the European Commission directives), which aim to collect all possible medical information before releasing tissue for transplantation (Van Geyt et al. 2010).

In this context, some reports emphasize the value of autopsy or of any histological examination other than autopsy to improve the safety of transplantation for all types of tissue: Visser et al. show that contraindications for tissue transplantation were found in 7.8 % Dutch donors who underwent autopsy (n. 220) or any histological examination of tissue remnants - including heart tissue - (n. 136) of 758 Dutch donors enlisted in a 6-month period and suitable for at least one tissue transplantation (Visser et al. 2012).

Specifically for the heart, the valve tissue banking program is crucial to create an opportunity to perform pathologic examination of the entire heart or of heart tissue remnants following valve donation: the valve removal procedure does not significantly impair cardiac pathologic examination, especially if adequate caution is taken (Mackey-Bojack et al. 2007).

Nowadays, heart valves can be obtained not only from deceased donors (brain death and cardiac death) but also from "live donors", i.e. recipients of transplanted hearts.

In this regard, the experience at the National Cardiovascular Homograft Bank of Singapore (Heng et al. 2014) is notable; pathologic examination of heart tissue became mandatory for valve deceased donors after routine pathology study of recipient native hearts revealed a case of cardiac sarcoidosis, which may be a possible contraindication to tissue retrieval as it can involve cardiac valves. In their work, aimed at increasing the safety of heart valve homografts, Heng et al. provided convincing data to support the importance of examining hearts not only for safe tissue donation but also for motivated exclusion.

In the setting of organ retrieval, a paper by Doroshow et al. (1995) emphasizes the potential role of myocardial pathology evaluation in brain-dead infant donors who have undergone autopsy, to define more accurate predictors in assessment of donor suitability. This report highlights the issue of lack of correspondence between pathology findings and current clinical selection criteria.

These data, although limited, emphasize that pathology evaluation of discarded hearts and anatomo-clinical correlation may be essential additional factors to identify donor features that may assist selection and potentially improve the number of organs accepted.

As summarized in Sect. 7.2, the criteria for heart acceptance rely mainly on the data provided by the intensive care units regarding patient history and current management. The donor heart case records are heterogeneous and incomplete, and it is often difficult to piece together standardized information regarding the refusal of a heart based on instrumental data from coronary angiography and echocardiography, as these tests are not routinely performed. Consequently subjectivity still plays a significant role in donor heart evaluation and more reproducible objective data would be desirable.

To illustrate the potential value of donor heart pathology evaluation, we will present some data from the Heart Transplant Center of Bologna (Italy), where pathology examination of a considerable number of donor hearts unsuitable for transplantation has been carried out for some 10 years, in the context of two major projects:

- The "valve tissue bank" project. Since 2006, throughout the Emilia-Romagna region, all hearts of multitissue donors excluded from donation for various reasons are explanted in order to collect valves for the tissue bank and sent to the Pathology Institute of the Sant'Orsola Hospital for centralized pathological examination.
- The Adonhers (Aged Donor Heart Rescue by Stress Echo) project, which uses pharmacological stress echocardiography screening for marginal donors to identify healthy donor hearts that would historically have been rejected due to patient age or transient left ventricular dysfunction.

7.4.1 Methodology of Pathology Examination

The pathological approach for gross and histological examination of these hearts should be very accurate and standardized in order to make data as comparable as possible.

The approach is as for explanted native hearts in terms of gross examination, sectioning, sampling for histology and staining, as detailed in Chap. 5, especially Sects. 5.1 and 5.2. The main limitation is the condition of the heart, which due to removal of semilunar valves for bank tissue, is often incomplete or fragmented (Figs. 7.1 and 7.2). An expert cardiovascular pathologist will

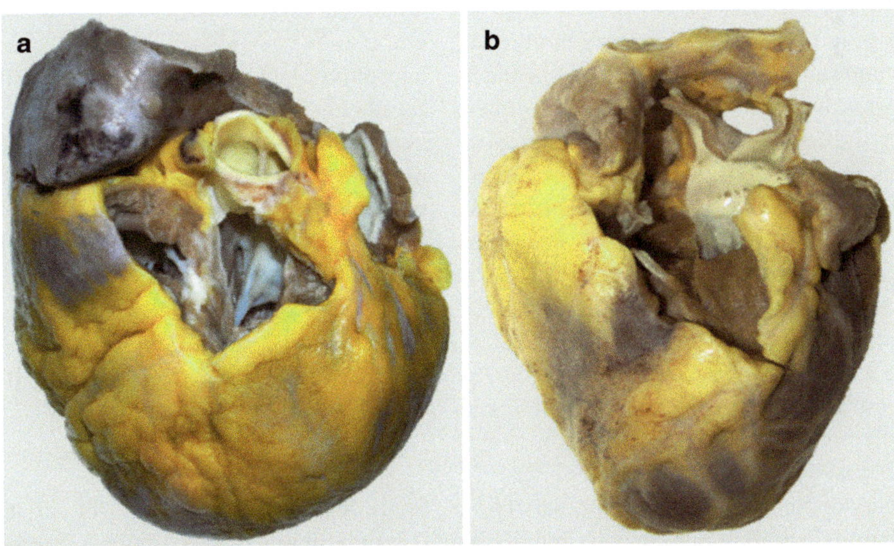

Fig. 7.1 (**a**, **b**) Multitissue donor hearts excluded from donation and explanted for the valve tissue bank. The hearts are almost complete: only the ventricle outflow tracts are missing due to semilunar valve removal

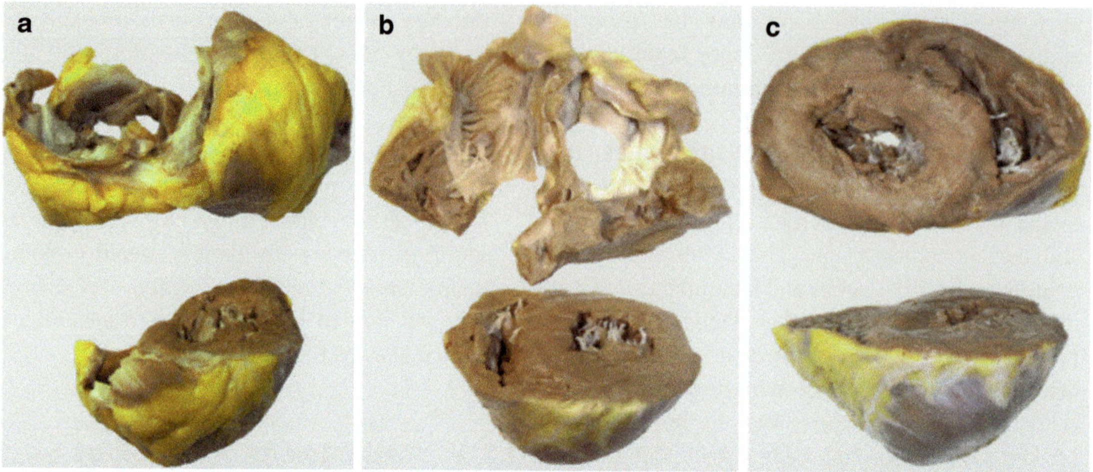

Fig. 7.2 Multitissue donor hearts excluded from donation and explanted for the valve tissue bank. In these cases hearts are incomplete and fragmented. (**a**, **b**) The middle part of the organs is lacking. (**c**) The base of the heart is lacking

however be able to reconstruct the heart, although parts of some epicardial main coronary arteries can inevitably be missed. Keeping in mind the current recommendations from the Association for European Cardiovascular Pathology and Society for Cardiovascular Pathology is a good rule (Stone et al. 2012).

After recording weight (entire or summing different fragments), dimensions, shape and chamber sizes, any external alterations should be noted.

Before sectioning the heart, the main subepicardial coronary arteries (left main, left anterior descending, left obtuse marginal and circumflex branches and right coronary) should be opened in situ with multiple transverse cuts at 3-mm intervals along the course and atherosclerotic plaques described. Then serial transverse sections along the short axis of the heart are obtained from the apex to the midventricular level (as far as the apex of papillary muscles) at 1-cm intervals.

Parietal myocardium thickness of the free wall of both ventricles and the interventricular septum should be measured at basal, medium and apical levels. Gross appearance of the myocardium should be carefully noted and detailed description of evident alterations be given: recent lesions, scars or fibrosis, fatty or fibro-fatty replacement, specifying their extent and localizations in both ventricular walls or septum and along the subepicardial-mediomural-subendocardium layers.

Sampling is extensive: an entire representative transverse slice at midventricular level; further specimens from each right and left ventricle and interventricular septum (one sample from the right ventricle, one from the left ventricle and one from the septum from both basal and apical segments); all macroscopically altered areas; stenotic or obstructed tracts of coronary artery (serial blocking) or, if these lesions are absent, randomized samples.

Standard Haematoxylin-Eosin, stains for collagen and elastic fibers (Masson or Mallory trichrome, Weigert–Van Gieson, etc.) and further appropriate histochemical and immunohistochemical staining are performed.

All the hearts were examined by an expert cardiovascular pathologist, blind in the first instance to clinical information or death circumstances. Pathology and clinical data were subsequently correlated.

7.4.2 Heart Pathology Findings in "Valve Tissue Bank" Project Pool

Preliminary data are available for 210 hearts, both from multitissue and multiorgan donors. It was a heterogeneous group of patients (72 % males and 28 % females, with a median age of 42 years – range

11–66): only about half were heart donors; the others were multitissue donors. The hearts were removed exclusively for valve tissue banking.

The causes of death are listed in Table 7.2, most frequently road accident and brain haemorrhage and the reasons for excluding a heart from donation in Table 7.3, where the most frequent reasons are cardiac arrest, heart pathology and exclusion due to positive echocardiography or altered ejection fraction.

Other factors influencing exclusion (9.4 %) were female gender, brain haemorrhage/ictus, diabetes, dislipidemia, inotropic drugs > 0.04 g/kg/min.

The hearts of this heterogeneous group fall into two main categories:

1. Hearts with significant disease/damage (78 %), where pathology alterations may be categorized as:
   - Pathologies preexisting donation (55 %)
   - Pathologies arising in the course of donation (23 %)
2. Hearts with no significant damage/pathologic findings (i.e. pathologically normal hearts) (22 %)

Table 7.2 Causes of death in donor pool (*Valve tissue bank project, Heart Transplant Centre of Bologna, Italy*)

Road accident: 32.2 %
Brain haemorrhage: 20.8 %
Cranial trauma: 13.9 %
Sudden death: 9.4 %
Cardiac arrest: 7.5 %
Suicide: 5.6 %
Ischemic ictus: 5 %
Subarachnoid haemorrhage: 2.5 %
Miscellaneous: 2.5 %

Table 7.3 Reasons for excluding a heart from donation (*Valve tissue bank project, Heart Transplant Centre of Bologna, Italy*)

Cardiac arrest: 51.2 %
Positive stress-echo/altered ejection fraction: 11.7 %
Heart pathology: 11 %
Age: 6.7 %
Haemodynamic instability: 5.5 %
Globally suboptimal donation: 1.2 %
Atrial fibrillation: 0.6 %
Lack of recipients: 1.2 %
Lack of information: 1.5 %

The major preexisting disease was coronary atherosclerosis (Fig. 7.3) associated with myocardial signs of ischemia/hypoperfusion in varying degrees and stages of evolution (Fig. 7.4). A few additional particular lesions such as hypertensive heart disease, cardiac trauma, lymphocytic myocarditis, myocardial bridging, anomalous origin of coronary arteries and an unusual case of diffuse microvascular thrombosis were also found (Fig. 7.5).

Focusing on coronary atherosclerosis, the degree of plaque stenosis was evaluated semi-quantitatively at histology, considering the reduction of cross-sectional luminal area between the luminal border of the plaque and the internal elastic lamina. Atherosclerosis was graded as mild (stenosis < 50 %), subcritical (50–75 %) and critical/significant (75–100 %) (Fig. 7.6). While taking into account the limitations of pathological examination of coronary atherosclerosis (nonphysiological conditions of nonpressure-distended arteries and nonpressure-fixed vessels, and the inevitable collapse of the medial layer where it is uninvolved by the eccentric plaque), 41.4 % of patients had coronary atherosclerosis – critical/significant in 33 %. In this last subgroup, the disease was prevalently (70 %) limited to a single coronary vessel (monovasal); double or triple vessel involvement was found in only 30 % of cases (22.5 % bivasal; 7.5 % trivasal). The median age of patients with significant CAD was 51.3 years (42 years for the entire group).

Damage attributable to events during donation can principally be attributed to cathecolamine-injury, due to both neurogenic stunned myocardium and inotropic therapy.

These lesions were present in a significant number of patients, both in isolation as the main lesion in non-altered hearts or in association with other diseases.

Donor hearts work in an extraordinary physiopathologic context, where many factors concur: processes related to brain death with endogenous autonomic/cathecolamine storm and

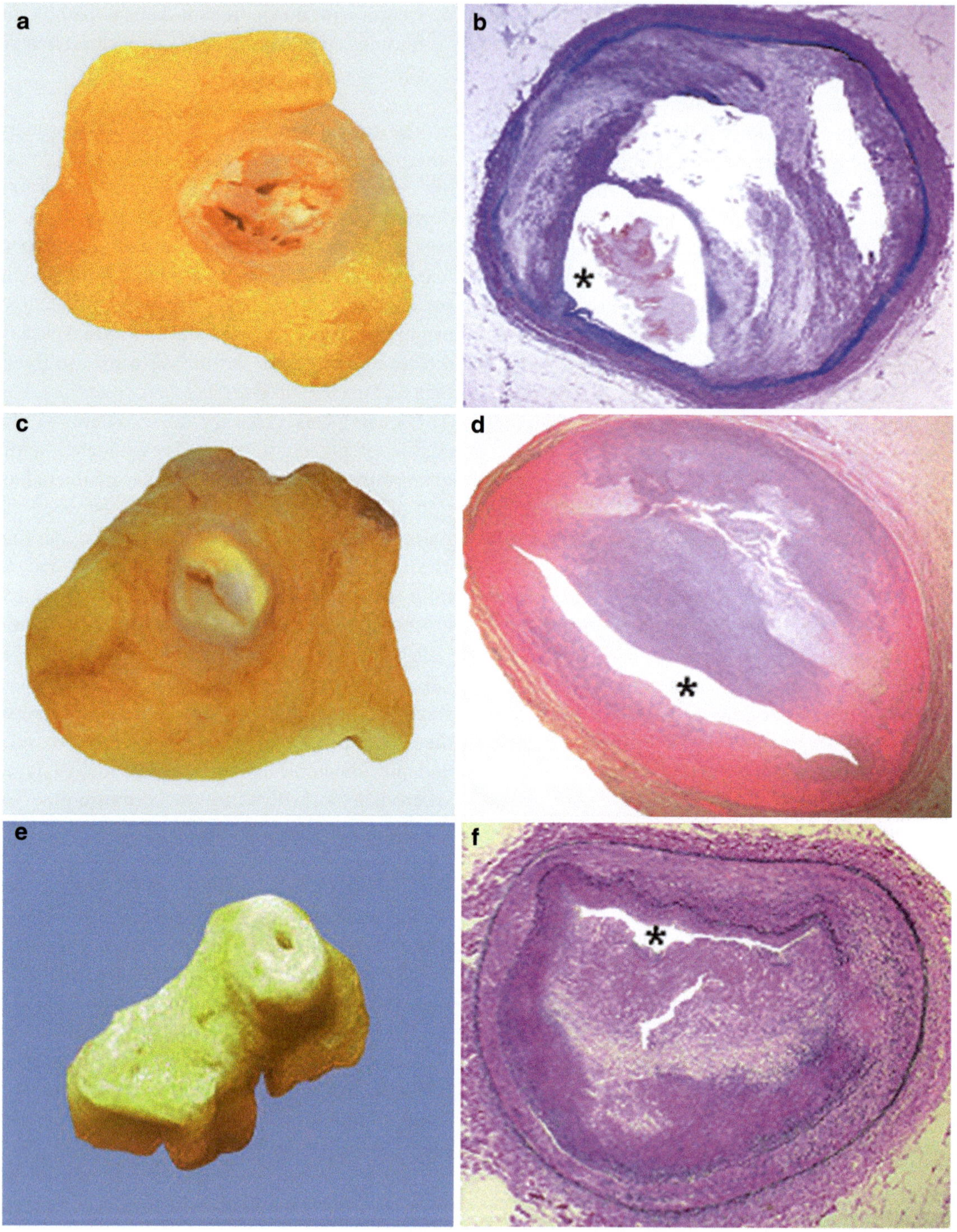

Fig. 7.3 Donor coronary artery atherosclerosis. Macroscopic specimens of left anterior descending coronary artery (**a**, **c**, **e**) and corresponding histologic sections (**b**, **d**, **f**), showing a fibrocalcific plaque (**a**, **b**, Weigert-Van Gieson, 25×), a fibrolipidic plaque (**c**, **d**, Haematoxylin-eosin, 25×) and a predominantly fibrous plaque with histiocytes and focal lipid deposits (**e**, **f**, Weigert-Van Gieson, 25×). All the atherosclerotic plaques severely narrow the lumina (*asterisks*), by 80–95 %

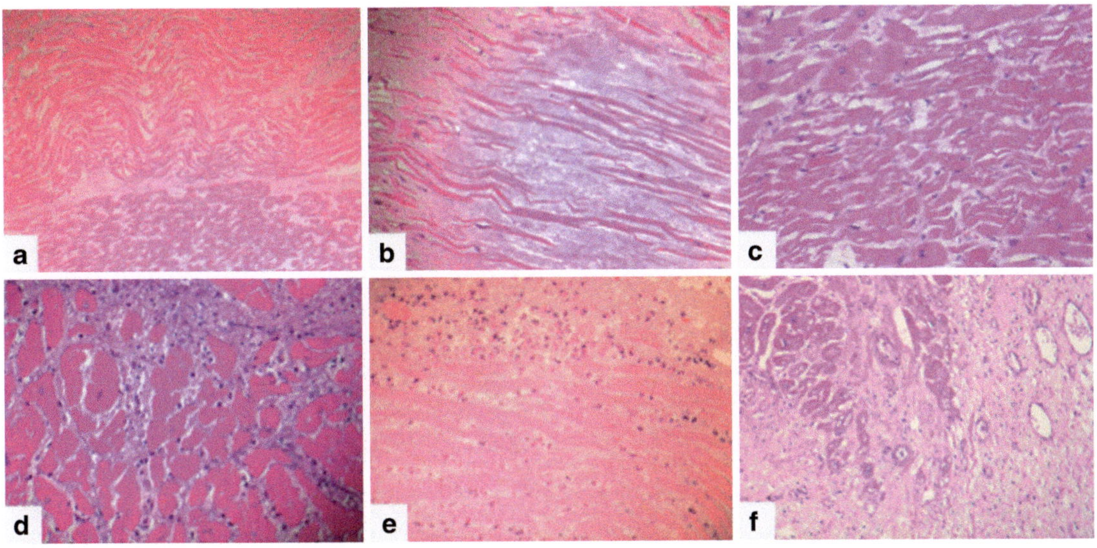

Fig. 7.4 Donor myocardial signs of ischemia/hypoperfusion in varying degrees and stages of evolution. (**a**) Myocell waving (Haematoxylin-eosin, 100×); (**b**) myocell thinning out and waving within oedematous and fibrotic myocardial interstitium (Haematoxylin-eosin, 100×); (**c**) area of early coagulative necrosis (Haematoxylin-eosin, 100×); (**d**, **e**) diffuse and advanced coagulative necrosis with neutrophilic interstitial infiltration (Haematoxylin-eosin, 200×); (**f**) reparative phase of ischemia with loose fibrous tissue and granulation tissue (Haematoxylin-eosin, 100×)

neurohormonal derangement, cathecolamine surge occurring in patients with subarachnoid haemorrhage and sustained pharmacologic inotropic support (Dronavalli et al. 2010). These profound changes, mainly related to intensive sympathetic and catecholamine activity, may result in severe myocardial injury and dysfunction (Zaroff et al. 2003). The histologic substrate underlying these changes, all due to adrenergic stress, is nowadays known, although investigated in different contexts: toxic myocardial damage, pheochromocytoma, stress cardiomyopathy/acute emotional distress, stunning myocardium, consequent on subarachnoid haemorrhage or traumatic head injury, exogenous administration of catecholamines or drugs with sympathomimetic mechanism (Sardesal et al. 1990; Giavarini et al. 2013; Burke et al. 2001; Pérez López et al. 2009; Berman et al. 2010).

In these conditions histology can show: contraction band necrosis with transverse eosinophilic homogeneous hypercontracted/cross bands or diffuse sarcoplasmic hypereosinophilia, real coagulative-type cardiomyocyte necrosis or foci of toxic myocarditis made up of small aggregates of eosinophilic/fragmented myocells surrounded by scarce inflammatory infiltrates (prevalently macrophages or granulocytes, sporadic lymphocytes or mixed inflammation) (Fig. 7.7).

These necrotic-inflammatory lesions are individually small and show typical focal/multifocal distribution. They probably result from both direct damage to the myocyte or acute necrosis secondary to acute hypoxia through vasoconstriction of small intramyocardial vessels.

Due to the heterogeneity of these cases, the pathology data cannot be used for detailed anatomoclinical correlation regarding hearts excluded from donation. But the essential message is that routine pathology examination can be useful to categorize pathologies present in hearts excluded from donation and also to identify hearts with structural versus potentially reversible abnormalities.

The main results to emphasize:

- A significant number of these hearts were pathologically normal and potentially suitable for acceptance: most of the damage seemed acquired during the process of brain death and

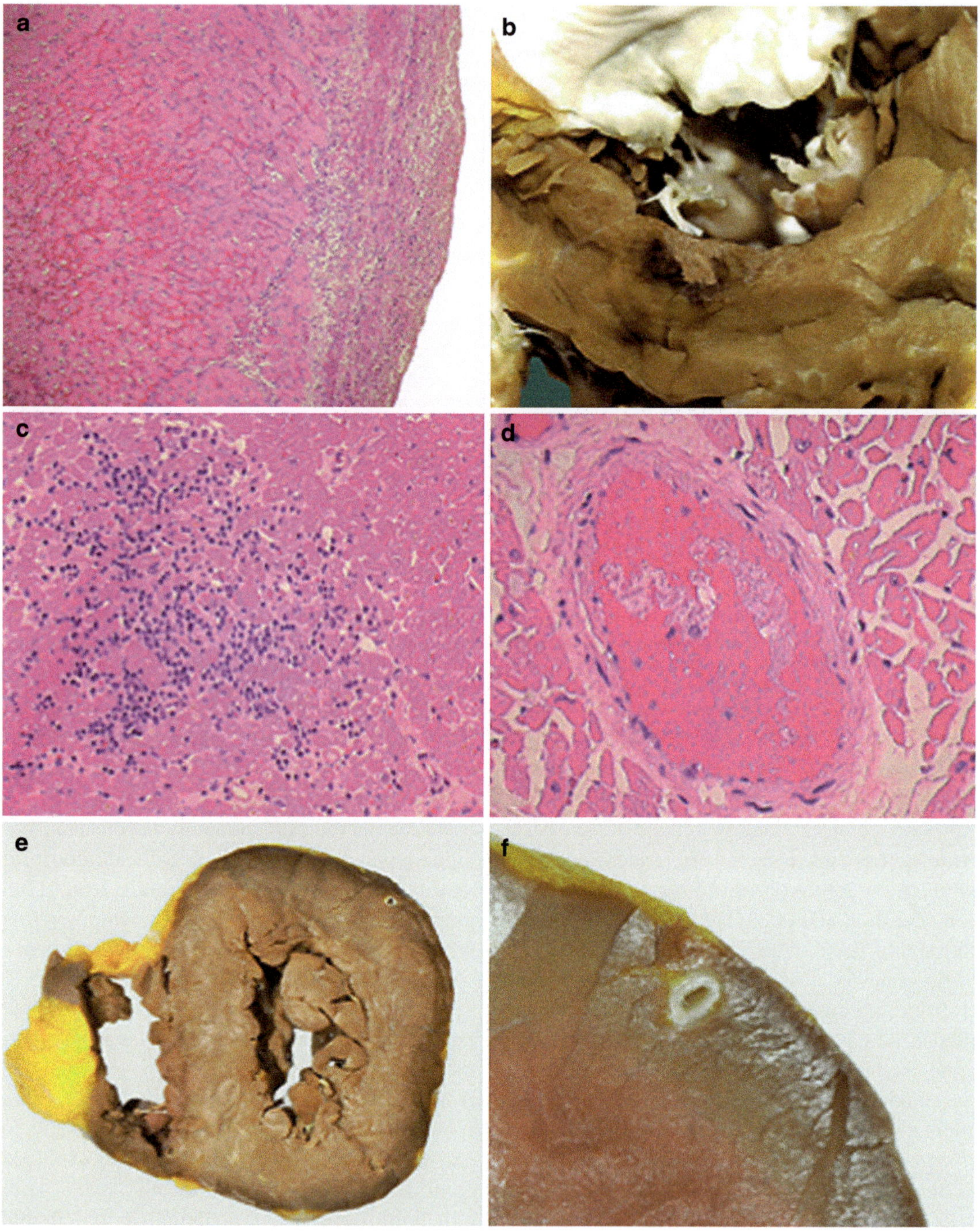

Fig. 7.5 Particular and rarer lesions/diseases found in donor hearts. (**a**) Subendocardial and interstitial haemorrhage, associated with myocyte damage, due to cardiac contusion trauma (Haematoxylin-eosin, 200×); (**b**) macroscopy of cardiac trauma in the interventricular septum; (**c**) active multifocal lymphocytic myocarditis (Haematoxylin-eosin, 200×); (**d**) an unusual case of diffuse myocardial microvascular thrombosis (Haematoxylin-eosin, 200×) – the main branches of coronary arteries were uninvolved; (**e**) myocardial bridging, an anatomical congenital variation of coronary circulation in which an epicardial artery lies in the myocardium for part of its course. In the image the left descending coronary artery is 'bridged' by the myocardium; (**f**) detail of myocardial bridging

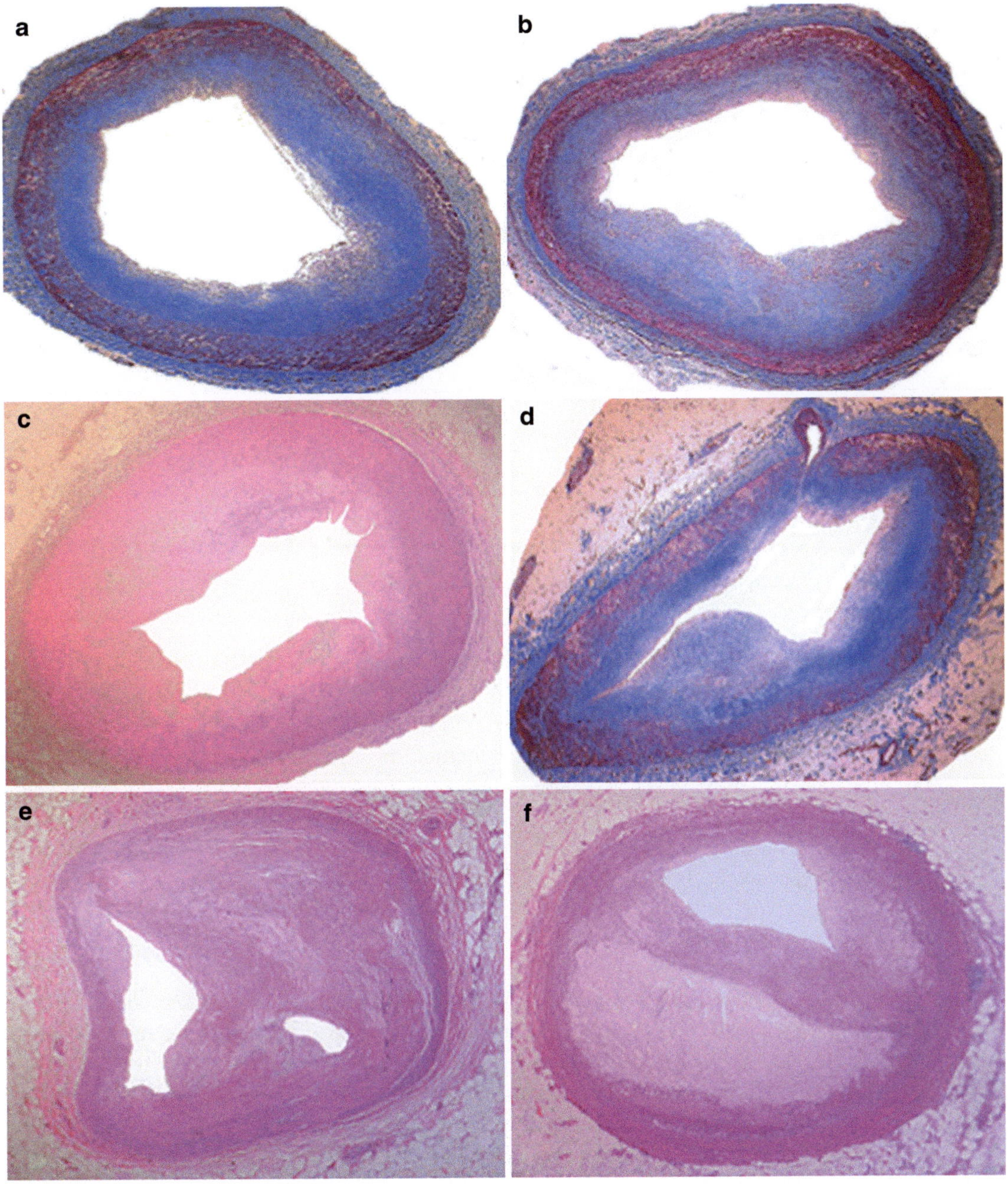

Fig. 7.6 (**a**, **b**) Donor mild (stenosis < 50 %) coronary artery disease: intimal thickening made up of collagen mixed with fibroblasts and mononuclear inflammatory cells (pathological intimal thickening/AHA type III intermediate lesion/preatheroma) (Azan Mallory trichrome, 25×). (**c**, **d**) Donor subcritical (stenosis 50–75 %) coronary artery atherosclerosis. (**c**) Pathological intimal thickening with focal extracellular lipid accumulation (Haematoxylin-eosin, 25×); (**d**) early fibroatheroma (AHAtype IV lesion/atheroma), where the plaque is formed by a central lipidic core and a luminal fibrous cap (Azan Mallory trichrome, 25×). (**e**, **f**) Donor significant critical (stenosis >75–100 %) coronary artery atherosclerosis. Advanced fibroatheroma (AHA type IV-V/fibroatheroma), which widely affects the intimal surface as a consequence of progressive depositions of lipidic and fibrous components. In **f** the central lipidic core is for the most part formed by cholesterol crystals, with some necrotic debris (Haematoxylin-eosin, 25×). *AHA* American Heart Association classification

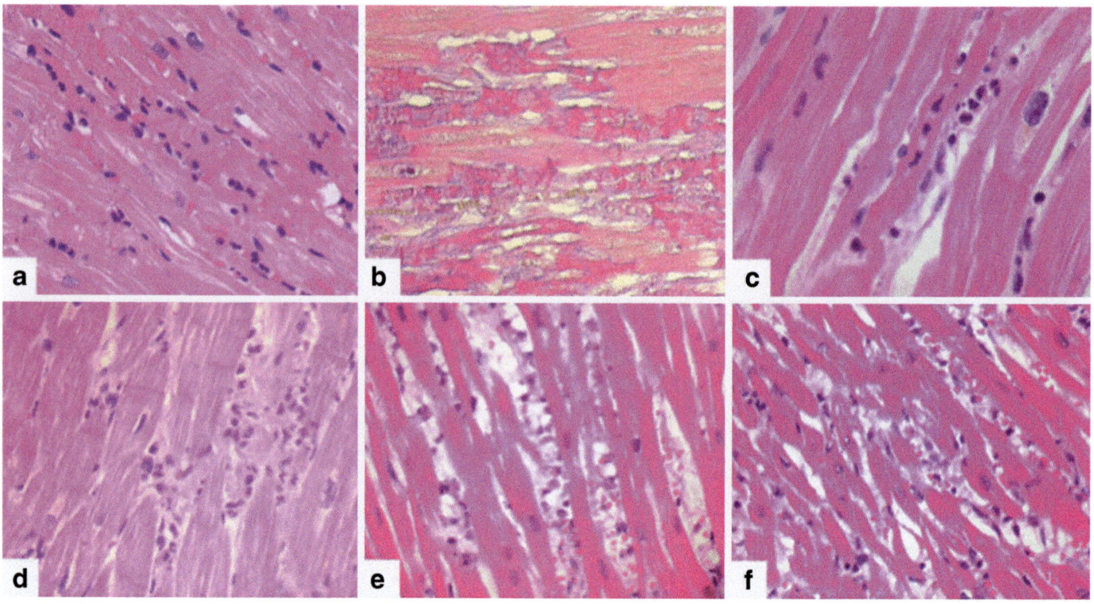

Fig. 7.7 Foci of myocardial damage related to cathecolamine-injury: contraction band necrosis in varying degrees or real cardiomyocyte coagulative-type necrosis (**a**, **b**); foci of toxic myocarditis made up of small aggregates of eosinophilic/fragmented myocells surrounded by scarce inflammatory infiltrates (prevalently macrophages or granulocytes, sporadic lymphocytes or mixed inflammation) (**c**–**f**) (Haematoxylin-eosin, 400×)

donor management. These organs came from younger donors with a low cardiovascular risk profile, high catecholamine doses and with a low ejection fraction, supporting the idea that special management might have improved eart function and acceptability in at least some cases.

- Coronary atherosclerosis was confirmed as a major issue in the older donors, but severity and distribution in the coronary tree needs careful evaluation with appropriate instrumental methods. The presence of atherosclerosis was more common in older donors with a significant cardiovascular risk profile.
- The need for better understanding of the phenomenon of cathecolamine-associated ventricular dysfunction and related myocardial damage, in order to recognize potentially reversible abnormalities and poorly functioning hearts potentially suitable for acceptance (Berman et al. 2010). Some of such abnormalities could be recuperated with appropriate treatment and some dysfunctional hearts become of clinical use for transplantation (Casartelli et al. 2012).

It is incumbent on us all to use every possible method to improve the number of usable hearts as waiting list mortality is increasing and donated hearts decreasing. We should probably abandon the simple idea of "a good or bad donor heart" and consider a wider spectrum of suitability of hearts for transplantation.

7.4.3 Adonhers (Aged Donor Heart Rescue by Stress Echo) Project

Here we want to describe the results of pathology evaluation of donor hearts excluded in the Adonhers project.

The Adonhers protocol uses marginal candidate donors, defined as those aged >50 years or <50 years with concomitant risk factors (history of cocaine use or three risk factors such as hypertension, diabetes, smoking history, dyslipidemia or family history of premature coronary artery disease).

After legal declaration of brain death, all marginal donors undergo baseline echocardiography for evaluation of regional wall motion, global ventricular function and ventricular mass. When the results of resting echocardiography are normal, pharmacologic stress echocardiography is performed, using either dipyridamole or dobutamine.

When stress echocardiography results are normal, the heart is accepted and transplanted. In this case, a coronary angiography or intravascular ultrasound (IVUS) is performed at 1-month posttransplant.

Those donor hearts that are excluded because of positive results on resting or stress echocardiography or eligible hearts not used due to lack of a suitable recipient undergo pathologic examination in order to evaluate the pathologic substrate underlying the stress-echo alterations (Fig. 7.8).

By coupling coronary flow and myocardial function, stress echocardiography allows simultaneous evaluation of inducible ischemia (evaluated by wall motion score index - WMSI), and contractile reserve of the left ventricle (evaluated by pressure volume relationship - PVR). When inducible ischemia is negative (WMSI = 1), the heart is accepted; when it is >1, the heart is excluded. Equally when the contractile reserve is abnormal, donation is contraindicated; when it is normal, the heart is accepted.

Leone et al. published the results of the first 18 cases examined with stress-echo, 6 of whom were successfully transplanted (Leone et al. 2009). Of the six hearts excluded from donation due to positive stress-echo, five had moderate to severe CAD and one a possible idiopathic dilated cardiomyopathy. This paper shows that pharmacologic stress echo can safely be performed on candidate heart donors and can correctly identify hearts with underlying transplant-limiting coronary and/or myocardial disease. Moreover it

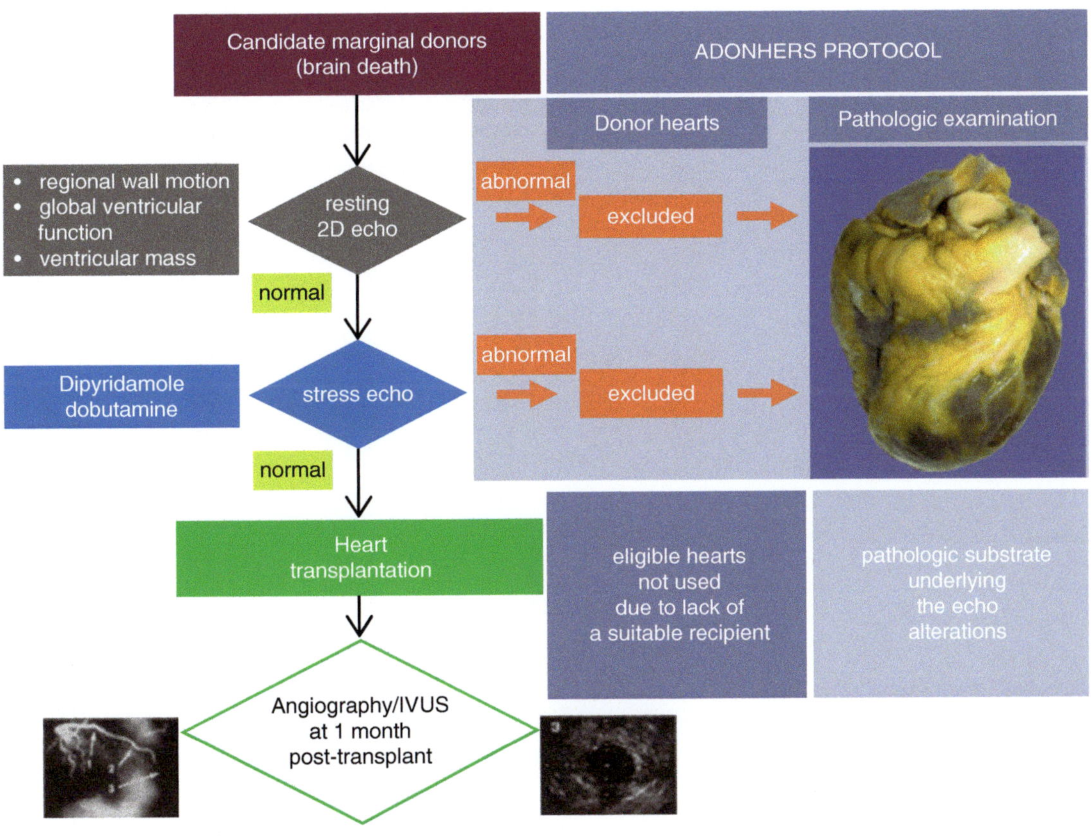

Fig. 7.8 Flow chart of the Adonhers protocol

may also serve to identify transient ventricular dysfunction detected on the rest echo and due to neurogenic stunning, which may be reversible.

Subsequent studies on short and medium-term outcome of recipients of marginal donor hearts selected with pharmacological stress-echocardiographic techniques showed favourable results with survival rates similar to that of recipients of standard donor hearts (Bombardini et al. 2011, 2014).

Pathology examination of the hearts excluded from donation on the basis of an abnormal stress echocardiograph or of eligible hearts not transplanted for various reasons has an important role in correlating pathologic findings with clinical instrumental data.

Although greater experience is needed to determine future optimal donor-to-recipient matching, some available studies show that early and late survival outcomes are more similar in older and younger donor groups and that there is a clear long-term survival benefit for recipients receiving older donor hearts in comparison with those waiting longer for a younger donor.

The heart donor pool we deal with today has a more complex profile and the most significant differences are:

- Older donors with comorbidities including a higher number of grafts with coronary atherosclerosis.
- The progressive shift from young and healthy trauma victims to brain death donors from intracranial haemorrhage, which may cause adverse haemodynamic cardiac events, endocrine or metabolic consequences and the development of a proinflammatory state.

The prevalence of significant coronary atherosclerosis in the donor pool is high and various studies have demonstrated that CAD may frequently although inadvertently be transmitted from donor to recipient. Donor-transmitted atherosclerosis may be a risk factor for early graft failure (Grauhan et al. 2007) and a contributing factor in an increased risk of developing accelerated allograft vasculopathy.

Pathology evaluation may add essential information in new recruitment strategies for donor hearts.

Illustrative Case 1 (Fig. 7.9)

Illustrative Case 2 (Fig. 7.10)

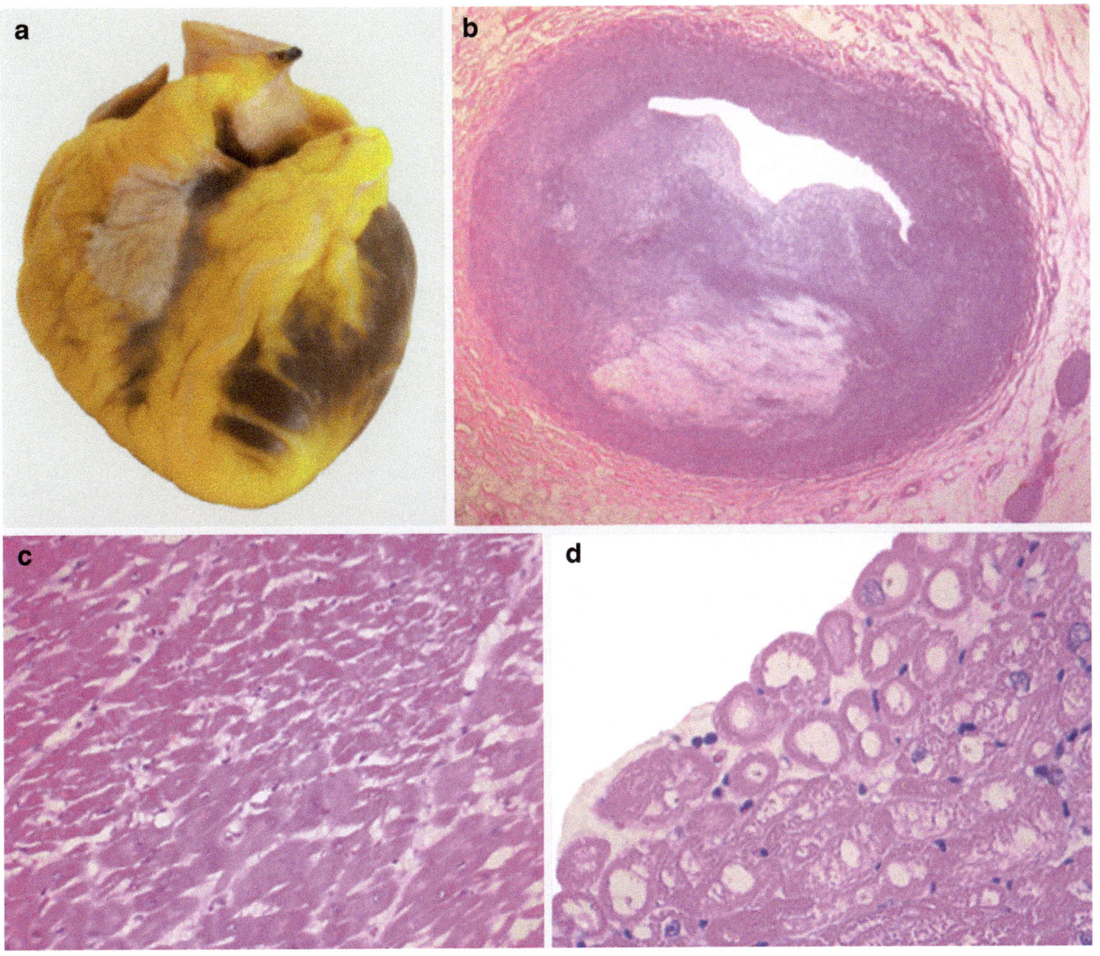

Fig. 7.9 Illustrative Case 1 Heart of a female donor of 50 years (**a**), in which stress-echo revealed a hypoakinesia of the medial-apical portion of the left ventricle. Pathological examination showed a fibrolipidic plaque narrowing around 90 % of LAD lumen (**b**, Haematoxylin-eosin, 25×) and multifocal myocardial coagulative necrosis irregularly distributed in the left ventricle and the interventricular septum (**c**, Haematoxylin-eosin, 200×), associated with diffuse coagulative subendocardial myocytolysis (**d**, Haematoxylin-eosin, 400×). *LAD* left anterior descending coronary artery

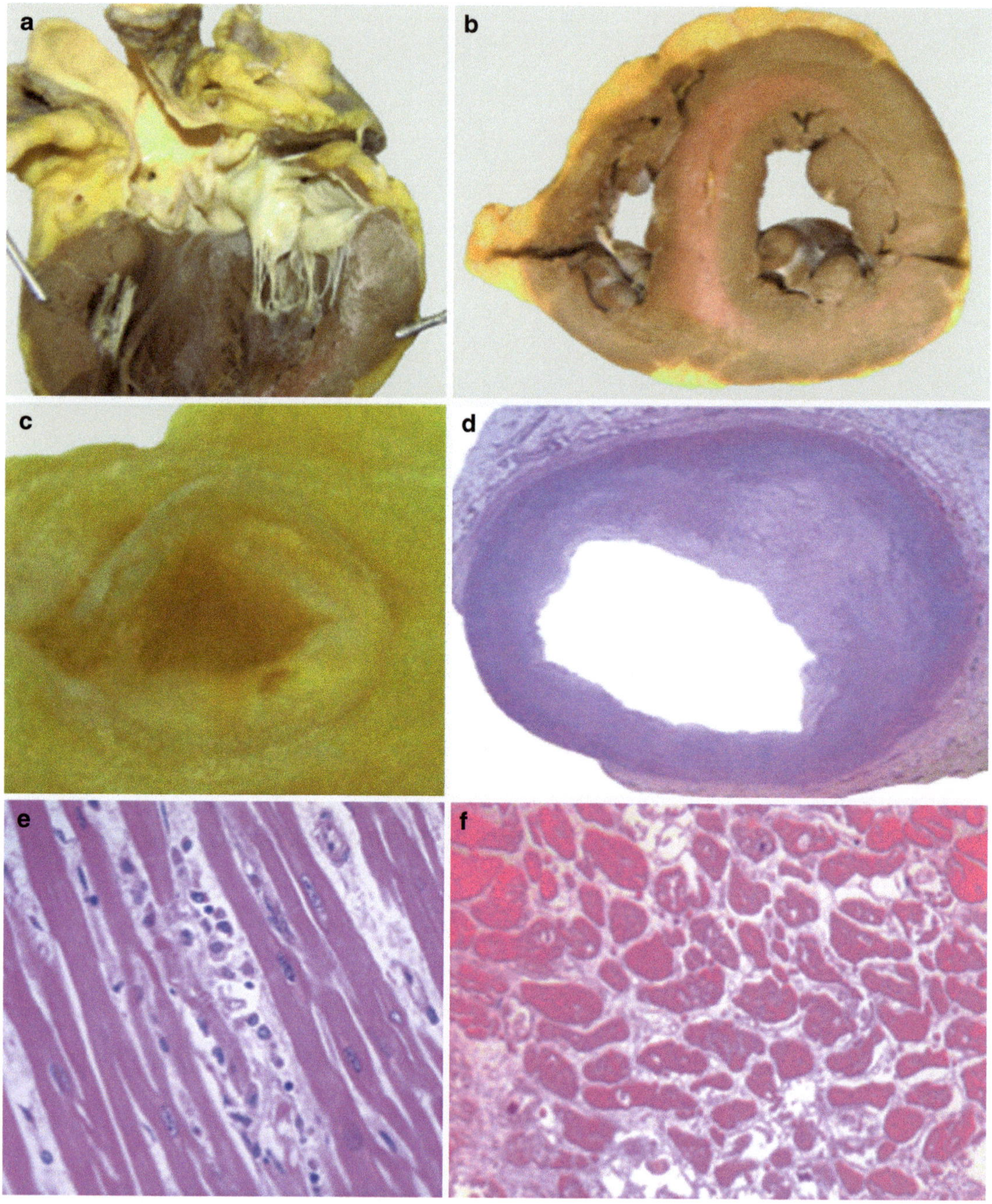

Fig. 7.10 Illustrative Case 2 Heart of a 59 year-old male donor (**a**, **b**). Stress echocardiography described stress-induced inferior wall motion and pathological examination showed 60% right coronary artery stenosis (**c**, **d**, Haematoxylin-eosin, 25×), diffuse cathecolamine necrosis (**e**, Haematoxylin-eosin, 400×) and ischemic necrosis in the inferior left ventricle papillary muscle (**f**, Haematoxylin-eosin, 200×)

Key Points

- Careful evaluation of donors and donor organs is essential for all solid organ transplantations, as their characteristics affect recipient outcome.
- In heart transplantation two further aspects are also crucial:
  1. Donor age, closely related to age-dependent risk of transmission of donor subclinical coronary artery atherosclerosis;
  2. Potentially reversible myocardial abnormalities consequent on brain death.
- Besides coronary artery atherosclerosis, arterial hypertension, diabetes mellitus, and left ventricular hypertrophy may also impact donor heart quality.
- General donor criteria to consider are: donor age; donor size and weight, donor history, cause of death, malignancies, donor infection status.
- In cardiac transplantation important information is derived from electrocardiography, echocardiography (now routinely performed in most hospitals), coronary angiography (should be performed whenever possible in cases with a high risk of CAD or signs of potential CAD at ECG or echocardiography, especially in older donors >55 years).
- Donor vasopressor (norepinephrine) and/or inotropic (dobutamin, dopamine) support is another essential issue for heart transplantation, as higher catecholamine dosage is associated with potential organ damage.
- Pathological assessment of heart biopsy is not part of the routine work-up as there are many limiting factors.
- Pathology abnormalities found in donor hearts can be subdivided as related to pathologies preexisting donation and pathologies arising in the course of donation.
- Some major points emerging from pathology examination of donor hearts are:
  - Coronary atherosclerosis is a major issue in older donors with a significant cardiovascular risk profile;
  - A significant number of the hearts from younger donors with a low cardiovascular risk profile are pathologically normal and potentially suitable for acceptance;
  - A need for better understanding of the phenomenon of cathecolamine-associated ventricular dysfunction and related myocardial damage which seems to be acquired during the process of brain death and donor management.

Acknowledgements Particular thanks go to Prof. Giorgio Arpesella, Head of Surgery Heart Transplant Unit of Bologna Sant'Orsola-Malpighi University Hospital until 2013, for his inspiration in creating the Adonhers project. Thanks also to Dr. Tonino Bombardini, Researcher of the Institute of Clinical Physiology-National Research Council, Pisa (Italy), for his assistance to Prof. Arpesella in setting up the project.

References

Abuanzeh R, Hashmi F, Dimarakis I, Khasati N, Machaal A, Yonan N, Venkateswaran RV. Early donor management increases the retrieval rate of hearts for transplantation in marginal donors. Eur J Cardiothorac Surg. 2015;47(1):72–7; discussion 77.

Ali AA, Lim E, Thanikachalam M, Sudarshan C, White P, Parameshwar J, Dhital K, Large SR. Cardiac arrest in the organ donor does not negatively influence recipient survival after heart transplantation. Eur J Cardiothorac Surg. 2007;31(5):929–33.

Balaz P, Rokosny S, Wohlfahrtova M, Wohlfahrt P, Bartonova A, Pokorna E, Honsova E, Viklicky O. Identification of expanded-criteria donor kidney grafts at lower risk of delayed graft function. Transplantation. 2013;96(7):633–8.

Berman M, Ali A, Ashley E, Freed D, Clarke K, Tsui S, Parameshwar J, Large S. Is stress cardiomyopathy the underlying cause of ventricular dysfunction associated with brain death? J Heart Lung Transplant. 2010;29(9):957–65.

Bombardini T, Gherardi S, Arpesella G, Maccherini M, Serra W, Magnani G, Del Bene R, Picano E. Favorable short-term outcome of transplanted hearts selected from marginal donors by pharmacological stress echocardiography. J Am Soc Echocardiogr. 2011;24(4):353–62.

Bombardini T, Arpesella G, Maccherini M, Procaccio F, Potena L, Bernazzali S, Leone O, Picano E. Medium-term outcome of recipients of marginal donor hearts selected with new stress-echocardiographic techniques over standard criteria. Cardiovasc Ultrasound. 2014;12:20–7.

Burke A, Tavora F, editors. Hypersensivity and toxic myocarditis, chap. 23. In: Practical cardiovascular pathology. Philadelphia: Lippincott Williams & Wilkins; 2001. p. 249.

Caforio AL, Tona F, Fortina AB, Angelini A, Piaserico S, Gambino A, Feltrin G, Ramondo A, Valente M, Iliceto S, Thiene G, Gerosa G. Immune and nonimmune predictors of cardiac allograft vasculopathy onset and severity: multivariate risk factor analysis and role of immunosuppression. Am J Transplant. 2004;4(6):962–70.

Casartelli M, Bombardini T, Simion D, Gaspari MG, Procaccio F. Wait, treat and see: echocardiographic monitoring of brain-dead potential donors with stunned heart. Cardiovasc Ultrasound. 2012;10:25–32.

Dark JH. Safe and effective use of the extended donor heart. Eur J Cardiothorac Surg. 2015;47(1):78–9.

Desai R, Collett D, Watson CJ, Johnson P, Evans T, Neuberger J. Estimated risk of cancer transmission from organ donor to graft recipient in a national transplantation registry. Br J Surg. 2014;101(7):768–74.

Doroshow RW, Ashwal S, Saukel GW. Availability and selection of donors for pediatric heart transplantation. J Heart Lung Transplant. 1995;14(1 Pt 1):52–8.

Dronavalli VB, Banner NR, Bonser RS. Assessment of the potential heart donor: a role for biomarkers? J Am Coll Cardiol. 2010;56:352–61.

Durand F, Renz JF, Alkofer B, Burra P, Clavien PA, Porte RJ, Freeman RB, Belghiti J. Report of the Paris consensus meeting on expanded criteria donors in liver transplantation. Liver Transpl. 2008;14:1694–707.

D'Alessandro AM, Kalayoglu M, Sollinger HW, Hoffman RM, Reed A, Knechtle SJ, et al. The predictive value of donor liver biopsies for the development of primary nonfunction after orthotopic liver transplantation. Transplantation. 1991;51:157–63.

Eskandary FA, Kohl M, Dunkler D, Aliabadi A, Grommer M, Schiferer A, Gokler J, Wieselthaler G, Laufer G, Zuckermann A. Lack of donor and recipient age interaction in cardiac transplantation. J Heart Lung Transplant. 2014;33(6):629–35.

Giavarini A, Chedid A, Bobrie G, et al. Acute cathecolamine cardiomyopathy in patients with phaeochromocytoma or functional paraganglioma. Heart. 2013;99:1438–44.

Goland S, Czer LS, Kass RM, Siegel RJ, Mirocha J, De Robertis MA, Lee J, Raissi S, Cheng W, Fontana G, Trento A. Use of cardiac allografts with mild and moderate left ventricular hypertrophy can be safely used in heart transplantation to expand the donor pool. J Am Coll Cardiol. 2008;51(12):1214–20.

Grauhan O, Siniawski H, Dandel M, Lehmkuhl H, Knosalla C, Pasic M, Weng YG, Hetzer R. Coronary atherosclerosis of the donor heart – impact on early graft failure. Eur J Cardiothorac Surg. 2007;32(4):634–8.

Hauptman PJ, O'Connor KJ, Wolf RE, McNeil BJ. Angiography of potential cardiac donors. J Am Coll Cardiol. 2001;37:1252–8.

Heng WL, Lai SH, Lim YP, Lim CH. The importance of histopathological examination for safety in heart valve transplantation – evaluation of histopathological findings in heart tissues from valve donors. J Cytol Histol. 2014;S4:003.

Hosenpud JD, Pantely GA, Morton MJ, Norman DJ, Cobanoglu AM, Starr A. Relation between recipient: donor body size match and hemodynamics three months after heart transplantation. J Heart Transplant. 1989;8(3):241–3.

Jochmans I, Pirenne J. Graft quality assessment in kidney transplantation: not an exact science yet! Curr Opin Organ Transplant. 2011;16(2):174–9.

Karamlou T, Shen I, Slater M, Crispell K, Chan B, Ravichandran P. Decreased recipient survival following orthotopic heart transplantation with use of hearts from donors with projectile brain injury. J Heart Lung Transplant. 2005;24(1):29–33.

Khush KK, Menza R, Nguyen J, Zaroff JG, Goldstein BA. Donor predictors of allograft use and recipient outcomes after heart transplantation. Circ Heart Fail. 2013;6(2):300–9.

Khush KK, Nguyen J, Goldstein BA, McGlothlin DP, Zaroff JG. Reliability of transthoracic echocardiogram interpretation in potential adult heart transplant donors. J Heart Lung Transplant. 2015;34(2):266–9.

Kransdorf EP, Stehlik J. Donor evaluation in heart transplantation: the end of the beginning. J Heart Lung Transplant. 2014;33:1105–13.

Kuppahally SS, Valantine HA, Weisshaar D, Parekh H, Hung YY, Haddad F, Fowler M, Vagelos R, Perlroth MG, Robbins RC, Hunt SA. Outcome in cardiac recipients of donor hearts with increased left ventricular wall thickness. Am J Transplant. 2007;7(10):2388–95.

Leone O, Gherardi S, Targa L, et al. Stress echocardiography as a gatekeeper to donation in aged marginal donor hearts: anatomic and pathologic correlations of abnormal stress echocardiography results. J Heart Lung Transplant. 2009;28:1141–9.

Li H, Tanaka K, Anzai H, Oeser B, Lai D, Kobashigawa JA, Tobis JM. Influence of pre-existing donor atherosclerosis on the development of cardiac allograft vasculopathy and outcomes in heart transplant recipients. J Am Coll Cardiol. 2006;47(12):2470–6.

Lietz K, John R, Mancini DM, et al. Outcomes in cardiac transplant recipients using allografts from older donors versus mortality on the waiting list. J Am Coll Cardiol. 2004;43:1553–61.

Lund LH, Edwards LB, Kucheryavaya AY, Benden C, Christie JD, Dipchand AI, Dobbels F, Goldfarb SB, Levvey BJ, Meiser B, Yusen RD, Stehlik J. The registry of the International Society for Heart and Lung Transplantation: thirty-first official adult heart transplant report – 2014; focus theme: retransplantation. J Heart Lung Transplant. 2014;33(10):996–1008.

Mackey-Bojack S, Roe S, Titus JL. Review of pathologic findings in remnant hearts following valve donation. J Forensic Sci. 2007;52(3):692–7.

Marelli D, Laks H, Fazio D, Moore S, Moriguchi J, Kobashigawa J. The use of donor hearts with left ventricular hypertrophy. J Heart Lung Transplant. 2000;19(5):496–503.

Markin RS, Wisecarver JL, Radio SJ, Stratta RJ, Langnas AN, Hirst K, et al. Frozen section evaluation of donor livers before transplantation. Transplantation. 1993;56:1403–9.

Mohamedali B, Bhat G, Tatooles A, Zelinger A. Neurogenic stress cardiomyopathy in heart donors. J Card Fail. 2014;20(3):207–11.

Patel ND, Weiss ES, Nwakanma LU, Russell SD, Baumgartner WA, Shah AS, Conte JV. Impact of donor-to-recipient weight ratio on survival after heart transplantation: analysis of the United Network for Organ Sharing Database. Circulation. 2008;118(14 Suppl):S83–8.

Pérez López S, Otero Hernández J, Vázquez Moreno N, Escudero Augusto D, Álvarez Menéndez F, Astudillo González A. brain death effects on catecholamine levels and subsequent cardiac damage assessed in organ donors. J Heart Lung Transplant. 2009;28:815–20.

Reed RM, Netzer G, Hunsicker L, Mitchell BD, Rajagopal K, Scharf S, Eberlein M. Cardiac size and sex-matching in heart transplantation: size matters in matters of sex and the heart. JACC Heart Fail. 2014;2(1):73–83.

Roig E, Almenar L, Crespo-Leiro M, Segovia J, Mirabet S, Delgado J, Perez-Villa F, Luis Lambert J, Teresa Blasco M, Muniz J, rest of the participants of the Spanish Heart Transplantation R. Heart transplantation using allografts from older donors: multicenter study results. J Heart Lung Transplant. 2015;34(6):790–6.

Sardesal SH, et al. Phaechromocytoma and catecholamine induced cardiomyopathy presenting as heart failure. Br Heart J. 1990;63:234–7.

Sethi GK, Lanauze P, Rosado LJ, Huston C, McCarthy MS, Butman S, Copeland JG. Clinical significance of weight difference between donor and recipient in heart transplantation. J Thorac Cardiovasc Surg. 1993;106(3):444–8.

Smits JM, De Pauw M, de Vries E, Rahmel A, Meiser B, Laufer G, Zuckermann A. Donor scoring system for heart transplantation and the impact on patient survival. J Heart Lung Transplant. 2012;31(4):387–97.

Stehlik J, Feldman DS, Brown RN, VanBakel AB, Russel SD, Ewald GA, Hagan ME, Folsom J, Kirklin JK. Interactions among donor characteristics influence post-transplant survival: a multi-institutional analysis. J Heart Lung Transplant. 2010;29(3):291–8.

Stone RJ, Basso C, Baandrup UT, Bruneval P, Butany J, Gallagher PJ, Halushka MK, Miller DV, Padera RF, Radio SJ, Sheppard MN, Suvarna K, Tan CD, Thiene G, van der Wal AC, Veinot JP. Recommendations for processing cardiovascular surgical pathology specimens: a consensus statement from the Standards and Definitions Committee of the Society for Cardiovascular Pathology and the Association for European Cardiovascular Pathology. Cardiovasc Pathol. 2012;21(1):2–16.

Van Geyt C, Van Wijk M, Bokhorst A, Beele H. Physical examination of the potential tissue donor, what do European tissue banks do? Clin Transplant. 2010;24(2):259–64.

Visser L, Holsboer E, Bokhorst AG, van Wijk MJ. The value of autopsy and other histological examinations for the safety of tissue transplantation. Cell Tissue Bank. 2012;13(1):37–46.

Warrens AN, Birch R, Collett D, Daraktchiev M, Dark JH, Galea G, Gronow K, Neuberger J, Hilton D, Whittle IR, Watson CJ, Advisory Committee on the Safety of Blood, Tissues and Organs, UK. Advising potential recipients on the use of organs from donors with primary central nervous system tumors. Transplantation. 2012;93(4):348–53.

Weiss ES, Allen JG, Patel ND, Russell SD, Baumgartner WA, Shah AS, Conte JV. The impact of donor-recipient sex matching on survival after orthotopic heart transplantation: analysis of 18 000 transplants in the modern era. Circ Heart Fail. 2009;2(5):401–8.

Wittwer T, Wahlers T. Marginal donor grafts in heart transplantation: lessons learned from 25 years experience. Transpl Int. 2008;21:113–25.

Young JB. Age before beauty: the use of 'older' donor hearts for cardiac transplantation. J Heart Lung Transplant. 1999;18:488–91.

Zaroff JG, Babcock WD, Shiboski SC. The impact of left ventricular dysfunction on cardiac donor transplant rates. J Heart Lung Transplant. 2003;22:334–7.

Donor Organ Harvesting and Preservation

8

Jonida Bejko, Giuseppe Feltrin, Annalisa Angelini, and Gino Gerosa

Contents

J. Bejko • G. Gerosa (✉)
Division of Cardiac Surgery, Department of Cardiac, Thoracic and Vascular Sciences, University of Padua, Padua, Italy
e-mail: gino.gerosa@unipd.it

G. Feltrin
Operative Unit of the Regional Center for Transplant Coordination, University of Padua, Padua, Italy

A. Angelini
Pathology of Cardiac Transplantation and Regenerative Medicine Unit, Department of Cardiac, Thoracic and Vascular Sciences, University of Padua, Padua, Italy

8.1 Background

Heart allograft preservation is essential to graft function and survival, and for long-term outcome (Demmy et al. 1997; Keck et al. 1994), but preservation injury and transplant ischemia–reperfusion injury (IRI) are unavoidable consequences of solid organ transplantation. Various strategies exist to overcome the problem (Breda et al 1989); currently, the most commonly used preservation method is static cold storage, although donor heart preservation is limited to 4–6 h of cold ischemia storage (Li et al. 2016). More than 150 preservation fluids, both intracellular or extracellular, based on their concentration of ions, exist, designed to attenuate the detrimental effects of cold storage and reperfusion (Jacobs et al. 2010; Jahania et al. 1999), but as yet no standard optimal solution has emerged.

Of course, as heart transplantations are relatively infrequent, there is a lack of high-quality randomized clinical trials that examine precise effects of the preservation fluids on graft function and survival. The main cause of primary graft dysfunction is IRI, which contributes to microvascular dysfunction and myocardial injury, thus activating proinflammatory and profibrotic processes and eventually leading to cardiac fibrosis and allograft vasculopathy (Stehlik et al. 2012). To cope with this, two basic strategies are combined to improve the results of donor heart preservation: shortening of cold ischemic time and refining preservation techniques.

O. Leone et al. (eds.), *The Pathology of Cardiac Transplantation*,
DOI 10.1007/978-3-319-46386-5_8

The shortage of donor organs is the other critical problem in heart transplantation. According to the Organ Procurement and Transplantation Network (OPTN), the number of registrations on the heart waiting list is approximately 3000 over a 3-year period, and 15% of patients die within 1-year waiting (Osaki et al. 2014). To maintain or increase the present transplantation rate, donation after cardiac death (DCD) has been proposed as another source, but there have been very few preliminary cases of hearts harvested from donors with cardiac death (Dhital et al. 2015), in combination with perfusion machines, like the Organ Care System (OCS) for ex-vivo perfusion of human donor hearts (Ardehali et al. 2015).

8.2 Principles of the Cold Ischemic Storage

The principle of cold ischemic storage is to maintain the heart graft at hypothermia between 4 and 8 °C to reduce metabolism. The chemical constituents of the fluid maintain viability of the structural components of the tissue and reduce the IRI, thus preserving graft function with rapid cessation of electrical activity (Belzer and Southard 1988). Cold storage solutions can be divided into two categories based on different concentrations of Na^+ and K^+ ions, as shown in Table 8.1. Other components such as impermeants, free radical scavengers, metabolic nutrients, and various acid buffers are added to reduce the negative effects of hypothermia and ischemia. Hypothermia per se does not stop metabolism, but it slows biochemical intracellular reactions and decreases the rate at which intracellular enzymes released by organelles can exert their effects (which can lead to cell death.) Most enzymes of hypothermic animals show a twofold decrease in activity for every 10 °C decrease in temperature (Jahania et al. 1999). Hypothermia remains one of the most important tools for organ preservation.

Preservation fluids can be grouped into "intracellular type" (e.g. University of Wisconsin Solution—UW standard, Roe Solution, Collins Solution, and Intracellular Stanford Solution) which mimic the interior cellular ionic milieu, and "extracellular type" (e.g. Celsior Solution, Krebs Solution, and St. Thomas Hospital Solution) where ionic concentrations are similar to those of extracellular fluids.

Table 8.1 Various preservation fluids and their potassium and sodium concentrations

Solution	Type	Na^+ (mmol/L)	K^+ (mmol/L)
Krebs	Extracellular	118	5
Bretschneider	Intracellular	15	8
Celsior	Extracellular	100	15
St. Thomas	Extracellular	100	16
Plegisol	Extracellular	110	16
Roe	Intracellular	27	20
UW (modified)	Extracellular	125	25
UW (standard)	Intracellular	25	125
NIH	Extracellular	77	30
Stanford	Intracellular	28	30
Collins	Intracellular	10	115
Collins–Sachs	Intracellular	10	115
EuroCollins	Intracellular	10	115

UW University of Wisconsin

Several clinical studies have found better results with intracellular solutions than with the extracellular type (Jahania et al. 1999). The benefits of intracellular type fluids may be due to their ability to induce more rapid and complete cardiac arrest and to prevent intracellular edema.

Although hypothermia and cold ischemic storage delay cell death, a number of processes are activated that can ultimately damage the preserved organ (Table 8.2) (Jahania et al. 1999). Cooling reduces glucose utilization, adversely alters intracellular hydrogen regulation, and slows tissue oxygen uptake. Under 12 °C, hemoglobin can no longer contribute to oxygen delivery, and activity of mitochondrial enzymes declines with the ultimate result of mitochondrial ATP depletion.

8.3 Preservation Solutions

In the 1990s, there were many attempts to find the best Heart Preservation Solutions (HPSs) (more than 167) (Demmy et al. 1997). Of the following three, two mainly intracellular types and

Table 8.2 Deleterious processes activated by hypothermia and cold ischemic storage and strategies to contrast them

Processes	Mechanism involved	Strategies to contrast them
Cellular swelling	Na–K ATPase pump suppression	Impermeants and colloids addition
Extracellular edema	Excessive hydrostatic force during flushing with the preservation solution	Impermeants addition and colloids addition
Intracellular acidosis	Lactic acid accumulation due to anaerobic glycolysis	Provision of glucose in large concentrations and/or addition of hydrogen ion buffers
Reperfusion injury	Production of free radicals via the hypoxanthine–xanthine oxidase reaction	Administration of exogenous antioxidants (glutathione), antioxidant, and free radical scavengers
Calcium overload	Compromised sarcoplasmic reticulum Ca^{2+} pumps	Addition of calcium channel blockers and enhancement of endogenous adenosine levels
Endothelial injury	Reduced production of endothelium-dependent nitric oxide (EDNO), endothelium-dependent hyperpolarization factor (EDHF) as side effect of hyperkalemic preservation	–

one of extracellular type are widely used: histidine–tryptophan–ketoglutarate (HTK) solution, the University of Wisconsin (UW) solution, and Celsior solution.

HTK (or Custodiol) was first proposed by Bretschneider in the 1970s as a cardioplegic solution and was later adopted for the preservation of solid organs too. In heart transplantation, a single dose of cold HTK is injected into the coronary vascular tree to ensure adequate protection from IRI for at least 2 h.

UW, first proposed by Belzer, has a low Na^+ concentration. Nowadays, an extracellular modification, which includes 125 mmol/l Na^+, is also used.

Other notable intracellular solutions are the Euro-Collins and the Stanford ones. The former has high glucose (194 mmol/l) and K^+ (115 mmol/l) concentrations as well as bicarbonate and phosphate buffer systems. The latter is similar to Euro-Collins but has an even higher glucose level (250 mmol/l) and a lower K^+ concentration (27 mmol/l), in order to prevent edema.

The most common extracellular HPS is Celsior, with its high Na+, low K+ concentrations, and 20 mmol/l glutamate components, which can be enriched with lactobionate and glutathione to contrast oxidative stress during reperfusion.

As large-scale clinical trials are lacking due to the relatively few numbers of cardiac transplants worldwide, an effective comparison of HPSs is difficult.

What studies exist are retrospective, with clinical data reported in various ways, with different inclusion criteria, nonrandomized trials of specific preservation solution.

Table 8.3 summarizes some of the more interesting studies and their results.

8.4 Improving Donor Heart Outcomes

There are many strategies to improve donor heart outcomes, such as reducing the ischemic time, optimizing the preservation solutions, improving heart perfusion, persufflating the heart with gaseous oxygen, and pre- and postconditioning of heart grafts.

The most effective way to increase donor heart viability would doubtless be to limit ischemia time, but in the vast majority of cases, this is impossible for technical and logistical reasons.

Hence, several new alternative approaches have been suggested and experimentally validated in recent decades to guarantee protection and extend time intervals. These include

Table 8.3 Comparison of different heart preservation solutions

Authors	Reference	Solutions	No of pts	Results
Stein et al.	*J Thorac Cardiovasc Surgery* 1991;102:657–65 (Randomized trial)	UW vs Stanford	29 (14/15)	Similar histological ischemic damage. Superiority of UW for improving end-ischemic ATP and creatine phosphate levels, and decreasing defibrillations and intraoperative pacing
George TJ	*J Heart Lung Transplant* 2011;30:1033–43. Retrospective study	UW vs Celsior	4910 (3107/1803)	UW better survival at 30 days and 1 year
Wildhirt SM	*Transpl Int* 2000; 13:S203–11. A single center, prospective randomized trial	UW vs Celsior	41 (20/21)	UW causes less IRI, and requires less vasodilator and catecholamine dosages ET and iNOS gene expression higher in Celsior
Cannata A	*Eur J Cardiothorac Surg* 2012;41:e48–52. Retrospective cohort study	HTK, Celsior, and STH2	133 (61/38)	No difference in outcomes (mortality and biventricular GF)
Lee KC	*Transplant Proc* 2012; 44:886–9.	Combined STH2 and HTK	31 pts	Short-term survival similar to other approaches
Li Y	*Artif Organs*. 2015 Nov 2. Review meta-analysis	UW, Celsior, and HTK	UW vs Celsior: 5301 heart UW vs HTK: 1091 heart HTK vs Celsior:147	UW: better survival and less ischemic damage on EMBs vs Celsior UW: better survival vs HTK HTK vs Celsior: no difference
Kur F	*Transplant Proc* 2009;41:2247–9	UW in extended ischemic time	34 > 5 h 103 < 5 h	UW better protection
Stringham JK	*J Heart Lung Transplant* 1999;18:587–96	UW vs HTK	1091	UW better survival and better graft function
Kofler S	*Transpl Int* 2009;22:1140–50. Retrospective single-center study	UW vs HTK	1000 (628/254)	UW decreased early mortality and better long-term survival: At 1 year, UW 80.1 % vs HKT 66.1 %; At 15 years, UW 46.4 % vs HTK 36.4 %
Reichenspuruer H	*Transpl Int* 1994;7:S481–4. Retrospective single-center study	UW vs HTK	209 (61/38)	UW better outcomes (better early survival at 30 days—90 % vs 81 %; at 6 months—88 % vs 78 %)

Table 8.4 Strategies to improve donor heart outcomes

Improvements of heart preservation solutions
Supplementation with anti-ischemic agents
New formulations of heart preservation solutions
Hyperpolarizing heart preservation solutions
Donor heart preservation at subzero temperature
Donor heart perfusion
TransMedics Organ Care System
Perfusion (persufflation) of donor heart with gaseous oxygen
Pre- and postconditioning of cardiac graft

improved heart preservation solutions, pre- and postconditioning of the cardiac graft, and most especially machine perfusion of donor hearts (Table 8.4),

8.4.1 Improvements in Heart Preservation Solutions

HPS have been modified to obtain better anti-ischemic effects. Besides the principal components of each (listed below), other substances have been added primarily to increase buffer capacity for cardioprotection and support ATP production, and also to prevent intracellular edema, favor endothelial function, and stabilize osmolality. These have been tested in preclinical models, and include: diadenosine tetraphosphate, cariporide and diazoxide, cyclosporin A, cariporide, U74389G: 16-desmethyl tirilazad, recombinant human hepatocyte growth factor, glyceryl trinitrate and cariporide, taurine, nucleoside–nucleotide mixture, tetrahydrobiopterin, INO-1153, hydrogen sulfide donor, bisindolylmaleimide derivative, carbon monoxide-releasing molecule (CORM-3), iloprost, Rho-kinase inhibitor, small interfering RNA, epoxomicin, pinacidil, neuregulin-1, glyceryl trinitrate, cariporide, levocarnitine, clusterin, hydrogen (1.27 ± 0.05 μg/l), erythropoietin (5 U/ml), doxycycline, levosimendan (from Minasian et al. 2015). Whether cardiac grafts from marginal donors can be protected against IRI to the same extent remains to be seen (Minasian et al. 2015).

Other new extracellular solutions are enriched with energy substrates, metabolic modulators, antioxidants, L-arginine, and phosphate and bicarbonate buffers, so producing better viability of cardiac myocytes and endothelial cells (Lowalekar et al. 2014; Desrois et al. 2008; Wakayama et al. 2012; Loganathan et al. 2010; Hoenicke et al. 2000; Snabaitis et al. 1997; Rudd and Dobson 2011).

Another technique to minimize cardiac energy demand by graft cooling to subzero temperatures has been experimented on animals. To prevent freezing-mediated irreversible cell injury, preservation solutions have been supplemented with antifreeze proteins with cryoprotective properties resulting in better LV function after ischemia (Balfoussia et al. 2012).

8.4.2 Pre- and Post-conditioning of Cardiac Graft

Ischemic preconditioning aims to protect the myocardium from prolonged ischemic injury by using brief episodes of nonlethal ischemia; ischemic postconditioning acts during the reperfusion phase by briefly interrupting reperfusion after ischemic episodes in order to reduce myocardial injury. A large body of experimental evidence suggests that preconditioning and postconditioning protocols are the most effective endogenous cardioprotective techniques to obtain improved postischemic left ventricle functional recovery, to suppress reperfusion arrhythmias, and to reduce superoxide anion production (Murry et al. 1986; Jennings et al. 1991; Kloner and Jennings 2001; Galagudza et al. 2008; Karck et al. 1996; Landymore et al. 1998; Kevelaitis et al. 2001; Lauzier et al. 2007). Even with these techniques and the encouraging experimental results, donor heart preconditioning and postconditioning have yet to be tested on humans.

8.4.3 Donor Heart Perfusion

The idea of ex vivo heart perfusion with blood or crystalloid perfusion fluid is not new, but dates from the early heart transplant era. Due to high costs and technical complexity, however, it was soon supplanted by cardiac arrest and static cold storage. More recently, the idea of machine perfusion has been revived. There are two different approaches: (1) continuous perfusion of the arrested heart by oxygenated cold CPS and (2) perfusion of the beating heart with blood at normothermia, which requires monitoring of heart viability.

In perfusion, the perfusate is a proprietary priming solution with the addition of insulin, antibiotics, methylprednisolone, sodium bicarbonate, multivitamins, and fresh donor blood. Pulsatile flow is generated by a diaphragmatic pump, and an integrated plate heater maintains normothermia. At present, two randomized clinical trials to evaluate new heart perfusion systems are underway: the Transmedics organ care system (Transmedics, Inc., USA) and the LifeCradle® system (Organ Transport Systems, Inc., USA) to support heart function during transportation (Minasian et al. 2015). Experiments on pig hearts have shown better preservation of myocardial ultrastructure and less endothelial dysfunction with 4 h ex vivo oxygenated hypothermic perfusion compared to SCS in Celsior solution (Michel et al. 2014).

Cold ischemia time in the Organ Care System group is limited to the obligatory initial retrieval (i.e. the time needed to harvest and instrument the heart into the Organ Care System) and final re-implantation phases. Keeping the cold ischemia time within a reasonable range (6 h) could favor long-distance procurements, increase sharing of donor hearts to balance differences in donor heart availability, and allow donor and recipient HLA matching. Other potential benefits might include resuscitation of unused or unacceptable hearts with expansion of the donor pool (Ardehali et al. 2015).

Another possible way to ensure adequate oxygen delivery to the heart during transportation and to avoid possible myocardial hypoxia during static cold storage is persufflation of the donor heart with humidified gaseous oxygen into the coronary vascular bed (Suszynski et al. 2013; Tsutsumi et al. 2001). However, despite the promising experimental data (Fischer et al. 2004), oxygen persufflation (PSF) is not currently a valid clinical option due to the threat of endothelial injury.

8.5 Cardiac Donation After Circulatory Death

The first human heart transplantation by Christian Barnard used a cardiac death (CD) donor (Barnard 1967). CD donors were used before the law permitted the use of brain dead donors. Now, CD donors have again been proposed to increase the donor organ pool.

According to 1995 Maastricht classification, cardiac donors after circulatory death are subdivided into uncontrolled and controlled donors based on circumstances of death. Uncontrolled donors are dead on arrival (category I) or were resuscitated without success (category II). Controlled donors are classed according to the circumstances of cardiac arrest: category III—an awaited cardiac arrest follows withdrawal of care; category IV—cardiac arrest develops after brain death (Kootstra et al. 1995). Withdrawal of donor treatment (usually in the intensive care unit or operating room) is a controlled CD technique and the only one currently used in the United States.

In 2000, a new category was added (category V—unexpected cardiac arrest in a hospital patient) which allows better evaluation of outcomes (Sanchez-Fructuoso et al. 2000; Morrissey and Monaco 2014). Category III CDs could potentially be used for clinical heart transplantation.

However, many of the pretreatments used in experimental animal models would be ethically unacceptable in humans.

The major cause of CD graft deterioration is warm ischemic injury which produces a more severe injury than does cold ischemia. Warm ischemia, commonly defined as the interval between withdrawal of therapy and start of cold perfusion for organ preservation, is unavoidable during donation after cardiac death or circulatory arrest (Osaki et al. 2014). Warm ischemia leads to a depletion of ATP, anaerobic metabolism, and development of intracellular acidosis, with myocyte death after reperfusion. Moreover, CD hearts support the entire circulatory load in an increasingly hypoxic environment.

In 2015, Dhital et al. published three cases of successful heart transplants from CD donors; the innovative aspect was that all transplants were performed following distant procurement with normothermic machine perfusion (Dhital et al. 2015).

Now, a multicenter program of heart transplantation from DCD donors has started in the United Kingdom (Macdonald 2016).

Portable ex vivo heart perfusion systems have the advantage of delivering pharmaceutical agents to support reparative processes in ischemic myocardium and of allowing assessment of graft function before transplantation. Although normothermic machine perfusion has dramatically changed organ procurement, many questions, both ethical and procedural, still remain on how best to manage the hearts from CD donors. (Macdonald 2016; White et al. 2013; Iyer et al. 2014) At present, most researchers agree that a warm ischemic time of 30 min is probably the upper limit before the heart starts to suffer irreversible ischemic injury.

Key Points

- Cold ischemic storage is based on two principles:
  - Preservation hypothermia at 4–8 °C (delays cell death)
  - Use of preservation solutions (facilitate rapid cessation of electrical activity and myocardial contraction)
- The formulation of the preservation solution is based on three principles:
  - Hypothermic arrest of metabolism
  - A physical and biochemical environment that maintains viability of the structural components of the tissue during hypothermic metabolic arrest
  - Minimization of the effects of reperfusion injury
- Cold storage solutions can be divided into:
  - Intracellular type: solutions which mimic the interior cellular ionic milieu (Bretschneider, Roe, Stanford, Collins, Collins-Sachs, EuroCollins, University of Wisconsin—UW Standard), thereby ensuring rapid cardiac mechanical arrest and less intracellular edema
  - Extracellular type with ionic concentrations similar to extracellular fluid (Krebs, Celsior, St. Thomas, Plegisol, UW (modified), NIH)
- Portable ex vivo heart perfusion systems may help to:
  - Facilitate the delivery of pharmaceutical agents that support reparative processes
  - Assess graft function before transplantation
- The major cause of CD graft deterioration is warm ischemic injury (commonly defined as the interval between extubation—definitive withdrawal of treatment—and the initiation of cold perfusion for organ preservation)
  - A warm ischemic time of 30 min is probably the upper limit before the heart starts to suffer irreversible ischemic injury
  - Other variables that may affect the extent of ischemia–reperfusion injury:
    - Temperature of the perfusate
    - Oxygen content of the perfusate
    - Initial perfusion pressure

References

Ardehali A, Esmailian F, Deng M, Soltesz E, Hsich E, Naka Y, Mancini D, Camacho M, Zucker M, Leprince P, Padera R, Kobashigawa J, PROCEED II trial investigators. Ex-vivo perfusion of donor hearts for human heart transplantation (PROCEED II): a prospective, open-label, multicentre, randomised non-inferiority trial. Lancet. 2015;385:2577–84.

Balfoussia D, Yerrakalva D, Hamaoui K, Papalois V. Advances in machine perfusion graft viability assessment in kidney, liver, pancreas, lung, and heart transplant. Exp Clin Transplant. 2012;10:87–100.

Barnard CN. The operation. A human cardiac transplant: an interim report of a successful operation performed at Groote Schuur Hospital, Cape Town. S Afr Med J. 1967;41:1271–4.

Belzer FO, Southard JH. Principles of solid organ preservation by cold. Overview. Transplantation. 1988;45: 673–6.

Breda MA, Drinkwater DC, Laks H, Bhuta S, Corno A. Prevention of reperfusion injury in the neonatal heart with leukocyte depleted blood. J Thorac Cardiovasc Surg. 1989;97:654–65.

Demmy TL, Biddle JS, Bennet LE, Walls JT, Schmaltz RA, Curtis JJ. Organ preservation solutions in heart transplantation—patterns of usage and related survival. Transplantation. 1997;63:262–9.

Desrois M, Caus T, Belles PM, Dalmasso C, Lan C, Cozzone PJ, Bernard M. Limitation of myocardial and endothelial injury of the rat heart graft after preservation with Centre de Resonance Magnetique Biologique et Medicale (CRMB) solution. Transpl Int. 2008;21:276–83.

Dhital KK, Iyer A, Connellan M, Chew HC, Gao L, Doyle A, Hicks M, Kumarasinghe G, Soto C, Dinale A, Cartwright B, Nair P, Granger E, Jansz P, Jabbour A, Kotlyar E, Keogh A, Hayward C, Graham R, Spratt P, Macdonald P. Adult heart transplantation with distant procurement and ex-vivo preservation of donor hearts after circulatory death: a case series. Lancet. 2015;385: 2585–91.

Fischer JH, Funcke C, Yotsumoto G, Jeschkeit-Schubbert S, Kuhn-Rǧgnier F. Maintenance of physiological coronary endothelial function after 3.3 h of hypothermic oxygen persufflation preservation and orthotopic transplantation of non-heart-beating donor hearts. Eur J Cardiothorac Surg. 2004;25:98–104.

Galagudza MM, Blokhin IO, Shmonin AA, Mischenko KA. Reduction of myocardial ischemia-reperfusion injury with pre- and postconditioning: molecular mechanisms and therapeutic targets. Cardiovasc Hematol Disord Drug Targets. 2008;8:47–65.

Hoenicke EM, Sun X, Strange Jr RG, Damiano Jr RJ. Donor heart preservation with a novel hyperpolarizing solution: superior protection compared with University of Wisconsin solution. J Thorac Cardiovasc Surg. 2000;120:746–54.

Iyer A, Gao L, Doyle A, Rao P, Jayewardene D, Wan B, Kumarasinghe G, Jabbour A, Hicks M, Jansz PC, Feneley MP, Harvey RP, Graham RM, Dhital KK, Macdonald PSL. Increasing the tolerance of DCD hearts to warm ischemia by pharmacological postconditioning. Am J Transplant. 2014;14:1744–52.

Jacobs S, Rega F, Meyns B. Current preservation technology and future prospects of thoracic organs. Part 2: heart. Curr Opin Organ Transplant. 2010;15:156–9.

Jahania MS, Sanchez JA, Narayan P, Lasley RD, Mentzer Jr RM. Heart preservation for transplantation: principles and strategies. Ann Thorac Surg. 1999;68:1983–7.

Jennings RB, Murry CE, Reimer KA. Preconditioning myocardium with ischemia. Cardiovasc Drugs Ther. 1991;5(5):933–8.

Karck M, Rahmanian P, Haverich A. Ischemic preconditioning enhances donor heart preservation. Transplantation. 1996;62:17–22.

Keck BM, White R, Breen TJ, Daily OP, Hosenpud JD. Thoracic organ transplants in the United States: a report from the UNOS/ISHLT Scientific Registry for Organ Transplants, United Network for Organ Sharing, International Society for Heart and Lung Transplantation. Clin Transplant. 1994;26:37–46.

Kevelaitis E, Oubenaissa A, Mouas C, Peynet J, Menaché P. Ischemic preconditioning with opening of mitochondrial adenosine triphosphate-sensitive potassium channels or Na/H exchange inhibition: which is the best protective strategy for heart transplants? J Thorac Cardiovasc Surg. 2001;121:155–62.

Kloner RA, Jennings RB. Consequences of brief ischemia: stunning, preconditioning, and their clinical implications: Part 1. Circulation. 2001;104:2981–9.

Kootstra G, Daemen JH, Oomen AP. Categories of non-heart-beating donors. Transplant Proc. 1995;27:2893–4.

Landymore RW, Bayes AJ, Murphy JT, Fris JH. Preconditioning prevents myocardial stunning after cardiac transplantation. Ann Thorac Surg. 1998;66:1953–7.

Lauzier B, Sicard P, Bouchot O, Delemasure S, Menetrier F, Moreau D, Vergely C, Rochette L. After four hours of cold ischemia and cardioplegic protocol, the heart can still be rescued with postconditioning. Transplantation. 2007;84:1474–82.

Li Y, Guo S, Liu G, Yuan Y, Wang W, Zheng Z, Hu S, Ji B. Three preservation solutions for cold storage of heart allografts: a systematic review and meta-analysis. Artif Organs. 2016;40(5):489–96.

Loganathan S, Radovits T, Hirschberg K, Korkmaz S, Koch A, Karck M, Szabó G. Effects of Custodiol-N, a novel organ preservation solution, on ischemia/ reperfusion injury. J Thorac Cardiovasc Surg. 2010;139: 1048–56.

Lowalekar SK, Cao H, Lu XG, Treanor PR, Thatte HS. Sub-normothermic preservation of donor hearts for transplantation using a novel solution, Somah: a comparative pre-clinical study. J Heart Lung Transplant. 2014;33:963–70.

Macdonald P. Heart transplantation from donation after circulatory death: the impact of global warming. Am J Transplant. 2016;16(3):737–8.

Michel SG, La Muraglia 2nd GM, Madariaga ML, Titus JS, Selig MK, Farkash EA, Allan JS, Anderson LM, Madsen JC. Preservation of donor hearts using hypothermic oxygenated perfusion. Ann Transplant. 2014;19:409–16.

Minasian SM, Galagudza MM, Dmitriev YV, Karpov AA, Vlasov TD. Preservation of the donor heart: from basic science to clinical studies. Interact Cardiovasc Thorac Surg. 2015;20:510–9.

Morrissey PE, Monaco AP. Donation after circulatory death: current practices, ongoing challenges and potential improvements. Transplantation. 2014;97:258–64.

Murry CE, Jennings RB, Reimer KA. Preconditioning with ischemia: a delay of lethal cell injury in ischemic myocardium. Circulation. 1986;74:1124–36.

Osaki S, Locher MR, Lushaj EB, Akhter SA, Kohmoto T. Functional evaluation of human donation after cardiac death donor hearts using a continuous isolated myocardial perfusion technique: potential for expansion of the cardiac donor population. J Thorac Cardiovasc Surg. 2014;148.

Rudd DM, Dobson GP. Eight hours of cold static storage with adenosine and lidocaine (Adenocaine) heart preservation solutions: toward therapeutic suspended animation. J Thorac Cardiovasc Surg. 2011;142:1552–61.

Sanchez-Fructuoso AI, Prats D, Torrente J, Perez-Contin MJ, Fernandez C, Alvarez J, Barrientos A. Renal transplantation from non-heart beating donors: a promising alternative to enlarge the donor pool. J Am Soc Nephrol. 2000;11:350–8.

Snabaitis AK, Shattock MJ, Chambers DJ. Comparison of polarized and depolarized arrest in the isolated rat heart for long-term preservation. Circulation. 1997;96:3148–56.

Stehlik J, Edwards LB, Kucheryavaya AY, Benden C, Christie JD, Dipchand AI, Dobbels F, Kirk R, Rahmel AO, Hertz MI. The Registry of the International Society for Heart and Lung Transplantation: 29th official adult heart transplant report—2012. J Heart Lung Transplant. 2012;31:1052–64, 1123–30.

Suszynski TM, Rizzari MD, Scott WE, Eckman PM, Fonger JD, John R, Chronos N, Tempelman LA, Sutherland DE, Papas KK. Persufflation (gaseous oxygen perfusion) as a method of heart preservation. J Cardiothorac Surg. 2013;8:105.

Tsutsumi H, Oshima K, Mohara J, Takevoshi I, Aizaki M, Tokumine M, Matsumoto K, Morishita Y. Cardiac transplantation following a 24-h preservation using a perfusion apparatus. J Surg Res. 2001;96:260–7.

Wakayama K, Fukai M, Yamashita K, Kimura T, Hirokata G, Shibasaki S, Fukumori D, Haga S, Sugawara M, Suzuki T, Taniguchi M, Shimamura T, Furukawa H, Ozaki M, Kamyama T, Todo S. Successful transplantation of rat hearts subjected to extended cold preservation with a novel preservation solution. Transpl Int. 2012;25:696–706.

White CW, Ali A, Hasanally D, Xiang B, Li Y, Mundt P, Lytwyn M, Colah S, Klein J, Ravandi A, Arora RC, Lee TW, Hryshko L, Large S, Tian G, Freed DH. A cardioprotective preservation strategy employing ex vivo heart perfusion facilitates successful transplant of donor hearts after cardiocirculatory death. J Heart Lung Transplant. 2013;32:734–43.

Perioperative Myocardial Damage to the Graft

9

Annalisa Angelini and Marny Fedrigo

Contents

A. Angelini (✉)
Pathology of Cardiac Transplantation and Regenerative Medicine Unit, Department of Cardiac, Thoracic and Vascular Sciences, University of Padua, Padua, Italy
e-mail: annalisa.angelini@unipd.it

M. Fedrigo
Cardiovascular Pathology Unit, Department of Cardiac, Thoracic and Vascular Sciences, Azienda Ospedaliera Padua, Padua, Italy

9.1 Background

Perioperative myocardial damage encompasses all the injuries to the cardiac allograft, which can be found up to 6 weeks after transplantation (Stewart et al. 2005) as the result of various noxae affecting the graft prior to transplantation, during procurement and transplantation of graft, and immediately after transplantation due to recipient's general condition (Table 9.1).

These injuries all produce ischemic or ischemic-like myocardial damage, which can

Table 9.1 Conditions which could produce perioperative myocardial damage

Prior to transplantation, donor related
Hypovolemia/hypoxia
Catecholamine storm
Vasoconstriction related to drugs
Fluctuation in hormones
Electrolyte imbalance
Donor native atherosclerotic coronary disease
At harvesting and transplantation
Warm ischemia
Cold ischemia with preservation solution
Warm ischemia at transplantation
Reperfusion process
Immediately posttransplantation
Drug-related if graft failure occurs
Recipient's general condition (catecholamines, proinflammatory status related to left ventricular assist device (LVAD), hormonal imbalance, etc.)

O. Leone et al. (eds.), *The Pathology of Cardiac Transplantation*,
DOI 10.1007/978-3-319-46386-5_9

affect graft integrity of varying severity. When extensive, they can have short- or long-term effects. A most undesirable result would be graft failure, even occasionally requiring mechanical circulatory support; there is still little data on long-term effects.

9.2 Epidemiological Data

There are little accurate data on the exact incidence of perioperative myocardial injury at endomyocardial biopsy (EMB) or at autopsy following early death after heart transplantation, because the causes are numerous and change over time.

In recent years, donor and recipient inclusion criteria have significantly changed: suboptimal grafts are increasingly used to expand the donor pool; patient management strategy in Intensive Care Unit (ICU) has improved; the introduction of the continuous perfusion machine during procurement allows better preservation of hearts. Finally, there are also new perfusion and preservation solutions and techniques, which have changed the extent and severity of ischemic damage.

In the past, the focus was on finding the best preservation solution for harvesting (see Chap. 8) (Livi et al. 1993; George et al. 2012).

In the late 1990s some degree of perioperative myocardial damage was reported in nearly 90 % of EMBs performed within the first 4 weeks, and cardiomyocyte necrosis in two-thirds of EMBs performed in the first week after orthotopic heart transplantation (Fyfe et al. 1996).

As different centers vary in their protocols and strategies for organ procurement and harvesting, and for donor management, large-scale data are really difficult to collect and compare.

9.3 Histopathological Substrates

Perioperative myocardial damage is heterogeneous and not always easily recognizable (Figs. 9.1 and 9.2). It is characterized by focal or diffuse interstitial edema, contraction band

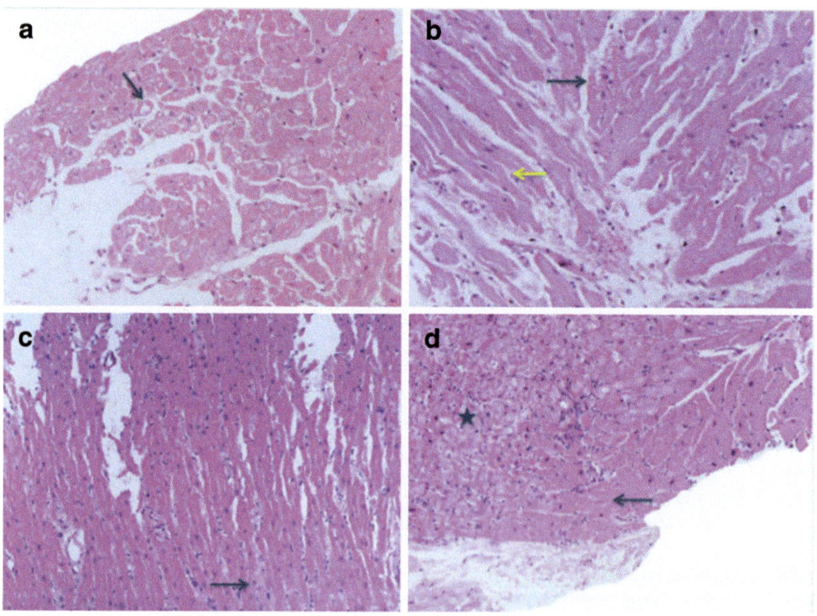

Fig. 9.1 (**a**) Diffuse interstitial edema dissociating the cardiomyocytes and vacuolization of cardiomyocytes (*arrow*). Hematoxylin–eosin staining; original magnification ×125. (**b**) Focal cardiomyocyte necrosis (*blue arrow*) and attenuated cardiomyocytes which appear elongated due to coagulative necrosis (*yellow arrow*). Hematoxylin–eosin staining; original magnification ×160. (**c**) Diffuse edema dissociating the cardiomyocytes may sometimes appear as loose connective tissue resembling early interstitial fibrosis (*arrow*). Hematoxylin–eosin staining; original magnification ×125. (**d**) Focal small subendocardial aggregates of cardiomyocytes with coagulative necrosis (*arrow*), contraction band necrosis (*asterisk*) and a few inflammatory cells encroaching on a few cardiomyocytes in the border zone between subendocardial coagulative necrosis and contraction band necrosis. Hematoxylin–eosin staining, original magnification ×160.

necrosis, foci of coagulative myocardial cell necrosis, either isolated or more often clustered in small groups, myocytolysis, and inflammation.

The inflammatory infiltrate consists mainly of polymorphonuclear leucocytes and macrophages, possibly including some lymphocytes and plasma cells, which enlarges the interstitium without encroaching on the adjacent viable myocardium, and normally separate from it. The inflammatory cell infiltrate is heterogeneously located, scattered in the interstitium, preferably perivascular, and mainly in the subendocardial regions, associated to cardiomyocyte necrosis or myocytolysis. Usually, a sharp border between the inflammatory cells and the viable myocytes is found.

Myocyte hypereosinophilia with pyknotic nuclei, stretched and vacuolated myocytes, loss of nuclei, and loss of cytoplasmic detail can easily be seen on hematoxylin–eosin; a trichrome stain can highlight these lesions as it stains the affected myocytes blue–gray.

Contraction band necrosis can be present in reperfusion injury areas (Baroldi et al. 2003): this lesion may sometimes be difficult to distinguish from hypercontracted myocytes, which are often seen at EMBs in viable myocardium.

Fyfe et al. proposed a four-point semiquantitative score (0: absent; 1: mild focal; 2: moderate multifocal; 3: severe confluent) to grade the severity and extent of coagulative myocyte necrosis related to perioperative injury.

Myocytolysis or myocyte vacuolization, especially when confined to the subendocardium or perilesional areas, is sometimes considered stunning myocardium in the sense that the myocytes may be recuperated.

Interstitial edema can be focal or diffuse and is characterized by an increase in interstitial empty space with separation of cardiomyocytes, but it is difficult to assess at EMBs because of technical artifacts.

Vascular damage can be present as well and characterized by endothelial swelling, leucocytes adhering to the endothelium, and clustered inside the vessel, sometimes infiltrating the vessel wall resulting in vasculitis, and, more rarely, by microthrombosis in intramyocardial arterioles and small arteries.

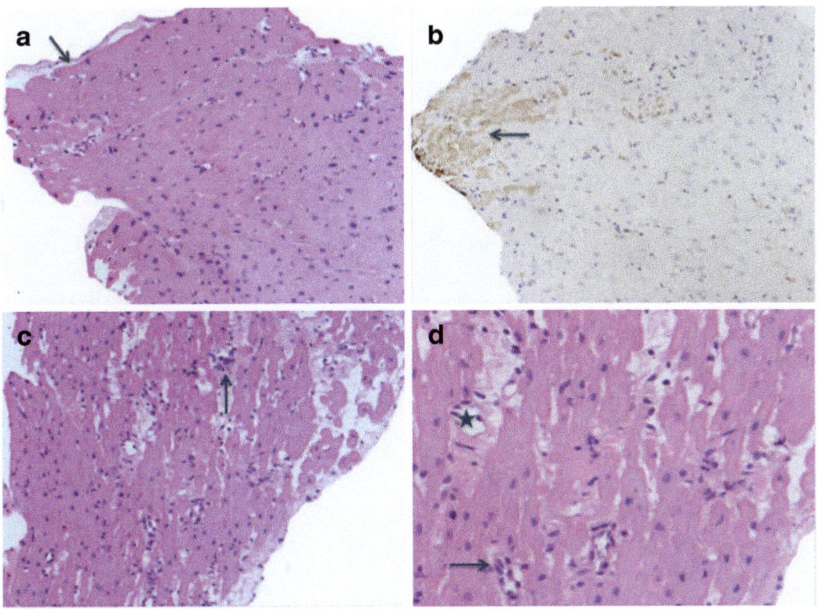

Fig. 9.2 (**a**) Focal subendocardial coagulative necrosis (*arrow*) difficult to see at hematoxylin–eosin staining. Original magnification ×125. (**b**) C4d antibody may be useful to highlight the area of ischemic injury. C4d antibody immunostaining, original magnification ×125. (**c**) Multifocal ischemic damage with endothelial injury. Hematoxylin–eosin staining, original magnification ×125. (**d**) High-power view of C to show the endothelial damage and adhesion of leucocytes (*arrows*)

As complement activation markers as a result of ischemic injury can be found, C4d and C3d can be positive at immunohistochemical staining on early EMBs: this finding should be evaluated as ischemic damage and not as a sign of AMR (Labarrere et al. 2012).

9.4 Temporal Evolution of Perioperative Myocardial Damage

Perioperative myocardial damage evolves, with contraction band necrosis (Fig. 9.3b), coagulative necrosis (Fig. 9.3a), and myocytolysis (Fig. 9.3d) appearing in the first 2 weeks after transplantation, and inflammation following at about 3–4 weeks. Perioperative myocardial damage can persist up to 6 weeks after transplantation, as mentioned in the ISHLT 2004 classification for acute cellular rejection among the criteria for perioperative damage (Stewart et al. 2005).

The next healing phase can be quite protracted (Fig. 9.3c): here the inflammatory cells are mainly composed of macrophages clearing the necrotic myocyte debris, with hemosiderin laden cytoplasm. Neoangiogenesis with dispersed fibroblasts and loose extracellular matrix and scant inflammation can be found in later EMBs. It has been reported that resolution of myocardial injury resolves slowly due to the anti-inflammatory effects of induction or maintenance immunosuppressive therapy.

The presence of perioperative myocardial damage both acute and in the healing phase does not preclude the coexistence of acute cellular rejection.

Within the first month following transplantation some two-thirds of EMBs show evidence of acute cellular rejection associated with histological signs of perioperative myocardial damage.

9.5 Source of Cardiac Graft, Severity of Myocardial Injury, and Outcomes

The majority of cardiac grafts for transplantation are still acquired from brain dead donors, and only a minority from nonbeating heart donors. In the latter case, a few studies report that EMBs

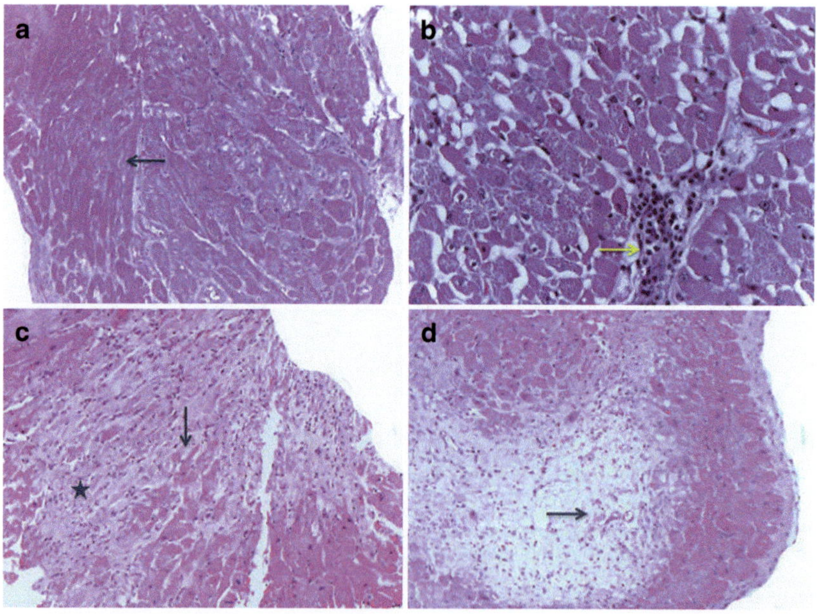

Fig. 9.3 (**a**) Diffuse band-like coagulative necrosis in the subendocardium (*arrow*). Hematoxylin–eosin staining, original magnification ×125. (**b**) Thrombus of a small intramyocardial vessel (*arrow*) in the context of single multifocal coagulated myocytes hematoxylin–eosin staining, original magnification ×160. (**c**) Healing phase of the ischemic damage (*star*) with persistence of some cardiomyocytes with coagulative necrosis (*arrow*). (**d**) Evolution of myocytolysis with neoangiogenesis (*arrow*) beside coagulative necrosis. Hematoxylin–eosin staining, original magnification ×160

show less myocardial damage and fewer episodes of acute cellular rejection.

Many studies have addressed the influence of brain death on cardiac allograft outcomes and show that brain death negatively affects graft function and is associated with a worse outcome. Brain death produces profound neurohormonal derangement causing hemodynamic fluctuations, global organ ischemia, hypothermia, coagulopathies, hormonal depletion, and electrolytic abnormalities and a proinflammatory status in donors, with the activation of complement factors in the graft and its reduced survival (Atkinson et al. 2013). A catecholamine storm leads to calcium overflow injury, in turn producing a decrease in heart rate, an increase in coronary artery resistance, and inhibition of the myocardial contractile mechanism. Myocardial damage during brain death may be further worsened by global hypothermic ischemia at the time of organ harvesting (Novitzky et al. 1987).

An acute rise in intracranial pressure increases the deleterious effect of brain death on heart function. Moreover, brain death produces an inflammatory response, with the upregulation of proinflammatory cytokines and adhesion molecules and rapid leukocyte infiltration, which in turn exacerbates myocyte injury.

There are, however, discordant data in the literature in relation to mode of donor death, the severity of graft injury and outcomes. Donor trauma was shown to influence number of rejection episodes treated in recipients, but not medium- or long-term survival. Donors spending more than 3 days in ICU were associated with worse outcomes suggesting that this can negatively impact on the effect of a prolonged catecholamine storm following brain death (Ganesh et al. 2005).

However, a recent nationwide UK study showed that the donor cause of death was no longer a significant predictor of recipient death, either early or late (Cantin et al. 2003).

Endothelial injury and activation really do seem to be the final common pathway of multiple damage including brain death, ischemic and hypothermic storage, reperfusion, allorecognition, and cardiopulmonary bypass, which all evoke a systemic proinflammatory status in the donor and inflammatory infiltrates in the cardiac allograft (Livi et al. 1993; Verrier 2004). Recently published data suggest that graft failure early after transplantation may depend upon the extent of very early posttransplant microvascular damage and the capacity of the transplanted heart to remove microthrombi through active fibrinolysis (Labarrere et al. 2012).

Clinicopathological correlations have shown that coagulative myocyte necrosis is associated with a longer ischemic time and higher rate of postoperative mortality, although mortality at 1 year or at longer follow-up seems unaffected by severity of damage.

In the literature there are varying results for identification of risk factors in development of severity of perioperative myocardial damage, such as increased vasopressor dosage, advanced age, or sex of donor (Livi et al. 1993). No correlation between perioperative myocardial damage and the number of rejection episodes during the first year posttransplantation has been reported.

9.6 Differential Diagnosis with Acute Rejection

The histological features of perioperative myocardial damage must be differentiated from hyperacute rejection (today rare), acute cellular, and humoral rejection.

The main differential features between acute cellular rejection and perioperative myocardial damage are the following:

- Acute cellular rejection is frequently characterized by the presence of eosinophils, usually lacking in perioperative myocardial damage, where the most prominent cells are T lymphocytes and macrophages.
- Unlike the acute cellular rejection, in perioperative myocardial damage there is disproportion between the extent of myocyte injury and that of lymphocyte inflammation (myocardial damage is more extensive than the inflammation).
- In perioperative myocardial damage there is a sharp border between the necrosis, in single cells, or mainly in clusters, and the nearby viable myocardium.

Key Points

- Perioperative myocardial damage includes all the injuries to the cardiac allograft, which can be found up to 6 weeks posttransplantation
- The damage may stem from insult prior to transplantation procedures during harvesting and transplantation and posttransplantation
- The histopathological substrate consists of interstitial edema, contraction band necrosis, foci of coagulative myocardial cell necrosis, myocytolysis, and inflammation.
- Vascular damage can be characterized by endothelial swelling, leucocytes adhering to the endothelium and clustered inside the vessel and, more rarely, by microthrombosis in intramyocardial small arteries.
- Brain death negatively affects graft function producing a profound neurohormonal derangement leading to a pro-inflammatory status in donors and an inflammatory response in the graft.
- Perioperative myocardial damage can coexist with acute cellular rejection.

References

Atkinson C, Floerchinger B, Qiao F, Casey S, Williamson T, Moseley E, Stoica S, Goddard M, Ge X, Tullius SG, Tomlinson S. Donor brain death exacerbates complement-dependent ischemi/reperfusion injury in transplanted hearts. Circulation. 2013;127(12):1290–9.

Baroldi G, Silver MD, De Maria R, Parolini M, Turillazzi E, Fineschi V. Frequency and extent of contraction band necrosis in orthotopically transplanted human hearts. A morphometric study. Int J Cardiol. 2003;88(2–3): 267–78.

Cantin B, Kwok BW, Chan MC, Valantine HA, Oyer PE, Robbins RC. Hunt SA The impact of brain death on survival after heart transplantation: time is of the essence. Transplantation. 2003;76(9):1275–9.

Fyfe B, Loh E, Winters GL, Couper GS, Kartashov AI, Schoen FJ. Heart transplantation-associated perioperative ischemic myocardial injury. Morphological features and clinical significance. Circulation. 1996;93(6): 1133–40.

Ganesh JS, Rogers CA, Banner NR, Bonser RS. Donor cause of death and medium-term survival after heart transplantation: a United Kingdom national study. J Thorac Cardiovasc Surg. 2005;129:1153–9.

George TJ, Arnaoutakis GJ, Beaty CA, Shah AS, Conte JV, Halushka MK. A novel method of measuring cardiac preservation injury demonstrates University of Wisconsin solution is associated with less ischemic necrosis than Celsior in early cardiac allograft biopsy specimens. J Heart Lung Transplant. 2012;31(4): 410–8.

Labarrere CA, Woods JR, Hardin JW, Campana GL, Ortiz MA, Jaeger BR, Baldridge LA, Pitts DE, Kirlin PC. Value of the first post-transplant biopsy for predicting long-term cardiac allograft vasculopathy (CAV) and graft failure in heart transplant patients. PLoS One. 2012;7(4), e36100.

Livi U, Milano A, Valente M, Cocco P, Angelini A, Casula R, Bortolotti U, Gambino A, Thiene G, Casarotto D. Ultrastructural correlation of endomyocardial biopsy findings with myocardial preservation in human cardiac allografts. Transplant Proc. 1993;25(6): 3199–200.

Novitzky D, Cooper DK, Reichart B. Hemodynamic and metabolic responses to hormonal therapy in brain-dead potential organ donors. Transplantation. 1987; 43(6):852–4.

Verrier ED. Activation of the endothelium in cardiac allografts. J Heart Lung Transplant. 2004;23(9 Suppl): S229–33.

Stewart S, Winters GL, Fishbein MC, Tazelaar HD, Kobashigawa J, Abrams J, Andersen CB, Angelini A, Berry GJ, Burke MM, Demetris AJ, Hammond E, Itescu S, Marboe CC, McManus B, Reed EF, Reinsmoen NL, Rodriguez ER, Rose AG, Rose M, Suciu-Focia N, Zeevi A, Billingham ME. Revision of the 1990 working formulation for the standardization of nomenclature in the diagnosis of heart rejection. J Heart Lung Transplant. 2005;24(11): 1710–20.

Part IV

Post-cardiac Transplantation: The Multiple Faces of Rejection

Graft Failure/Dysfunction: Clinical Issues and Role of Endomyocardial Biopsy

10

Luciano Potena, Valentina Manfredini, and Ornella Leone

Contents

L. Potena (✉) • V. Manfredini
Heart Failure and Heart Transplant Program, Cardiology Unit, S. Orsola-Malpighi University Hospital, Bologna, Italy
e-mail: luciano.potena2@unibo.it

O. Leone
Cardiovascular and Cardiac Transplant Pathology Program, Department of Pathology, Sant'Orsola-Malpighi University Hospital, Bologna, Italy

10.1 Background

Despite progressive improvements in surgical and medical management, failure of the transplanted graft is still the major cause of death after heart transplantation (HTx) (Lund et al. 2014). Clinical presentation, aetiologies, and possible treatments for heart allograft failure vary within a wide spectrum, preventing a clear-cut definition of the phenomenon.

In this chapter, we will discuss the main clinical scenarios leading to graft failure in heart recipients, to clinically contextualize the main pathological diagnoses (cardiac rejection, infections, etc.), which are treated in-depth in subsequent dedicated chapters. An overview of the role of endomyocardial biopsy (EMB) in these various clinical conditions is also given.

In this setting, we will use the term "graft failure" to indicate the terminal state of irreversible loss of graft function causing death or retransplantation, and the term "graft dysfunction" to indicate a potentially reversible and partial loss of function, often preceding but not necessarily leading to graft failure and death. The aetiologies and clinical presentations of graft dysfunction will be dealt with according to time of onset after transplantation (Fig. 10.1).

O. Leone et al. (eds.), *The Pathology of Cardiac Transplantation*,
DOI 10.1007/978-3-319-46386-5_10

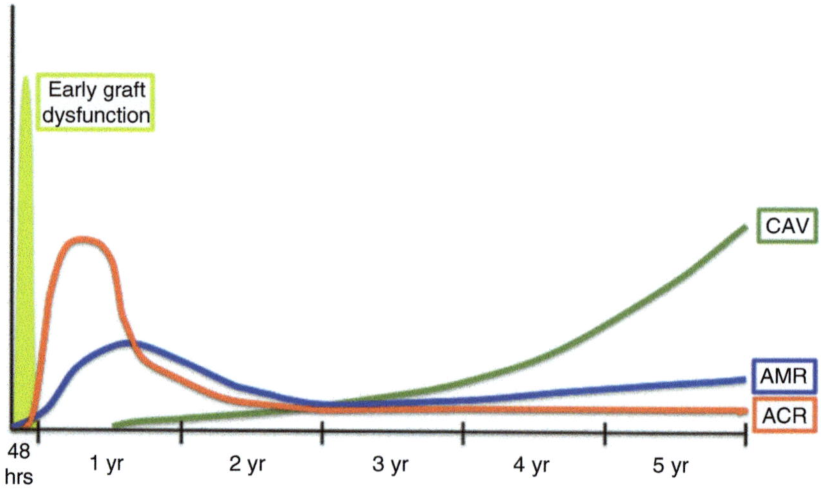

Fig. 10.1 The graph shows the trend of the main causes of acute and chronic graft dysfunction according with time post-transplantation. Primary and secondary early graft dysfunction occurs within the 24–48 h after surgery. (ACR: acute cellular rejection; AMR: antibody-mediated rejection; CAV: cardiac allograft vasculopathy)

10.2 Postoperative Graft Dysfunction

A recent survey of the International Society of Heart and Lung Transplantation (ISHLT) showed that up to 66 % of 30 days mortality after HTx is reported as related to graft failure and subsequent multiorgan dysfunction. Most of these events are probably the result of primary and secondary graft dysfunction (Kobashigawa et al. 2014).

Early graft dysfunction is a threatening complication occurring during the initial 24–48 hours after surgery characterized by the inability of the graft to sustain adequate hemodynamic and organ perfusion. Epidemiology of this condition is highly variable, depending on its definition, which is not consistent across multiple studies where incidence varies from 2.3 to 28 %. In this context, the definition of graft dysfunction includes several parameters, e.g. time of onset, echocardiographic and haemodynamic findings, need for inotropic support, or need for mechanical support. Only recently, a consensus document from ISHLT has set clear standards to recognize and define post-operative graft dysfunction, with a clear distinction between "primary" and "secondary" graft dysfunction (Table 10.1) (Kobashigawa et al. 2014). We can use "secondary" to describe graft dysfunction related to identifiable causes, the most common being recipient pulmonary hypertension; while hyperacute rejection, technical surgical failures, and unrecognized donor heart disease (see Chap. 7) are currently rare possibilities. The term "primary" graft dysfunction (PGD) encompasses all those cases in which a single cause cannot be identified, although a series of combined risk factors have been reported (Cosio et al. 2013).

Pathological findings from autopsies or from explanted hearts of patients undergoing retransplant are essential to understand the pathophysiology of PGD and to identify possible causes not originally clear at clinical presentation. Published reports state that in cases of PGD the pathologist may find rejection, oedema and/or haemorrhage, or reperfusion injury and ischemia (Kobashigawa et al. 2014). EMB on patients with PGD may be useful to rule out hyperacute rejection, but this is not recommended in these critically ill patients unless the suspicion of hyperacute rejection is supported by sound evidence, such as positive immunological crossmatch. However, it is important to emphasize that PGD in clinical practice is a diagnosis made with the use of imaging and haemodynamic data, not with the aid of pathologic information, as any delay in therapy is inadvisable in this dramatic and life-threatening event.

Pathogenesis of PGD is multifactorial, including characteristics of the recipient, donor, and surgical procedure, with several single-centre reports identifying a large array of factors

Table 10.1 Classification of graft dysfuntion

Definition of Severity Scale for Primary Graft Dysfunction (PGD)		
1. PGD-Left ventricle (PGD-LV):	*Mild PGD–LV*: *One* of the following criteria must be met:	LVEF ≤ 40 % by echocardiography, *or* Hemodynamics with RAP > 15 mmHg, PCWP > 20 mmHg, CI < 2.0 L/min/m² (lasting more than 1 h) requiring low-dose inotropes
	Moderate PGD-LV: Must meet one criterion from I*and* another criterion from II:	I. *One* criteria from the following: Left ventricular ejection fraction ≤ 40 %,*or* Hemodynamic compromise with RAP > 15 mmHg, PCWP > 20 mmHg, CI < 2.0 L/min/m², hypotension with MAP < 70 mmHg (lasting more than 1 h)
		II. *One* criteria from the following:
		(i) High-dose inotropes—Inotrope score > 10[a] *or*
		(ii) Newly placed IABP (regardless of inotropes)
	Severe PGD–LV	Dependence on left or biventricular mechanical support including ECMO, LVAD, BiVAD, or percutaneous LVAD. Excludes requirement for IABP.
2. PGD-right ventricle (PGD-RV):	Diagnosis requires either both i and ii, or iii alone:	(i) Hemodynamics with RAP > 15 mmHg, PCWP < 15 mmHg, CI < 2.0 L/min/m² (ii) TPG <15 mmHg and/or pulmonary artery systolic pressure < 50 mmHg, *or* (iii) Need for RVAD

From Kobashigawa et al. (2014)
BiVAD biventricular assist device, *CI* cardiac index, *ECMO* extracorporeal membrane oxygenation, *IABP* intra-aortic balloon pump, *LVAD* left ventricular assist device, *PCWP* pulmonary capillary wedge pressure, *RAP* right atrial pressure, *RVAD* right ventricular assist device, *TPG* transpulmonary pressure gradient
Inotrope score = dopamine (×1) + dobutamine (×1) + amrinone (×1) + milrinone (×15) + epinephrine (×100) + norepinephrine (×100)[67] with each drug dosed in μg/kg/min

associated with the development of PGD. Among these, however, we can identify some general categories and common points.

10.2.1 Donor Factors and Periprocedural Factors

- *Brain death* in the donor is associated with a series of events that may impair myocardial contractility and sensitize the heart to ischemia-reperfusion injury. Brain death induces an intense release of myocardial norepinephrine that results in mitochondrial and cytosolic calcium overload, which may activate autophagy, apoptosis or necrosis if this process is extensive. Calcium overload in contractile proteins leads to contracture and is associated with characteristic histologic features (see Chap. 7) (Mohamedali et al. 2014; White et al. 1995).
- The use of *exogenous catecholamine* during patient and then donor management in intensive care units, in addition to the endogenous catecholamine storm after brain death, desensitize myocardial beta-receptor signalling, disrupting myocyte contractile ability (6), and activate multiple proinflammatory mediators, including complement (Novitzky et al. 2006).
- *Donor age* can influence the ability of the organ to tolerate the period of cold and warm ischemia. This is partly due to unrecognized coronary artery disease or pathologic left ventricular hypertrophy in elderly donors with a history of hypertension. Moreover there is an age related decline in endogenous cardioprotective mechanisms such as ischemic preconditioning and postconditioning (Boengler et al. 2009).
- *Ischaemic time* is the period from arrest of donor heart to time of graft reperfusion in the recipient: 1-year mortality risk after heart transplantation increases steadily with the increase of ischaemic time over 3 h. Donor hearts are usually stored in cold *preservation solutions* and transported on ice. Hypothermic storage slows but does not completely arrest cellular metabo-

lism. Consequently, progressive ischemic injury is an inevitable consequence of prolonged static storage. The loss of the normal aerobic metabolism paralyzes the transmenbrane Na+/K+ adenosine triphosphatase pump, leading to cellular swelling and development of lactic acidosis (Hicks et al. 2006). The kind of preservation solution used in this setting may play a role, although clear-cut data allowing us to recommend one over the many available are inconsistent. A recent retrospective study comparing two commonly used solutions (University of Winsconsin and Celsior) found that there was increased ischemia damage in bioptic specimens when Celsior had been used, although this finding did not correlate with different clinical outcomes. There is a clear need to develop more effective preservation – either by improving the cardioprotective efficacy of the storage solution or through use of an oxygenated ex vivo perfusion system. In the future the development of organ care systems allowing the transportation of the heart perfused by warm donor blood may revolutionize the concept of organ preservation (Ardehali et al. 2015). Donor recipient weight mismatching and female donor to male recipient are associated with increased PGD. A possible link to immunological process and increased rejection episodes have also been described (Khush et al. 2012).

10.2.2 Recipient Factors

Age, poor clinical conditions, renal insufficiency, obesity, and diabetes represent general risk factors for complications in any cardiac surgical procedure. In the specific setting of heart transplantation, a major factor influencing early dysfunction of the graft is recipient pulmonary hypertension. The presence of *high pulmonary vascular resistance* in the recipient may lead to early failure of the right ventricle. However, even when pulmonary pressures and resistances are within the commonly accepted range for heart transplantation, pulmonary pressure correlates with the incidence of PGD (Butler et al. 2005). Donor recipient size mismatch has also been identified as a significant contributing factor of PGD. In one study, the combination of donor-recipient weight ratio of less than 0.8 with pulmonary hypertension in the recipient (>4 Wood Units) was associated with PGD (Russo et al. 2010). In the presence of *fixed pulmonary vascular resistance* in the recipient, the right ventricle of the donor heart may be unable to overcome the afterload imposed and selective or predominant right ventricle failure frequently occurs, often needing mechanical circulatory support (Oto et al. 2008).

10.3 Hyperacute Rejection

This cause of postoperative graft dysfunction and failure is currently rare but threatening and often fatal. Hyperacute rejection is mediated by preexisting complement fixing antibodies which, upon cross clamp removal, enter the vasculature and bind to the vascular endothelium. They then activate complement cascade, which causes direct lysis of endothelial cells on the graft vasculature. The histologic picture of this uncommon form of rejection consists of diffuse interstitial oedema and/or haemorrhage, massive infiltration of neutrophils, macrophage inflammation, and widespread myocell damage. Fibrin thrombi and platelet aggregates may be found in small vessels (capillary, arterioles and venules) (Stewart et al. 2005). Hyperacute rejection can be safely prevented by careful screening of transplant candidates for preformed anti-HLA antibodies. When reacting against over 10% of the local blood donor lymphocyte panel, organ allocation should be subjected to direct cross-match only. This procedure may not be feasible in certain areas where highly urgent cases may receive long-distance organs, thus exposing patients to the risk of immediate transplant failure (Nwakanma et al. 2007).

Modern solid phase techniques, such as single antigen bead assay, allow detection of non-cytotoxic antibodies, which may however react with the graft, even if not immediately. Detection of these antibodies should flag out the patient as high risk for early antibody-mediated rejection (see below) and, when possible, allocation of organs non-compatible with detected antibodies should be avoided (Potena et al. 2013).

Presence of anti HLA antibodies is more common in multiparous women, subjects with prior blood transfusion, prior transplantation, or insertion of a ventricular assist device.

10.4 Acute Graft Dysfunction

By "acute" graft dysfunction we mean a rapid reduction of graft function as measured by ultrasound or right heart catheterization, with or without accompanying symptoms of heart failure (dizziness, shortness of breath, etc.). It is more frequent during the first year post-transplantation, although it can occur later.

Clinical presentation of acute graft dysfunction is not usually specific for one aetiology, and the likelihood of different aetiologies varies during the course of post-transplant follow up, with cellular rejection being more frequent during the first year and antibody-mediated rejection or cardiac allograft vsculopathy (CAV) later on. Of note, mixed rejection should be regarded as important, associated with acute graft dysfunction and, when occurring late after transplant, may be a marker of inadequate drug adherence (Sellares et al. 2012; Fedrigo et al. 2015).

Acute cellular rejection (ACR) mostly occurs in the first 6–12 months after HTx and is characterized by varying extents of predominantly lymphocytic inflammation in the myocardium, with or without signs of myocyte injury (see Chap. 13). Typically, moderate to severe ACR is treated by pulse steroid, with or without adjustment of chronic immunosuppression (e.g. shifting cyclosporine to tacrolimus or maintaining higher drug through levels).

Antibody-mediated rejection (AMR) is characterized by a microvascular injury mediated by graft-specific antibodies, which can be directed against Human Leucocyte Antigen (HLA) or non-HLA antigens (see Chap. 14). Aside from hyperacute rejection occurring in the context of postoperative graft dysfunction, which has a dramatic clinical and pathological presentation, AMR has been reported to be a cause both of early and late graft dysfunction. It is associated with poor outcome factors such as the increased incidence of hemodynamic compromise rejection, greater development of CAV, and high incidence of death (Michaels et al. 2003; Kfoury et al. 2006). The pathogenesis of acute AMR is related to complement-mediated endothelial injury, endothelial dysfunction, microvascular coagulation, myocardial ischemia and, ultimately, allograft dysfunction. Its diagnosis is complex, requiring an articulated set of histological and immunopathological criteria on EMB, detection of circulating donor specific antibodies (DSAs), and signs of graft dysfunction, which, as already mentioned, are often subtle and are hard to detect. Treatment is not standardized and comprises a stepwise approach based on off-label treatments from high-dose intravenous immunoglobulines and plasma exchange to monoclonal antibodies such as rituximab or eculizumab (Table 10.2) (Kobashigawa et al. 2011; Nair et al. 2011).

Table 10.2 Targets of therapy in antibody-mediated rejection

Targets of therapy				
Elimination of circulating antibodies	Inhibition of circulating antibodies	Suppression of B cells	Plasma cell depletion	Complement inhibition
Plasma exchange	Intravenous immunoglobulin	Rituximab	Bortezomib	Eculizumab
Double filtration plasmapheresis	Cytomegalovirus hyperimmunoglobulin	Splenectomy		
Immunoadsorption plasmapheresis		Calcineurin inhibitors (antiproliferative/ apoptotic effects)		
		Belimumab (anti-Blys antibody)?		
		Epratuzumab (anti-CD22 antibody)?		

From Nair et al. (2011)

Risk factors for AMR include presence of pre-transplant HLA antibodies, detection of de-novo DSAs, female sex, poor drug adherence. In particular, non-adherence, as well as need to over-reduce the immunosuppressive drug burden, have been associated with late development of DSAs and onset of graft dysfunction due to AMR, usually several years after transplantation (Sellares et al. 2012).

An important and still unresolved issue, however, is the definition of cardiac "graft dysfunction". Clearly, if we consider "dysfunction" only acute reduction of ejection fraction and/or clinical signs of heart failure, it is a rare event, especially in the context of patients monitored with scheduled EMB and pathology-guided treatment. On the other hand, studies investigating non-invasive methods to diagnose myocardial rejection (see Chap. 17) revealed that in most cases histological signs of acute rejection are accompanied by subclinical signs of diastolic dysfunction that can be detected by cardiac ultrasound, or by right heart catheterization. It is important to note, however, that diastolic abnormalities are often subtle, and need to be actively sought. For these methodologies to be sufficiently sensitive, measurements need to be compared serially to a basal condition state with proven absence of acute rejection: in this context these signs of graft dysfunction may indicate EMB performance, the results of which are of key importance in guiding treatment (Badano et al. 2015).

EMB is the key element to diagnose aetiology of acute graft dysfunction. This strategy, developed following the pivotal studies of Caves et al. (1974), helped to reveal many of the mechanisms leading to myocardial graft injury and prompted the histological grading for pathological classification of rejection severity, further detailed in Chap. 13 (Billingham et al. 1990; Stewart et al. 2005). EMB findings have long defined the phenomenology of acute cardiac rejection and, independently of the presence of clinical signs of graft dysfunction, routine surveillance with EMB has been the cornerstone of monitoring ACR. However, as mentioned, cardiac rejection is no longer identified only with ACR: in recent years AMR came to the fore as the other main form of cardiac rejection, either alone or in association with ACR, in the as yet not fully explored phenomenon of mixed rejection. Consequently, the value of EMB in cardiac rejection diagnosis is today much enhanced, especially now that agreed pathological criteria for AMR are available. Noninvasive methods for detection of rejection, although promising, have low sensitivity in terms of assessing grades of ACR – especially mild or borderline but clinically significant – and do not detect AMR or differentiate it from ACR, at the present stage of research at least. The major limit of EMB is its invasiveness. Sampling error is a minor problem in recognizing significant grades of rejection. Interobserver variation among pathologists is also a well-known issue in the literature and although less of an issue within a single center, where pathologists share cross-reading and similar grading criteria, it may be more serious across different centers.

The role of EMB is different when performed in scheduled protocols from when a systolic or diastolic graft dysfunction is present.

In the former situation, EMB is mainly required to monitor for initial pathological signs of rejection that may precede overt graft dysfunction in order to allow pre-emptive treatment and avoid a potentially harmful clinical syndrome. In the latter, the situation is more complex because EMB is also involved in resolving possible differential diagnosis within an unclear clinical scenario: in this case EMB can identify the clear cause of allograft dysfunction (rejection or other) and give a positive diagnosis or can exclude recognizable pathologies thus opening the way for further investigation. A negative/exclusion diagnosis is also an essential tool.

The pathologist should be aware that in cardiac patients there is a wide spectrum of myocardial inflammation findings, whether associated with myocyte damage or not, and these findings should always be carefully evaluated and interpreted (see Chap. 16).

The first point in *acute graft dysfuntion* is undoubtedly to recognize cardiac rejection findings, and identify the different forms of ACR, AMR or mixed rejection, and grade them, in order to tailor therapy.

The absence of ACR or AMR in biopsy findings in presence of cardiac dysfunction (unless a sampling error) has been recognized as a rare phenomenon, a different form of rejection not apparent at biopsy and more severe and difficult to treat than classic forms (Tang et al. 2013). Although this is possible, not all cases of acute systolic heart dysfunction with negative biopsy are necessarily a consequence of rejection (Boilson et al. 2008) and a clinical approach focusing only on rejection may be limiting.

The other important points are:

- To distinguish rejection from peritransplant injury, which may be evident in biopsies in the first month after transplantation and show myocell damage associated with various degrees of inflammatory infiltrates.
- To recognize reparative inflammation associated with real ischemic focal damage as different from rejection.
- To identify cardiac localization of infections, rare but possible. Cellular rejection is indeed an allo-immune myocarditis that on histological grounds can be indistinguishable from a viral myocarditis. Thus, viral post-transplant myocarditis is an important differential diagnosis with cellular rejection in heart transplant recipients with steroid resistant rejections or worsening clinical syndromes despite adequate immunosuppression: Cytomegalovirus and Parvovirus are the most common viruses that may be implicated in allograft myocarditis. In some cases histologic findings can be sufficiently indicative and identification of the microorganism possible; in other cases, especially in viral myocarditis other than Cytomegalovirus, histologic findings are indistinguishable from those of rejection and only an atypical clinical course might suggest infection (see Chap. 16).

Acute Coronary Syndromes
Acute coronary syndromes (ACS) are a rare clinical presentation of coronary artery disease in heart transplant recipients, despite the high incidence of coronary lesions in long-term survivors. Nevertheless, myocardial infarction can be a cause of acute graft dysfunction that may have heart failure symptoms or atypical chest pain as clinical presentation: to be considered in a differential diagnosis with acute rejection. Clinical judgement based on ECG changes and wall motion abnormalities with coronary distribution should raise the suspicion of ACS in these patients, suggesting coronary angiography before EMB.

10.5 Chronic Graft Dysfunction

Late post-transplantation acute graft dysfunction is rare. Patients with chronic graft malfunction present slow and progressive onset of diastolic abnormalities accompanied by slight decrease in ejection fraction and worsening heart failure symptoms. These clinical-ultrasound changes may be associated with low voltages on surface ECG, increased QRS duration and rhythm disturbances (more frequent in patients operated with the Shumway technique with bi-atrial anastomosis) (Fig. 10.2).

The most common and typical cause of this clinical scenario is CAV, which can be considered a form of chronic vascular rejection. Typically, CAV development is triggered by metabolic risk factors – as well as native coronary atherosclerosis – and by immune-mediated injury, including antibody-mediated endothelial injury (indeed, CAV may be a chronic phenotype of AMR). CAV is characterized by diffuse intimal hyperplasia arising from peripheral vessels and spreading to proximal tracts of arteries and veins, thus determining diffuse luminal narrowing, often without focal luminal stenoses. Although this pattern leads coronary angiography to underestimate the disease, it remains the basic imaging tool to diagnose and classify CAV (Mehra et al. 2010). Intravascular ultrasound allows the morphology of graft arteries to be studied in detail, by detection of changes in vascular wall morphology and progression of intimal thickening, which provides more prognostic information than angiography does (Potena et al. 2015; Cheng et al. 2015).

EMB is not a typical diagnostic tool for CAV, although it is often indicated at the onset of clinical symptoms, even late after transplant, to

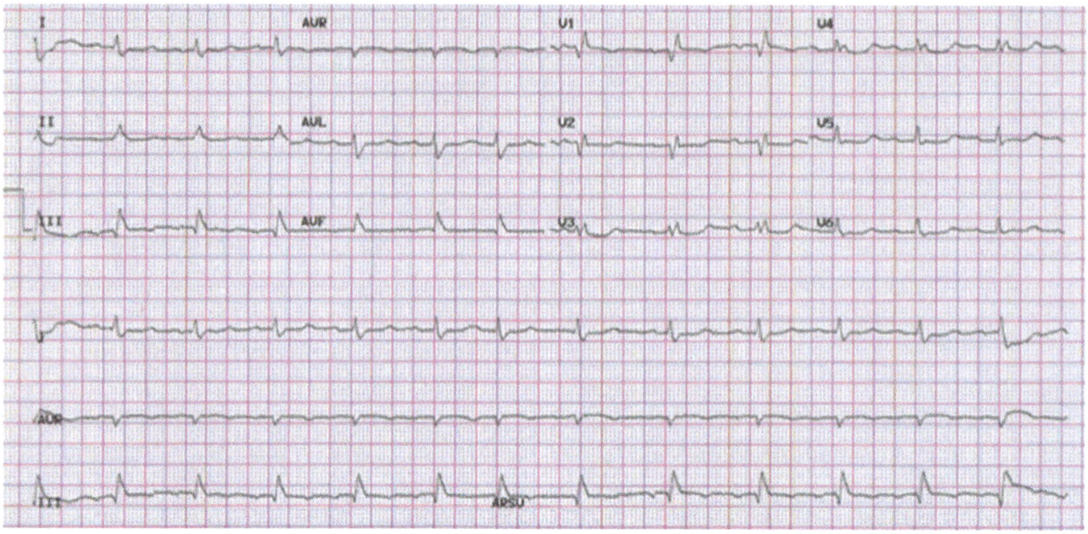

Fig. 10.2 12-lead electrocardiogram of a patient 13 years after transplantation who suffered from heart failure symptoms. Significant widening of QRS, with a right bundle branch block morphology, is accompanied by diffuse low voltages, in particular in the precordial leads, and diffuse repolarization abnormalities. Note that no-q waves are present, indicating absence of transmural necrosis. Cardiac ultrasound shows a mildly dilated left ventricle with diffuse ipokinesia, 35 % ejection fraction, and restrictive filling pattern

rule out possible acute immune injuries that may require targeted treatment (i.e. ACR or AMR). It is however important in routine biopsies to describe the presence and histologic findings of microvasculopathy, which goes hand in hand with epicardial vasculopathy and is characterized by a concentric thickening of small vessels, for both intimal and medial disease. Evidence of stenotic microvasculopathy in EMB has been found to be a negative prognostic marker in these patients (Hiemann et al. 2007). Regardless of known CAV, in these patients EMB may also reveal pathology findings compatible with AMR. However, specific treatment of AMR in patients with chronic syndromes may be associated with poor clinical and histological response and the risk-benefit ratio of aggressive anti-AMR therapies in these often old and frail patients needs careful evaluation (Gupta et al. 2014). Clinics and pathology of CAV are described in Chap. 18.

Although CAV is the most frequent complication expected in *late graft dysfunction*, causes may be more unclear and intricate and be the result of concurrent alterations. In this context, the role of EMB is again to recognize possible late episodes of acute rejection, both ACR and AMR, but even simply to exclude significant rejection is important, so that clinicians can turn their attention to alternatives. EMB can also show concurrent findings, such as a mild form of rejection, CAV-related microvasculopathy or significant interstitial fibrosis, which can reinforce each other and cause graft compromise or impaired performance.

10.6 Illustrative Cases

Case 1

Primary early graft failure (Figs. 10.3, 10.4, and 10.5)

A woman of 61 was transplanted for end-stage idiopathic dilated cardiomyopathy but underwent a second heart transplantation 4 days later due to failure of the graft.

The first donor was a 26-year-old woman who had died of post-anoxic encephalopathy. Ischemic time was 160 min; panel reactive antibody was negative.

It was impossible to wean the patient off from the cardiopulmonary by-pass and therefore she

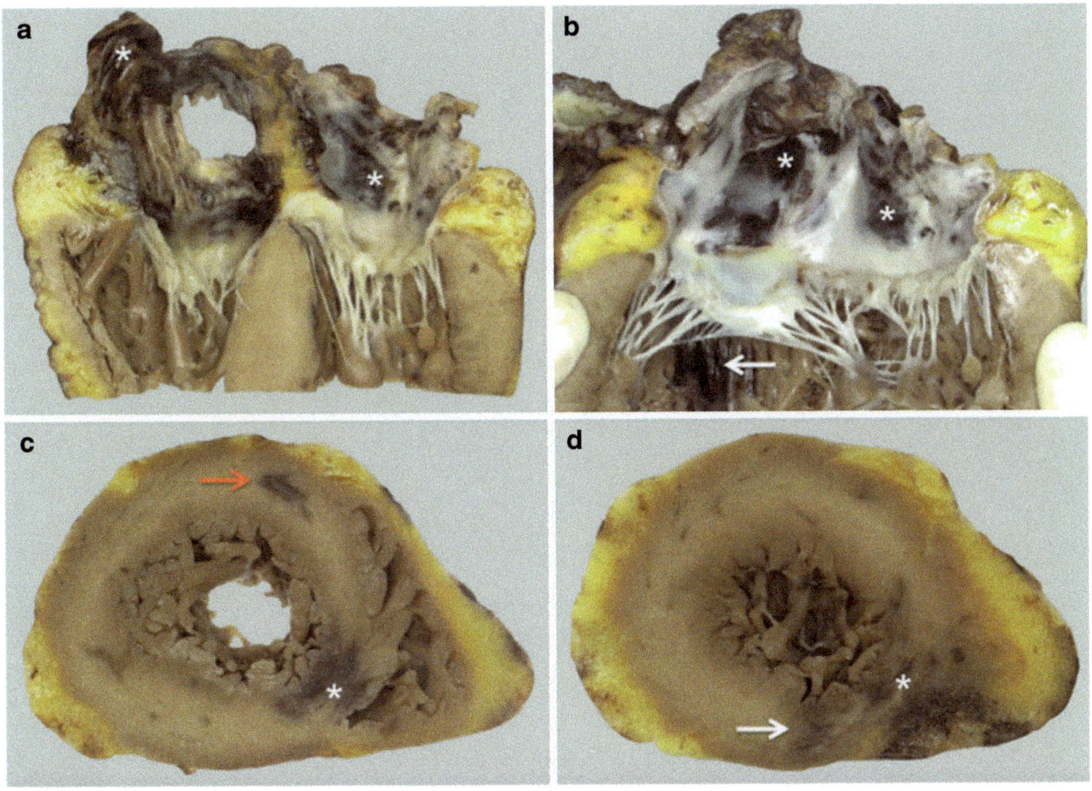

Fig. 10.3 Primary early graft failure: macroscopy of the grafted heart. (**a, b**) Extensive subendocardial haemorrhagic areas are present in the atria (*asterisks*) and in the basal septum (*arrow*). (**c, d**) The transverse slices of the heart show multiple necrotic-haemorrhagic areas in the mid-apical septum (*asterisks*), in both ventricle inferior walls (*white arrow*) and in left ventricle anterior wall (*red arrow*)

was implanted with a total cardiocirculatory assistance – right atrium and left atrium to aorta – based on an extracorporeal circulatory membrane oxygenation (ECMO). Subsequently graft function failed to recover and the patient was then retransplanted.

Pathology of the first grafted heart

The weight was regular (280 g) and it was dilated (7 cm along the longitudinal axis and 11.5 along the transverse one). The epicardial surface showed multiple haemorrhagic areas and fibrin deposition.

At macroscopy, after opening and sectioning the heart, there were:

- Multiple subendocardial haemorrhagic areas in both the atria (Fig. 10.3a, b).
- Extensive area of haemorrhage and necrosis in the basal septum (arrow) (Fig. 10.3b).
- Other multiple haemorragic areas in the mid-apical septum, in both ventricle inferior walls and in left ventricle anterior wall (Fig. 10.3c, d).

Left ventricular cavity was not significantly dilated and wall thickness quite regular. There were no significant alterations in the coronary arteries.

The main histologic findings were:

- Multiple and extensive areas of myocardial coagulative necrosis distributed throughout the subendocardial, midmural, and subepicardial myocardial layers. These areas were sharply demarcated from the non-altered myocardium by the interposition of a coagulative myocytolisys zone (Fig. 10.4).
- Marked multifocal inflammatory infiltrates, associated or not with the coagulative

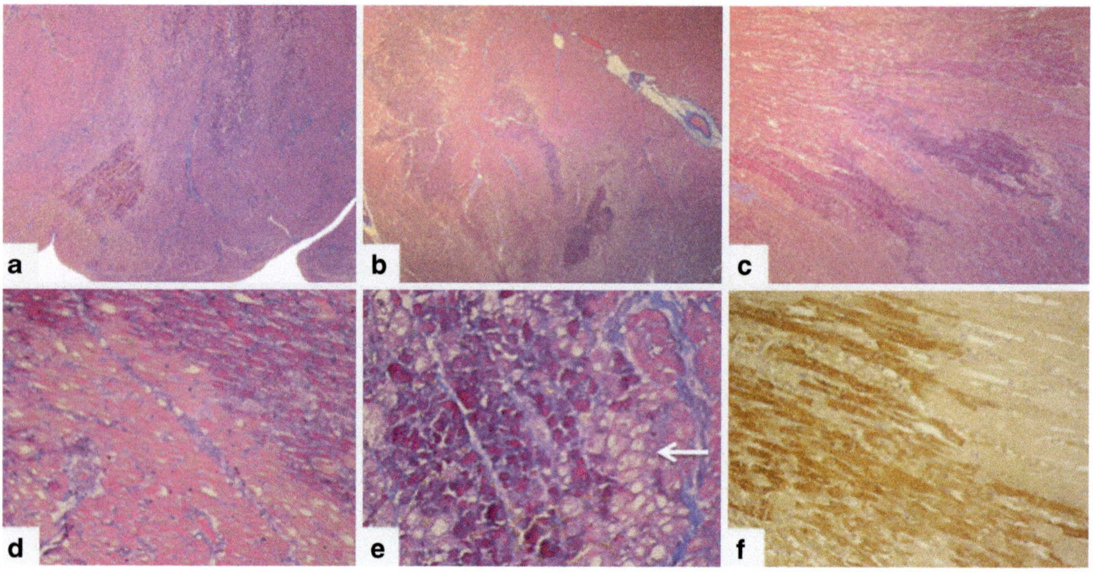

Fig. 10.4 Primary early graft failure: histology of left ventricular myocardium showing multifocal irregularly distributed areas of coagulative necrosis in the subendocardium and midmural layers (**a–c**). At high power, these areas are sharply demarcated from the non-altered myocardium (**d**) and zones of interposed coagulative myocytolisys are evident (**e**, *arrow*) (Azan Mallory trichrome; **a**, **b**: ×25; **c**: ×100; **d**, **e**: ×200). (**f**) C4d immunostaining is strongly positive in necrotic myocytes (×200)

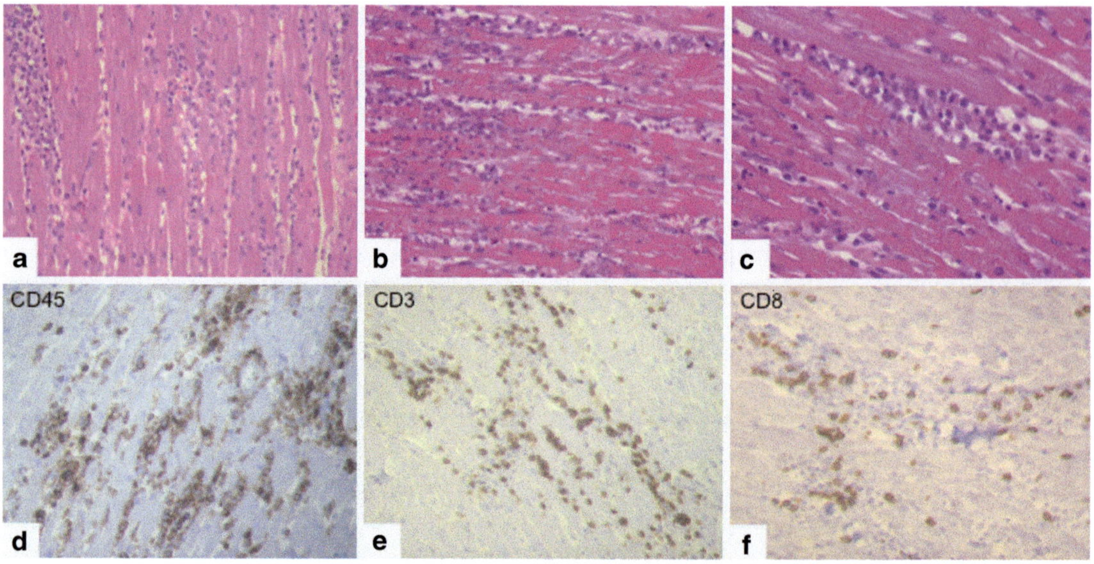

Fig. 10.5 Primary early graft failure. (**a–c**) Histology also reveals multiple and extensive interstitial inflammatory infiltrates, which in some areas are associated with the coagulative myocardial necrosis (**b**) or with myocyte band necrosis (**c**) (Haematoxylin-Eosin, ×200). (**d–f**) Immunohistochemical typing of inflammatory infiltrates showing CD45+ cells (**d**), CD3 T-lymphocytes (**e**) and a significant component of cytotoxic CD8-lymphocytes (**f**) (original magnification ×200)

myocardial necrosis, of mixed composition (lymphocytes, granulocytes, and a minor component of macrophages and plasmacells). Interestingly the lymphocytic component was rich in cytotoxic CD8-lymphocytes (Fig. 10.5).

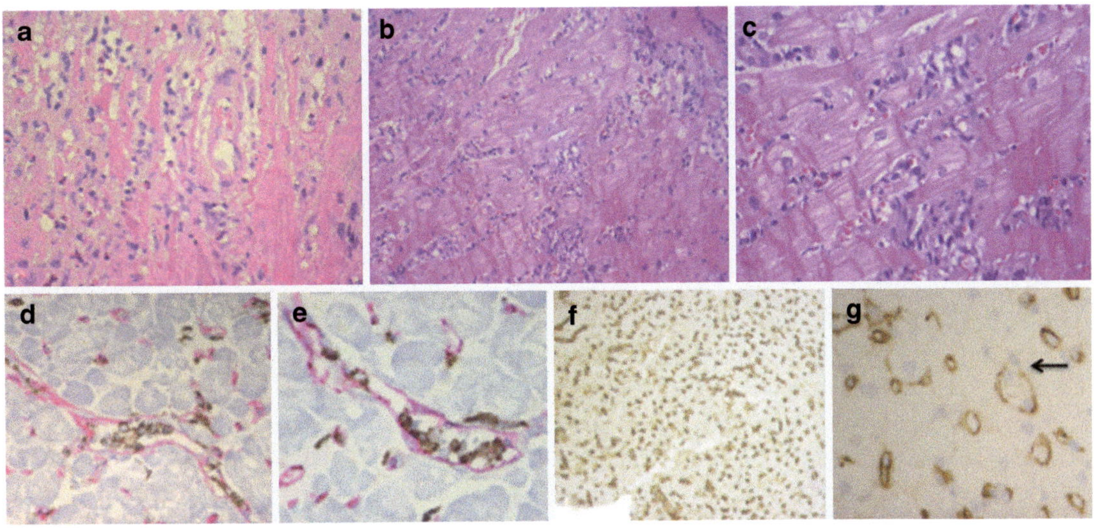

Fig. 10.6 Early graft dysfunction. Endomyocardial biopsy shows widespread interstitial inflammatory infiltrates, mostly lymphocytes and macrophages but with a significant number of neutrophils and eosinophils, especially where associated with myocyte necrosis and damage (**a**: Haematoxylin-eosin, ×200). In many areas the venules and capillaries are engorged (**b**, **c**: Haematoxylin-eosin, **b**: ×100; **c**: ×200) and have many macrophages within their lumens (**d**, **e**: CD34 (*red*)-CD68 (*brown*) double immunostaining; **d**: ×250; **e**: ×400). C4d immunostaining shows strong diffuse positivity of capillaries and venules (**f**, ×100) and CD34 immunohistochemistry for endothelial cells highlights the discontinous outline of some capillaries (*arrow*) (**g**: ×400)

No histologic and immunopathologic findings of antibody-mediated rejection were found.

Discussion/Conclusion

As is frequently the case with primary early graft failure, this case too is difficult to interpret. Although the donor heart was excellent, the organ was unable to wean itself from cardiopulmonary bypass (CPB) pump.

We can exclude the most frequent causes of secondary graft failure/dysfunction, such as:

- Pulmonary hypertension.
- Hyperacute rejection (no significant interstitial oedema, massive infiltration of neutrophils, fibrin-platelet microthrombi in small vessels or evident endothelial damage were present).
- ACR (inflammatory infiltrate is atypical for ACR and coagulative necrosis is the most striking lesion).
- AMR (no histologic and immunopathology findings).
- Technical surgical problems.

The most probable cause was poor preservation of the heart: this caused extensive and irregularly distributed areas of necrosis which prevented weaning of the heart from CPB pump. In the next 4 days, the necrosis attracted the inflammatory cells many of which were CD8-cytotoxic lymphocytes directed against the damaged myocells.

Case 2

Early graft dysfunction (Fig. 10.6)

A 45-year-old woman was transplanted because of dilated cardiomyopathy due to a frameshift mutation of the lamin A/C gene.

Eight days after transplantation, the patient had severe acute graft dysfunction with hypotension and low ejection fraction (25 %).

An EMB was perfomed (Fig. 10.6) and showed severe rejection with a mixed pattern made up of widespread diffuse inflammation, both extravascular and intravascular, associated with oedema and foci of haemorrhage. The inflammatory infiltrates were mostly made up of mononuclear cells (lymphocytes and macrophages), with a significant number of neutrophils and eosinophils and were associated with diffuse myocyte damage, suggesting a high grade ACR. In addition, the venules and capillaries were engorged, some with an indistinct outline suggesting injury. Immunohistochemistry for AMR was performed and showed strong, diffuse C4d staining of capillaries and venules (around 90 %) with many macrophages within the lumen (around 25 % of the specimens), together with interstitial macrophages. CD34 immunohistochemistry for endothelial cells confirmed that the capillaries were damaged.

The final diagnosis was mixed rejection pattern: severe ACR and full pathologic AMR.

Patient was treated with thymoglobulines, plasmapheresis, IV immunoglobulins, and rituximab.

The subsequent biopsies showed a rapid and complete resolution of ACR histologic findings (15 days). AMR histologic and immunopathological findings persisted longer in EMBs: the histological findings had disappeared 40 days later and C4d positivity 80 days later.

One year later this important episode, graft function is normal and patient is well.

Histopathology and diagnostic criteria for ACR, AMR, and mixed rejection are treated in Chaps. 13, 14, and 15.

Case 3
Late graft dysfunction (Figs. 10.7 and 10.8)

A man of 51 years underwent heart transplantation in 2003 for ischemic heart disease. The donor was a woman of 55 years; cold ischemia time was 165 min. The total mismatch was 4 and the donor-recipient CMV mismatch was negative.

In the first year post-transplant, the patient developed two episodes of mild rejection (both grade 1B/1R); 4 years-6 months later he had a moderate (3A/3R) rejection episode, treated with corticosteroids. The total ACR rejection score (Σ grading of each EMB/number of total EMBs) was 1.1, with a very low ACR severe rejection score (Σ EMB>= 3A/total EMBs) of 0.2. He developed mild CAV (ISHLT grade 1) after 5 years post-transplantation

In May 2011, 7 years 8 months after transplant, he returned to us with mild dyspnoea and severe fluid retention (NYHA class 2). ECG showed sinus rhythm with low voltages and right heart catheterization showed increased filling pressure with low cardiac output and wedge capillary pressure of 23 mmHg, despite normal ejection fraction (65 %).

An EMB was performed (Fig. 10.7). Histologically, at low power assessment, the myocardial interstitium appeared more cellular than normal. At high power, mild inflammatory mononuclear infiltrates were present in the extravascular interstitial compartment, not associated with significant myocyte damage; the capillaries and small venules had enlarged and prominent endothelial cells and lumina filled with aggregates of mononuclear cells. The inflammatory burden was high and inflammatory cells were prevalently extravascular. Immunohistochemistry for AMR revealed C4d positive in more than 50 % of capillaries and intravascular macrophages in less than 10 % of capillaries and small venules.

Histologic and immunopathologic findings were diagnostic of mixed rejection pattern: mild ACR (1B/1R grade) and full pathologic AMR (pAMR2).

Inflammatory infiltrates were evaluated in more detail: besides the expected inflammatory cells (CD3+ lymphocytes – total 25 % – and CD68+ macrophages – total 37 %) a significant number of CD138+ plasmacells were found (total 28 %: extravascular 71 %; intravascular 29 %) (Fig. 10.8).

DSA assessment with Luminex technique showed the presence of B40 class I antibody with MFI of 2278 and DQ2 class II with MFI of 3694. A DR7 class II nonspecific antibody was also found with MFI of 4381.

The patient was treated for both ACR (metilprednisolone 1 g ×3) and AMR (plasmapheresis and intravenous immunoglobulins).

In the following 4 months, C4d positivity dropped below 50 % although there were still histological findings of AMR. ACR was negative. In January 2012, the patient had another episode of pathologic AMR (pAMR2), in absence of ACR. The patient was again treated with plasmapheresis and intravenous immunoglobulins and also with rituximab.

Monitoring continued until December 2014: EMBs showed persistence of histologic findings of AMR and progressive lowering of C4d positivity.

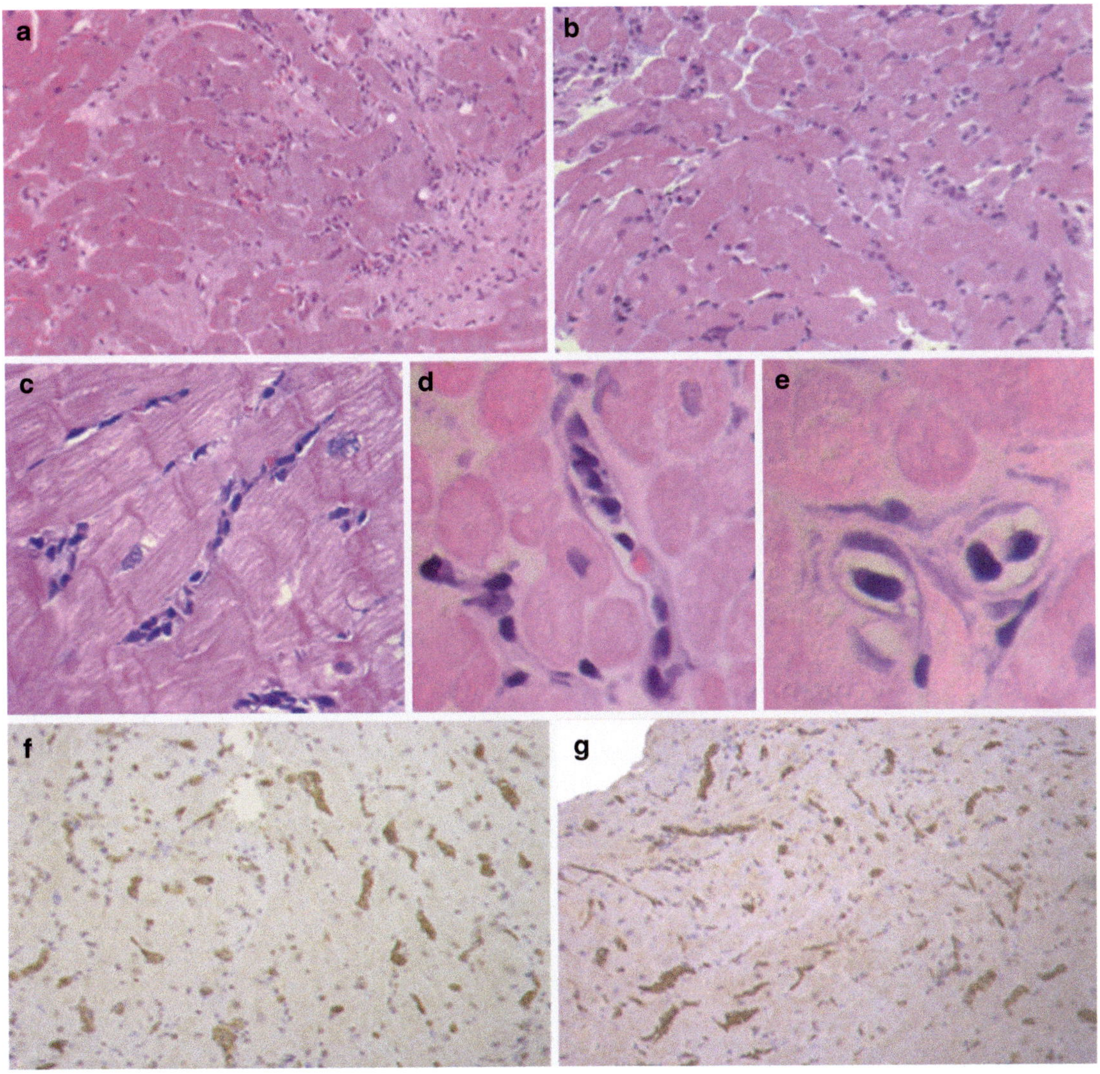

Fig. 10.7 Late graft dysfunction: Endomyocardial biopsy. (**a**, **b**) The myocardial interstitium is more cellular than normal due to the presence of mild extravascular inflammatory mononuclear infiltrates not associated with significant myocyte damage (**a**, Haematoxylin-eosin; ×200) and also to microvascular inflammation (**b**, Haematoxylin-eosin; ×200) with prominent endothelial cells and lumina of capillary and small venules filled with aggregates of mononuclear cells (**c**–**e**, Haematoxylin-eosin; ×400) (Fig. 10.3). (**f**, **g**) C4d immunostaining showing positivity in capillaries and small venules (×200)

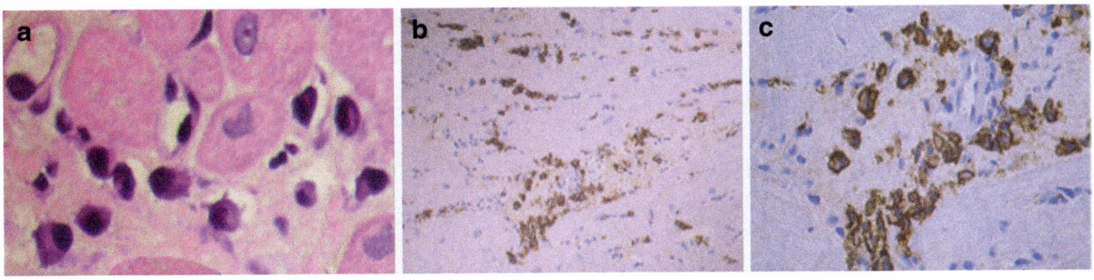

Fig. 10.8 Late graft dysfunction: The inflammatory infiltrates are rich in plasmacells: (**a**) Haematoxylin-eosin, ×400; (**b**, **c**): CD138 immunostaining for plasmacells (**b**: ×200; **c**: ×400)

Key Points

- Graft failure indicates the terminal state of irreversible loss of graft function causing retransplantation or death.
- Graft dysfunction indicates a potentially reversible and partial loss of function, often preceding but not necessarily leading to graft failure and death.
- Acute graft dysfunction is more frequent during the first year post-transplantation, but can occur later: the most common cause is cardiac rejection (cell-mediated, antibody mediated or mixed).
- Chronic graft dysfunction occurs later and the most common cause is CAV.
- Clinical presentation of acute/chronic graft dysfunction is not usually specific for one aetiology.
- EMB is the key element to diagnose the aetiology of acute graft dysfunction, where the main pathologic differential diagnoses are:
  - Rejection
  - Peritransplant injury
  - Ischemic damage
  - Cardiac localization of infections (rare event)
- The role of EMB in chronic late graft dysfunction is:
  - To recognize late episodes of ACR or AMR or to exclude them
  - To show concurrent findings (mild form of rejection, CAV-related microvasculopathy or significant interstitial fibrosis), which together can cause graft compromise or impaired performance.

References

Ardehali A, Esmailian F, Deng M, Soltesz E, Hsich E, Naka Y, Mancini D, Camacho M, Zucker M, Leprince P, Padera R, Kobashigawa J. Ex-vivo perfusion of donor hearts for human heart transplantation (PROCEED II): a prospective, open-label, multicentre, randomised non-inferiority trial. PROCEED II trial investigators. Lancet. 2015;385(9987):2577–84.

Badano LP, Miglioranza MH, Edvardsen T, Colafranceschi AS, Muraru D, Bacal F, Nieman K, Zoppellaro G, Marcondes Braga FG, Binder T, Habib G, Lancellotti P. European Association of Cardiovascular Imaging/Cardiovascular Imaging Department of the Brazilian Society of Cardiology recommendations for the use of cardiac imaging to assess and follow patients after heart transplantation. Eur Heart J Cardiovasc Imaging. 2015;16(9):919–48.

Billingham M, Cary N, Hammond E. A working formulation for the standardisation of nomenclature in the diagnosis of heart and lung rejection: heart rejection study group. J Heart Lung Transplant. 1990;8:587–93.

Boengler K, Schulz R, Heusch G. Loss of cardioprotection with ageing. Cardiovasc Res. 2009;83(2):247–61.

Boilson BA, Miller DV, Pereira NL. Late allograft failure after heart transplantation: 2 unusual cases. J Heart Lung Transplant. 2008;27(9):1050–4.

Butler J, Stankewicz MA, Wu J, et al. Pre-transplant reversible pulmonary hypertension predicts higher risk for mortality after cardiac transplantation. J Heart Lung Transplant. 2005;24:170–7.

Oto T, Excell L, Griffiths AP, Levvey BJ, Bailey M, Marasco S, Macdonald P, Snell P, Snell GI. Association between primary graft dysfunction among lung, kidney and heart recipients from the same multiorgan donor. Am J Transplant. 2008;8(10):2132–9.

Caves PK, Stinson EB, Billingham ME, Shumway NE. Serial transvenous biopsy of the transplanted human heart. Improved management of acute rejection episodes. Lancet. 1974;1(7862):821–6.

Cheng R, Azarbal B, Yung A, Chang DH, Patel JK, Kobashigawa JA. Elevated immune monitoring early after cardiac transplantation is associated with increased plaque progression by intravascular ultrasound. Clin Transplant. 2015;29(2):103–9.

Cosio C, Gomez Bueno M, Almenar L, Delgado JF, Arizon JM, Gonzalez Vilchez F, Crespo-Leiro MG, Mirabet S, Roig E, Perez Villa F, Fernandez-Yanez JF, Lambert JL, Manito N, Fuente L, Sanz Julve ML, Pascual D, Rabago G, Millan I, Alonso-Pulpon LA, Segovia J. Primary graft failure after heart transplantation: characteristics in a contemporary cohort and performance of the RADIAL risk score. J Heart Lung Transplant. 2013;32(12):1187–95.

Fedrigo M, Leone O, Burke MM, Rice A, Toquet C, Vernerey D, Frigo AC, Guillemain R, Pattier S, Smith J, Lota A, Potena L, Bontadini A, Ceccarelli C, Poli F, Feltrin G, Gerosa G, Manzan E, Thiene G, Bruneval P, Angelini A, Duong Van Huyen JP. Am J Transplant. Inflammatory cell burden and phenotype in endomyocardial biopsies with antibody-mediated rejection (AMR): a multicenter pilot study from the AECVP. 2015;15(2):526–34.

Gupta G, Abu Jawdeh BG, Racusen LC, Bhasin B, Arend LJ, Trollinger B, Kraus E, Rabb H, Zachary AA, Montgomery RA, Alachkar N. Late antibody-mediated rejection in renal allografts: outcome after conventional and novel therapies. Transplantation. 2014;97(12):1240–6.

Hicks M, Hing A, Gao L, Ryan J, Macdonald PS. Organ preservation. Methods Mol Biol. 2006;333:331–74.

Hiemann NE, Wellnhofer E, Knosalla C, Lehmkuhl HB, Stein J, Hetzer R, Meyer R. Prognostic impact of microvasculopathy on survival after heart transplantation: evidence from 9713 endomyocardial biopsies. Circulation. 2007;116(11):1274–82.

Kfoury AG, Stehlik J, Renlund DG, et al. Impact of repetitive episodes of antibody-mediated or cellular rejection on cardiovascular mortality in cardiac transplant recipients: defining rejection patterns. J Heart Lung Transplant. 2006;25:1277–82.

Khush KK, Kubo JT, Desai M. Influence of donor and recipient sex mismatch on heart transplant outcomes: analysis of the International Society for Heart and Lung Transplantation Registry. J Heart Lung Transplant. 2012;31(5):459–66.

Kobashigawa J, Crespo-Leiro MG, Ensminger SM, et al. Report from a consensus conference on antibody-mediated rejection in heart transplantation. J Heart Lung Transplant. 2011;30(3):252–69.

Kobashigawa J, Zuckermann A, Macdonald P, Leprince P, Esmailian F, Luu M, Mancini D, Patel J, Razi R, Reichenspurner H, Russell S, Segovia J, Smedira N, Stehlik J, Wagner F, Consensus Conference participants. Report from a consensus conference of primary graft dysfunction after cardiac transplantation. J Heart Lung Transplant. 2014;33(4):327–40.

Lund LH, Edwards LB, Kucheryavaya AY, Benden C, Christie JD, Dipchand AI, Dobbels F, Goldfarb SB, Levvey BJ, Meiser B, Yusen RD, Stehlik J. The registry of the International Society for Heart and Lung Transplantation: thirty-first official adult heart transplant report – 2014; focus theme: retransplantation. J Heart Lung Transplant. 2014;33(10):996–1008.

Mehra MR, Crespo-Leiro MG, Dipchand A, Ensminger SM, Hiemann NE, Kobashigawa JA, Madsen J, Parameshwar J, Starling RC, Uber PA. International Society for Heart and Lung Transplantation working formulation of a standardized nomenclature for cardiac allograft vasculopathy-2010. J Heart Lung Transplant. 2010;29:717–27.

Michaels PJ, Espejo ML, Kobashigawa JA, et al. Humoral rejection in cardiac transplantation: risk factors, hemodynamic consequences and relationship to transplant coronary artery disease. J Heart Lung Transplant. 2003;22:58–69.

Mohamedali B, Bhat G, Tatooles A, Zelinger A. Neurogenic stress cardiomyopathy in heart donors. J Cardiac Fail. 2014;20:207–11.

Nair N, Ball T, Uber PA, Mehra MR. Current and future challenges in therapy for antibody-mediated rejection. J Heart Lung Transplant. 2011;30(6):612–7.

Novitzky D, Cooper DK, Rosendale JD, Kauffman HM. Hormonal therapy of the brain-dead organ donor: experimental and clinical studies. Transplantation. 2006;82(11):1396–401.

Nwakanma LU, Williams JA, Weiss ES, Russell SD, Baumgartner WA, Conte JV. Influence of pretransplant panel-reactive antibody on outcomes in 8,160 heart transplant recipients in recent era. Ann Thorac Surg. 2007;84(5):1556–62; discussion 1562–3.

Potena L, Bontadini A, Iannelli S, Fruet F, Leone O, Barberini F, Borgese L, Manfredini V, Masetti M, Magnani G, Fallani F, Grigioni F, Branzi A. Occurrence of fatal and nonfatal adverse outcomes after heart transplantation in patients with pretransplant noncytotoxic HLA antibodies. J Transplant. 2013;2013:519680.

Potena L, Masetti M, Sabatino M, Bacchi-Reggiani ML, Pece V, Prestinenzi P, Dall'Ara G, Taglieri N, Saia F, Fallani F, Magnani G, Rapezzi C, Grigioni F. Interplay of coronary angiography and intravascular ultrasound in predicting long-term outcomes after heart transplantation. J Heart Lung Transplant. 2015;34(9):146–53.

Russo MJ, Iribarne A, Hong KN, et al. Factors associated with primary graft failure after heart transplantation. Transplantation. 2010;90:444–50.

Sellares J, de Freitas DG, Mengel M, Reeve J, Einecke G, Sis B, Hidalgo LG, Famulski K, Matas A, Halloran PF. Understanding the causes of kidney transplant failure: the dominant role of antibody-mediated rejection and nonadherence. Am J Transplant. 2012;12(2):388–99.

Stewart S, Winters GL, Fishbein MC, Tazelaar HD, Kobashigawa J, Abrams J, Andersen CB, Angelini A, Berry GJ, Burke MM, Demetris AJ, Hammond E, Itescu S, Marboe CC, McManus B, Reed EF, Reinsmoen NL, Rodriguez ER, Rose AG, Rose M, Suciu-Focia N, Zeevi A, Billingham ME. Revision of the 1990 working formulation for the standardization of nomenclature in the diagnosis of heart rejection. J Heart Lung Transplant. 2005;24(11):1710–20.

Tang Z, Kobashigawa J, Rafiei M, Stern LK, Hamilton M. The natural history of biopsy-negative rejection after heart transplantation. J Transplant. 2013;2013:236720.

White M, Wiechmann RJ, Roden RL, Hagan MB, Wollmering MM, Port JD, Hammond E, Abraham WT, Wolfel EE, Lindenfeld J, et al. Cardiac beta-adrenergic neuroeffector systems in acute myocardial dysfunction related to brain injury. Evidence for catecholamine-mediated myocardial damage. Circulation. 1995;92(8):2183–9.

Clinical Management of Transplant Recipients

11

Marco Masetti and Francesco Grigioni

Contents

11.1 Background

Heart transplantation (HTx) is regarded as the most effective therapeutic strategy for patients with end-stage heart failure, with an overall 1- and 5-year survival of 85 % and 70 %, respectively, according to the Registry of the International Society for Heart and Lung Transplantation (ISHLT) (Stehlik et al. 2013). Despite these encouraging data, the marked discrepancy between the need for and availability of donor organs limits access to HTx, and thus its overall success. Advances in medical and interventional treatments (including drug optimization, electrostimulatory devices, and implantable mechanical assist devices) have also improved the outcomes of patients with heart failure (Kirklin et al. 2014; Yancy et al. 2013), leading to an increased number reaching an advanced stage with multiple comorbidities, and thus increasing the number of patients needing heart

M. Masetti, PhD • F. Grigioni, MD, PhD (✉)
Heart Failure and Heart Transplant Program, Cardiology Unit, S. Orsola Malpighi University Hospital, Bologna, Italy
e-mail: francesco.grigioni@unibo.it

O. Leone et al. (eds.), *The Pathology of Cardiac Transplantation*,
DOI 10.1007/978-3-319-46386-5_11

transplantation, but with a predicted more complicated posttransplant course. In this context, the most common cause of death remains graft failure, whose etiology usually varies with time from transplant and can be related to cardiac allograft vasculopathy (CAV), rejection (both in the cellular-mediated rejection (CMR) or antibody-mediated rejection (AMR) forms or even mixed) (see Chap. 10). Posttransplant malignancies are the second most common cause of death, followed by infections and renal failure. These adverse events as well as other comorbidities may arise as a consequence of long-term immunosuppression, which may exacerbate preexisting conditions and favor new-onset noncardiac diseases (e.g., diabetes, renal insufficiency).

In this chapter we will review patient management strategies to reduce the risk of acute and chronic graft failure, as well as the onset of noncardiac comorbidities, which are often related to immunosuppressive drug side effects.

11.1.1 Evaluation Criteria for Heart Transplantation

The first step toward an optimal posttransplant outcome is adequate patient selection. The evaluation of a patient for a HTx is an ongoing, longitudinal process, aiming both to carefully assess the real need for HTx, through evaluation of clinical and instrumental parameters, and to exclude potential contraindications. Eligibility for HTx must be assessed after a period of optimized medical therapy; the main indications were recently redefined by ISHLT Guidelines (Mehra et al. 2016). Indications and contraindications for HTx are discussed in detail in Chap. 4.

11.2 Early Postoperative Management

Early postoperative management focuses on two major goals: (1) recovery of graft function after myocardial and endothelial injuries related to donor brain death and ischemia during organ transportation and (2) acute immunosuppression to avoid or at least delay immune system priming against graft antigens. As early graft dysfunction is the first cause of death in the postoperative period (Kobashigawa et al. 2014), control of potential factors influencing delayed recovery of hemodynamic function is crucial. The task starts with careful organ protection strategies during donor management, organ retrieval, and transportation (Jahania et al. 1999) (see also Chaps. 7 and 8). After organ implantation, circulatory function usually needs to be supported by inotropes with (adrenaline, dobutamine, noradrenaline) or without (milrinone, levosimendan) vasoconstrictive properties, balancing, as much as possible, the catecholamine-mediated positive effect on circulatory support and peripheral organ perfusion with the injury that these drugs may further cause.

With an uneventful postoperative period, inotropes are gradually withdrawn and the patient is usually weaned from the ventilator within 24 h. A major threat in this phase is recipient's pulmonary hypertension (PH). Postcapillary PH is a common finding in patients with advanced heart failure and may be associated with a precapillary component reactive to chronic left-side elevated filling pressures (Grigioni et al. 2006; Vachièry et al. 2013). After graft implantation, even if normal left ventricular function and adequate cardiac output are restored, elevated pulmonary resistance may not decrease promptly, so causing increased post-load in pulmonary circulation, which can severely impair right ventricular function. To avoid this, careful pretransplant periodic assessment of changes in pulmonary pressures and resistances is performed; post-Htx PH therapeutic strategy includes direct pulmonary vasodilators such as inhaled nitric oxide, oral sildenafil, or even intravenous prostaglandin, in association with inotropes. There have been reports of success with this in single-center observational experiences, but it must be emphasized that randomized studies are lacking (Singh et al. 2014; Stobierska-Dzierzek et al. 2001).

When drugs are not sufficient to restore or support ventricular function after transplantation, mechanical circulatory devices may help to bridge the patient to recovery. The most frequent approach is an extracorporeal membrane oxygenator (ECMO) pump, an extracorporeal device that can totally or partially substitute heart and lung function. According to the recent ISHLT consensus classification, the need for ECMO identifies severe early graft dysfunction. Incidences of reported ECMO use vary, but in all cases, related mortality is rather high, ranging from 30 to 60 %.

As mentioned, clinical complexity and patient deterioration are major risk factors for early graft dysfunction and associated postoperative complications; compromised posttransplant conditions are associated with renal and hepatic failure with need of dialysis or ultrafiltration. Compromised multi-organ function, in turn, increases the risk of systemic or respiratory infections: of note, in our Center's experience, 50 % of deaths of patients needing ECMO support after transplantation are related to infectious complications.

Arrhythmias can also occur after surgery, so temporary epicardial pacing wires are usually put in place at the time of HTx, even if the initial rhythm is sinus, in order to maintain heart rates of >90 beats/min. Supraventricular arrhythmias, including atrial fibrillation, are not uncommon after HTx, particularly as a consequence of surgical anastomosis,

Other early surgical complications can be surgical wound problems, mediastinitis, and pleural and pericardial effusions, which often require drainage (i.e., pericardiocentesis or thoracentesis). For this reason, pleural and pericardial drainages are maintained in the first 2–4 days after surgery and removed after X-ray documentation of the absence of pleural effusions.

During the first days following surgery, a physical training program is gradually started, aiming to improve respiratory mechanics and to limit the occurrence of pulmonary infections.

Immunosuppression is started in the early postoperative phase (in the operating theater as an induction therapy in most centers) then maintenance immunosuppression is progressively tapered, initially through intravenous drugs then orally, after the patient is extubated. At the beginning of immunosuppression, acute rejection episodes (typically ACR) can occur, as well as bacterial or fungal infections, especially in the lung or urinary tract, as a consequence of immune system depression. These aspects of rejection and immunosuppression will be discussed in further detail below.

11.3 Early Problems After Heart Transplantation

The clinical follow-up is very strict in the first weeks after hospital discharge. In this period, the main complications are acute myocardial rejection, both cell mediated (ACR) and antibody mediated (AMR), and clinically significant infections related to immunosuppressive therapy.

11.3.1 Rejection

Myocardial rejection is routinely monitored with scheduled endomyocardial biopsies (EMB).

EMB protocols might differ among centers and also according to predicted risk of rejection (higher in young people, women with previous pregnancies, African-Americans, and patients with other prior surgical operations or blood transfusions). Scheduled EMBs are usually performed until the first or second year after HTx (more rarely up to 5 years in some centers) and are more frequent in the first 3–6 months. Additional biopsies are performed in case of clinical suspicion of rejection; however, most cases of cellular rejection are asymptomatic without any graft or hemodynamic impairment. Cellular rejection (ACR) or mixed scenarios with both ACR and antibody-mediated rejection (AMR) can lead to clinical signs of graft dysfunction or symptoms that can vary from supraventricular or ventricular arrhythmias to mild dyspnea or asthenia or even signs of heart failure. The clinical picture of graft dysfunction is treated in detail in Chap. 10.

Treatment of acute rejection is discussed later in this chapter.

11.3.2 Infections

Infections are usually more frequent during the first months after HTx due to the high immunosuppressive burden associated with postoperative frailty, especially in high-risk patients (i.e., older, with renal failure, COPD), but can occur even in the late postoperative period. As depicted in Fig. 11.1, in the early phase, wound infections and *Candida albicans* infections are the most frequent complications, whereas in the midterm pneumonia (bacterial, *Pneumocystis carinii*), urinary tract infections (often bacterial), *Cytomegalovirus* (CMV) infections, herpes virus or varicella-zoster infections, and mycosis (*Candida albicans*) might occur.

Prophylaxis for *Pneumocystis carinii* and for oral candidiasis is usually delivered for at least 6 months after HTx. In case of a severe infection, global immunosuppression is generally reduced, as long as no significant recent rejection episodes have occurred.

11.3.3 CMV Infection

Given the high prevalence of *Cytomegalovirus* (CMV) latent infection in the general population, CMV reactivation frequently occurs after HTx, favored by immunosuppression and postoperative inflammation. The risk of virus reactivation or infection is highest in seronegative patients receiving hearts from positive donors (CMV mismatch, R–/D+) and moderately frequent in positive recipients (R+). Therefore, the CMV serologic status of both donor and recipient is evaluated to stratify patient risk for developing a CMV infection and to manage anti-CMV strategy (Kotton et al. 2010).

CMV infection can be completely asymptomatic, especially when viral load is low; occasionally it may lead to flu-like symptoms: fatigue, low-grade fever, leukopenia (CMV syndrome). More severe clinical scenarios with organ

	<1 month *(mainly nosocomial)*	1–6 months *(mainly oportunisitc)*	>6 months *(mainly community acquired)*
Viral	HSV	CMV EBV Zoster HBV/HCV reactivation	CMV Papillomavirus
Fungal	Candida	Pneumocystis Aspergillus Cryptococcus	
Bacterial	Wound and urinary tract infections Bacterial pneumonias	Nocardia Listeria Tubercolosis	Community acquired pneumonias and urinary infections
Parasitosis		Toxoplasma Leishmania Tripanosoma	

Fig. 11.1 Course of infection according to time from HTx

involvement can however occur, including hepatitis, gastroenteritis, and pneumonia (CMV disease) (Griffiths et al. 1999). Strategies to prevent CMV infection and disease should be planned, because of CMV impact on organ function in cases of overt CMV disease, and because of its indirect effects on graft function: even subclinical low-grade CMV infection may trigger immune-mediated endothelial damage, and so possibly even cardiac allograft vasculopathy (Griffiths et al. 1999; Potena et al. 2006). The impact of CMV on the graft appears to be mediated by innate and adaptive immune systems, rather than by a direct in situ viral cytotoxic effect. The more aggressively CMV infection is treated and prophylaxis used, the less intimal hyperplasia develops.

Using specific anti-CMV agents such as (val) ganciclovir, two strategies are recommended to prevent CMV infection and disease: universal prophylaxis and preemptive therapy. While prophylaxis consists of administrating the antiviral agent to all patients at risk, with the preemptive strategy, only patients who develop a "certain" threshold of subclinical infection receive treatment (Kotton et al. 2010; Potena et al. 2009).

Immunosuppressive agents also influence CMV infection: inhibitors of the mammalian target of rapamycin (mTOR), tested for prevention of acute rejection in solid organ transplant recipients, appear to have anti-CMV properties and to reduce CAV progression when started early post HTx (Eisen et al. 2013).

11.4 Immunosuppressive Drugs

A complete description of the various immunosuppressive drugs and their respective treatments goes beyond the purposes of this textbook (see Table 11.1). These drugs act at various levels in the pathways involved in cellular proliferation, as depicted in Fig. 11.2. Immunosuppressive drugs may be administered at the induction phase, as maintenance therapy or to treat rejection.

"Induction" consists in the administration of a high immunosuppressive burden by polyclonal or monoclonal antibody preparations (described below) at the time of transplant and for a few days after. Not all transplant centers currently use this approach and the efficacy of induction strategy over noninduction is debated (Costanzo et al. 2010; Whitson et al. 2015).

This approach is related to the need to monitor for the effect of inflammatory stimuli such as donor brain death, ischemia/reperfusion, and surgical trauma, which increase donor antigen expression and thus recipient immune response.

In this phase, the not fully recovered renal function and low levels of hemoglobin may disturb the beginning of the immunosuppression maintenance regimen, especially of calcineurin inhibitors (CNI).

Induction therapy (with thymoglobulin, or alternatively with basiliximab) allows the introduction of other immunosuppressive agents, particularly CNI (either tacrolimus or cyclosporine) to be delayed, in order to avoid CNI-related exacerbation of renal dysfunction and to preserve renal function in the postoperative period. Disadvantages of induction therapy are the increased risk of infection, malignancies, and elevated costs.

"Maintenance therapy" consists in a long-term immunosuppressive regimen to monitor immune system activity against graft antigens and so prevent acute and chronic rejection.

We will now provide a brief description of the mechanism of action of the main compounds used for induction and maintenance therapy, and of treatments for acute rejection.

11.4.1 Polyclonal and Monoclonal Antilymphocyte Antibody Preparations

Polyclonal antibody preparations are ATGAM (derived from horses) and thymoglobulin (from rabbits); they act against surface T- and B-cell molecules, including HLA, leading to lymphocyte depletion by complement-dependent opsonization and eventual cell lysis and apoptosis. They may also bind granulocytes and platelets, potentially causing leucopenia and thrombocytopenia, thus requiring either a reduction in dose or

Table 11.1 Antirejection drugs and their use in various immunosuppression phases

Induction	Maintenance	Acute rejection
Polyclonal antilymphocytes antibodies *ATGAM (horses)* *Thymoglobulin (rabbits)*	Steroids (prednisone)	Steroids (methylprednisolone)
Anti-cytokine receptor antibodies *Basiliximab* *Daclizumab*	Calcineurin inhibitors *Cyclosporine* *Tacrolimus*	Thymoglobulin
	Antiproliferative agents *Azathioprine* *Mycophenolate mofetil* *mTOR inhibitors (everolimus, sirolimus)* *Cyclophosphamide*	Intravenous immunoglobulin
		Pheresis treatments *Plasma exchange* *Plasmapheresis* *Immunoadsorption*

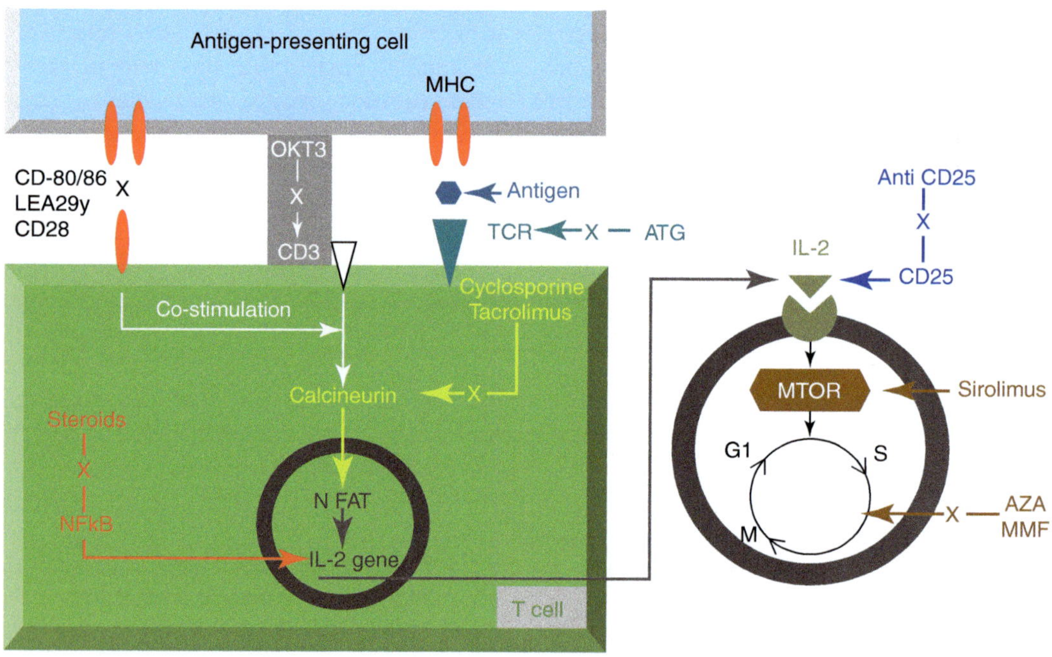

Fig. 11.2 Different action points of immunosuppressive drugs. *CD80* protein found on activated B cells and monocytes providing a co-stimulatory signal for T-cell activation, *CD86* protein expressed on antigen-presenting cells, *CD28* protein expressed on T cells, *LEA29y* (*belatacept*) fusion protein crucial in the regulation of T-cell co-stimulation, *NFAT* nuclear factor of activated T cells, *NF-kB* nuclear factor kappa-light-chain-enhancer of activated B cells, *MHC* major histocompatibility complex, *TCR* T-cell receptor

termination of therapy. Monitoring of T cells with flow cytometry is used to assess efficacy and to adjust dosage. The xenogeneic origin of these polyclonal antibodies can induce a hypersensitivity response characterized by urticaria, fever, chills, and rash, especially after the first dose, so premedication with steroids is often prescribed (Aliabadi et al. 2016).

11.4.2 Anti-cytokine Receptor Antibodies

The only anti-cytokine receptor antibody still available is basiliximab (daclizumab is no longer on the market). This is a chimeric (mouse/human) anti-IL-2R monoclonal antibody that binds CD25, a subunit of IL-2R expressed on antigen-activated T cells, preventing the binding of IL-2 to IL-2R and inhibiting T-cell proliferation. The drug is intravenously injected in two doses: the first in the operating room, the second after 4 days; its activity is maintained up to 4–6 weeks. Basiliximab is used as induction therapy in many heart transplantation centers, although recent registry analysis suggests lower efficacy than thymoglobulins (Ansari et al. 2015; Martin et al. 2015; Campara et al. 2010). Belatacept (LEA29y) and muronomab (OKT3) are not currently used in the setting of heart transplantation.

11.4.3 Corticosteroids (Steroids)

Steroids are a historic cornerstone in all phases of immunosuppression: induction, maintenance, and acute therapy. The glucocorticoid receptor–steroid complex translocates into the nucleus, where by binding to DNA, it influences the expression of genes involved in immune and inflammatory response and affects the number, distribution, and function of all types of leukocytes (T and B lymphocytes, granulocytes, macrophages, and monocytes), as well as endothelial cells. High-dose steroids are usually given intravenously at the time of operation and in the first days after HTx, and then orally, with gradual dose tapering over months or years, according to rejection surveillance. Pulse steroids, either oral or intravenous, are usually the first treatment for moderate rejection (ISHLT grade 3A/2R) without hemodynamic impairment, with efficacy in 80–85 % of cases. Current guidelines suggest weaning from steroids within the first year after transplant, to avoid long-term adverse events (Costanzo et al. 2010). Main side effects are hypertension, emotional lability, cataracts, gastric ulcer, poor wound healing, and proximal myopathy. Cosmetic effects include hirsutism, acne, easy bruising, skin fragility, moon face, buffalo hump, weight gain, and truncal obesity. Major metabolic effects are hyperlipidemia, salt and water retention, diabetes mellitus, osteopenia, avascular necrosis, and growth retardation in children. Long-term administration of steroids may result in chronic adrenal suppression, and adrenal insufficiency can follow steroid tapering, with fever, asthenia, and hypotension (Lindenfeld et al. 2004).

11.4.4 Calcineurin Inhibitors (CNI)

The currently available CNIs are cyclosporine (CSA) and tacrolimus (TAC). Since its discovery in 1982, when it led to an improvement in post-transplant survival, CSA (derived from *Tolypocladium inflatum*) has remained a cornerstone of maintenance therapy. Both drugs bind to immunophilins (CSA to cyclophilin and TAC to FK binding protein 12, FKBP-12); the complex binds calcineurin, a phosphatase that dephosphorylates multiple molecules, including NF-AT (NF of activated T cells). Dephosphorylated NF-AT binds the promoter regions of IL-2, inhibiting IL-2 transcription (Lindenfeld et al. 2004). The CNI dose is adjusted according to blood levels, and depending on distance from transplant and occurrence of rejection. Their main adverse effect is renal toxicity. This dose-related side effect may be acute or chronic. According to the literature, CNI-related renal failure occurs in 40–70 % of transplant recipients; 33 % mean reduction of creatinine clearance at 6 months after HTx is reported; 7 % of patients require hemodialysis due to end-stage renal failure. Other frequent adverse effects are hypertension, hyperlipidemia, neurological problems (tremor, paresthesias, headache, seizures, mental status changes, visual symptoms, and insomnia), cholestasis, diabetes (more frequently in TAC), hypertrichosis, and gingival hyperplasia (only in CSA), alopecia (only TAC). TAC, previously known as FK506, is a macrolide produced by the fungus *Streptomyces tsukubaensis*. A clinical trial showed that TAC is more effective than CSA in preventing biopsy-proven cellular rejection when associated with mycophenolate mofetil (Kobashigawa et al. 2006); therefore, TAC/MMF is currently considered the standard of care in modern maintenance immunosuppressive regimens.

11.4.5 Antiproliferative Agents

Azathioprine (AZA) AZA is an oral prodrug that is converted to a purine analog and incorporated into DNA, inhibiting its synthesis and the proliferation of both T and B lymphocytes. The major side effects of AZA are myelosuppression (leukopenia, anemia, and thrombocytopenia) and skin cancers. More modern compounds (see below) have shown greater efficacy than AZA in preventing cellular rejection, thus confining the use of this drug to long-term maintenance patients, or to those not tolerating either mycophenolate or mTOR inhibitors (Kobashigawa et al. 1998; Eisen et al. 2003).

Mycophenolate mofetil (MMF) MMF is a noncompetitive inhibitor of inosine monophosphate dehydrogenase. Proliferating lymphocytes are dependent on this pathway as the only mechanism for purine synthesis and DNA replication, whereas other cells also use other salvage pathways for purine synthesis. MMF selectively inhibits lymphocyte proliferation in response to allogeneic stimulation without inhibiting other cell lines. MMF is given orally, usually twice a day, and in a prospective randomized trial proved superior to AZA for graft survival and in preventing rejection, even when used with reduced CSA doses. It is currently the standard antiproliferative drug. Major side effects are nausea, vomiting, and diarrhea, usually dose dependent (Lindenfeld et al. 2004; Kobashigawa et al. 1998).

mTOR inhibitors Sirolimus (SIR) and its analog everolimus (EVE), first isolated in soil samples from Rapa Nui (Easter Island), is a natural product of the actinomycetes *Streptomyces hygroscopicus*. These drugs bind to the same family of immunophilins as TAC, but rather than blocking calcineurin-dependent T-cell activation, inhibit the mammalian target of rapamycin (mTOR). This kinase phosphorylating protein is involved in the regulation of the cell cycle and plays a critical role in signals from the growth factor receptors to the cell nucleus, to stimulate growth and proliferation of T and B lymphocytes, smooth muscle cells, and endothelial cells. The frequent involvement of the mTOR system in various biological pathways (endothelial cells and smooth muscle cell proliferation, cancerogenesis, healing repair) explains both its adverse effects and its potentially positive effect in various pathological processes (Zuckermann et al. 2013). Both sirolimus and everolimus proved superior to AZA in prevention of cellular rejection, and everolimus proved noninferior to MMF. A peculiar clinical effect of this class of drugs is to reduce coronary intimal thickness, a major feature of early CAV development. In addition, antiproliferative properties of everolimus have been studied in general oncology (Baselga et al. 2012; Motzer et al. 2010) or in transplanted patients developing a tumor (Epailly et al. 2011; Stallone et al. 2005; Salgo et al. 2010).

On the same basis, these drugs can lead to a slower wound healing repair process, particularly in diabetic and obese patients (Zuckermann et al. 2013), and to a higher susceptibility to infection, particularly bacterial. The synergic effect with CSA allows a reduction in CSA dose, with the aim of reducing the CNI-related nephrotoxic effect. It must be noted, however, that sirolimus use in heart transplant is off-label and that, in the United States and Canada, everolimus is not registered for heart transplant.

11.5 Treatment of Acute Rejection

Acute cellular rejection episodes Although rejection treatment can vary slightly among centers, therapeutic protocols are more or less established. Biopsy-proven cellular rejection ≥2R (3A) is usually treated by intravenous methylprednisolone (normally 1 g for 3 days), sometimes followed by an increase in oral maintenance dosage. With higher grades of rejection (>2R) or a 2R rejection with compromised graft (i.e., low cardiac output or high ventricular filling pressures, reduced ejection fraction) or in symptomatic patients, thymoglobulins are used in addition to steroids. Any clinically symptomatic rejection must be treated regardless of histological grade. Treatment of low-grade (1R) rejection varies among centers, it is not usually treated if it occurs late after HTx; whereas in the earlier phases, background immunosuppression is usually increased. Recurrent rejections can be treated with thymoglobulin and a change in background immunosuppression.

Patients with severe hemodynamic impairment due to rejection can develop heart failure; in this case, they should be transferred to ICU for the standard heart failure treatment, including diuretics, inotropic drugs, or even temporary ventricular assist devices (intra-aortic balloon pump, ECMO). In these more severe cases, especially when occurring late after HTx, a mixed scenario characterized by coexistence of cellular and antibody-mediated rejection and graft vasculopathy may occur, thus complicating clinical management. A more detailed description of graft failure management is described in the correspondent Chapter in this book Chapter 11.

Antibody-mediated rejection (AMR) and mixed rejection forms There is as yet no standard treatment for AMR due to the lack of large sample prospective trials investigating this issue; although general recommendations were recently provided by ISHLT, treatment varies according to the local protocols. There is no agreed time to start treatment nor which specific drugs to choose. Current ISHLT guidelines and consensus on AMR recommend high-dose corticosteroids, plasmapheresis, and IVIg as first-line therapies. Currently secondary therapies include rituximab, bortezomib, and anti-complement antibodies. While there is general consensus in treating AMR with any sign of graft dysfunction, whether to treat (and how) pAMR findings with or without donor specific antibodies, in absence of graft dysfunction, is still under debate.

Typical pathological findings of AMR are extensively described in Chap. 14. Here we must emphasize the clinical importance of a differential diagnosis between cellular and antibody-mediated rejection, which is currently only possible with pathological analysis of EMB, because of the different therapeutic approaches.

11.6 Strategies for Antibody-Mediated Rejection

Mechanical removal of antibodies These methods are used to remove circulating alloantibodies mechanically, and have the advantage of being inexpensive. The general principle is to separate plasma from cellular blood components by centrifugation or membrane filtration, which removes the alloantibody. The reconstituted blood is then reinfused into the patient.

There are three different techniques (Kobashigawa et al. 2011):

1. Plasma exchange (PE): the plasma-depleted blood is reconstituted with fresh-frozen plasma or albumin, which usually gives no anaphylactic reactions.
2. Double-filtration plasmapheresis (DF-PP): after removal of plasma, the low-molecular-weight fraction of plasma is obtained by a second physical separation and then infused into the patient.
3. Immunoabsorption (IA) plasmapheresis: here the second separation is immunochemical and allows removal of only immunoglobulins, through binding them to immune absorbents, which are typically porous beads covalently coupled to polyclonal antihuman IgG antibody or to protein A, a natural component of *Staphylococcus aureus* with high affinity for circulating immune complex and IgG.

The first two techniques remove nonselectively (or only partially) all plasma components, such as proteins, leading to an increased risk of bleeding and infection; these require fluid replacement with fresh-frozen plasma or albumin, with possible allergic reactions and infections. They are not selective enough to remove all antibodies, and administration of immunosuppressive agents is then needed. IA avoids fluid replacement, but is more expensive than the other techniques and does not allow the removal of cytokines, which often play a role in AMR. Before HTx, plasmapheresis can be used in highly sensitized waiting list patients to reduce their circulating antibodies, so increasing their chances of finding a donor with negative crossmatch. After HTx, PP or IA are used to treat symptomatic AMR. Duration of plasmapheretic treatment varies between centers and ranges from a few days to 3–4 weeks.

Drugs to decrease antibody activity Intravenous immunoglobulin (IVIG) is currently the primary method used to inhibit, often used in combination with plasmapheresis, to reduce the reactivity of eventual residual circulating alloantibodies. Major adverse events are allergic reaction and, rarely, thromboembolic events and renal insufficiency (Jordan et al. 2009).

Drugs suppressing B-cell lines Rituximab is a chimeric monoclonal anti-CD20 antibody. It binds to CD20, which is involved in B-cell activation and differentiation, and leads to B-cell depletion by antibody-dependent cell cytotoxicity (ADCC). This drug has been approved for treatment of B-cell lymphomas and rheumatoid arthritis; it is currently used in AMR treatment, but in studies or in clinical series has often been used in combination with other immunosuppressive agents and PP, thus limiting the reliability of its evaluation as a single agent. Drugs targeting proteasomes show potential in reducing plasma cell activity and protein synthesis: *bortezomib* is a proteasome inhibitor approved for multiple myeloma and mantle cell lymphoma; it binds the catalytic site of the 26S proteasome. Adverse effects can be gastrointestinal toxicity, thrombocytopenia, and paresthesias (Kaczmarek et al. 2007; Kittleson and Kobashigawa 2012).

11.7 Long-Term Complications After Heart Transplantation

The major long-term complications after heart transplantation include cardiac allograft vasculopathy, renal insufficiency, and malignancies. Because of their clinical importance and complexity, they are dealt with in Chaps. 18, 20, and 21. We shall now describe additional complications often seen after heart transplant, mainly related to side effects of immunosuppressive therapy, and which may significantly affect morbidity and quality of life.

11.7.1 Hypertension

Hypertension occurs frequently after HTx (up to 90% of cases), as a side effect of steroids and CNIs (Lindenfeld et al. 2005). Some patients, particularly those with ischemic cardiomyopathy, were already hypertensive prior to HTx. Antihypertensive therapy is the same as for the general population: beta blockers, ACE inhibitors, angiotensin-receptor blockers, calcium blockers, alpha-antagonists, diuretics, and nitrates are the drugs commonly used. High doses of beta blockers, given the denervation of the transplanted heart; possible higher incidence of lower limb edema in patients taking calcium blockers and mTOR inhibitors; and effects of ACE inhibitors or sartans on renal function, particularly in diabetic patients, all require extra caution.

11.7.2 Noncardiac Surgery

Often HTx recipients may need noncardiac surgery, most frequently oncological and vascular surgery, general abdominal surgery (i.e., gallbladder), followed by orthopedic (i.e., hip prosthesis after steroid-induced aseptic necrosis), and minor surgery (i.e., hernias, dermatological, ocular). In the presence of a normal graft function, most of the surgical risk is related to kidney function and to infections; cardiac complications or graft failure episodes after surgery are rare. For this reason, depending on the type of surgery, immunosuppression is generally reduced before, during, and after the operation, to allow wound healing and tissue repair and to decrease the incidence of infections. Aggressive intra- and postsurgical antibiotic prophylaxis is given. In patients undergoing respiratory and gastrointestinal surgery, after which oral alimentation is not possible for a certain period, intravenous immunosuppressants are used (steroids, CSA, and in certain countries MMF and TAC). A myocardial biopsy before surgery can be considered in patients with recent or recurrent rejection episodes. The use of blood products (filtrated and irradiated) must be limited, in order to contain sensitization and avoid arising new antibodies, which could trigger rejection. mTOR inhibitors are interrupted before and after surgery to limit wound healing problems. Coronary angiography is not usually done before surgery, except in selected high-risk cases (Lyons et al. 1995).

11.7.3 Osteoporosis

Osteoporosis and osteopenia are quite frequent after HTx, for two main reasons: (1) a 30–50 % reduction in bone mass prior to HTx, caused by heart failure (hypocalcemia is related to high doses of diuretics, renal failure, and low levels of physical activity) and (2) high doses of steroids, especially in the first 6 months after HTx, leading to a reduction in bone density, especially in the vertebral column and hips. For these reasons, all adult HTx candidates should be screened for preexisting bone disease, with a dual energy X-ray absorptiometry scan of the lumbar spine and femoral neck. Aggressive treatment of osteoporosis is mandatory to prevent bone and hip fractures; bisphosphonates are the treatment of choice and are used to reduce bone turnover (with caution in presence of renal insufficiency), even in patients with osteopenia. All patients must have the recommended daily dose of calcium and vitamin D, if necessary with oral implementation, often used in patients with osteopenia. Regular physical activity must be encouraged to prevent fractures and osteoporosis (Jeon et al. 2015).

11.7.4 Diabetes Mellitus

Prevalence and incidence of diabetes increase after HTx (35–40 % of patients), due to steroid therapy. In a diabetic patient, glycemia worsens after HTx, due to steroids; a steroid-induced form of diabetes can reveal itself after HTx, which in some cases can be at least partially reversed with steroid tapering. The worsening of glycemia levels after HTx can accelerate vascular and nonvascular complications of diabetes: neuropathy, diabetic nephropathy, retinopathy, and peripheral vascular disease are a frequent cause of morbidity and mortality after HTx. For this reason, vascular damage related to diabetes must be carefully assessed before HTx. Claudicatio intermittens, repeated peripheral revascularizations, or even limb amputations and strokes are not rare after HTx, especially in former smokers and in patients with severe renal failure. Overall, the prevalence of vascular diseases related to diabetes is high after HTx; in these patients, a tapering of steroids can be considered, when possible. Diabetes is an independent predictor of mortality and a frequent cause of renal insufficiency; poor glycemia levels accelerate renal failure; 7 % of patients are on long-term dialysis after HTx, and diabetes is the prevalent cause in a consistent percentage of cases. As a renal-sparing strategy, CNI minimization or even elimination, together with avoidance of ACE inhibitors, is generally used with these patients. The topic of renal failure is treated elsewhere in this book.

11.7.5 Pregnancy and Sexual Health

Sexual reproduction in transplanted patients is challenging. When approaching this issue, the clinician must take several factors into account, and explain them to the patient: (1) the personal wishes of the patient, especially for pregnancy, and their associated psychological background, (2) graft function and the risk of sensitization and of rejection during pregnancy, (3) the potential teratogenicity of immunosuppressive agents, that can be transmitted both by placenta and by sperm, (4) the risk of transmitting familial heart disease (i.e., some forms of hypertrophic and dilated cardiomyopathy). Male transplant recipients may have reduced fertility, due to impaired spermatogenesis, and sometimes, erectile dysfunction. However, no malformations of newborns have been reported, despite a slight increase in the risk of preeclampsia (Morken et al. 2015).

In general, pregnancy should not be attempted sooner than 1 year after HTx. For a woman considering pregnancy, a global graft and rejection assessment, coronary angiography (if not performed within the previous 6 months), together with urine cultures and serological and microbiological tests should be made. For a pregnant woman, CNI can be continued, but with closer monitoring of blood levels, as they can fluctuate considerably due to changes in plasma volume. MMF however should be discontinued; the use of AZA can be considered, but is still controversial; steroids can be continued. No teratogenic effects have been reported in a single case of unplanned pregnancy with everolimus (Fiocchi et al. 2016). Hormonal contraception can be taken only after a hypercoagulability state has been excluded and should not be given to patients with severe hypertension, CAV, or history of estrogen-sensitive malignancies. Sexually active patients with or without multiple partners should be educated to use condoms and to undergo regular screening for sexually transmitted infections. Women should receive the quadrivalent human papillomavirus (HPV) vaccine for infection prevention before HTx. Intrauterine devices (IUD) are not generally recommended because of concerns regarding increased risk of pelvic inflammatory infection and infertility. Erectile dysfunction (ED) is frequent after HTx and can be related to diabetes, drugs, and psychological problems; phosphodiesterase inhibitors can be considered with caution when there is concomitant nitrate therapy, as in the general population.

11.7.6 Psychological and Psychiatric Disorders

Psychological and psychiatric problems are common after HTx for various reasons: the consequences of the stress of waiting for transplant, the frequent medical controls after HTx, fear of rejection, and also the psychological difficulty of accepting an organ from another person. Steroids too can induce or exacerbate humor problems, causing anxiety, or even depression and aggressive behavior. Even with a careful psychological screening before HTx, these problems can sometimes arise unexpectedly after HTx; for this reason, regular psychological counseling is crucial even after surgery, also with the view to preventing nonadherence to medication and to identify behavior problems. Nonadherence is a major and underestimated problem and may lead to adverse outcomes; it must be identified by carefully analyzing patient attitude and relationship with the transplant center medical personnel (Dobbels et al. 2010; Schafer-Keller et al. 2008). Serotonin reuptake inhibitors, particularly citalopram, and new-generation antidepressants are the most frequently used medication, whereas caution must be used with tricyclic antidepressants and MAO inhibitors, because of their cardiovascular toxicity (conduction delay, orthostatic hypotension, and anticholinergic affects the former, hypotension the latter). Psychological discomfort may represent a significant marker of adverse prognosis (Sirri et al. 2010).

Key Points

- Clinical management of heart transplant recipients is centered on multidisciplinary longitudinal evaluation.
- Management of infections and rejection characterizes the first phase after transplant.
- Immunosuppression therapy is effective in preventing rejection but exposes patients to a wide array of adverse events.
- Long-term management is mainly focused on preventing and controlling the medical side effects of chronic immunosuppressive therapy.

References

Aliabadi AZ, Grömmer M, Dunkler D, Eskandary F, Salameh O, Gökler J, Hutschala D, Steinlechner B, Opfermann P, Laufer G, Zuckermann AO. Impact of rabbit antithymocyte globulin dose on long-term outcomes in heart transplant patients. Transplantation. 2016;100(3):685–93.

Ansari D, Lund LH, Stehlik J, Andersson B, Höglund P, Edwards L, Nilsson J. Induction with anti-thymocyte globulin in heart transplantation is associated with better long-term survival compared with basiliximab. J Heart Lung Transplant. 2015;34(10):1283–91.

Baselga J, Campone M, Piccart M, et al. Everolimus in postmenopausal hormone-receptor-positive advanced breast cancer. N Engl J Med. 2012;366:520.

Campara M, Tzvetanov IG, Oberholzer J. Interleukin-2 receptor blockade with humanized monoclonal antibody for solid organ transplantation. Expert Opin Biol Ther. 2010;10(6):959–69.

Costanzo MR, Dipchand A, Starling R, et al. The International Society of Heart and Lung Transplantation guidelines for the care of heart transplant recipients. J Heart Lung Transplant. 2010;29:914–56.

Dobbels F, Berben L, De Geest S, Drent G, Lennerling A, Whittaker C, Kugler C. The psychometric properties and practicability of self-report instruments to identify medication nonadherence in adult transplant patients: a systematic review. Transplantation. 2010;90(2):205–19.

Eisen HJ, Tuzcu EM, Dorent R, Kobashigawa J, Mancini D, Valantine-von Kaeppler HA, Starling RC, Sorensen K, Hummel M, Lind JM, Abeywickrama KH, Bernhardt P. Everolimus for the prevention of allograft rejection and vasculopathy in cardiac-transplant recipients. N Engl J Med. 2003;349(9):847–58.

Eisen HJ, et al. Everolimus versus mycophenolate mofetil in heart transplantation: a randomized, multicenter trial. Am J Transplant. 2013;13:1203–16.

Epailly E, Albanell J, Andreassen A, et al. Proliferation signal inhibitors and post-transplant malignancies in heart transplantation: practical management questions. Clin Transplant. 2011;25:E475–86.

Fiocchi R, D'Elia E, Vittori C, Sebastiani R, Strobelt N, Eleftheriou G, Introna M, Freddi C, Crippa A. First report of a successful pregnancy in an everolimus-treated heart-transplanted patient: neonatal disappearance of immunosuppressive drugs. Am J Transplant. 2016;16(4):1319–22.

Griffiths PD, Cope AV, Hassan-Walker AF, et al. Diagnostic approaches to cytomegalovirus infection in bone marrow and organ transplantation. Transpl Infect Dis. 1999;1(3):179–86.

Grigioni F, Potena L, Galiè N, Fallani F, et al. Prognostic implications of serial assessments of pulmonary hypertension in severe chronic heart failure. J Heart Lung Transplant. 2006;25(10):1241–6.

Jahania MS, Sanchez JA, Narayan P, Lasley RD, Mentzer RM. Heart preservation for transplantation: principles and strategies. Ann Thorac Surg. 1999;68:1983–7.

Jeon HJ, Kim H, Yang J. Bone disease in post-transplant patients. Curr Opin Endocrinol Diabetes Obes. 2015;22(6):452–8.

Jordan SC, Toyoda M, Vo AA. Intravenous immunoglobulin a natural regulator of immunity and inflammation. Transplantation. 2009;88(1):1–6.

Kaczmarek I, Deutsch MA, Sadoni S, Brenner P, Schmauss D, Daebritz SH, Weiss M, Meiser BM, Reichart B. Successful management of antibody-mediated cardiac allograft rejection with combined immunoadsorption and anti-CD20 monoclonal antibody treatment: case report and literature review. J Heart Lung Transplant. 2007;26(5):511–5.

Kirklin JK, Naftel DC, Pagani FD, Kormos RL, Stevenson LW, Blume ED, Miller MA, Baldwin JT, Young JB. Sixth INTERMACS annual report: a 10000-patient database. J Heart Lung Transplant. 2014;33:555–64.

Kittleson MM, Kobashigawa JA. Antibody-mediated rejection. Curr Opin Organ Transplant. 2012;17(5):551–7.

Kobashigawa J, Miller L, Renlund D, Mentzer R, Alderman E, Bourge R, Costanzo M, Eisen H, Dureau G, Ratkovec R, Hummel M, Ipe D, Johnson J, Keogh A, Mamelok R, Mancini D, Smart F, Valantine H. A randomized active-controlled trial of mycophenolate mofetil in heart transplant recipients. Mycophenolate Mofetil Investigators. Transplantation. 1998;66(4):507–15.

Kobashigawa JA, Miller LW, Russell SD, Ewald GA, Zucker MJ, Goldberg LR, Eisen HJ, Salm K, Tolzman D, Gao J, Fitzsimmons W, First R, Study Investigators. Tacrolimus with mycophenolate mofetil (MMF) or sirolimus vs. cyclosporine with MMF in cardiac transplant patients: 1-year report. Am J Transplant. 2006;6(6):1377–86.

Kobashigawa J, Zuckermann A, Macdonald P, Leprince P, Esmailian F, Luu M, Mancini D, Patel J, Razi R, Reichenspurner H, Russell S, Segovia J, Smedira N, Stehlik J, Wagner F, Consensus Conference Participants. Report from a consensus conference on antibody-mediated rejection in heart transplantation. J Heart Lung Transplant. 2011;30:252–69.

Kobashigawa J, Zuckermann A, MacDonald P, Leprince P, et al. Report from a consensus conference on primary graft dysfunction after cardiac transplantation. J Heart Lung Transplant. 2014;33:327–40.

Kotton CN, Kumar D, Caliendo AM, et al. International consensus guidelines on the management of cytomegalovirus in solid organ transplantation. Transplantation. 2010;89:779.

Lindenfeld J, Miller GG, Shakar SF, Zolty R, Lowes BD, Wolfel EE, Mestroni L, Page 2nd RL, Kobashigawa J. Drug therapy in the heart transplant recipient. Part II: immunosuppressive drugs. Circulation. 2004;110(25):3858–65.

Lindenfeld J, Page 2nd RL, Zolty R, Shakar SF, Levi M, Lowes B, Wolfel EE, Miller GG. Drug therapy in the heart transplant recipient. Part III: common medical problems. Circulation. 2005;111(1):113–7.

Lyons JB, Chambers FA, MacSullivan R, Moriarty DC. Anaesthesia for non-cardiac surgery in the post-cardiac transplant patient. Ir J Med Sci. 1995;164(2):132–5.

Martin ST, Kato TS, Farr M, McKeen JT, Cheema F, Ji M, Ross A, Yerebakan H, Naka Y, Takayama H, Restaino S, Mancini D, Schulze PC. Similar survival in patients following heart transplantation receiving induction therapy using daclizumab vs. basiliximab. Circ J. 2015;79(2):368–74.

Mehra MR, Canter CE, Hannan MM, Semigran MJ, Uber PA, Baran DA, Danziger-Isakov L, Kirklin JK, Kirk R, Kushwaha SS, Lund LH, Potena L, Ross HJ, Taylor DO, Verschuuren EAM, Zuckermann A. The 2016 International Society for Heart Lung Transplantation listing criteria for heart transplantation: a 10-year update. J Heart Lung Transplant. 2016;35(1):1–23.

Morken NH, Diaz-Garcia C, Reisaeter AV, Foss A, Leivestad T, Geiran O, Hervás D, Brännström M. Obstetric and neonatal outcome of pregnancies fathered by males on immunosuppression after solid organ transplantation. Am J Transplant. 2015;15(6):1666–73.

Motzer RJ, Escudier B, Oudard S, et al. Phase 3 trial of everolimus or metastatic renal cell carcinoma: final results and analysis of prognostic factors. Cancer. 2010;116:4256.

Potena L, Holweg CT, Chin C, Luikart H, Weisshaar D, Narasimhan B, Fearon WF, Lewis DB, Cooke JP, Mocarski ES, Valantine HA. Acute rejection and cardiac allograft vascular disease is reduced by suppression of subclinical cytomegalovirus infection. Transplantation. 2006;82(3):398–405.

Potena L, Grigioni F, Magnani G, et al. Prophylaxis versus pre-emptive anti-cytomegalovirus approach for prevention of allograft vasculopathy in heart transplant recipients. J Heart Lung Transplant. 2009;28:461–7.

Salgo R, Gossmann J, Schofer H, et al. Switch to a sirolimus-based immunosuppression in long-term renal transplant recipients: reduced rate of (pre)-malignancies and non melanoma skin cancer in a prospective, randomized, assessor-blinded, controlled clinical trial. Am J Transplant. 2010;10:1385.

Schafer-Keller P, Steiger J, Bock A, Denhaerynck K, De Geest S. Diagnostic accuracy of measurement methods to assess non-adherence to immunosuppressive drugs in kidney transplant recipients. Am J Transplant. 2008;8(3):616–26.

Singh RK, Richmond ME, Zuckerman WA, Lee TM, et al. The use of oral sildenafil for management of right ventricular dysfunction after pediatric heart transplantation. Am J Transplant. 2014;14(2):453–8.

Sirri L, Potena L, Masetti M, Tossani E, Magelli C, Grandi S. Psychological predictors of mortality in heart transplanted patients: a prospective, 6-year follow-up study. Transplantation. 2010;89(7):879–86.

Stallone G, Schena A, Infante B, et al. Sirolimus for Kaposi's sarcoma in renal-transplant recipients. N Engl J Med. 2005;352:1317.

Stehlik J, Hosenpud JD, Edwards LB, Hertz MI, Mehra MR. ISHLT International Registry for Heart and Lung Transplantation – into fourth decade, from strength to strength. J Heart Lung Transplant. 2013;32(10):941–50.

Stobierska-Dzierzek B, Award H, Michler RE. The evolving management of acute right-sided heart failure in cardiac transplant recipients. J Am Coll Cardiol. 2001;38(4):923–31.

Vachièry JL, Adir Y, Barbera JA, Champion H, Coghlan JG, Cottin V, De Marco T, Galiè N, Ghio S, Gibbs JS, Martinez F, Senigram M, Simonneau G, Wells A, Seeger W. Pulmonary hypertension due to left heart diseases. J Am Coll Cardiol. 2013;62(25 Suppl):D100–8.

Whitson BA, Kilic A, Lehman A, Wehr A, Hasan A, Haas G, Hayes Jr D, Sai-Sudhakar CB, Higgins RS. Impact of induction immunosuppression on survival in heart transplant recipients: a contemporary analysis of agents. Clin Transplant. 2015;29(1):9–17.

Yancy CW, Jessup M, Bozkurt B, Butler J, Casey DE, Drazner MH, et al. 2013 ACCF/AHA guideline for the management of heart failure: a report of the American College of Cardiology Foundation/American Heart Association Task Force on Practice guidelines. Circulation. 2013;128:e240–327.

Zuckermann A, Wang SS, Epailly E, Barten MJ, Sigurdardottir V, Segovia J, Varnous S, Turazza FM, Potena L, Lehmkuhl HB. Everolimus immunosuppression in de novo heart transplant recipients: what does the evidence tell us now? Transplant Rev (Orlando). 2013;27(3):76–84.

Practical Immunology for Pathologists

12

John D. Smith and Marlene L. Rose

Contents

J.D. Smith, FRCPath (✉)
Tissue Tying Laboratory, Harefield Hospital, Harefield, Middlesex, UK
e-mail: j.smith@rbht.nhs.uk

M.L. Rose, BSc, MSc, PhD
National Heart and Lung Institute, Imperial College, Heart Science Centre, Harefield Hospital, Harefield, Middlesex, UK
e-mail: Marlene.Rose@imperial.ac.uk

12.1 Background

The main role of immunologists in cardiac transplant programmes is to prevent antibody-mediated rejection (AMR). The immunosuppressive drugs currently used (such as calcineurin inhibitors and mTOR inhibitors) mainly target T lymphocytes, which are needed for production of antibodies, but once antibodies are made, currently used immunosuppressive drugs have no effect on circulating antibody. It is thus imperative to prevent the production of antibodies to donor antigens.

The most important antibodies are antigens encoded by genes of the major histocompatibility complex (MHC), which in humans is known as the human leukocyte antigen (HLA) system and is located on chromosome 6. The protein products of genes within the HLA system can be classified as either HLA class I (HLA-A,HLA-B,HLA-C), HLA class II (HLA-DR,HLA-DP,HLA-DQ) or other immune-related gene products such as components of the complement cascade, cytokines such as tumour necrosis factor (TNF)-α, nonclassical MHC genes (MIC-A and MIC-B) as well as heat-shock proteins. Histocompatibility & Immunogenetics (H&I) scientists have to determine the HLA type of both donors and recipients and to determine whether patients have preformed antibodies to donor HLA antigens. Hence, all patients on the transplant waiting list are screened for antibodies to HLA antigens.

O. Leone et al. (eds.), *The Pathology of Cardiac Transplantation*,
DOI 10.1007/978-3-319-46386-5_12

When a potential donor becomes available for a sensitised patient, care is taken to ensure that either they do not receive a donor heart bearing those particular HLA antigens or, if they do, the level of antibodies are too low to be clinically relevant. This procedure is known as the virtual crossmatch.

At our institution approximately 30–40 % of patients waiting for a heart or lung transplant have preformed antibodies to HLA antigens. Production of antibodies to HLA antigens can be caused by multiple pregnancies, blood transfusions or transplantation. There are also patients who have preformed HLA antibodies for unknown reasons. The number of sensitised patients awaiting transplantation has increased in recent years, due to the introduction of more sensitive assays for HLA antibody detection.

12.2 Nomenclature, Structure and Tissue Distribution of MHC Antigens

There are six loci-coding HLA antigens relevant to solid organ transplantation, HLA-A, HLA-B, HLA-C, HLA-DR, HLA-DP and HLA-DQ. When these antigens were first discovered in mice, immunologists thought they were antigens which regulated the immune response, and the antigens coded for by the Ia gene (in mice) were called class II genes, and those coded by the Ie gene were called class I genes. The equivalents in human are HLA-DR, HLA-DP and HLA-DQ known as class II antigens and HLA-A, HLA-B and HLA-C which are known as class I genes or antigens.

12.2.1 Structure of HLA Molecules

The class I molecule is a transmembrane glycoprotein consisting of two polypeptide chains. The heavy chain is a 44kD protein which is associated with β2 microglobulin, a molecule which is coded for outside the HLA region on chromosome 15. The heavy chain has three extracellular domains, α1, α2 and α3, as well as a transmembrane region and a cytoplasmic tail. The variability between class I molecules is found largely within the α1 and α2 domains, with different alleles of the class I genes varying by as many as 30 residues. The α1 and α2 domains constitute the functional site of the HLA molecule, where the molecules fold to form a groove. This groove is filled by a peptide for contact/presentation with the T cell receptor.

The class II molecule is a heterodimer comprised of a heavy chain (the alpha chain) of approximately 33KD and a light chain (beta chain) of approximately 28KD. Each chain has two extracellular domains (α1, α2, β1 and β2), as well as a transmembrane region and cytoplasmic tail. The polymorphisms of class II molecules reside within the β1 domain, which in combination with the invariant α1 domain folds to form the peptide-binding groove.

12.2.2 Tissue Distribution of HLA Molecules

Class I antigens are constitutively expressed on the surface of all nucleated cells in humans including endothelial cells. Nonnucleated cells such as erythrocytes or syncytial tissue such as the myocardium and skeletal muscle do not constitutively express class I antigens but can be induced to express class I by inflammatory cytokines such as tumour necrosis factor (TNF). Hence, immunocytochemical staining of cardiac biopsies not showing rejection shows the absence of MHC class I on the membranes of myocardial cells, but MHC class I is induced on the myocardium during acute cellular rejection (Fig. 12.1).

MHC class II antigens have a more restricted tissue distribution; they are constitutively present on antigen-presenting cells of the immune system such as dendritic cells, monocytes, macrophages and B lymphocytes. HLA-DR antigens are also constitutively expressed on human endothelial cells within the heart (Rose et al. 1986) (Fig. 12.2), and HLA-DQ and HLA-DP are induced by inflammatory responses (Suitters et al. 1987). HLA-DR is also constitutively expressed on endothelial

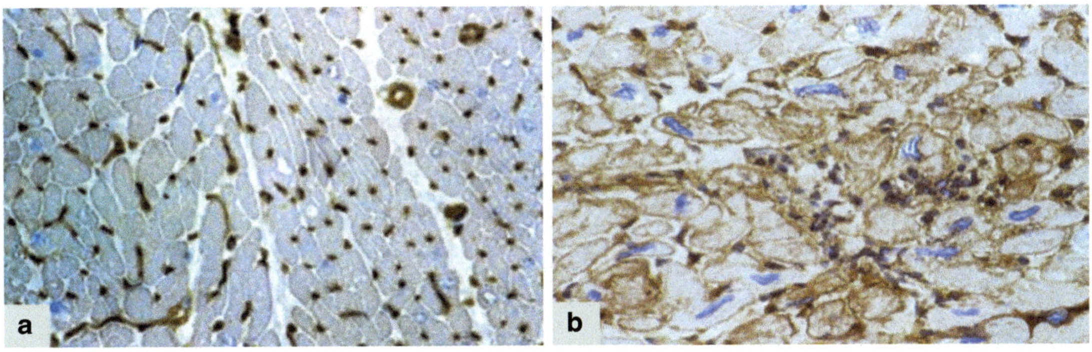

Fig. 12.1 Frozen sections of human endomyocardial biopsy (6 um) stained with mouse monoclonal antibody to MHC class I antigen (W6/32) followed by biotin-labelled secondary antibody to murine IgG, followed by incubation in avidin–biotin peroxidase complex. Immersion in a mixture of diaminobenzidine tetrahydrochloride and hydrogen–peroxide allows visualisation of peroxidase activity. It can be seen that MHC class I antigen is present on interstitial structures (such as dendritic cells and endothelial cells) in biopsy not showing rejection (**a**), but myocardial membranes are negative for class I. In contrast in the biopsy showing cellular rejection, (**b**) myocardial cells are MHC class I positive (From Rose et al. (1986))

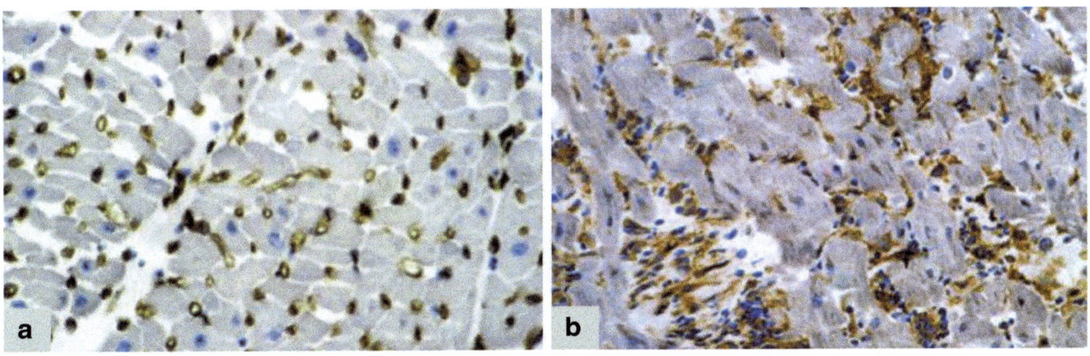

Fig. 12.2 Frozen sections of human endomyocardial biopsy (6 um) stained with mouse monoclonal antibody to MHC class II antigen (L243, against DR) followed by biotin-labelled secondary antibody to murine IgG, followed by incubation in avidin–biotin peroxidase complex. Immersion in a mixture of diaminobenzidine tetrahydrochloride and hydrogen–peroxide allows visualisation of peroxidase activity. It can be seen that DR antigen is constitutively expressed on interstitial structures (such as dendritic cells and endothelial cells) in biopsy not showing rejection (**a**) and is expressed on infiltrating lymphocytes in biopsy showing cellular rejection (**b**). Myocardial cell membranes do not express DR antigen (From Rose et al. (1986))

cells in the lung (Taylor et al. 1989) and kidney (Fuggle et al. 1986). The constitutive expression of MHC class I and HLA-DR antigens on human endothelial cells of transplanted organs (i.e. hearts, lungs and kidneys) makes these organs a target if transplanted into patients with preformed donor-specific HLA antibodies. Attachment of complement-fixing HLA antibodies to donor endothelial cells results in lysis of the endothelial layer and rapid thrombotic events.

The function of MHC molecules is to present antigen to cells of the immune system. Cells are continually degrading cellular proteins, either self-proteins or proteins derived from viruses. Peptides from degraded proteins are exported to the cell surface, and they reside within the groove of the MHC antigens. Class I antigens present peptides to CD8+T lymphocytes, whereas class II molecules present peptides to CD4+T lymphocytes. Hence, presentation of peptides from alloantigens, by class II-presenting cells which have originated within the donor organ (i.e. dendritic cells), initiates transplant rejection. Polymorphism of HLA antigens is caused by amino acid differences in the helical part of the molecule forming the base of the groove.

The HLA system is extremely polymorphic. To date over 8000 class I and over 3000 class II alleles have been described encoding almost 9000 proteins (Robinson et al. 2015). The nomenclature for HLA alleles is complex; each HLA allele is uniquely numbered with at least a four-digit name (e.g. HLA*02:01), although longer names can be assigned up to four sets of digits separated by colons (e.g. HLA-A*02:01:01:01). Many of the described alleles have 'serological' equivalents which are generally used for analysis of HLA matching/antibody identification in solid organ transplantation (HLA-A*02:01 is HLA-A2). At this level of resolution, analysis of HLA antigens is limited to approximately 20 HLA-A, 46 HLA-B, 15 HLA-C, 15 HLA-DR and 7 HLA-DQ antigens.

Prospective selection of recipients based on HLA matching with the donor does not occur in cardiac transplantation. It has been shown that matching or minimising the HLA mismatch between donor and recipient, especially at the HLA-DR locus, results in less frequent and less severe cellular rejection episodes in both renal and heart transplantation (Opelz et al. 1992; Dyer et al. 1989; Smith et al. 1995). However, it is not logistically possible to select patients by HLA mismatch in heart transplantation due to a number of factors which include numbers of donors, size of waiting lists and the relative short cold ischaemic time tolerated by hearts for transplantation. Early AMR can be prevented by ensuring recipients do not have donor-specific HLA antibodies at the time of transplantation and by carefully monitoring patients for AMR after transplantation.

12.2.3 Antibody Subclasses

The focus of HLA antibody testing in solid organ transplantation is on the detection of circulating immunoglobulin (Ig)G HLA-specific antibodies. Detection of IgM anti-HLA antibodies is generally thought not to be a risk factor for AMR although some evidence does suggest that IgM HLA-specific antibodies detected by solid-phase assays may have deleterious effects on graft outcome (Stastny et al. 2009).

There are four IgG subclasses in humans, IgG1, IgG2, IgG3 and IgG4 (Table 12.1). The Fc receptor of the antibody molecule determines the different functions such as binding to phagocytic cells or fixing complement.

12.3 Methods of Detecting IgG HLA Antibodies

12.3.1 Complement-Dependent Cytotoxicity Test (CDC Test)

The complement-dependent cytotoxicity assay can be used to perform serological HLA typing; HLA antibody screening or donor/recipient crossmatching was first introduced in 1964 (Terasaki and McClelland 1964). Serological HLA typing, which has been superseded by molecular methodologies, involves incubation of peripheral blood mononuclear cells (PBMC) of unknown HLA type with alloantisera containing antibodies to known HLA antigens. During this stage antibodies which are specific for the HLA molecules on the cell surface bind to the target antigen. Following the addition of an exogenous source of complement, usually rabbit serum, the bound antibody activates the classical complement pathway leading to the formation of the membrane attack complex (C5b-9) which causes lysis of the cells (Fig. 12.3). Viability is assessed using a staining procedure. The pattern of reactivity of cell death allows identification of the HLA type of the cells.

HLA antibody screening is performed using a panel of PBMC of known HLA type (usually at least 50 different cells) which are incubated with patient sera. Any positivity is assessed and the pattern of reactivity aligned to specific HLA antigens if possible. Careful consideration of the panel composition is required to cover the majority of the HLA antigens in the population. The percentage panel reactive antibodies (PRA) is calculated as the frequency of the panel to which

Table 12.1 Properties of human IgG isotypes

Name	Percent (%)	Crosses placenta easily	Complement activator	Binds to Fc receptor on phagocytic cells
IgG1	66	Yes	Yes (++)	High affinity
IgG2	23	No	Yes (+)	Extremely low affinity
IgG3	7	Yes	Yes (+++)	High affinity
IgG4	4	Yes	No	Intermediate affinity

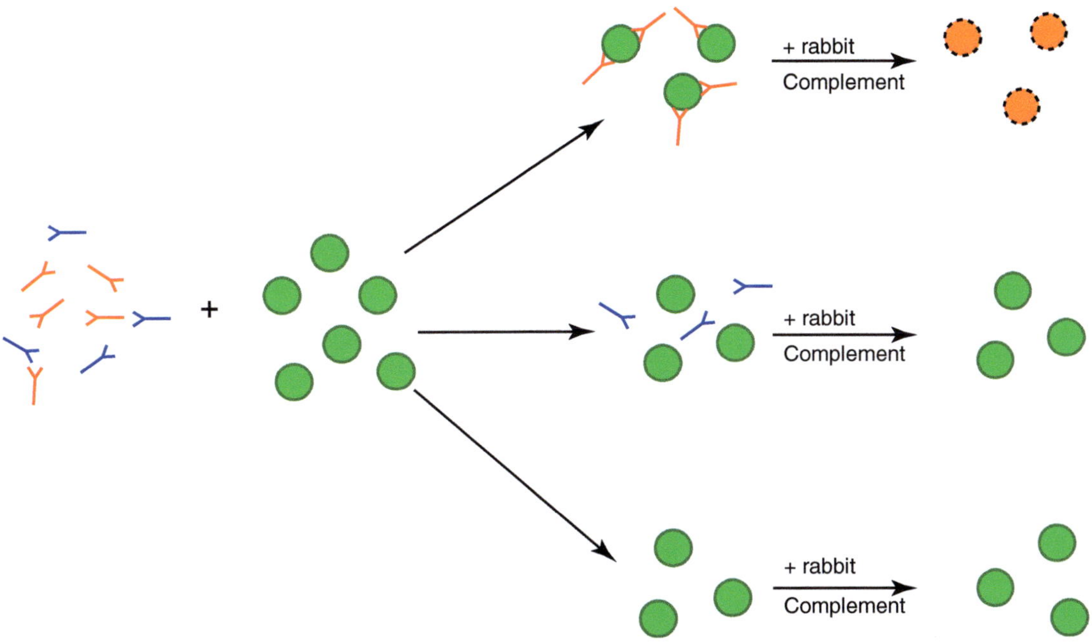

Fig. 12.3 CDC methodology. Patient serum containing HLA antibodies is incubated with the target cell during which time antibodies specific for the target cell HLA antigens will bind. Rabbit complement is then added, and where specific binding has occurred, lysis will occur which can be visualised with a staining procedure

reactivity has been detected and was considered a reflection of the frequency of reactivity against the donor population, although this may not be the case with selected cell panels.

CDC crossmatching which is still in use in solid organ transplantation involves the incubation of donor leukocytes with recipient serum, in the presence of exogenous complement. Any 'killing' of donor cells above background levels by the recipient sera is classified as a positive crossmatch. It is generally accepted that a positive crossmatch is associated with hyperacute rejection of the allograft. This was first described in renal transplantation by Patel and Terasaki where 80 % of grafts with a positive crossmatch failed within 2 days compared to just 2 % of grafts with a negative crossmatch (Patel and Terasaki 1969).

Various modifications have been made to the assay to enhance sensitivity including increased incubation periods, using purified T and B lymphocytes, and addition of antihuman globulin (AHG method) (Fuller et al. 1982). Additionally, with the addition of dithiothreitol into the assay, it is possible to distinguish between IgM and IgG antibodies. This is a relatively crude determination, but dithiothreitol breaks down disulphide bonds, and as IgM has significantly more than IgG, IgM antibodies are degraded preferentially over IgG (Chapman et al. 1986).

Whilst this method is simple and relatively inexpensive, there are a number of disadvantages and limitations for routine antibody screening and crossmatching as follows:

(a) The method only detects complement-fixing antibodies and is insensitive. It will only detect complement-fixing antibodies of high affinity (i.e. sufficient strength to cause cell lysis).
(b) Whereas MHC class I antigens are abundantly expressed on circulating leukocytes (such as neutrophils), MHC class II antigens are only expressed on monocytes and B cells. Hence this method is much more efficient at detecting C'-fixing antibodies to MHC class I antigens than to MHC class II, which may be poorly expressed.
(c) Antibody screening by CDC can be time-consuming and may result in delays to reporting.
(d) Viable leukocytes express many determinants other than HLA molecules, and false-positive results owing to the presence of IgM non-HLA autoreactive antibodies can be misleading.
(e) The method relies on the quality of the isolated cells which express many more proteins than HLA, and some positive reactions may not be due to HLA-specific antibodies.
(f) Therapeutic antibodies such as rituximab (anti-CD20) and anti-thymocyte globulin can cause positive reactivity in CDC tests masking any HLA-specific antibodies present.

12.3.2 Flow Cytometry

Flow cytometry assays are more sensitive than conventional CDC and do not rely on complement fixation but rather measure binding of antibody to targets and are used for both HLA antibody screening and donor crossmatching. For antibody screening, pools of cells selected to cover the majority of HLA specificities are used, whilst for donor crossmatching, donor lymphocyte preparations are used. The assay involves incubating patient serum with the target cell preparation, followed by a series of washes and then incubation with fluorescent-conjugated antibody directed against human IgG. The fluorescent channel shift against negative controls is often used as a measure of a positive reaction.

12.3.3 Solid-Phase Assays

These assays have greatly increased the ability of the immunologist to detect and define the nature of HLA antibodies in patient serum. The assays arose as a consequence of technical innovations which enabled purification of HLA molecules and/or production of recombinant HLA molecules, which can be bound to solid surfaces. Hence, HLA molecules can be bound to plastic plates or beads, these are incubated with patient sera, and the binding of patient IgG to the molecules is detected (Kao et al. 1993; Pei et al. 1998; Gibney et al. 2006).

The basic principle for solid-phase assays is similar for all techniques. Purified or recombinant HLA molecules are bound to the solid surface (enzyme-linked immunosorbent assay (ELISA) plate or microbeads); patient serum and control sera are added, followed by antihuman IgG monoclonal antibody conjugated for either fluorometric or colorimetric detection. Quantification of binding of antibodies to ELISA plates or beads is measured as mean fluorescent intensity (MFI).

The different methods are described below.

12.3.3.1 Enzyme-Linked Immunosorbent Assay (ELISA)

ELISA methods employ a colorimetric detection stage. Purified or recombinant HLA molecules are coated in wells of an ELISA plate. ELISA methods are considered to be less sensitive than assays utilising microbeads.

12.3.3.2 FlowPRA Assay

This uses pooled panels of different microparticles coated with different purified HLA class I and HLA class II antigens to detect HLA-specific antibodies using a fluorescein isothiocyanate (FITC)-conjugated antihuman IgG monoclonal antibody in a standard flow cytometer. These assays can utilise up to 30 different bead populations in each assay. Single-antigen assays are also available for definition of the antibody specificities.

12.3.3.3 Luminex X-Map-Based Assays

Luminex X-map assays use microbeads which are coated with purified class I or class II HLA antigens or recombinant single HLA antigens. In this way an initial screening test can be performed to detect antibodies to MHC class I or class II antigens; should this be positive, further tests are performed using the single-antigen beads to determine specificity of the antibodies. Detection of human immunoglobulin binding to beads is done using a phycoerythrin-conjugated monoclonal antibody to human IgG. Binding of antibodies to the microbeads is measured as mean fluorescent intensity (MFI) (Fig. 12.4). Luminex assays utilise the Luminex® 100/200 fluoroanalyser for analysis of up to 100 different bead sets in a single test (Fig. 12.5). Luminex assays are now in widespread use in H&I laboratories and are considered the most sensitive assays available.

12.3.3.4 Modification of Solid-Phase Bead Assays to Detect C′-Fixing Antibodies

Both FlowPRA and Luminex-based bead assays have been modified to detect complement-fixing antibodies in patient sera. This was first demonstrated by Wahrmann et al. (Wahrmann et al. 2005) using FlowPRA microbeads, in which the antihuman IgG secondary antibody was replaced with antihuman C4d or antihuman C1q antibodies. Modifications to the Luminex-based assays to measure C4d deposition on the microbeads (Smith et al. 2007) or C1q binding (Chen et al. 2011) have also been described. Donor HLA-specific antibodies (DSA) causing C4d fixation on HLA-coated microbeads in patient sera prior to heart transplantation have been shown to have a strong correlation with poor survival post-transplantation (Smith et al. 2011). Similarly, C1q-fixing antibodies have been shown to correlate with antibody-mediated rejection in cardiac transplant recipients (Chin et al. 2011).

The advantages and disadvantages of bead assays are as follows:

(a) Solid-phase assays utilise purified HLA molecules and do not have a requirement for viable cells or complement and therefore should detect only antibodies specific for HLA molecules.
(b) They can detect both complement-fixing and non-complement-fixing antibodies.
(c) They are commercially available and can be automated.
(d) Have increased sensitivity over CDC and flow cytometric assays.

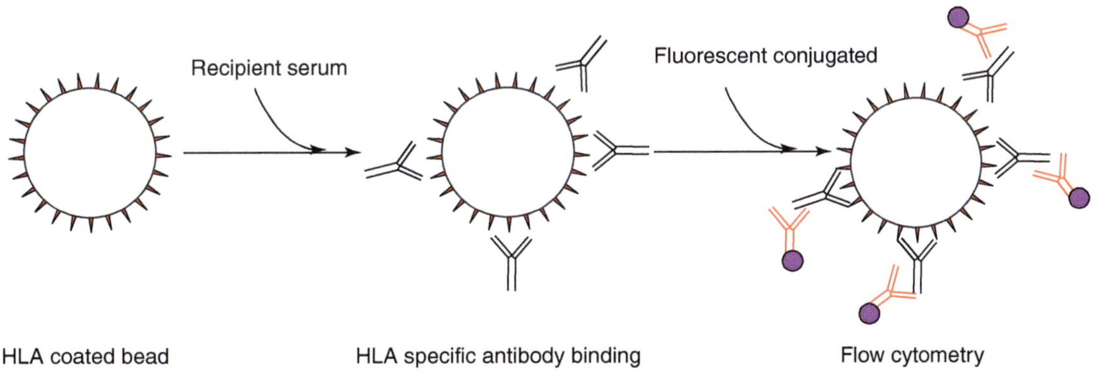

Fig. 12.4 Patient sera are incubated with pools of microbeads, each coated with a single HLA molecule in a single well of a 96-well plate during which time any HLA antigen-specific antibodies will bind to the relevant antigen on the beads. After washing, the binding of any IgG to the molecules is detected by the addition of a fluoresceinated antihuman IgG secondary antibody. The fluorescence signal of each bead is analysed in a Luminex fluoroanalyser

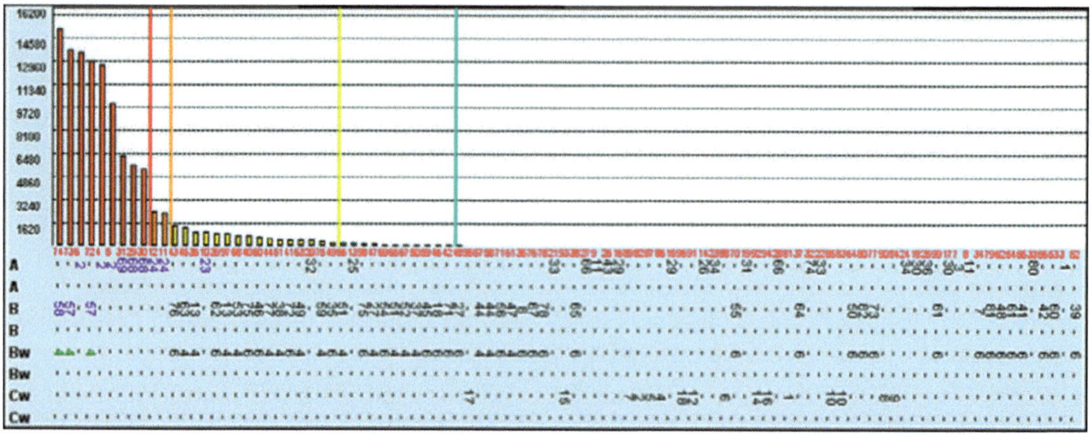

Fig. 12.5 Histogram of Luminex MFI data from patient sample showing antibody binding to microbeads bearing HLA antigens A2, A24, A68, A69, B57 and B58 but no binding to all other HLA antigens. The *y*-axis shows MFI levels, whilst the *x*-axis shows the HLA antigens bound to the different microbeads in the assay

(e) Tests are rapid with a complete antibody identification available in 3 h.
(f) Extremely expensive.

12.4 Role of Preformed HLA-Specific Antibodies in Cardiac Transplantation

It is well established that preformed HLA-specific antibodies directed against donor HLA antigens correlate with poor outcomes in heart transplantation (Smith et al. 1993; Przybylowski et al. 1999; Tambur et al. 2000). The introduction of solid-phase assays with increased sensitivity allowed the detection of low-level HLA antibodies that were previously undetectable. The situation currently facing clinicians and laboratory scientists is to determine if transplantation can be successfully performed against low-level DSA. In cardiac transplantation, Luminex-detected DSA, particularly, those which fix complement have been shown to have a significant impact on patient survival (Smith et al. 2007) (Fig. 12.6). Similarly, in lung transplantation it has been shown that preformed DSA lead to early graft failure in the majority of cases, particularly if the antibodies fix complement in the assay (Smith et al. 2014).

It is unclear whether all Luminex-detected DSA are associated with poor survival after transplantation. In renal transplantation, evidence would suggest that low-level DSA detected by Luminex-based assays do not correlate with early rejection (Aubert et al. 2009) or long-term graft outcomes (van den Berg-Loonen et al. 2008).

It has also been reported in heart transplantation that patients with low-level DSA (MFI <1500) were not associated with cellular or antibody-mediated rejection post-transplant (Gandhi et al. 2011). MFI levels produced by Luminex assays do not accurately measure the amount of antibody binding or titre; it is used by all centres and is an easy measure to use to attempt to stratify risk both before and after transplantation. Despite efforts to standardise the solid-phase assays, there is a degree of variability between centres (Reed et al. 2013), and therefore each transplant centre should determine the level of risk they are willing to accept. The identification of unacceptable donor HLA antigens prior to transplant should be patient specific. HLA antibodies should be identified, after which the risk for a particular patient should be assessed by a multidisciplinary approach. It is necessary to stratify risk using not just MFI but other factors including

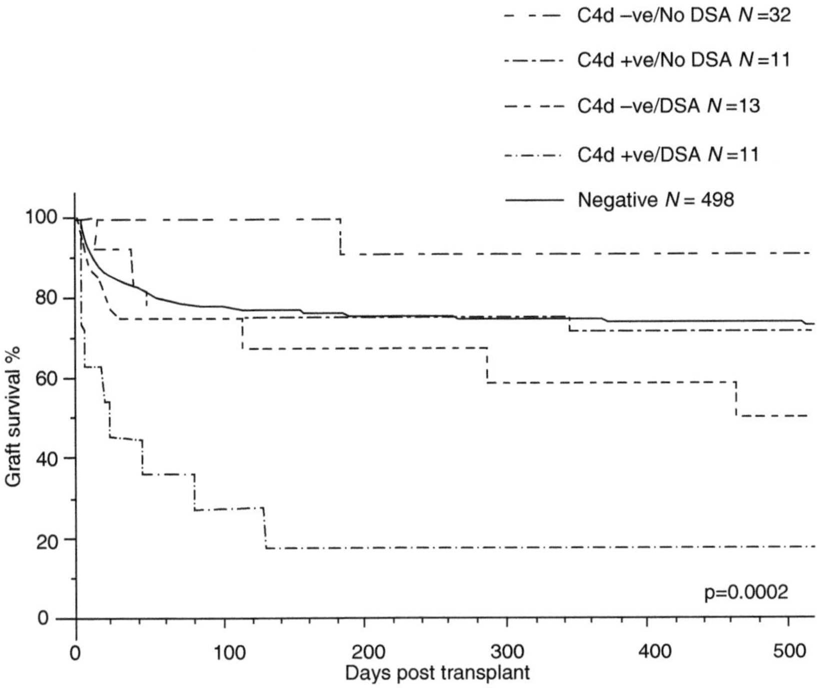

Fig. 12.6 Effect of C4d-depositing DSA on graft survival. Actuarial graft survival according to antibody status of pre-transplant sera; sera contained C4d +ve DSA ($n = 11$), C4d +ve non-DSA ($n = 11$), C4d –ve DSA ($n = 13$), C4d –ve non-DSA ($n = 32$) and no detectable HLA antibodies ($n = 498$), $p = 0.0002$ (From Smith et al. (2007))

biologic properties such as complement fixation, titre and nature of the target antigen (denatured/cryptic epitopes). Decisions as to whether accept transplanting against DSA are also influenced by clinical considerations including patient characteristics such as time of waiting list and chance of obtaining another donor.

Studies have reported a wide range of MFI levels ranging from 300 to 2000 for identification of antibodies pre- and post-transplantation (Brugiere et al. 2013; Morrell et al. 2014; Zeevi et al. 2013; Willicombe et al. 2014; Witt et al. 2013). In conclusion, for some sensitised patients, their DSA levels are considered unacceptable, and the relevant antigens must be avoided in the donor HLA type, but for others the level of DSA may be considered an acceptable risk. Some centres are known to transplant against DSA with MFI levels up to 8000 if the antibodies do not fix complement, whilst others may not go against MFI levels above 1000, depending on the risk assessment of clinical teams in conjunction with immunologists.

12.5 Virtual Crossmatch Procedures

In the era of single-antigen Luminex testing, the 'virtual crossmatch' is the name of the procedure which begins when a heart donor becomes available. The HLA type of the donor is checked with the HLA antibody profile of potential recipients (i.e. deemed suitable by other criteria such as blood group and size). If a potential recipient has HLA antibodies against the donor, either the transplant will not go ahead or, if the antibodies are at a low level, a clinical decision must be made whether the risk of rejection is manageable. The test is virtual, because the actual tests have been done before a donor becomes available and only records have to be checked at the time of transplant.

12.6 Post-Transplant Monitoring of HLA Antibodies

In the modern era, patients are transplanted either in the absence of detectable DSA or in the presence of low levels of detectable DSA (as described above). Despite these policies, a number of patients produce DSA after transplantation. For example, the study by Smith et al. in 2011 demonstrated that 57 of 224 (25%) of patients made DSA after transplantation (Smith et al. 2011).

Numerous studies have shown de novo DSA to be associated with worsening outcomes. There is increasing evidence that de novo DSA after heart transplantation is associated with increased incidence of AMR, graft vasculopathy and poor survival. Hodges et al. (Hodges et al. 2012) reported on a series of patients diagnosed with late AMR following development of DSA. Similarly, others have reported increased prevalence of DSA in patients with AMR (Chin et al. 2011; Nath et al. 2010a; Zhang et al. 2005; Ho et al. 2011; Zhang et al. 2011). In a series of 168 heart transplant recipients, Zhang et al. described 37 patients with AMR, of which 22 (60%) had DSA compared to six (5%) of the 131 patients with no evidence of AMR. Furthermore, recent evidence suggests that high titre, complement-fixing DSA are strongly correlated with an increased incidence of AMR in cardiac transplant recipients (Zeevi et al. 2013). Should the pathologist suspect AMR, it is very useful to take blood samples to investigate the presence of DSA, to confirm the diagnosis. This centre performs regular monitoring for DSA in the first year after transplantation as recommended by International Society for Heart and Lung Transplantation (ISHLT) guidelines (Kobashigawa et al. 2011; Frank et al. 2014).

De novo DSA have also been implicated in the development of cardiac allograft vasculopathy (Frank et al. 2014) and decreased patient survival (Smith et al. 2011) (Table 12.2). The Smith study did not show a significant correlation between DSA and development of Coronary artery vasculopathy (CAV), but it did show that patients who had CAV and DSA had shorter survival than CAV alone. In a large single-centre study, Smith et al. have shown that the development of DSA after heart transplantation is an independent predictor of poor patient survival following cardiac transplantation.

A number of therapeutic models have been used to remove or reduce HLA antibody levels both pre- and post-transplant, including plasma exchange, intravenous immunoglobulin (IVIg), immunoadsorption and monoclonal therapies such as rituximab and bortezomib (Hodges et al. 2012; Bierl et al. 2006; Everly et al. 2009; Morrow et al. 2012; Stegall et al. 2006). It is important that when undertaking such therapies, the HLA antibodies are monitored to determine if antibody levels are reducing. This can be easily performed using single-antigen bead analysis and has been used to monitor antibody removal in patients treated with immunoadsorption following a diagnosis of AMR (Hodges et al. 2012).

12.7 Non-HLA Antibodies

Many clinical studies have demonstrated that patients make autoantibodies following solid organ transplantation (Rose 2013; Besarani et al. 2014; Nath et al. 2010b; Haque et al. 2002). Following cardiac transplantation, autoantibodies to vimentin and myosin are produced – commonly IgM antibodies. De novo production of autoantibodies represents exposure of cryptic antigens following tissue damage caused by either reperfusion injury or the alloimmune response. Anti-myosin antibodies are found in some patients with dilated cardiomyopathy and myocarditis so will be present in some patients prior to transplantation. Our own studies of heart transplant patients have revealed that only 10% have IgM anti-vimentin antibodies before transplantation (Smith and Rose (2014) unpublished results).

The question arises whether autoimmune antibodies are directly damaging to the new heart or a sign of previous damage. Experimental studies have demonstrated that high titre IgG anti-vimentin antibodies cause accelerated acute

Table 12.2 Impact of persistent de novo DSA on patient survival in a multivariable Cox proportional hazards model

	Estimated hazard ratio	95 % confidence interval for hazard ratio	*P* value
De novo and persistent DSA	4.331	1.922–9.7600	<0.0004
HLA-DR mismatch	2.334	1.0782–5.0539	0.0315
Donor age	1.034	1.0048–1.0762	0.0256
Haemodynamic compromise	2.363	1.0003–5.5804	0.0499
Treated rejection in the first year	0.417	0.1825–0.9535	0.0382

From Smith et al. (2011)

rejection (Mahesh et al. 2007) but only in the presence of an existing alloimmune response. Nath et al. reported that production of anti-vimentin antibodies is associated with AMR in the first year after transplantation (Nath et al. 2010b) and that these antibodies preceded AMR by several months. Our own studies of AMR in heart transplant recipients investigated 17 patients with late AMR (Smith and Rose (2014) unpublished); in 15 cases donor-specific HLA antibodies were found at the time of diagnosis of AMR, and in two patients IgG anti-vimentin antibodies were detected at the same time. It is interesting that in another two patients, IgG anti-vimentin antibodies were detected at the time of diagnosis of AMR, but in the absence of donor-specific HLA antibodies. Other autoantibodies were not investigated. The possibility that autoantibodies contribute to pathogenesis of AMR following heart transplantation cannot be excluded.

One of the drawbacks of monitoring the presence of autoantibodies (such as vimentin or myosin autoantibodies) in patients is the lack of standardised reagents and assays. Currently assays use either whole human recombinant vimentin or whole human or pig myosin as antigens. Evidence from the autoimmune literature suggests that assays for antibodies to specific epitopes of autoantigens or to autoantigens modified by oxidation/glycosylation are needed to obtain clinical correlations (Bang et al. 2007). Such studies have not yet been performed after solid organ transplantation. Hence, further studies need to be done to improve the quality of reagents and sensitivity of assays before one could recommend routine monitoring autoantibody responses after cardiac transplantation.

Conclusion

Scientists in the H&I Laboratories have an essential role in monitoring the presence of antibodies to HLA antigens, both in patients prior to their transplant and in patients after transplantation. The use of leukocytes to detect complement-dependent cytotoxicity has been superseded by solid-phase assays using purified or recombinant HLA molecules. The Luminex method which uses microbeads coated with purified HLA molecules or recombinant single HLA molecules is probably the most common methodology. The method can be modified to detect complement-fixing antibodies to single HLA antigens. This method is very sensitive compared to CDC and detects more sensitised patients. Used prior to transplantation, it is known as the 'virtual crossmatch', and it means hearts are not transplanted into patients with 'clinically relevant' levels of pre-existing antibodies to donor HLA antigens. The major question now to be addressed by scientists and clinicians is what level of pre-existing HLA antibodies are clinically relevant and what levels are safe. Antibody-mediated rejection (AMR) sometimes occurring late after transplantation is strongly associated with production of donor-specific HLA antibodies; conceivably such antibodies may have been present before the transplant, but de novo production of DSA has also been reported. It is recommended that patients are monitored regularly post-transplant for DSA to aid diagnosis of AMR. Methods of treating AMR are improving, and monitoring the presence of DSA should allow early detection and removal of DSA, hence mitigating damage to the donor heart.

Key Points

- Approximately 40 % of cardiothoracic waiting list patients are sensitised to HLA antigens.
- The HLA system comprises six loci-coding HLA antigens relevant to solid organ transplantation, HLA-A, HLA-B and HLA-C (known as MHC class I antigens) and HLA-DR, HLA-DP and HLA-DQ (known as MHC class II antigens).
- MHC class I antigens are constitutively expressed on the surface of all nucleated cells in humans.
- MHC class II antigens have a more restricted tissue distribution, being constitutively present on dendritic cells, monocytes, macrophages, B lymphocytes and endothelial cells.
- It is of paramount importance that patients are not transplanted with an organ expressing HLA antigens to which the patient is highly sensitised, since this is likely to lead to hyperacute rejection or early antibody-mediated rejection.
- Solid-phase assays for the detection and identification of antibodies to HLA antigens are the best way of screening potential transplant recipients for the presence of HLA antibodies.
- All patients on the waiting list are initially screened for HLA antibodies. Those that are positive are investigated in more detail to determine the precise specificity of their HLA antibodies. Solid-phase assays can also be used with C4d and C1q to distinguish between complement-fixing and non-complement-fixing antibodies.
- Individual laboratories have to determine their own level of pre-transplant donor-specific HLA antibodies (DSA, using MFI values) against which it is acceptable or 'safe' to transplant.
- At the time of transplantation, the HLA typing of the donor is known, as is the HLA antibody status of potential recipients. Cardiothoracic organs are allocated to patients who do not have clinically relevant levels of DSA. This procedure is known as the virtual crossmatch.
- Even when patients are transplanted in the absence of detectable DSA, de novo DSA may be produced after transplantation leading to antibody-mediated rejection, poor survival and in the case of lung transplantation increased incidence of Bronchiolitis Obliterans Syndrome (BOS).
- Patients should be monitored regularly post-transplant for DSA to aid diagnosis of AMR.

References

Aubert V, Venetz JP, Pantaleo G, Pascual M. Low levels of human leukocyte antigen donor-specific antibodies detected by solid phase assay before transplantation are frequently clinically irrelevant. Hum Immunol. 2009;70:580–3.

Bang H, Egerer K, Gauliard A, Luthke K, Rudolph PE, Fredenhagen G, Berg W, Feist E, Burmester GR. Mutation and citrullination modifies vimentin to a novel autoantigen for rheumatoid arthritis. Arthritis Rheum. 2007;56:2503–11.

Besarani D, Cerundolo L, Smith JD, Procter J, Barnardo MC, Roberts IS, Friend PJ, Rose ML, Fuggle SV. Role of anti-vimentin antibodies in renal transplantation. Transplantation. 2014;98:72–8.

Bierl C, Miller B, Prak EL, Gasiewski A, Kearns J, Tsai D, Jessup M, Kamoun M. Antibody-mediated rejection in heart transplant recipients: potential efficacy of B-cell depletion and antibody removal. Clin Transpl. 2006;2006:489–96.

Brugiere O, Suberbielle C, Thabut G, Lhuillier E, Dauriat G, Metivier AC, Gautreau C, Charron D, Mal H, Parquin F, Stern M. Lung transplantation in patients with pretransplantation donor-specific antibodies detected by luminex assay. Transplantation. 2013;95(5):761–5.

Chapman JR, Taylor CJ, Ting A, Morris PJ. Immunoglobulin class and specificity of antibodies causing positive T cell crossmatches. Relationship to renal transplant outcome. Transplantation. 1986;42:608–13.

Chen G, Sequeira F, Tyan DB. Novel C1q assay reveals a clinically relevant subset of human leukocyte antigen antibodies independent of immunoglobulin G strength on single antigen beads. Hum Immunol. 2011;72:849–58.

Chin C, Chen G, Sequeria F, Berry G, Siehr S, Bernstein D, Rosenthal D, Reinhartz O, Tyan D. Clinical usefulness of a novel C1q assay to detect immunoglobulin G antibodies capable of fixing complement in sensitized pediatric heart transplant patients. J Heart Lung Transplant. 2011;30:158–63.

Dyer PA, Johnson RW, Martin S, Bakran A, Gokal R, Harris R, Mallick NP, Manos J, Orr WM, Pearson RC, et al. Evidence that matching for HLA antigens significantly increases transplant survival in 1001 renal transplants performed in the northwest region of England. Transplantation. 1989;48:131–5.

Everly JJ, Walsh RC, Alloway RR, Woodle ES. Proteasome inhibition for antibody-mediated rejection. Curr Opin Organ Transplant. 2009;14:662–6.

Frank R, Molina MR, Goldberg LR, Wald JW, Kamoun M, Lal P. Circulating donor-specific anti-human leukocyte antigen antibodies and complement C4d deposition are associated with the development of cardiac allograft vasculopathy. Am J Clin Pathol. 2014;142:809–15.

Fuggle SV, McWhinnie DL, Chapman JR, Taylor HM, Morris PJ. Sequential analysis of HLA-class II antigen expression in human renal allografts. Induction of tubular class II antigens and correlation with clinical parameters. Transplantation. 1986;42:144–50.

Fuller TC, Phelan D, Gebel HM, Rodey GE. Antigenic specificity of antibody reactive in the antiglobulin-augmented lymphocytotoxicity test. Transplantation. 1982;34:24–9.

Gandhi MJ, DeGoey SR, Bundy K, Kremers WK, Knauer R, Pereira N, Edwards B, Kushwaha S, Daly RC. Effect of pretransplant human leukocyte antigen antibodies detected by solid-phase assay on heart transplant outcomes. Transplant Proc. 2011;43:3840–6.

Gibney EM, Cagle LR, Freed B, Warnell SE, Chan L, Wiseman AC. Detection of donor-specific antibodies using HLA-coated microspheres: another tool for kidney transplant risk stratification. Nephrol Dial Transplant. 2006;21:2625–9.

Haque MA, Mizobuchi T, Yasufuku K, Fujisawa T, Brutkiewicz RR, Zheng Y, Woods K, Smith GN, Cummings OW, Heidler KM, Blum JS, Wilkes DS. Evidence for immune responses to a self-antigen in lung transplantation: role of type V collagen-specific T cells in the pathogenesis of lung allograft rejection. J Immunol. 2002;169:1542–9.

Ho EK, Vlad G, Vasilescu ER, de la Torre L, Colovai AI, Burke E, Deng M, Schwartz J, Marboe C, Mancini D, Opelz G, Suciu-Foca N. Pre- and posttransplantation allosensitization in heart allograft recipients: major impact of de novo alloantibody production on allograft survival. Hum Immunol. 2011;72:5–10.

Hodges AM, Lyster H, McDermott A, Rice AJ, Smith JD, Rose ML, Banner NR. Late antibody-mediated rejection after heart transplantation following the development of De Novo donor-specific human leukocyte antigen antibody. Transplantation. 2012;93(6):650–6.

Kao KJ, Scornik JC, Small SJ. Enzyme-linked immunoassay for anti-HLA antibodies – an alternative to panel studies by lymphocytotoxicity. Transplantation. 1993;55:192–6.

Kobashigawa J, Crespo-Leiro MG, Ensminger SM, Reichenspurner H, Angelini A, Berry G, Burke M, Czer L, Hiemann N, Kfoury AG, Mancini D, Mohacsi P, Patel J, Pereira N, Platt JL, Reed EF, Reinsmoen N, Rodriguez ER, Rose ML, Russell SD, Starling R, Suciu-Foca N, Tallaj J, Taylor DO, Van BA, West L, Zeevi A, Zuckermann A. Report from a consensus conference on antibody-mediated rejection in heart transplantation. J Heart Lung Transplant. 2011;30:252–69.

Mahesh B, Leong HS, McCormack A, Sarathchandra P, Holder A, Rose ML. Autoantibodies to vimentin cause accelerated rejection of cardiac allografts. Am J Pathol. 2007;170:1415–27.

Morrell R, Pilewski JM, Gries CJ, Pipeling MR, Crespo MM, Ensor CR, Yousem SA, D'Cunha J, Shigemura N, Bermudez CA, McDyer JF, Zeevi A. De novo donor-specific HLA antibodies are associated with early and high-grade bronchiolitis obliterans syndrome and death after lung transplantation. J Heart Lung Transplant. 2014;33:1288–94.

Morrow WR, Frazier EA, Mahle WT, Harville TO, Pye SE, Knecht KR, Howard EL, Smith RN, Saylors RL, Garcia X, Jaquiss RD, Woodle ES. Rapid reduction in donor-specific anti-human leukocyte antigen antibodies and reversal of antibody-mediated rejection with bortezomib in pediatric heart transplant patients. Transplantation. 2012;93:319–24.

Nath DS, Angaswamy N, Basha HI, Phelan D, Moazami N, Ewald GA, Mohanakumar T. Donor specific antibodies to HLA are associated with and precede antibodies to MICA in antibody mediated rejection and cardiac allograft vasculopathy following human cardiac transplantation. Hum Immunol. 2010a;71(12):1191–6.

Nath DS, Ilias BH, Tiriveedhi V, Alur C, Phelan D, Ewald GA, Moazami N, Mohanakumar T. Characterization of immune responses to cardiac self-antigens myosin and vimentin in human cardiac allograft recipients with antibody-mediated rejection and cardiac allograft vasculopathy. J Heart Lung Transplant. 2010b;29(11):1277–85.

Opelz G, Mytilineos J, Wujciak T, Schwarz V, Back D. Current status of HLA matching in renal transplantation. The Collaborative Transplant Study. Clin Investig. 1992;70:767–72.

Patel R, Terasaki PI. Significance of the positive crossmatch test in kidney transplantation. N Engl J Med. 1969;280:735–9.

Pei R, Wang G, Tarsitani C, Rojo S, Chen T, Takemura S, Liu A, Lee J. Simultaneous HLA Class I and Class II antibodies screening with flow cytometry. Hum Immunol. 1998;59:313–22.

Przybylowski P, Balogna M, Radovancevic B, Frazier OH, Susskind B, Van BC, Katz S, Kahan BD, Kerman R. The role of flow cytometry-detected IgG and IgM anti-donor antibodies in cardiac allograft recipients. Transplantation. 1999;67:258–62.

Reed EF, Rao P, Zhang Z, Gebel H, Bray RA, Guleria I, Lunz J, Mohanakumar T, Nickerson P, Tambur AR, Zeevi A, Heeger PS, Gjertson D. Comprehensive assessment and standardization of solid phase multiplex-bead arrays for the detection of antibodies to HLA-drilling down on key sources of variation. Am J Transplant. 2013;13:1859–70.

Robinson J, Halliwell JA, Hayhurst JD, Flicek P, Parham P, Marsh SG. The IPD and IMGT/HLA database: allele variant databases. Nucleic Acids Res. 2015;43:D423–31.

Rose ML. Role of anti-vimentin antibodies in allograft rejection. Hum Immunol. 2013;74:1459–62.

Rose ML, Coles MI, Griffin RJ, Pomerance A, Yacoub MH. Expression of class I and class II major histocompatibility antigens in normal and transplanted human heart. Transplantation. 1986;41:776–80.

Smith JD, Danskine AJ, Laylor RM, Rose ML, Yacoub MH. The effect of panel reactive antibodies and the donor specific crossmatch on graft survival after heart and heart-lung transplantation. Transpl Immunol. 1993;1:60–5.

Smith JD, Rose ML, Pomerance A, Burke M, Yacoub MH. Reduction of cellular rejection and increase in longer-term survival after heart transplantation after HLA-DR matching. Lancet. 1995;346:1318–22.

Smith JD, Hamour IM, Banner NR, Rose ML. C4d fixing, luminex binding antibodies – a new tool for prediction of graft failure after heart transplantation. Am J Transplant. 2007;7(12):2809–15. Epub 2007 Oct 1.

Smith JD, Banner NR, Hamour IM, Ozawa M, Goh A, Robinson D, Terasaki PI, Rose ML. De novo donor HLA-specific antibodies after heart transplantation are an independent predictor of poor patient survival. Am J Transplant. 2011;11:312–9.

Smith JD, Ibrahim MW, Newell H, Danskine AJ, Soresi S, Burke MM, Rose ML, Carby M. Pre-transplant donor HLA-specific antibodies: characteristics causing detrimental effects on survival after lung transplantation. J Heart Lung Transplant. 2014;33:1074–82.

Stastny P, Ring S, Lu C, Arenas J, Han M, Lavingia B. Role of immunoglobulin (Ig)-G and IgM antibodies against donor human leukocyte antigens in organ transplant recipients. Hum Immunol. 2009;70(8):600–4. Epub 2009 Apr 15.

Stegall MD, Gloor J, Winters JL, Moore SB, Degoey S. A comparison of plasmapheresis versus high-dose IVIG desensitization in renal allograft recipients with high levels of donor specific alloantibody. Am J Transplant. 2006;6:346–51.

Suitters A, Rose M, Higgins A, Yacoub MH. MHC antigen expression in sequential biopsies from cardiac transplant patients – correlation with rejection. Clin Exp Immunol. 1987;69:575–83.

Tambur AR, Bray RA, Takemoto SK, Mancini M, Costanzo MR, Kobashigawa JA, D'Amico CL, Kanter KR, Berg A, Vega JD, Smith AL, Roggero AL, Ortegel JW, Wilmoth-Hosey L, Cecka JM, Gebel HM. Flow cytometric detection of HLA-specific antibodies as a predictor of heart allograft rejection. Transplantation. 2000;70:1055–9.

Taylor PM, Rose ML, Yacoub MH. Expression of MHC antigens in normal human lungs and transplanted lungs with obliterative bronchiolitis. Transplantation. 1989;48:506–10.

Terasaki PI, McClelland JD. Microdroplet assay of human serum cytotoxins. Nature. 1964;204:998–1000.

van den Berg-Loonen EM, Billen EV, Voorter CE, van Heurn LW, Claas FH, van Hooff JP, Christiaans MH. Clinical relevance of pretransplant donor-directed antibodies detected by single antigen beads in highly sensitized renal transplant patients. Transplantation. 2008;85:1086–90.

Wahrmann M, Exner M, Haidbauer B, Schillinger M, Regele H, Kormoczi G, Bohmig GA. [C4d]FlowPRA screening – a specific assay for selective detection of complement-activating anti-HLA alloantibodies. Hum Immunol. 2005;66:526–34.

Willicombe M, Roufosse C, Brookes P, McLean AG, Galliford J, Cairns T, Cook TH, Taube D. Acute cellular rejection: impact of donor-specific antibodies and C4d. Transplantation. 2014;97:433–9.

Witt CA, Gaut JP, Yusen RD, Byers DE, Iuppa JA, Bennett BK, Alexander PG, Mohanakumar T, Trulock EP, Hachem RR. Acute antibody-mediated rejection after lung transplantation. J Heart Lung Transplant. 2013;32:1034–40.

Zeevi A, Lunz J, Feingold B, Shullo M, Bermudez C, Teuteberg J, Webber S. Persistent strong anti-HLA antibody at high titer is complement binding and associated with increased risk of antibody-mediated rejection in heart transplant recipients. J Heart Lung Transplant. 2013;32:98–105.

Zhang Q, Liang LW, Gjertson DW, Lassman C, Wilkinson AH, Kendrick E, Pham PT, Danovitch GM, Gritsch HA, Reed EF. Development of posttransplant antidonor HLA antibodies is associated with acute humoral rejection and early graft dysfunction. Transplantation. 2005;79:591–8.

Zhang Q, Cecka JM, Gjertson DW, Ge P, Rose ML, Patel JK, Ardehali A, Kobashigawa JA, Fishbein MC, Reed EF. HLA and MICA: targets of antibody-mediated rejection in heart transplantation. Transplantation. 2011;91:1153–8.

Pathology of Acute Cellular Rejection

13

Desley A.H. Neil and Alexandra J. Rice

Contents

13.1 Background

In the language of the heart transplant community, "acute cellular rejection" (ACR) indicates cell-mediated form of cardiac rejection (i.e. cellular rejection). Histological assessment of an endomyocardial biopsy (EMB) sample has for the last four decades been the only reliable way to determine whether a patient has rejection (Miller et al. 2013). Each transplant unit has developed a protocol of when to take biopsies to look for rejection, biopsies being more frequent early post-transplant and gradually decreasing in frequency with time and eventually stopping, generally at some point 1–3 years post-transplant. These protocol biopsies are designed to pick up rejection at earlier stages prior to significant clinical dysfunction (Miller et al. 2013). Indication biopsies are performed if there is a clinical change between these time points and further surveillance biopsies are performed regularly during periods when immunosuppressive treatment is being modified.

D.A.H. Neil, MD (✉)
Department of Histopathology,
Medical School University Hospitals Birmingham NHS Foundation Trust, Birmingham, UK
e-mail: desley.neil@uhb.nhs.uk

A.J. Rice, BA, MB, BChir, MRCPath
Department of Histopathology, Royal Brompton Hospital, Royal Brompton and Harefield NHS Trust, London, UK
e-mail: A.Rice@rbht.nhs.uk

O. Leone et al. (eds.), *The Pathology of Cardiac Transplantation*,
DOI 10.1007/978-3-319-46386-5_13

Prior to 1990, many "homegrown" grading schemes for cardiac rejection were developed and used, many being modifications of the Billingham grading system (Billingham 1979). As each was different, it was not possible to accurately compare results between centres or assess the impact of immunosuppressive agents. In 1990, under the direction of the International Society for Heart and Lung Transplantation (ISHLT), a standardised grading system was agreed by pathologists from large transplant centres (Billingham et al. 1990). This system was satisfactorily used worldwide for many years until 2004, when a multidisciplinary working group for ISHLT updated it to create the revised working formulation for the standardisation of nomenclature in the diagnosis of heart rejection (Stewart et al. 2005).

13.2 Histologic Features of Cellular Rejection

ACR is an immune-mediated inflammation of the myocardium where the immune response primarily targets cardiac myocytes and vascular cells. Host response aims to destroy the allografted hearts, which are recognised as foreign. ACR occurs within weeks or months after transplantation and may also recur after many years for a number of reasons which can reduce the immunologic tolerance which has gradually been established.

The key histologic findings of ACR are myocardial inflammation and myocyte injury (Fig. 13.1).

13.2.1 Myocardial Inflammation

The inflammatory infiltrates are typically composed of mononuclear cells, mainly activated lymphocytes and macrophages (Michaels et al. 2001), and are predominantly distributed within the interstitium, in perivascular spaces or amongst and around the myocytes. Lymphocytes are the predominant cells and are characteristically T cells. The extent and distribution of myocardial inflammation are related to the severity of rejection (see Sect. 13.3).

Eosinophils and/or neutrophils are seen in moderate/severe grades, where they are closely related to myocyte damage. A significant presence of neutrophils is strongly suggestive of some other pathologic process such as ischaemic injury, both recent and healing, and mixed cellular and antibody-mediated severe rejection or infections.

Plasma cells are not typical ACR cells and, when more than occasional, would be related to the healing process, especially when associated with fibrosis, some infections (i.e. parvovirus infection), chronic AMR or lymphoproliferative disorders.

Vascular involvement is not prominent in ACR: the nearby vessels are not usually significantly involved by inflammation and do not show the microvascular inflammation typically seen in antibody-mediated rejection. In a limited number of cases, vasculitis of small arteries and venules may coexist with interstitial inflammation.

To the best of our present knowledge, the prevalent interstitial extravascular distribution of inflammatory infiltrates and lack of significant endothelialitis/microvascular inflammation versus intravascular localisation are of major significance in distinguishing cell-mediated from antibody-mediated rejection (see Chap. 14).

It should be emphasised that ACR diagnosis is based purely on histologic findings and immunohistochemical characterisation of inflammatory infiltrates is not required.

CD3, CD68, CD20 or other markers might be used in differential diagnosis with other pathologic processes, although they are rarely the only elements of diagnosis, except for lymphoproliferative disorders.

13.2.2 Myocyte Injury

Identification of myocyte injury is the key to discriminating low and high grades of rejection. Myocyte damage, previously termed "myocyte necrosis", is always associated with mononuclear inflammation and may be difficult to define, as its aspect varies resulting in heterogeneous findings and a combination of subtle features:

- Distortion of the normal architecture of the myocardium on low power with apparent loss of myocytes at higher magnification (a "space-

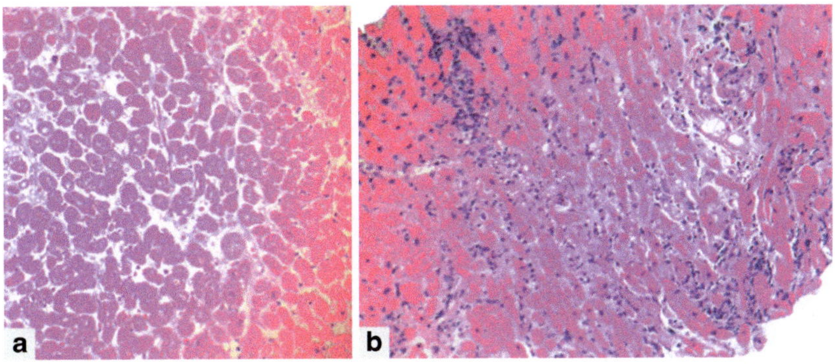

Fig. 13.1 (**a**) Normal myocardium. (**b**) Acute cellular rejection with inflammation and myocyte damage. Haematoxylin-eosin, 200× (Courtesy of Dr. O. Leone, Bologna, Italy)

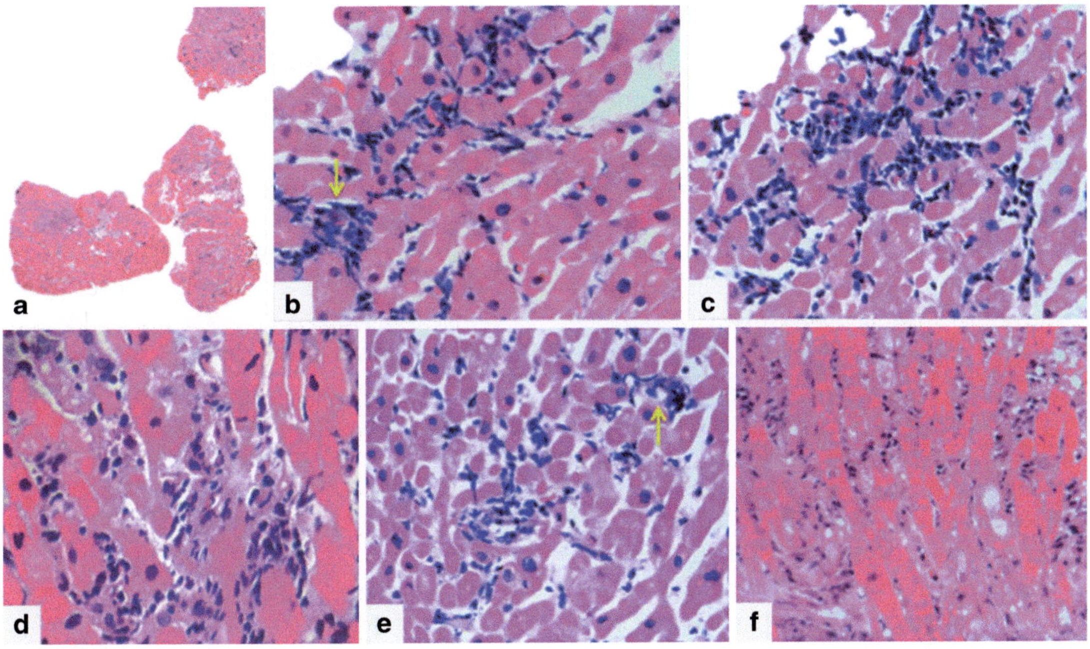

Fig. 13.2 (**a**) Low-power image of moderate rejection where myocyte injury is suggested by distortion of the architecture of the myocardium with apparent loss of myocytes (haematoxylin-eosin, 25×). (**b, c**) High power: encroachment of inflammatory cells on the cell membrane of myocytes with irregular cytoplasmic borders and free-lying myocyte nuclei admixed with mononuclear cells (*arrow*) (haematoxylin-eosin, 200×). (**d**) In a focus of moderate/severe ACR, myocytes are distorted and fragmented due to aggression of inflammatory cells (haematoxylin-eosin, 200×. (**e**) In this image a perinuclear halo indicates myocyte injury (*arrow*) (haematoxylin-eosin, 100×). (**f**) Extensive myocytolysis (cytoplasmic clearing) is seen in this image of ACR (haematoxylin-eosin, 200×)

occupying lesion" due to inflammatory infiltrate) (Fig. 13.2a).

- Inflammatory encroachment into myocytes: the mononuclear cell infiltrate surrounds and separates myocytes, with encroachment of the cell membranes giving an irregular appearance to the edge of some myocytes. Free-lying myocyte nuclei admixed with mononuclear cells may also be seen (Fig. 13.2b, c).
- Other findings such as fragmentation, perinuclear halo and myocytolysis with clearing/vacuolisation of the cytoplasm (Fig. 13.2d–f).

Nuclear enlargement and occasionally prominent nucleoli may also be seen.

Sarcoplasmic coagulation (hypereosinophilia), nuclear pyknosis and loss of nuclei are features of coagulative necrosis and not of ACR: these findings may occur in relation to previous biopsy sites, peritransplant injury and later ischaemic injury in the form of micro-infarcts or zonal infarcts. Coagulative necrosis stains with complement 9 (C9) and to lesser extents with C3d and C4d antisera (Neil 2013), whilst myocyte injury related to acute cellular rejection and contraction band necrosis does not stain with complement in the early stages.

13.2.3 Other Findings

Although minor and less specific, other histologic findings may accompany the basic histologic picture of ACR.

Myocardial interstitial oedema, both perivascular and perimyocytic, may be focally present or in high-grade rejection more extensive, although it is more commonly seen in antibody-mediated rejection. Oedema is seen as separation of myocytes on low power, and at higher power, wisps of eosinophilic material are identified between the myocytes (Fig. 13.3a). This latter feature helps to differentiate artefactual separation of myocytes related to the biopsy procedure (Fig. 13.3b).

Significant interstitial haemorrhage is seen only in severe grades of ACR; more subtle findings with individual red blood cells, which often degenerate, scattered throughout the interstitium (Fig. 13.3c), may be seen in association to oedema.

Histologically ACR may be confused with many other non-rejection lesions (see Chap. 15) or may overlap with some findings of AMR, especially in severe forms (see Chap. 14), or really coexist with these findings in mixed rejection (see Chap. 16).

13.3 Grading Systems

ACR appears in general as mild, moderate and severe. Grading systems aim to identify histologic patterns of progressively increasing severity in order to allow assessment of the clinical significance of different patterns and subsequent therapy.

13.3.1 1990 ISHLT Grading System

In 1989 the ISHLT urged pathologists to agree on a standardised grading system for ACR that should be easy to interpret and highly reproducible, which should replace the many grading systems currently used in transplant centres worldwide.

The result was the 1990 ISHLT standardised grading system (Billingham et al. 1990) in which a 7-point grading system was defined (Table 13.1) based on around three main categories of rejection, mild, moderate and severe, with grade 1-mild subdivided into focal (A) and diffuse (B) and grade 3-moderate subdivided into multifocal (A) and diffuse (B) based on the pattern of inflammatory cell infiltration.

Grade 0 (No Acute Rejection)
This grade implies no features of acute rejection or myocyte damage. Biopsy specimens with equivocal findings should be graded as zero. Non-rejection findings such as Quilty lesions and peritransplant ischaemic changes may be seen.

Grade 1A (Focal, Mild Acute Rejection)
Focal, perivascular or interstitial infiltrates of large lymphocytes in the absence of myocyte damage and with one or more pieces involved.

Grade 1B (Diffuse, Mild Acute Rejection)
More diffuse infiltrates of large lymphocytes and absence of myocyte damage, again with one or more pieces of biopsy tissue involved.

Grade 2 (Focal, Moderate Acute Rejection)
One focus only of aggressive infiltrate of lymphocytes (with or without eosinophils) sharply circumscribed, associated with focal myocyte damage. Architectural distortion with myocyte damage within the single focus should be present.

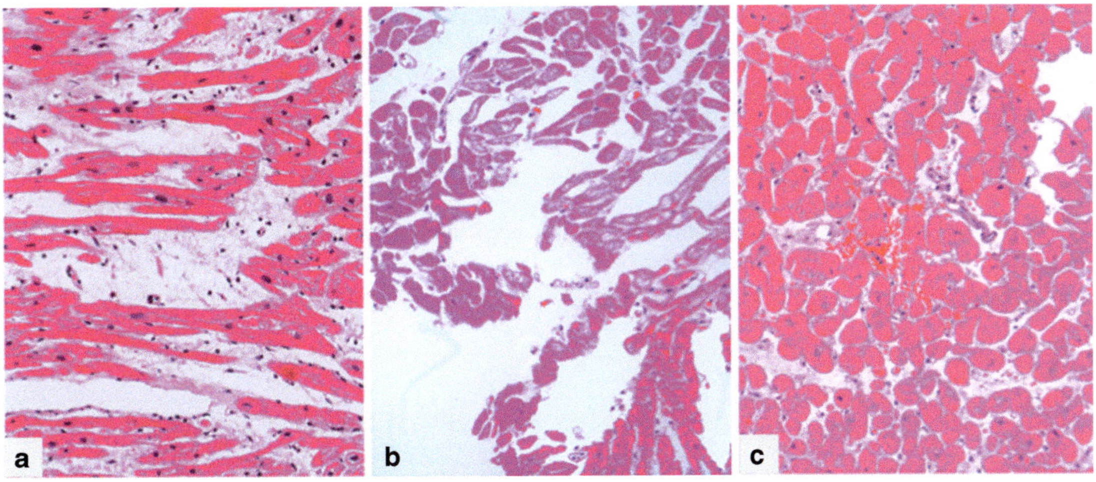

Fig. 13.3 (**a**) Oedema is seen as separation of the myocytes, which is relatively uniform throughout the biopsy and in the setting of rejection may be associated with an inflammatory cell infiltrate. At high power the extracellular matrix is apparent and has a frothy/bubbly look and the red cells are dispersed, often as one or a few cells throughout this oedematous interstitium, together with inflammatory cells. (**b**) Myocyte separation occurs with damage to the tissues during the biopsy procedure, and the myocytes are pulled away from each other with clear holes, with no bubbly/oedematous extracellular matrix between the myocytes. (**c**) As the biopsies tend to be in similar places, the haemorrhage can be the result of a previous biopsy during the same procedure due to tissue injury with damage to blood vessels by the bioptomes when they are torn from the adjacent tissues. The red cells tend to be quite obvious and clumped together, usually readily apparent at low power. There is nearby artefactual separation of myocytes (*top right*) and also some interstitial oedema (*lower left*), which can be seen at the edges of previous biopsy sites

Grade 3A (Multifocal Moderate Rejection)
Multifocal inflammatory infiltrates of large aggressive lymphocytes with or without eosinophils, associated with myocyte damage. The foci may be present in one piece or scattered across several pieces.

Grade 3B (Diffuse, Borderline Severe Acute Rejection)
Diffuse inflammatory process within several pieces, with myocyte damage. The aggressive inflammatory process is characterised by large lymphocytes and eosinophils with occasional neutrophils.

Grade 4 (Severe Acute Rejection)
Diffuse polymorphous inflammatory infiltrate that includes aggressive lymphocytes, eosinophils and neutrophils with myocyte necrosis and damage, with or without oedema, haemorrhage and vasculitis. The infiltrate is more diffuse and intense than in 3B and myocyte damage is conspicuous. Neutrophils and haemorrhage are often seen but are not required for classification as grade 4.

The virtue of this unified grading system was the creation of a common language amongst pathologists, which allowed centres throughout the world to compare results.

In time however various problems emerged:

- Very poor reproducibility of grades between centres (Stewart et al. 2005; Tan et al. 2007).
- Grades 1A, 1B and 2 were found to behave in a similar manner, with no clinical signs or symptoms (Stewart and Cary 1996) and only a 10–15 % risk of progressing to high-grade rejection (Stewart et al. 2005).
- Many grade 2 "rejections" were in fact found to be tangentially cut Quilty lesions.
- Grades 3B and 4 were generally aggressively treated, so sub-differentiation was unnecessary.

A number of papers discussed the issues concerning the system, and as a result, a working

Table 13.1 1990 ISHLT grading scheme for acute cellular rejection

Grade 0	No rejection
Grade 1, mild	
A: focal	Focal, perivascular or interstitial infiltrates of large lymphocytes without myocyte damage and with one or more pieces involved
B: diffuse	Diffuse infiltrates of large lymphocytes without myocyte damage with one or more pieces of biopsy tissue involved
Grade 2 moderate (focal)	One focus only of aggressive infiltrate of lymphocytes sharply circumscribed, associated with focal myocyte damage
Grade 3, moderate/borderline severe	
A: multifocal	Multifocal inflammatory infiltrates of large aggressive lymphocytes with or without eosinophils, associated with myocyte damage. The foci may be present in one piece or scattered across several pieces
B: diffuse	Diffuse inflammatory process (large lymphocytes and eosinophils with occasional neutrophils) within several pieces, with myocyte damage
Grade 4, severe	Diffuse polymorphous infiltrate with extensive myocyte damage ± oedema, ± haemorrhage + vasculitis

party for ISHLT simplified the grading system to a four-grade system by merging several grades (Stewart et al. 2005).

However it should be emphasised that many centres still continue to use both the "old" 1990 and "new" 2005 grade of rejection (Maleszewski et al. 2011), so today it is still essential to know it in detail.

13.3.2 2005 ISHLT Grading System

In this grading system, the basic no, mild, moderate and severe rejection hierarchy is maintained, but there are four levels of rejection (0R, 1R, 2R, 3R) with an R following the number grade to indicate it is the new revised grading and to avoid confusion with the previous 1990 grading.

Grade 0R remains the same, whilst grade 1R "mild" amalgamates 1990 grades 1A, 1B and 2; grade 2R "moderate" replaces the old grade 3A; grade 3R "severe" rejection amalgamates previous grades 3B and 4 (Table 13.2).

Table 13.2 2005 ISHLT grading scheme for acute cellular rejection

Grade 0R	No rejection
Grade 1R, mild	Interstitial and/or perivascular infiltrate with up to 1 focus of myocyte damage
Grade 2R, moderate	Two or more foci of infiltrate with associated myocyte damage
Grade 3R, severe	Diffuse infiltrate with multifocal myocyte damage ± oedema, ± haemorrhage ± vasculitis

The main differences between the 1990 and 2005 grading schemes are:

- The distinction between a focal and diffuse infiltrate is now not taken into account.
- Myocyte damage is still a discriminating parameter but one focus of myocyte injury does not condition a shift to moderate rejection and subsequent treatment.

Grade 0R (No Acute Cellular Rejection)

This grade implies no evidence of rejection. There is no mononuclear inflammation (lymphocytes/macrophages) or myocyte damage within the myocardium. Non-rejection infiltrates may be present such as Quilty lesions, previous biopsy sites or peritransplant injury.

Grade 1R (Mild, Low-Grade, Acute Cellular Rejection)

This grade corresponds to mild or low-grade rejection and includes two main pictures:

1. Perivascular and/or interstitial mononuclear (lymphocytes/macrophages) infiltrates which "respect" myocytes
2. One focus of mononuclear cells with associated myocyte damage

The degree and the pattern may vary, so it may be difficult to identify at low power and may only be present in some levels. Inflammatory cells do not usually encroach on myocytes and do not distort the normal architecture although a maximum of one focus of myocyte damage related to the infiltrate may be present. When there is a single focus, care must be taken to exclude a mimic of rejection such as a tangentially cut Quilty lesion (see Chap. 16). Macrophages can be part of the infiltrate, but neutrophils are not a feature, and interstitial oedema or haemorrhage is also not seen.

Grade 2R (Moderate, Intermediate-Grade, Acute Cellular Rejection)

Grade 2R rejection identifies moderate/intermediate grade of rejection and is defined as two or more foci of mononuclear cells (lymphocytes/macrophages) with associated myocyte damage. The infiltrate is usually multifocal and moderate in extent and easy to identify on low power. Foci of rejection may involve one or more fragments with intermixed uninvolved areas of myocardium. Foci of mild rejection may coexist. Similar to grade 1R rejection, lymphocytes are the predominant cell type with some macrophages; a few eosinophils/neutrophils may be seen. Oedema and interstitial haemorrhage are not a usual feature.

Grade 3R (Severe, High-Grade, Acute Cellular Rejection)

Grade 3R is a severe rejection characterised by a diffuse, often mixed, inflammatory infiltrate easily seen at low power, with extensive myocyte injury. Multiple fragments are usually involved, although with different degrees of intensity. The infiltrate can include neutrophils and eosinophils as well as lymphocytes and macrophages and is associated with interstitial oedema, and there is often interstitial haemorrhage, which must be differentiated from artefactual haemorrhage related to trauma from the biopsy procedure. Vasculitis may be present. Grade 3R rejection is very uncommon with current immunosuppressive protocols, and noncompliance with medication is the most common cause.

Table 13.3 compares ISHLT 1990 and 2005 grading schemes.

Figures 13.4, 13.5, 13.6 and 13.7 show different grades of ACR according to both ISHLT grading systems.

13.3.3 Reliability of Grading Systems

Essentially, an ideal grading system for acute rejection should accurately stratify patients into treatment groups; it should also be easy to apply and highly reproducible.

Grading simplicity is not however the only parameter for improving interobserver reproducibility: it is essential that the basic histologic criteria (type and site of inflammatory infiltrates, spectrum of myocyte damage, extension of fragment involvement, etc.) be clearly defined. Moreover simplification does not necessarily go with tapering of the immunosuppressive therapy.

In any case the simplified 2005 grading scheme was brought in to increase reproducibility and more readily identify patients for whom augmented immunosuppression was required. It was anticipated that a reduced number of rejection grades would improve interobserver variation; however, studies in the literature have so far failed to demonstrate this. In 2009 Yang et al. found there was no significant improvement in kappa values with the 2005 classification over the 1990 classification (Yang et al. 2009): the main areas of difficulty were subjective assessment of the degree of inflammation and myocyte injury.

In 2009 the Association for European Cardiovascular Pathology (AECVP) transplant working group undertook an assessment of the 2005 ISHLT classification at a European level using digitised images, and the findings were published in 2011 (Angelini et al. 2011). They demonstrated a small improvement in kappa values of the 2005 over the 1990 classification in the assessment and grading of biopsies for ACR, but this was not statistically significant. Again difficulties were noted in the assessment of inflammatory cell infiltrates and myocyte injury. In this study agreement amongst pathologists was better for features of chronic rejection and non-rejection-related findings.

Table 13.3 Comparison of ISHLT 1990 and 2005 grading schemes for cellular rejection

ISHLT 1990		ISHLT 2005	
Grade 0	No/minimal inflammation	Grade 0R	No/minimal inflammation
Grade 1A	Focal perivascular/interstitial inflammatory infiltrates. No myocyte damage	Grade 1R	Inflammatory infiltrates with no myocyte damage or with a single focus of myocyte damage
Grade 1B	Diffuse interstitial inflammatory infiltrates. No myocyte damage		
Grade 2	Single focus of aggressive inflammatory infiltrate with myocyte damage		
Grade 3A	Multifocal inflammatory infiltrates associated with myocyte damage	Grade 2R	Two or more foci of inflammatory infiltrates with myocyte damage
Grade 3B	Diffuse inflammatory infiltrates associated with myocyte damage	Grade 3R	Diffuse inflammatory infiltrate with myocyte damage and often with oedema, haemorrhage and/or vasculitis
Grade 4	Diffuse polymorphous inflammatory infiltrates associated with extensive myocyte damage, oedema, haemorrhage and vasculitis		

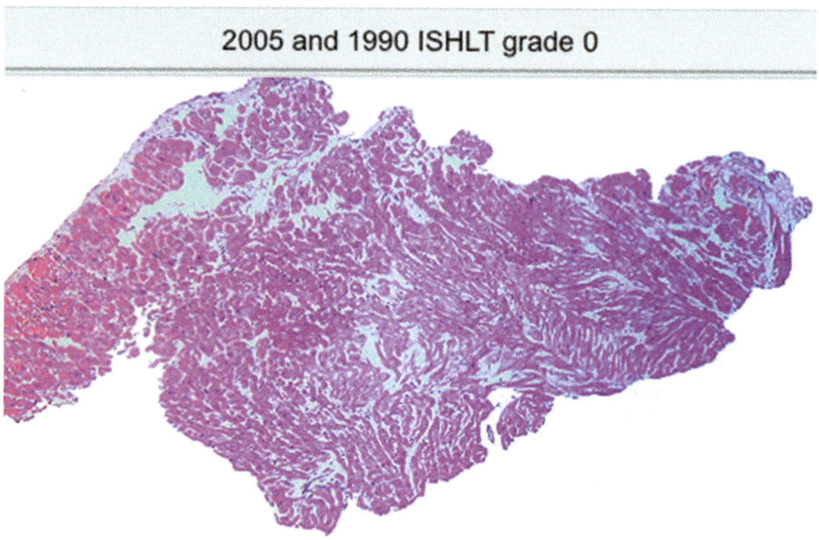

Fig. 13.4 2005 and 1990 ISHLT ACR grade 0. No rejection. Haematoxylin-eosin, 100×

Both studies show limitations: that of Yang et al. was performed in a single institution with a biopsy cohort in which there was a high percentage of cases of ACR compared to daily practice; the European study included pathologists with varied experience in reporting cardiac allograft biopsies and the use of digitised slides which pathologists were not used to assessing. It is hoped that increased centralisation of expertise within transplantation centres, ready access to online teaching resources and increased ease of inter-institutional referral via digital slides will result in improved rates of concordance between pathologists. However falling rates of heart transplantation and numbers of cardiac allograft biopsies reported by pathologists may limit any potential improvement.

Probably the best practice is to mention both 1990 and 2005 ISHLT grading systems in the pathology report, as it allows clinicians to modulate therapy within the clinical course of patients

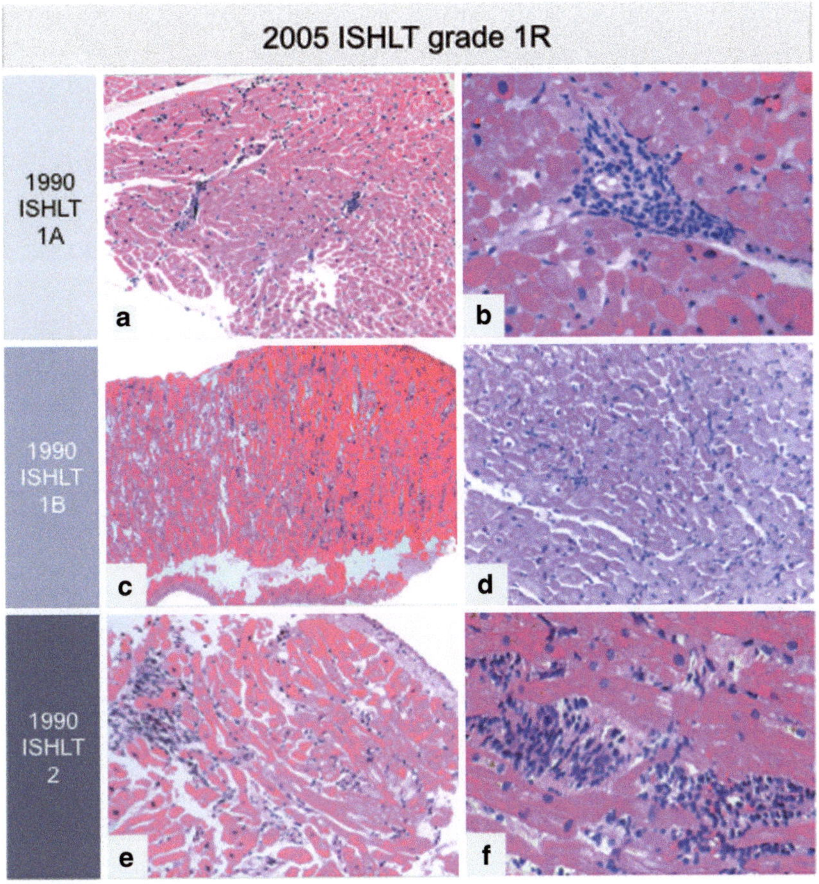

Fig. 13.5 2005 ISHLT 1R mild-low-grade ACR = 1990 ISHLT 1A-1B-2 grades. (**a**) Haematoxylin-eosin, 100×; (**b**) haematoxylin-eosin, 200×; (**c**) haematoxylin-eosin, 25×; (**d**) haematoxylin-eosin, 100×; (**e**) haematoxylin-eosin, 100×; (**f**) haematoxylin-eosin, 200×. (**b**, **d**, **f**: Courtesy of Drs. O. Leone (Bologna, Italy) and A. Angelini (Padua, Italy))

and better identify progression of some grades of low/borderline rejections.

13.4 Technical Aspects

In assessing cardiac rejection, technical issues are as essential as histopathology criteria in reproducibility of results.

The infiltrate in rejection is patchy, so to reduce missing rejection due to inadequate sampling, the ISHLT documents specify criteria for standardisation of sampling, with requirements for minimum numbers of biopsies and minimum numbers of sections for each biopsy.

13.4.1 Biopsy Sampling and Fragment Adequacy

With three biopsy samples, there is 5 % chance of missing a mild rejection but negligible risk of missing moderate or severe rejection (Spiegelhalter and Stovin 1983), and if there are four samples, the chance of missing mild rejection falls to 2 %. As the number of pieces containing a mild rejection infiltrate increases, the risk of missing a higher grade rejection increases (Sharples et al. 1992).

The minimum requirement is 3 "evaluable" fragments of myocardium, although 4 are considered preferable (4 were required in the 1990 ISHLT publication) and increasing sample size to

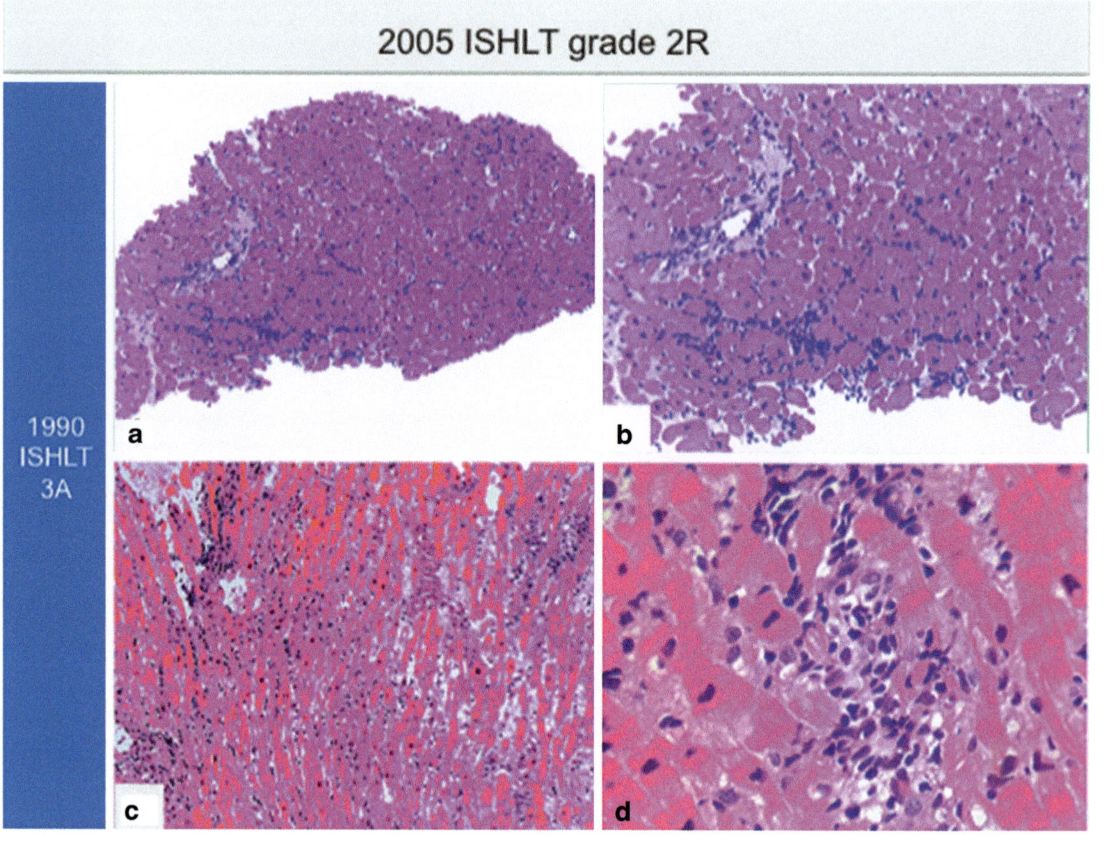

Fig. 13.6 2005 ISHLT 2R moderate/intermediate grade ACR = 1990 ISHLT 3A multifocal moderate grade. (**a**) Haematoxylin-eosin, 100×; (**b**) haematoxylin-eosin, 200×; (**c**) haematoxylin-eosin, 200x; (**d**) haematoxylin-eosin, 400× (Courtesy of Drs. O. Leone (Bologna, Italy) and A. Angelini (Padua, Italy))

5 has been shown to increase the sensitivity for detecting rejection. It is also recommended that fragments should never be subdivided to increase the number of fragments.

An evaluable fragment is defined as a biopsy which contains at least 50 % myocardium free of a previous biopsy site.

If the biopsy is inadequate based on containing fewer than three evaluable pieces, there are two outcomes:

- Rejection cannot be diagnosed, so no grade is given and the biopsy should be called inadequate, prompting a further biopsy to assess for rejection.
- Rejection is identified so the biopsy can be reported as rejection, but as more severe rejection may be missed the caveat of "at least" should be put before the grade, and a comment within the text of the report should indicate that the biopsy is inadequate/suboptimal and cannot exclude a higher grade of rejection.

How an inadequate/suboptimal biopsy is handled will depend on the time post-transplant, if very early and another biopsy is scheduled in 1–2 weeks and the patient is well, then it is likely that they will just stick to protocol. However if the next scheduled biopsy is not for some time, it is likely that a repeat biopsy to exclude rejection or higher-grade rejection will be organised sooner.

13.4.2 Sections

The biopsies should be embedded at a single level and ideally arranged so that it is easy to

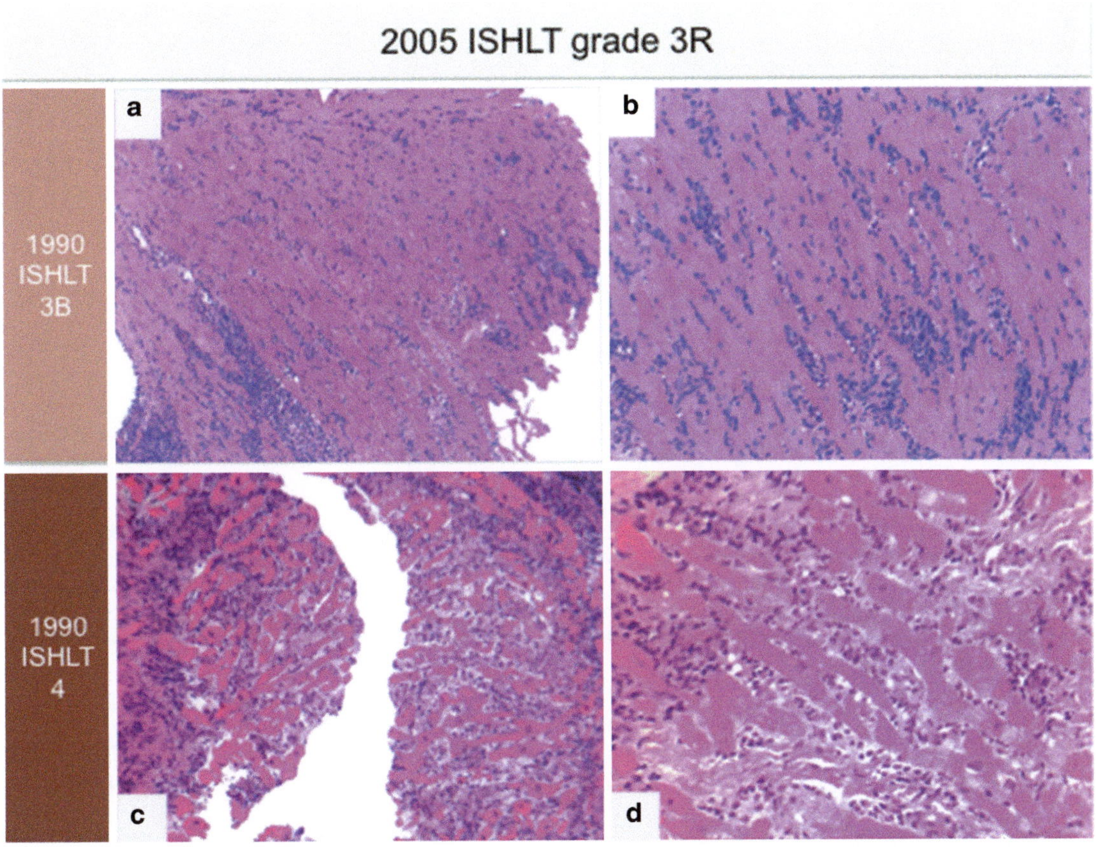

Fig. 13.7 2005 ISHLT 3R severe/high-grade ACR = 1990 ISHLT 3B diffuse – borderline severe grade and 4 severe grade. In grade 4 the inflammatory infiltrate is more polymorphous, diffuse and intense than in 3B, and myocyte damage is conspicuous. (**a**) Haematoxylin-eosin, 100×; (**b**) haematoxylin-eosin, 200×; (**c**) haematoxylin-eosin, 200×; (**d**) haematoxylin-eosin, 400× (Courtesy of Drs. O. Leone (Bologna, Italy) and A. Angelini (Padua, Italy))

assess them all without the risk of missing a piece, e.g. in a linear arrangement. Biopsies should be cut at multiple levels to minimise the risk of missing focal inflammatory infiltrates and to allow better appreciation of the position of the infiltrate. Rejection features are not uniform throughout the myocardium so this will improve detection and accuracy of rejection grading. ISHLT recommends at least three levels stained with haematoxylin and eosin (H&E) with spare sections between levels kept for more detailed assessment as required (Stewart et al. 2005). Spare sections or additional sections can be stained with H&E to try to confirm a Quilty lesion and/or immunohistochemistry for CD3, CD20, CD68 and CD21 to attempt to differentiate a Quilty lesion from a rejection infiltrate (Michaels et al. 2001; Sattar et al. 2006).

13.5 Assessment of Rejection at Microscope

13.5.1 Low Power

At scanning/low-power magnification (4×, 10×), biopsy adequacy (required number of pieces), overall biopsy cellularity, pattern and site of inflammatory infiltrates and worst areas of infiltration are determined.

13.5.1.1 Biopsy Adequacy

First the number of pieces of evaluable myocardium is determined for adequacy as defined above.

13.5.1.2 Cellularity

An assessment of overall cellularity is then made with particular emphasis on the location and pat-

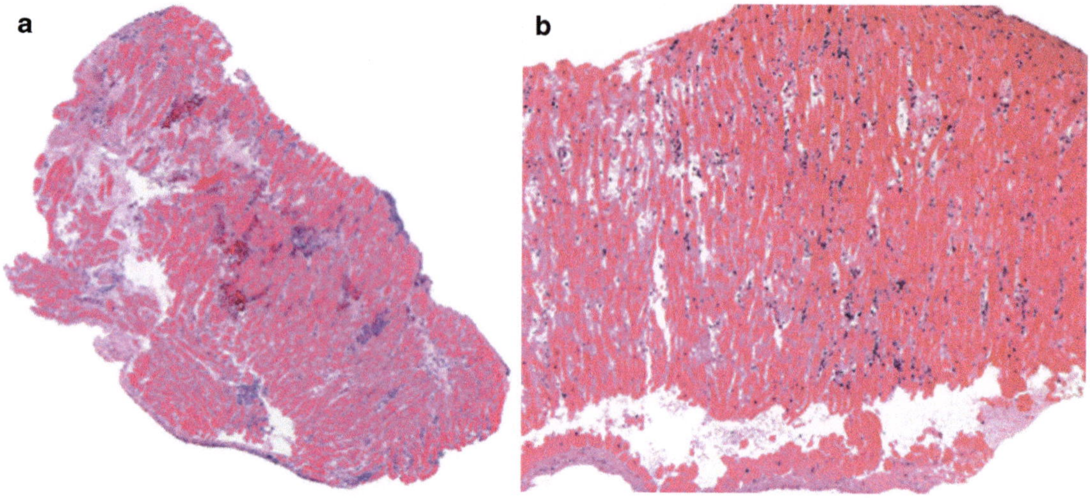

Fig. 13.8 (**a**) Focal infiltrates. At low power the focal infiltrates are often readily apparent as the inflammatory cells are aggregated with relatively pink areas with minimal inflammation between. A linear low-density endocardial infiltrate is also seen. In this biopsy artefactual tears in the tissue and aggregates of red blood cells are also seen related to the biopsy procedure (haematoxylin-eosin, 25×). (**b**) Diffuse infiltrates. At low power these can be difficult to spot as there are no discrete blue areas with pink areas between; however there are usually some areas where the infiltrate is more marked (haematoxylin-eosin, 40×)

tern of inflammatory cell infiltration. Whether the infiltrate is focal or diffuse and its relationship to the myocytes and endocardium can provide clues as to the underlying pathology. Rejection may be seen as bluer areas in focal areas of inflammatory infiltration (Fig. 13.8a), easy to spot on low power, or as a more diffuse infiltrate, which is often harder to pick up on scanning power (Fig. 13.8b). The position of the infiltrate is determined; this may require looking at the sequential levels, to see if the infiltrate is endocardially based with or without extension into the myocardium, myocardial or within areas or fibrosis or fat (see Sect. 13.7). Nodular endocardial inflammatory infiltrates, often with a pushing border, are more likely to be Quilty lesions (Fig. 13.9a), whilst less dense linear endocardial infiltrates may be part of rejection, warranting a closer search for myocardial infiltrates (Fig. 13.9b). If the infiltrate is within the myocardial layer, assess whether it is predominantly separating/surrounding the myocytes or in a perivascular distribution. These features may be better appreciated on a higher power. Perimyocytic inflammatory infiltrates should be examined at high power for the presence of myocyte injury.

13.5.1.3 Myocytes and Interstitium

Assess the myocytes for proximity to each other: are they close or are they separated? If separated is the interstitial space between myocytes pale in which case it might indicate tissue oedema or artefactual separation (Fig. 13.3), or are they separated by blue inflammatory cells (Fig. 13.2)? Do there appear to be any myocytes missing, which can be an indication of myocyte damage (Fig. 13.10)? Is there any haemorrhage apparent? Haemorrhage seen at low power is usually related to the biopsy procedure rather than a feature of severe rejection. These features should then be assessed in more detail at a higher power.

13.5.1.4 Other

Other features which can be identified include ischaemic injury, previous biopsy site reaction, fibrous scars, fat and thrombus (Fig. 13.11a, b). If mesothelium is identified, it indicates perforation, and this should be notified together with the biopsy grade, so that the patient can be

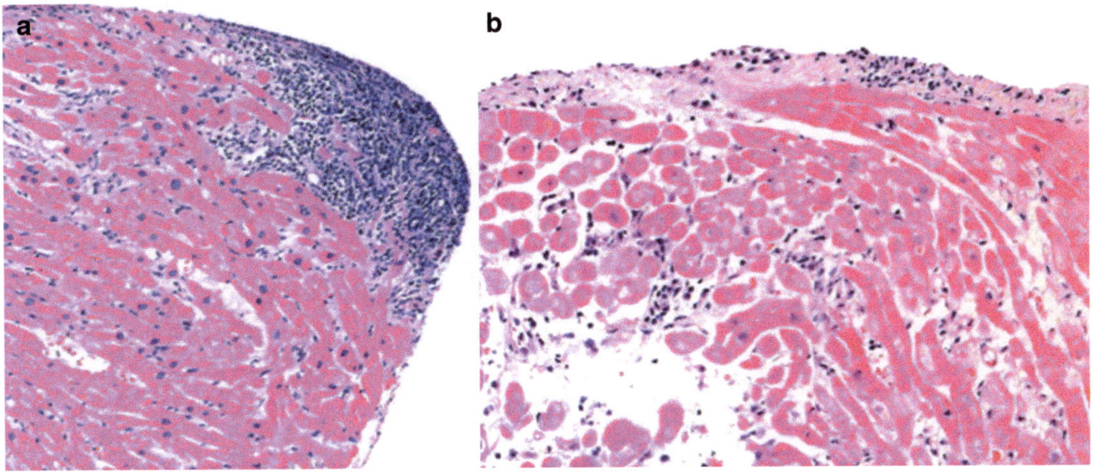

Fig. 13.9 (**a**) At low power a well-oriented Quilty lesion jumps out as a dense endocardially based infiltrate (haematoxylin-eosin, 200×). (**b**) A rejection inflammatory infiltrate can involve the endocardium; it tends to be linear and less dense than the nodular endocardial Quilty lesion. Mononuclear cell inflammatory infiltrates can be seen in the adjacent myocardium as part of rejection (haematoxylin-eosin, 200×)

more closely monitored for complications (Fig. 13.11c).

13.5.2 High Power

At high power the features on low power are examined in more detail, in particular to assess:

- Evidence of myocyte injury, particularly in the worst areas of inflammation
- Composition and distribution of inflammatory infiltrates
- Interstitium with microvessels

13.5.2.1 Myocyte Injury

Assess the myocytes within/associated with the areas of inflammatory infiltration for evidence of rejection looking at the type of myocyte injury, necrosis or loss (see illustrative Case 1). In rejection injured myocytes may appear moth eaten or fragmented with tiny fragments together with larger more normal-sized myocytes, there may be myocyte missing with gaps where a myocyte should be and the injured myocyte cytoplasm may appear granular and there may be a perinuclear halo zone and free-lying myocyte nuclei (Fig. 13.12). Hypereosinophilic myocytes usually indicate ischaemic type of coagulative necrosis (see Chap. 16), which is not part of cellular rejection and may occur as part of a previous biopsy site injury and peritransplant injury or could indicate an infarct due to an upstream vascular process.

13.5.2.2 Inflammatory Infiltrates

The composition and position/distribution of the inflammatory infiltrate are assessed. A rejection infiltrate is composed of mononuclear cells comprising mixed lymphocytes and macrophages. Occasional eosinophils may be present in moderate or severe grades of rejection (Fig. 13.12).

More diffuse infiltrates are more readily apparent at high power than low power.

Occasional lymphocytes and macrophages may be seen in normal myocardium.

13.5.2.3 Interstitium and Microvessels

Apart from interstitial inflammation, other interstitial changes such as oedema, haemorrhage or fibrosis are also carefully looked for.

Infiltrates which appeared to be perivascular at low power should be assessed in more detail

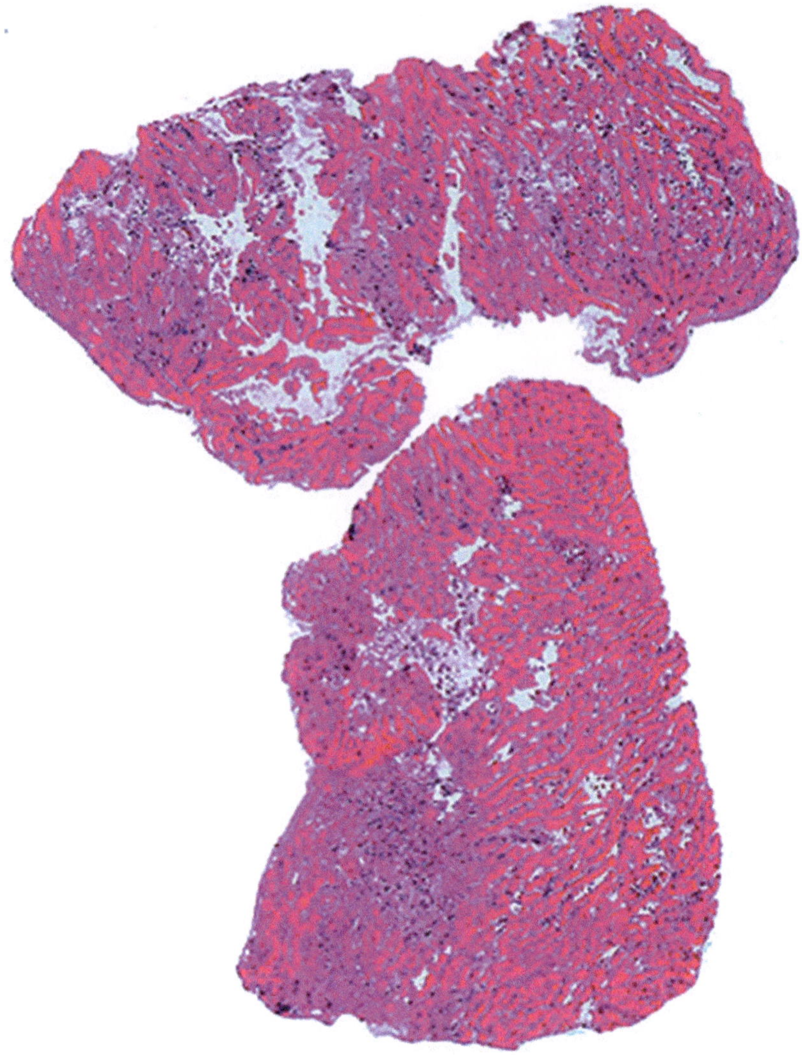

Fig. 13.10 A low-power image of acute cellular rejection where myocyte injury is suggested by distortion of the architecture of the myocardium with apparent loss of myocytes (haematoxylin-eosin, 25×)

to determine their relationship with microvessels, i.e. whether they are truly perivascular or associated with plump endothelial cells and cells within capillaries or small venules (a microvasculitis). If a microvascular inflammation is relatively prominent, then this may indicate either antibody-mediated rejection (see Chap. 14) or mixed cellular and antibody-mediated rejection, thus requiring immunohistochemistry (see Chap. 15). Intraluminal inflammatory cells in less than 10 % of the myocardium are permissible in pure acute cellular rejection; over 10 % and the diagnosis of mixed rejection or antibody-mediated rejection should be considered. Oedema, haemorrhage and karyorrhectic debris may be an indirect sign of microvasculitis.

At high power, small vessel disease due to chronic rejection should also be checked (see Chap. 18) as well as possible chronic degenerative changes in myocytes, such as vacuolisation, subendocardial myocytolysis, etc.

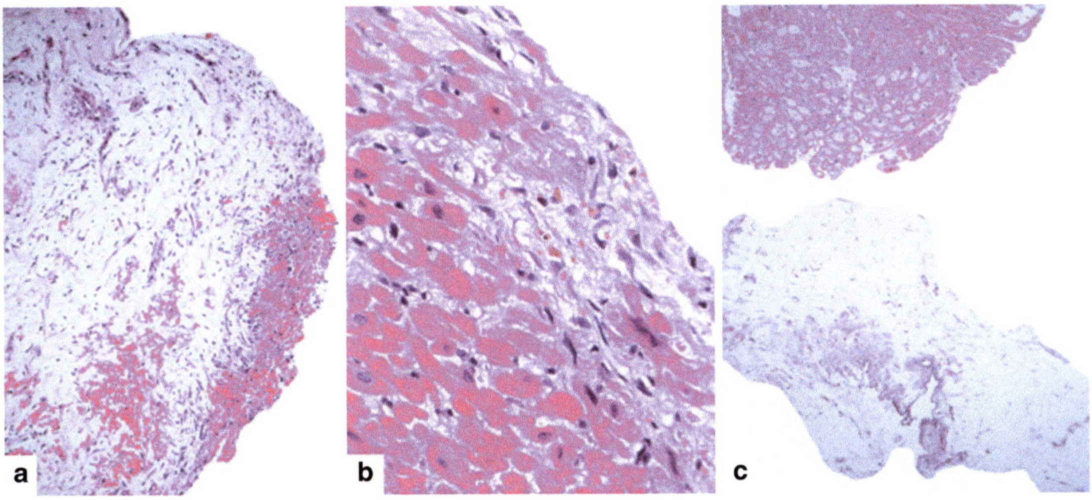

Fig. 13.11 (**a**) Previous biopsy site with fibrinous surface exudate overlying underlying fibrous granulation tissue (haematoxylin-eosin, 200×). (**b**) Healing peritransplant ischaemia/reperfusion injury with myocyte loss, lipofuscin laden macrophages and early loose fibrosis (haematoxylin-eosin, 200×). (**c**) The presence of mesothelium indicates perforation during the biopsy procedure. (Haematoxylin-eosin, 25×)

13.6 Changes in Rejection Over Time with Improvement in Immunosuppressive Agents

Immunosuppressants have improved over the years, with rejection becoming less common and of lesser severity. Since ciclosporin became available in the 1980s and tacrolimus in the 1990s, grade 4 (ISHLT-1990) is now virtually never seen, and the 1990 3B rejection is also uncommon. Most rejections seen now which require treatment are 2R (old 3A) rejections and tend to be down at the milder end of the spectrum, with less inflammatory infiltration, and careful searching over the levels is required to confirm myocyte injury.

13.7 Assessment of Biopsy

The best method to approach an EMB from heart transplanted patients is to form a first impression of all the pathologic features and then to reach a more precise assessment on the basis of a series of essential data:

- Time post-transplant (recent or late biopsy)
- How long since the last biopsy
- Sequence of previous rejections
- Any clinical symptoms
- Clinical information about other possible concurrent disease, such as infections
- Any change in medication either noncompliance or modification of immunosuppression by the clinical team

The relevant information may not be readily available, and discussion with the transplant surgeons or cardiologists may be required, particularly if the diagnosis is difficult. This is particularly important when the specimen is inadequate or suboptimal to convey the degree of uncertainty and allow them to make a decision as to the requirement and timing for a re-biopsy.

Illustrative Case: Early Rejection

(Figs. 13.13, 13.14, 13.15, and 13.16) First protocol biopsy day 8 post-transplant, doing well.

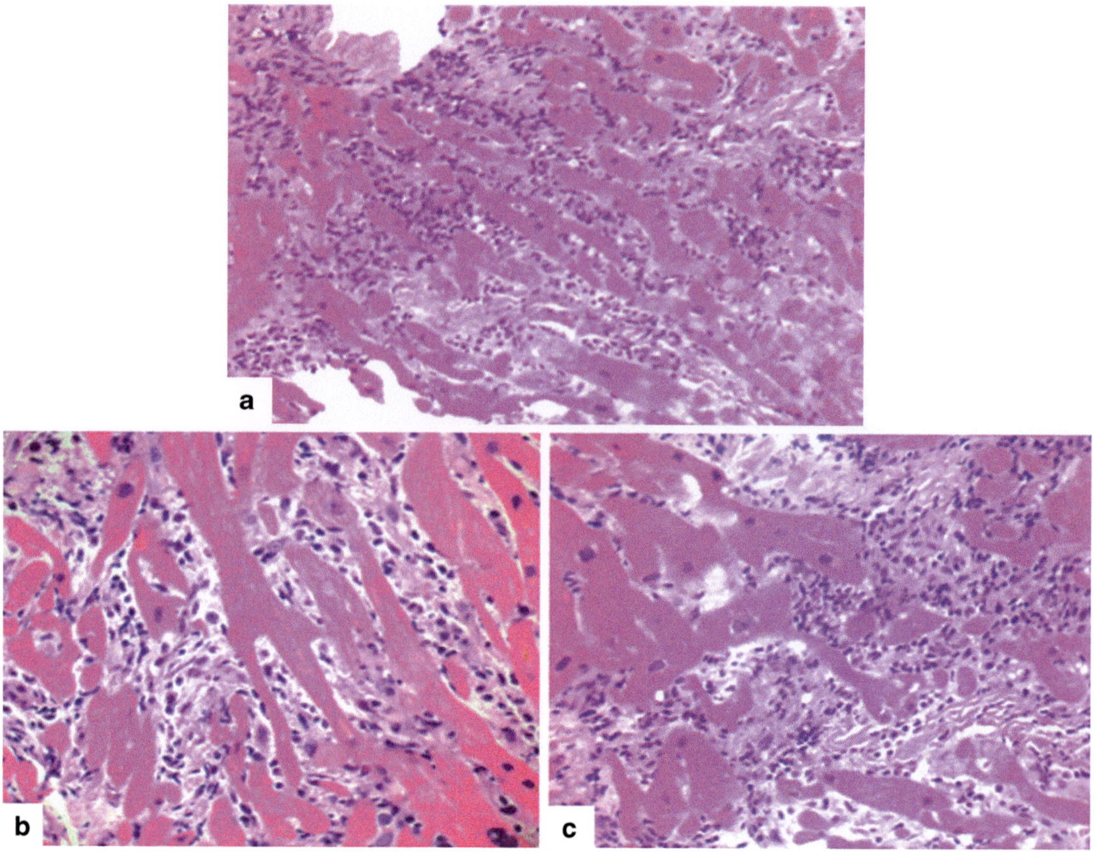

Fig. 13.12 High-power images of severe ACR foci. There is a diffuse mononuclear cell infiltrate separating and encroaching on myocytes with distortion of myocyte architecture and myocyte damage. Nature of inflammatory infiltrates can be easily recognised at this magnification. (**a**) Haematoxylin-eosin, 250×. (**b**, **c**) Haematoxylin-eosin, 400× (Courtesy of Dr. O. Leone, Bologna, Italy)

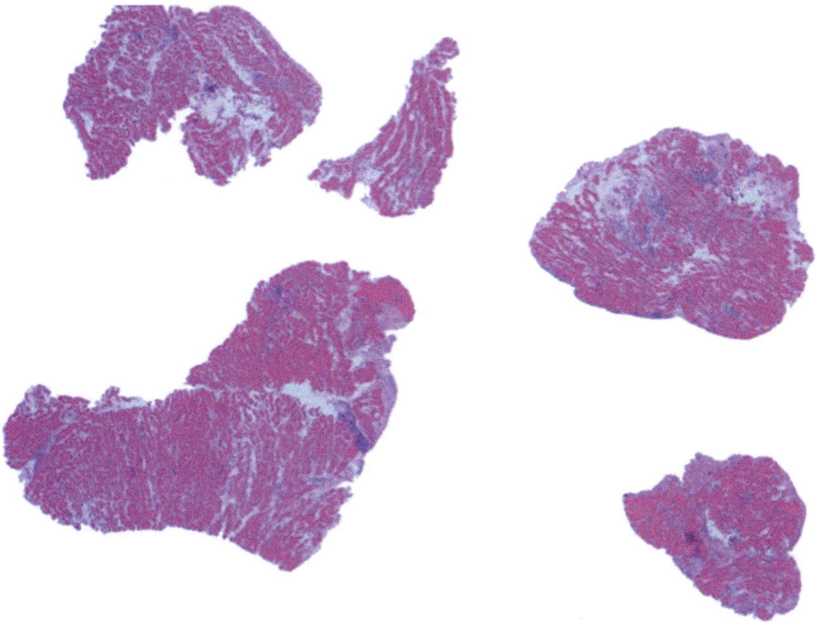

Fig. 13.13 Illustrative case. At low power, numerous focal *blue* areas are apparent

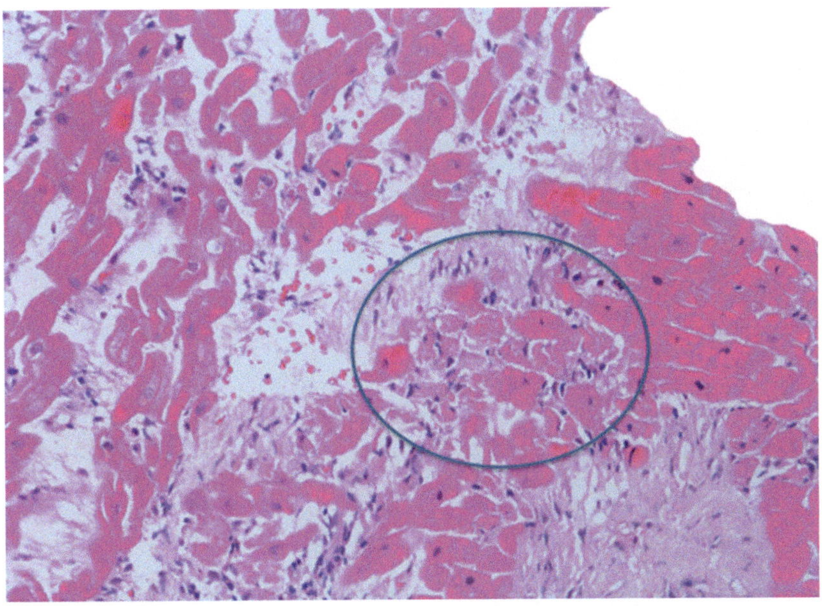

Fig. 13.14 Illustrative case. Areas of peritransplant injury are present (within *oval*). These were relatively sparse, had a generally very mild inflammatory infiltrate and showed is chaemic type coagulative necrosis and sarcoplasmic hypereosinophilia/coagulation of involved myocytes, which have a different appearance to the pattern of infiltration and look of the damaged myocytes which is much more subtle in areas of rejection

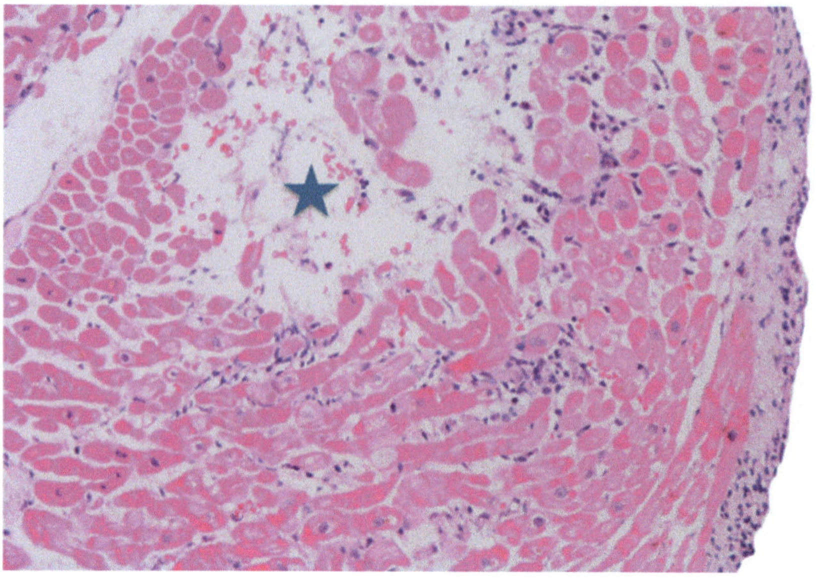

Fig. 13.15 Illustrative case. In this figure artefactual areas of separation of the myocytes (*star*) are seen. Adjacent to this is a focus of inflammation extending between and around myocytes with some linear involvement of the overlying endocardium. Even at this power, there is a suggestion of muscle damage, related to the relatively light mononuclear cell infiltrate, with some perinuclear clearing seen and an area in which there is inflammation and appears to lack a myocyte

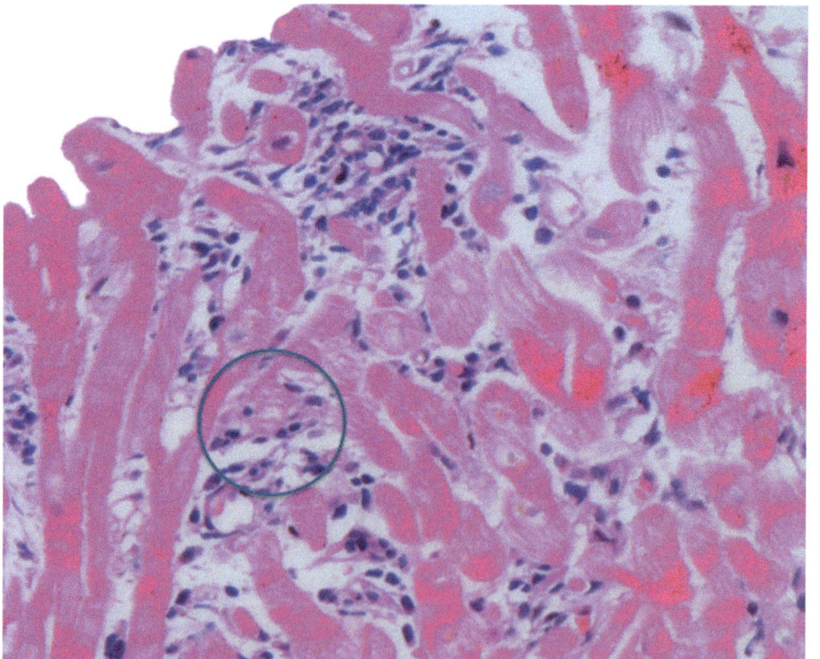

Fig. 13.16 Illustrative case. At higher power and with assessment of all areas of injury, myocyte damage is confirmed. There are fragments of myocytes, perinuclear clearing of damaged myocytes and mononuclear cells impinging on the outer aspects of the myocyte (*circle*)

The cytoplasm appears granular, nuclei are absent and the cells seem to be breaking up. The muscle damage is out of proportion to the inflammatory infiltrate.

The multifocal infiltrate with muscle damage related to a rejection type of inflammatory infiltrate was seen in several areas amounting to grade 2R (1990 grade 3A) rejection. Areas of peritransplant injury could be seen over the levels but they had a different appearance.

Key Points

- Cell-mediated rejection is an immune-mediated inflammation of the myocardium where the immune response primarily targets cardiac myocytes and vascular cells.
- ACR occurs within weeks or months after transplantation and may also recur after many years for a number of reasons which can reduce the immunologic tolerance which has gradually been established.
- The key histologic findings of ACR are myocardial inflammation and myocyte injury.
- An understanding of both the 1990 and 2005 ISHLT grading schemes is required.
- There are three basic grades of rejection: mild, moderate and severe.
- Biopsy adequacy should be assessed as this in fact determines the risk of missing rejection due to sampling error.
- The biopsy should first be examined at low power for features suggestive of rejection then at high power to confirm rejection and grade it accurately.

References

Angelini A, Andersen CB, Bartoloni G, Black F, Bishop P, Doran H, et al. A web-based pilot study of inter-pathologist reproducibility using the ISHLT 2004 working formulation for biopsy diagnosis of cardiac allograft rejection: the European experience. J Heart Lung Transplant. 2011;30(11):1214–20.

Billingham ME. Some recent advances in cardiac pathology. Hum Pathol. 1979;10(4):367–86.

Billingham ME, Cary NR, Hammond ME, Kemnitz J, Marboe C, McCallister HA, et al. A working formulation for the standardization of nomenclature in the diagnosis of heart and lung rejection: Heart Rejection Study Group. The International Society for Heart Transplantation. J Heart Transplant. 1990;9(6):587–93.

Maleszewski JJ, Kucirka LM, Segev DL, Halushka MK. Survey of current practice related to grading of rejection in cardiac transplant recipients in North America. Cardiovasc Pathol. 2011;20(5):261–5.

Michaels PJ, Kobashigawa J, Laks H, Azarbal A, Espejo ML, Chen L, et al. Differential expression of RANTES chemokine, TGF-beta, and leukocyte phenotype in acute cellular rejection and quilty B lesions. J Heart Lung Transplant. 2001;20(4):407–16.

Miller CA, Fildes JE, Ray SG, Doran H, Yonan N, Williams SG, et al. Non-invasive approaches for the diagnosis of acute cardiac allograft rejection. Heart. 2013;99(7):445–53.

Neil D. Transplant pathology. In: Suvarna SK, editor. Cardiac pathology. London: Springer; 2013. p. 163–81.

Sattar HA, Husain AN, Kim AY, Krausz T. The presence of a CD21+ follicular dendritic cell network distinguishes invasive Quilty lesions from cardiac acute cellular rejection. Am J Surg Pathol. 2006;30(8):1008–13.

Sharples LD, Cary NR, Large SR, Wallwork J. Error rates with which endomyocardial biopsy specimens are graded for rejection after cardiac transplantation. Am J Cardiol. 1992;70(4):527–30.

Spiegelhalter DJ, Stovin PG. An analysis of repeated biopsies following cardiac transplantation. Stat Med. 1983;2(1):33–40.

Stewart S, Cary NRB. The pathology of heart and lung transplantation. Curr Diagn Pathol. 1996; 3(2):69–79.

Stewart S, Winters GL, Fishbein MC, Tazelaar HD, Kobashigawa J, Abrams J, et al. Revision of the 1990 working formulation for the standardization of nomenclature in the diagnosis of heart rejection. J Heart Lung Transplant. 2005;24(11):1710–20.

Tan CD, Baldwin III WM, Rodriguez ER. Update on cardiac transplantation pathology. Arch Pathol Lab Med. 2007;131(8):1169–91.

Yang HM, Lai CK, Gjertson DW, Baruch-Oren T, Ra SH, Watts W, et al. Has the 2004 revision of the International Society of Heart and Lung Transplantation grading system improved the reproducibility of the diagnosis and grading of cardiac transplant rejection? Cardiovasc Pathol. 2009;18(4): 198–204.

Pathology of Antibody-Mediated Rejection

14

Samuel Rotman, Dylan V. Miller, Claire Toquet, and Gerald J. Berry

Contents

S. Rotman
Institute of Pathology, University Hospital of Lausanne, Lausanne-CHUV, Switzerland
e-mail: samuel.rotman@chuv.ch

D.V. Miller
Intermountain Central Lab, University of Utah, Salt Lake City, UT, USA
e-mail: Dylan.Miller@imail.org

C. Toquet, MD, PhD (✉)
Department of Pathology, Hôpital Hôtel-Dieu, Nantes, France
e-mail: claire.toquet@chu-nantes.fr; claire.toquet@gmail.com

G.J. Berry
Department of Pathology, Stanford University, Stanford, CA, USA
e-mail: gjberry@stanford.edu

14.1 Background

The concept of cardiac antibody-mediated rejection (AMR) emerged in the late 1980s and early 1990s and was initially termed "acute vascular rejection" or "acute humoral rejection" (Hammond et al. 1989; Ratliff et al. 1995). Clinically, AMR usually presented in the first few weeks after transplantation with allograft

O. Leone et al. (eds.), *The Pathology of Cardiac Transplantation*,
DOI 10.1007/978-3-319-46386-5_14

dysfunction, occurring in close to half of patients in some programs. The primary histopathologic findings consisted of prominent endothelial cells lining the myocardial vessels and/or vasculitis. Immunofluorescence (IF) staining performed on posttransplant EMB revealed immunoglobulin and complement deposition. The constellation of findings was associated with a diminished survival compared to patients with acute cellular rejection (ACR) or mixed ACR and AMR. Subsequent studies showed an association of AMR with the accelerated development of transplant-associated vasculopathy (TAV) of the coronary arteries (Hammond et al. 1992). Reports from other transplant centers identified patients with allograft dysfunction in the absence of ACR, and descriptive terms such as "biopsy-negative rejection" appeared in the literature (Costanzo-Nordin et al. 1993). The members of the 1990 International Society for Heart and Lung Transplantation (ISHLT) Working Formulation Consensus group briefly addressed the concept of AMR indicating the need for additional investigation but did not provide detailed criteria (Billingham et al. 1990). Wider acknowledgment of its existence and its clinical significance for cardiac allograft recipients evolved over the ensuing two and a half decades. AMR was formally recognized by the 2005 ISHLT Working Formulation Consensus group as part of the revision of ISHLT criteria for cardiac allograft rejection (Stewart et al. 2005; Reed et al. 2006), and histopathologic and immunophenotypic criteria were proposed. The characteristic morphologic findings included enlarged, "swollen" interstitial endothelial cells and intravascular aggregates of macrophages within the interstitial capillaries and venules. The key immunopathologic findings by IF were immunoglobulin (IgG, IgM, and/or IgA) and complement degradation product (C3d, C4d, and/or C1q) deposition on the endothelium of the interstitial capillaries. Utilizing an alternative methodology such as formalin-fixed paraffin section immunohistochemistry (IHC) required the demonstration of C4d deposition on the capillary endothelium and the presence of CD68-positive macrophages within the microvasculature. A provisional grading scheme was introduced that was limited to the presence (AMR1) or absence (AMR 0) of antibody-mediated rejection. A definitive diagnosis of AMR required the combination of clinical dysfunction, histopathologic and immunophenotypic findings, and the presence of circulating anti-HLA antibodies. The proposed criteria represented a substantial advancement in the recognition of pathologic components of AMR. However, a number of technical and interpretative issues remained unresolved. Detailed surveys of clinical practices sponsored by the Society of Cardiovascular Pathology (SCVP) and the Association of European Cardiovascular Pathologists (AECVP) highlighted the variability of methodologies, interpretative thresholds, and reporting approaches. Some centers utilized IF, while many others used IHC techniques, and a limited number of centers applied both approaches. Some centers employing frozen section IF applied broad panels of immunoglobulin, complement, and HLA-DR, while others advocated a restricted panel of complement activation markers, C4d and C3d. Centers using the IHC approach reported a variety of antibody panels that included some combination of C4d (with or without C3d) and macrophage markers such as CD68. A number of grading schemes for the distribution and intensity of antibody staining were applied, including adoption of the Banff system for renal transplant rejection, but these generally remained center-specific. The results of the surveys highlighted the lack of uniformity among transplant centers and the difficulty in assessing or comparing the results from different centers (Burke et al. 2010; Kucirka et al. 2011). The findings were discussed at the 10th Banff Allograft Pathology Conference in August 2009. Among the important findings discussed there were the results of a multicenter IHC study of C4d and C3d staining of AMR cases captured in a tissue array sample that demonstrated remarkable reproducibility among centers. At the pathology breakout session of the ISHLT AMR Consensus Conference held in conjunction with the ISHLT 30th Annual Meeting and Scientific Sessions in Chicago, Illinois, in April 2010, the recommendations from the Banff Conference, a detailed literature review and the experience of the transplant pathologists attending the session formed the nidus for technical and interpretative recommendations and a preliminary grading scheme reported in 2011 (Kobashigawa et al. 2011; Berry et al. 2011). Additional work by the working group of pathologists was carried out over the next few years culminating in the 2013 ISHLT Working Formulation for the diagnosis and reporting of cardiac AMR (Berry et al. 2013). While controversies still exist and challenges and unanswered questions remain, AMR is now a fully recognized entity that is defined and classified solely by pathologic findings. A few multicenter cooperative studies are underway, and more are needed to further refine thresholds for therapeutic interventions and better understand its short- and long-term clinical implications.

It should be emphasized that the ISHLT WF is not evidence-based and does not purport to be scientifically definitive of *all* the key pathologic events in AMR. The clinical significance of each pAMR grade has not yet been fully established. The goal of this effort was primarily to establish a framework and basis for characterizing features of AMR that could be more meaningfully and reliably compared between centers and aggregate multicenter research studies. Substantial progress has been made concerning cardiac AMR since the controversial single-center reports 30 years ago. The consensus guideline-defined criteria in the 2013 ISHLT WF attest to this. However, as in the rest of science and medicine, each answered question leads to even more questions to be answered and issues to be resolved. There is still much remaining to be clarified, especially with regard to therapies and long-term consequences of this disease.

14.2 Histopathologic Features of Cardiac AMR

According to the 2013 ISHLT WF, the histopathologic features of AMR on routine hematoxylin- and eosin (H&E)-stained sections reflect interstitial capillary injury with swollen, enlarged, hyperplastic endothelial cells and intravascular macrophages. Since it is often difficult to distinguish endothelial cells from macrophages (both may have oval nuclei with delicate dispersed chromatin) and indeed from other cell types like transformed lymphocytes, the descriptive term "activated mononuclear cells" was proposed to account for this ambiguity (Berry et al. 2013). Having said that, the manifestations of AMR encompass a broad morphologic spectrum ranging from very subtle changes in some cases to florid alterations in others. The salient features are described in detail below.

14.2.1 Intravascular Activated Mononuclear Cells

The normal myocardium is characterized by a rich network of capillaries (lined by endothelial cells) within the interstitial spaces, admixed with occasional interstitial macrophages and T-cells. In the quiescent state the endothelial cells remain barely discernable (Fig. 14.1). However, in AMR the capillaries are usually diffusely and uniformly altered, although occasionally the changes may only be observed in some biopsy pieces and not others or even focally in a given piece. At scanning magnification (×10–20), the interstitial changes generate a "busy" look – the interstitium appears more cellular than normal (Fig. 14.1). High-power magnification (×200–400) confirms that the network of capillaries (and to some extent the associated post-capillary venules) shows enlarged and prominent "swollen" endothelial cells. The nuclei of activated endothelial cells protrude into the lumens, and their cytoplasm creates narrowing of the luminal space sometimes rendering the appearance of luminal obstruction (Fig. 14.1). In advanced stages of activation and injury, endothelial cells may undergo pyknosis and/or karyorrhexis (now reported as severe AMR or pAMR3).

Resident interstitial macrophages can be found in the normal heart in limited numbers,

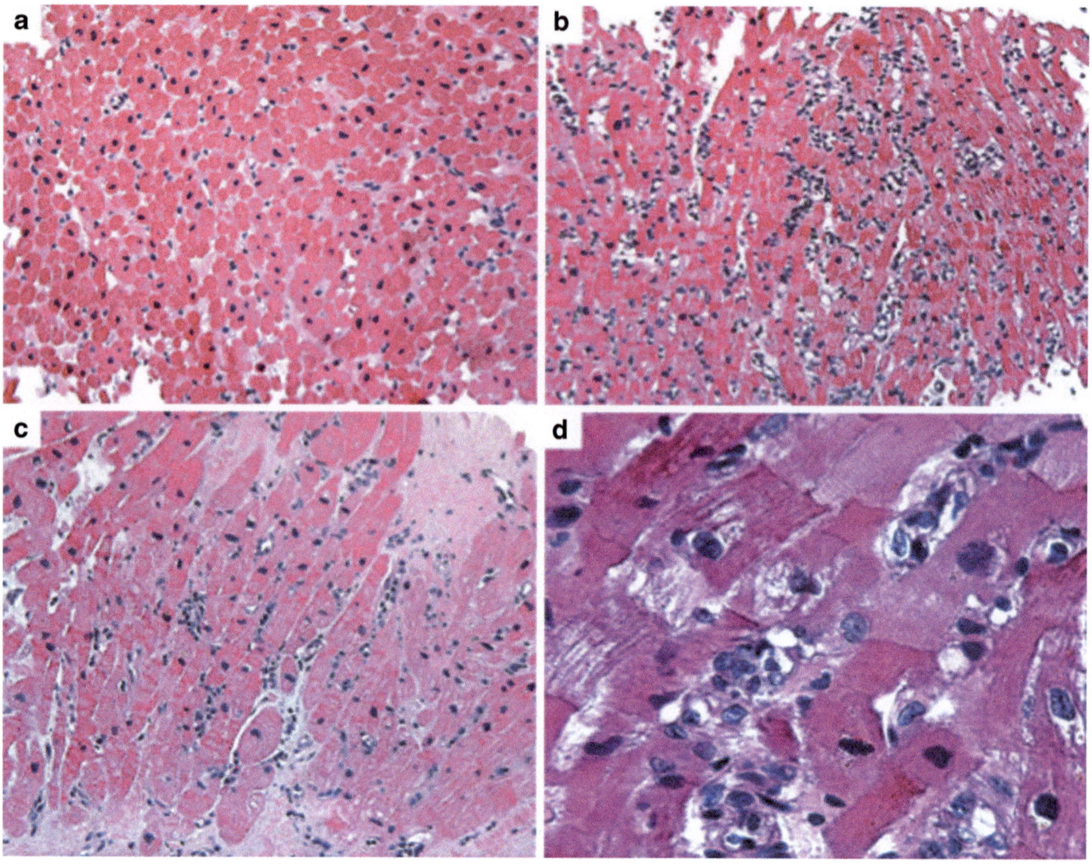

Fig. 14.1 Activated mononuclear cells in AMR. (Panel **a**) Quiescent endomyocardial biopsy showing normal microvasculature without cellular or antibody-mediated rejection (H&E ×250). (Panel **b**) "Busy" appearance of the myocardial interstitium (H&E ×100). (Panel **c**) High-power magnification showing activated mononuclear cells in the interstitial capillaries (H&E ×200). (Panel **d**) Interstitial capillaries are narrowed by plump mononuclear cells that could be swollen endothelial cells, intravascular macrophages, or both (H&E ×400)

but immune mechanisms associated with AMR lead to recruitment of additional monocyte/macrophage lineage cells. The presence of these cells in appreciable numbers within capillaries is another hallmark of AMR (Fig. 14.1). These macrophages may distend and even fill capillary and venular lumens. Mononuclear cells within arterioles and large venules are not taken into account in the evaluation of light microscopy findings according to the ISHLT WF. As mentioned previously, unless completely detached from the vessel wall and demonstrating classic morphologic features of macrophages, they can be difficult to distinguish from endothelial cells (which have similar nuclear size and chromatin pattern) without the assistance of immunophenotypic studies. Indeed in some cases, the number of CD68-positive macrophages highlighted by IHC is unexpected because the macrophages are subtly embedded within capillaries in routine histology (Berry et al. 2013). Intravascular macrophages help contribute to the "busy" appearance of the myocardial interstitium. The relative proportions of hyperplastic endothelial cells and intravascular macrophages may vary from case to case.

Since AMR is a morphologic and immunologic continuum potentially involving several immunological mechanisms, the correlation of intravascular activated mononuclear cells with other morphologic findings (e.g., complement staining by immunopathology) and serum indicators (e.g., circulating DSA by single-antigen bead flow cytometry) can be variable from case to case. In terms of correlating histologic and immunopathologic features of AMR (i.e., using histologic findings to predict immunopathologic findings), Hammond et al. found acceptable specificity, but poor sensitivity for this approach. For biopsies showing endothelial swelling by histology, the sensitivity for predicting positive immunofluorescence was 63 % (specificity 80 %). For biopsies showing intravascular macrophages by histology, the sensitivity was 30 % (specificity 99 %) (Hammond et al. 2005). Fedrigo and colleagues reported that combining both the endothelial and macrophage parameters in C4d + biopsy specimens yielded a sensitivity of 31 %, a specificity of 71 %, and a likelihood ratio of 1.08 (Fedrigo et al. 2013). These studies highlight the limited utility of histologic criteria alone as screening criteria for AMR. An approach incorporating both histopathology and immunopathology is needed for effective AMR screening. If immunopathologic analysis of every biopsy specimen is not practical, the ISHLT WF recommends a screening strategy in the first months after transplantation with periodic monitoring until the 1-year mark. Thereafter, immunopathology may be omitted if histopathologic AMR features are absent (Berry et al. 2011). That said, cases of late AMR are often encountered in clinical practices, and AMR should always be considered in the differential diagnosis of late-onset allograft dysfunction.

Concerning the specificity of intravascular activated mononuclear cells for AMR, it is recognized that endothelial activation and macrophage recruitment can occur in other processes such as ACR, ischemic injury, infection, healing biopsy sites, and at the edges of Quilty lesions. Thus, these findings should always be interpreted in their appropriate context. A threshold of "more than occasional focal aggregates or scattered isolated foci of intravascular activated mononuclear cells" is recommended for assessing histopathologic AMR (Berry et al. 2013). Above this threshold, the finding should trigger immunopathologic consideration for DSA testing.

14.2.2 Interstitial Edema

Edema is defined as the presence of a pale basophilic or occasionally eosinophilic extracellular matrix in perivascular and/or interstitial spaces. It is typically associated with activated intravascular mononuclear cells and rarely, if ever, represents a solitary finding in AMR. The finding of edema may vary from sparse patchy accumulations to prominent widespread collections, especially in cases of more advanced AMR (Fig. 14.2).

Edema should not be confused with artifacts due to technical issues with biopsy processing and histology preparation, which can lead to tissue separation characterized by empty clear spaces between myocytes and around vessels. Edema should be also distinguished from interstitial fibrosis. Noticing the wavy, pale eosinophilic fibrillar character of collagen fibrils on routine histology or confirmation by connective tissue stains, such as Masson or Azan-Mallory trichrome, will avoid confusing subtle fibrosis with edema. Like intravascular mononuclear cells, edema is not specific to AMR. It can be seen in the setting of ischemic and perioperative "harvesting" injury, at the edge of recent biopsy sites, infectious myocarditis, and in advanced ACR.

14.2.3 Inflammation

Mononuclear inflammatory cells other than macrophages may also be conspicuous in some cases of AMR. These are often present in the interstitium and occasionally within vascular lumens. When seen, the possibility of "mixed" rejection (AMR plus definitive features of ACR) should be considered. In the setting of pure AMR, the inflammatory composition can also include scattered neutrophils and eosinophils as well as occasional lymphocytes (especially NK cells). Mixed interstitial inflammation is more prominent in

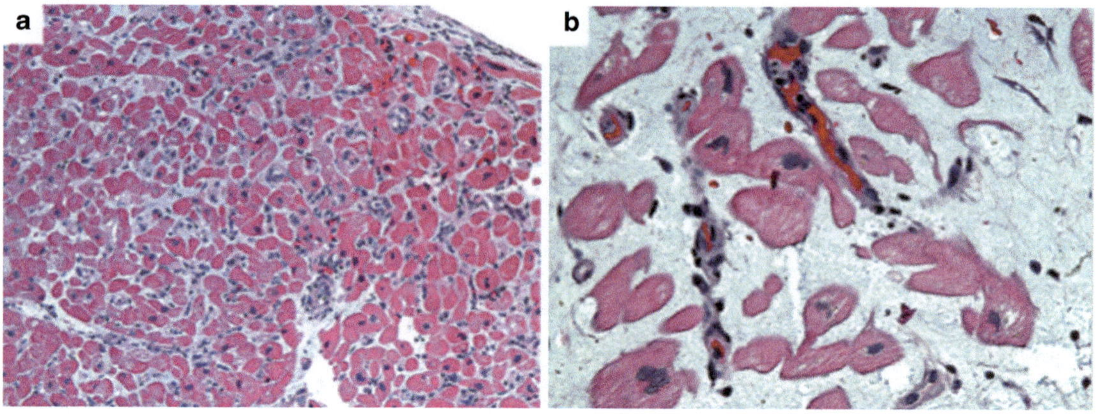

Fig. 14.2 Interstitial edema. (Panel **a**) Mild interstitial edema creating separation of myocytes throughout the sample. Note the pale basophilic appearance of the edema fluid (H&E ×200). (Panel **b**) Marked edema in association with activated mononuclear cells (H&E ×400)

severe AMR, in combination with edema, hemorrhage, endothelial cell pyknosis/karyorrhexis, and myocyte damage (Berry et al. 2013).

14.2.4 Severe AMR (pAMR3)

This form of AMR is now rarely encountered in most clinical practices. The first descriptions of this extreme manifestation of AMR (in the setting of high-titer preformed antibody) arose from cases of hyperacute or otherwise early and overwhelming rejection at time before highly sensitive histocompatibility testing and effective immunosuppressive regimens were available (Kemnitz et al. 1991). These findings were associated with profound allograft dysfunction and poor clinical outcomes. Since this pattern is thought to represent the extreme end of the AMR spectrum, it is designated as severe AMR. In more recent years, severe AMR typically occurs in the setting of a history of presensitization or cessation of immunosuppressive therapy (e.g., noncompliance).

In severe AMR, the capillaries, venules, and small arterioles are distorted, and the lumens appear occluded or severely narrowed by cellular and acellular debris. Degenerated/necrotic endothelial cells with pyknosis and/or karyorrhexis are present as well as necrosis of surrounding myocytes (Fig. 14.3). Inflammatory infiltrates are seen within the lumens and walls of the vessels and in the perivascular spaces. These include intravascular and extravascular macrophages but also neutrophils, eosinophils, and lymphocytes. Platelet-fibrin thrombi may be present. Perivascular and interstitial edema are usually present, and interstitial hemorrhage may be conspicuous (though in biopsies true hemorrhage can be difficult to distinguish from procedure-related extravasation of blood).

14.3 Immunopathology of Cardiac AMR

14.3.1 Screening Strategies and Technical Aspects

Although AMR occurs more frequently during the first year following transplantation (Yerly et al. 2015), late AMR can also occur. Careful histopathologic screening of each biopsy sample is imperative, and there is a strong recommendation for serial immunopathologic testing during this period. Because the levels of complement split products generated from AMR may fluctuate over time, serial assessment at various time points after transplantation has been recommended in the 2013 ISHLT WF. Except in highly sensitized patients deemed at extreme risk for early AMR, the first

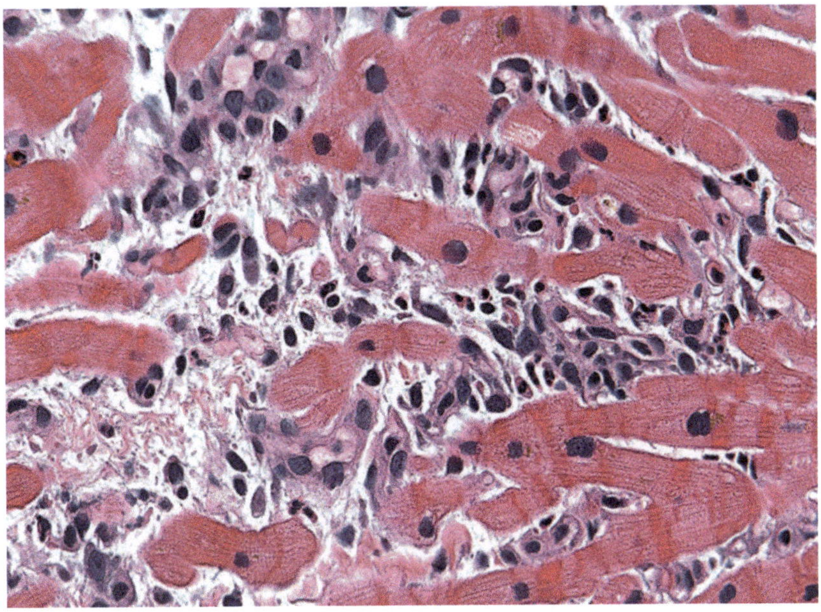

Fig. 14.3 Histopathology of severe AMR. High-power magnification showing mixed inflammatory cell infiltrates, pyknotic debris, activated mononuclear cells, edema, and patchy myocyte damage (H&E ×400)

immunopathologic study is initiated at 2 weeks to allow resolution of ischemic and other perioperative forms of injury. The protocol mirrors the clinical recommendations for DSA testing with immunopathologic studies at 2 and 4 weeks and then testing at 3, 6, and 12 months (Kobashigawa et al. 2011). Modifications by individual centers could reflect research protocols, at-risk patient populations, and financial or other considerations.

Two immunopathologic techniques are generally used in the laboratory: immunohistochemistry (IHC) performed on formalin-fixed paraffin-embedded tissue and immunofluorescence (IF) on snap-frozen fresh tissue samples. Since the reagent antibody clones differ between these methods and antigen retrieval steps to disrupt formalin-generated peptide cross-links are required for IHC (but not IF), there is a theoretic basis for differing sensitivity and specificity for each approach. Despite this, both techniques seem to be highly comparable when the assay parameters are optimized and run with appropriate controls (Miller et al. 2010). In most centers IHC is performed by automated staining techniques. The IF method requires enhanced logistical organization, in terms of obtaining an extra biopsy piece, transporting fresh tissue in saline or other media like Zeus (avoiding formalin fixation of the biopsy sample), and the need for cryostat microtomes, fluorescence-capable microscopes, and experienced technicians.

Antibodies to several different proteins of interest are used in both IHC and IF techniques to identify the immunopathologic features of AMR (principally complement deposition by both IHC and IF and intravascular macrophages by IHC). Several different sources are commercially available. It should also be noted that at present there are some proteins that are optimally assessed by only one of the techniques. The prognostic and predictive experience with C3d is currently limited to IF, as there were no IHC clones commercially available until recently. Conversely, CD68 immunostaining is currently restricted to IHC methods. Regardless of the specific clone chosen, it should always be optimized and validated thoroughly before clinical use against appropriate control tissues (*both known positive and negative samples*) in each immunopathology laboratory. Partnering with another laboratory that has

Table 14.1 Recommended and optional antibody panels

	Primary or mandatory panel	Secondary or optional panel
Paraffin section immunohistochemistry	C4d and CD68	CD3, CD20, C3d, CD31, CD34, complement regulators
Frozen section immunofluorescence	C4d, C3d HLA-DR (to assess vascular integrity as needed)	Fibrin, immunoglobulins

Table 14.2 Interpretive criteria for IHC

	Scoring system	Result/interpretation
Capillary C4d distribution:	0: < 10 % negative 1: 10–50 % "focal" staining 2: > 50 % "multifocal or diffuse" staining	Negative: 0, 1 Positive: 2 (assuming intensity is at least weak positive)
Capillary C4d intensity	0: negative/equivocal 1: faint positive staining 2: strong positive staining	Negative: 0 Positive: 1, 2
Intravascular CD68 macrophage distribution	0: < 10 % negative 1: 10–50 % "focal" macrophages 2: > 50 % "multifocal or diffuse" macrophages	Negative: 0 Positive: 1, 2 (intensity irrelevant for CD68)

already validated a particular antibody is helpful in this endeavor. Importantly, positive and negative control slides should always be generated daily and negative control slides prepared with each case.

The 2013 ISHLT WF provides careful interpretative guidelines for histopathologic and immunopathologic criteria. That said, there is always concern for possible interpretative variability by pathologists and the need for optimizing standardization in this regard. In developing the diagnostic criteria, the 2013 ISHLT WF incorporated the results of a reproducibility exercise utilizing a survey of 25 cases with both histopathology and immunostains (Berry et al. 2013). The interpretative recommendations are summarized in Tables 14.1, 14.2, and 14.3 and will be discussed in detail.

14.3.2 Antibody Panels for Immunopathology

The 2005 ISHLT WF was not prescriptive as to panels and interpretive criteria for immunopathology. Evidence supporting the recommendations were (and to extent some still are) lacking. In the 1980s some centers adopted an IF approach similar to renal biopsy immunopathology (IgG, IgM, C3, etc.). After reports of C4d in AMR emerged in the renal literature in the 1990s, centers began using C4d (by IF or IHC). Some began to include CD68 in their diagnostic panel as well. Correlation with other signs of AMR emerged as well as an impact of graft outcomes, but these studies varied widely with respect to antibodies selection, techniques, and interpretive criteria. The 2013 ISHLT WF elucidates a standardized approach based on available published evidence and expert recommendations.

Both primary and secondary panels were proposed for each modality. For IHC, the recommended primary panel includes C4d and CD68. For IF the recommended stains are C4d and C3d (Table 14.1).

14.3.3 Anticomplement Antibody C4d (IF and IHC)

The assessment of C4d staining by IHC or IF is often challenging, and there are potential pitfalls

Table 14.3 Interpretive criteria for IF

	Scoring system	Result/interpretation
Capillary C4d or C3d distribution:	0: < 10 % negative 1: 10–50 % "focal" staining 2: > 50 % "multifocal or diffuse" staining	Negative: 0, 1 Positive: 2 (assuming intensity is at least faint positive)
Capillary C4d or C3d intensity	0: negative/equivocal 1: faint or trace positive staining 2: strong positive staining	Negative: 0 Positive: 1, 2

that can lead to either overinterpretation or underinterpretation of the findings. The 2013 ISHLT WF specifies that only staining of interstitial capillaries should be considered in the evaluation. Staining of the venules, arterioles, arteries, elastic tissue, and vessels associated with Quilty lesions, scars, or necrotic/ischemic areas should not be considered the in diagnostic interpretation of AMR but instead serve as useful internal controls for the technical quality of the stain (Berry et al. 2013). A positive C4d staining pattern is defined as linear endothelial staining producing a "donut" pattern in cross-sectional vessels and an "elliptical" pattern in vessels arranged in longitudinal alignment (Fig. 14.4).

The spectrum of C4d staining intensity and the distribution can be considerable from case to case. This is especially true for IHC techniques compared to IF techniques. IHC stains also frequently show artifactual serum staining within capillary lumens and incomplete granular staining of the endothelium, resulting from fixation of congealed serum (which contains complement factors) to the capillary wall during tissue fixation and processing (Fig. 14.5). This artifact can be distinguished from true C4d staining by its asymmetric and non-circumferential disposition in a vessel. Serum artifactual staining is less commonly encountered in IF staining.

C4d evaluation criteria are described in Tables 14.2 (IHC) and 14.3 (IF).

The *distribution* of C4d staining is reported as follows:

- <10 %: no staining
- 10–50 %: focal staining
- >50 %: multifocal/diffuse staining

The *intensity* of the staining is usually graded from 0 to 2 as follows:

- 0: negative/equivocal staining.
- 1 (faint/weak): not readily appreciated on low magnification but discernible as distinct, although still weak in intensity and on medium- and high-power magnification.
- 2 (strong): capillary structures are delineated even on low-power magnification.

Moderate intensity may also be seen as staining readily appreciated on low magnification and more intense on medium and high-power magnification.

A *positive C4d staining result* is defined in the 2013 ISHLT WF as multifocal/diffuse (>50 %) capillary staining of weak or strong intensity of the interstitial capillaries evaluated in intact myocardium.

A more limited *distribution* (focal, <50 %) is considered technically negative but warrants communication with clinicians because of the possibility of an incipient, evolving, or resolving episode of AMR. In cases of severe AMR (pAMR 3) or following repeated episodes of AMR, the loss of endothelial integrity may alter C4d deposition, and the assessment of microvasculature with vascular markers such as CD31 or CD34 (part of the optional panel for IHC) may be useful. Weak staining may also warrant direct communication to correlate with the clinical picture and guide appropriate clinical studies and follow-up. Neither weak nor focal staining has been studied extensively and needs further experience and outcome studies before a clearer recommendation can be made. False-negative staining outcomes are also a concern and should be assessed

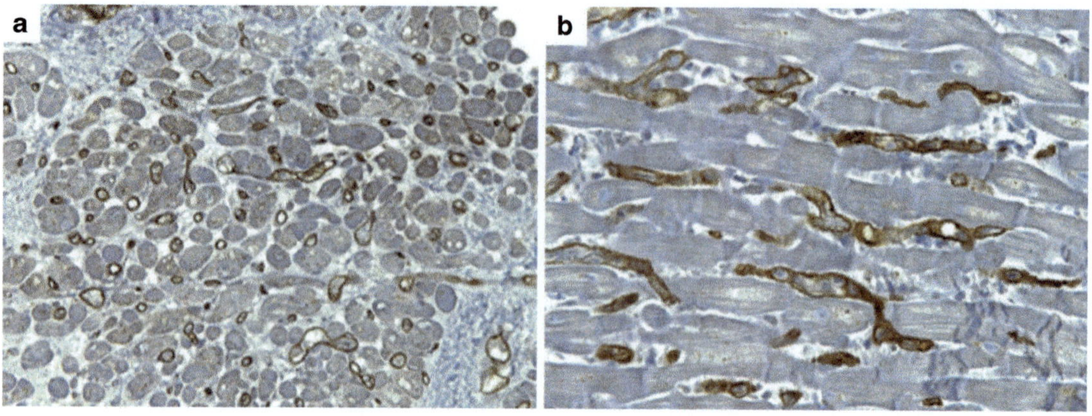

Fig. 14.4 C4d staining profiles by IHC. (Panel **a**) Interstitial capillary captures in cross section show round-to-"doughnut" staining. Note the continuous linear staining pattern in each vessel (×200). (Panel **b**) In longitudinal plane, the outline of the capillaries, including branching points, is readily observed (×400)

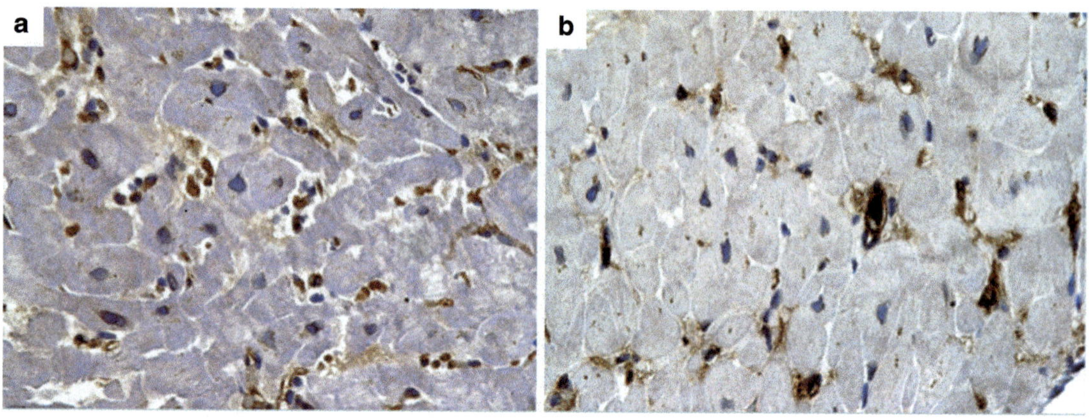

Fig. 14.5 Artifactual C4d staining patterns. (Panel **a**) Luminal clumps of serum throughout the microvasculature (×400). (Panel **b**) In addition to serum staining, there is patchy incomplete endothelial staining indicative of artifactual effect (×400)

by regularly reviewing batch controls and daily positive and negative controls.

14.3.4 Macrophage Antibody CD68 (IHC)

One of the earliest and most reliable histologic observations in AMR was the accumulation of macrophages within capillaries and small venules (Lones et al. 1995; Ratliff et al. 1995). As discussed previously intravascular macrophages cannot always be reliably differentiated from swollen endothelial cells. Staining for macrophage antigen CD68 was adopted by some centers and endorsed (along with C4d) in the 2005 ISHLT WF (Stewart et al. 2005). CD68 staining is part of the 2013 ISHLT WF primary panel for IHC.

Because a small number of resident macrophages and circulating monocytes can be present in the heart in the absence of rejection, quantitative criteria were needed for the number and distribution of macrophages seen by CD68 staining. The 2013 ISHLT WF defines convincing positive staining for CD68 as a chain-like, linear, or beading arrangement of macrophages within interstitial capillaries and venules (for vessels aligned in longitudinal orientation) and clusters or beading within lumens (for vessels observed in cross section) (Fig. 14.6).

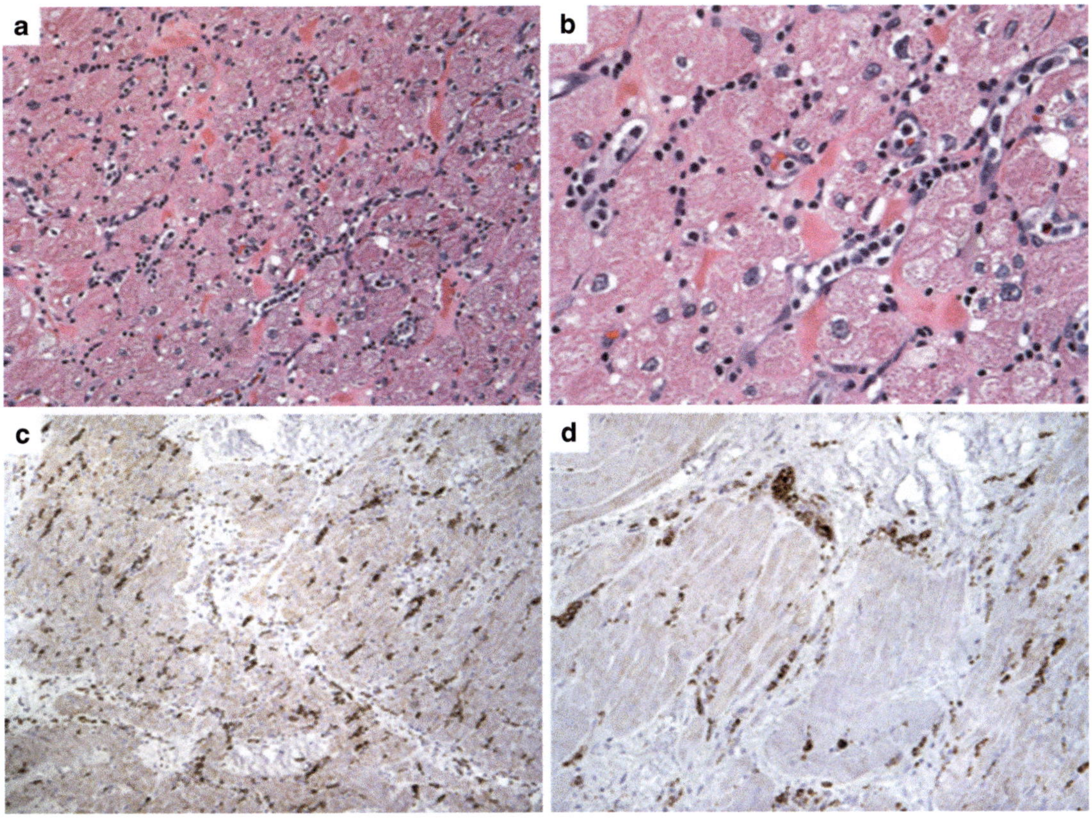

Fig. 14.6 Intravascular macrophages and CD68 staining patterns. (Panel **a**) Scanning magnification showing numerous intravascular cells creating a busy pattern of activated mononuclear cells (H&E ×200). (Panel **b**) At high-power magnification, the linear arrangement of intravascular macrophages is confirmed (H&E ×400). (Panel **c**) Low-power CD68 staining by IHC shows linear, bead-like profiles throughout the biopsy (×100). (Panel **d**) CD68 staining at higher magnification shows intravascular localization within capillaries and venules of macrophages (×200)

The *distribution* of CD68+ macrophages, similar to C4d, is graded semiquantitatively according to percent involvement of the intact biopsy surface area (Table 14.2). Focal staining is defined as prominent intravascular staining in 10–50 % of the area, less than that is considered negative and more than that is considered multifocal/diffuse. Intensity of CD68 does not vary appreciably, so it is not a consideration. A positive CD68 staining result is reported when beads or clusters of CD68+ macrophages within interstitial capillaries occupy more than 10 % (focal) of the specimen surface area. It is recognized that this threshold is arbitrary but was selected to emphasize the diagnostic experience that the macrophage distribution in AMR is more than an occasional intravascular presence. Further, its prognostic significance has not yet been established. A negative CD68 staining result is reported when less than (<10 %) of the specimen surface area contains intravascular macrophages as described above. Any equivocal or confusing result should prompt a discussion with the clinical team to generate a plan for current clinicopathologic interpretation and follow-up.

There is ongoing debate whether confirming that intravascular activated mononuclear cells are indeed macrophages holds the same prognostic significance as the demonstration of complement deposition. Since intravascular mononuclear cells can be appreciated on light microscopy, but complement activation cannot, some consider the ISHLT WF grading criteria that allow intravascular activated mononuclear cells and positive

CD68 immunopathology as separate factors to be "double counting" the same biologic phenomenon. The rationale for this, ostensibly, is that the additive value and specificity of CD68 justify separate scoring since in some cases intravascular macrophages may be present in significant numbers but not readily apparent on H&E sections. Furthermore, distinguishing interstitial versus intravascular macrophages is aided considerably by CD68. In fact, toggling slides under the microscope between the H&E and CD68 can be very helpful in localizing macrophages, and there are often more CD68-positive cells than expected when a careful comparison is made.

A recent study provided some reassurance as to the validity of CD68 staining. Fedrigo and colleagues correlated C4d and CD68 staining in serial transplant biopsies and found that early after transplantation intravascular macrophages predict capillary C4d deposition, circulating DSAs, and clinical symptoms (Fedrigo et al. 2013). Interestingly, the correlation and predictive ability diminished later in the posttransplant course.

Lastly, the significance of CD68+ intravascular macrophages in the absence of morphologic features (pAMR1-I+) is unknown, but this pattern is less frequent and warrants follow-up clinical and serologic evaluation and continued immunostaining of subsequent cardiac specimens.

14.3.5 Anticomplement Antibody C3d

Staining for complement component C3d is not widely used in practice currently but is gaining implementation. Technically, the C3d immunostaining by paraffin section IHC commonly produces extensive nonspecific background that renders interpretation and staining assessment unreliable. For this reason, its use has been largely restricted to frozen tissue IF, and published clinical correlation experience is limited to a few centers (Moseley et al. 2010; Tan et al. 2009). Tan and colleagues have reported that there is diminished overall survival in patients with clinical dysfunction, positive DSA, and both C3d and C4d deposition. This suggests that progression down the complement cascade was not impeded by complement regulators after C4 cleavage (which precedes C3 cleavage) and likely resulted in membrane attack complex formation and cell damage.

For IHC methods, the 2013 ISHLT WF currently places C3d in the secondary/optional panel group, pending further experience by transplant centers. A recommendation was made to each center that was interested in elaborating the potential diagnostic and prognostic utility of C3d by IHC to optimize their protocols and evaluate results in structured scientific studies. For centers utilizing the IF technique, C3d is listed in the primary panel of antibody selection. The diagnostic criteria for staining intensity and distribution are similar to the C4d thresholds for both IHC and IF (Fig. 14.7).

14.3.6 HLA-DR

HLA-DR is part of the primary recommended IF panel in the 2013 ISHLT WF. HLA-DR is constitutively expressed by myocardial capillary endothelial cells in cardiac allografts. As such, this stain aids in assessing capillary integrity, particularly in the setting of recurrent AMR episodes and in severe AMR, and is comparable to vascular markers, CD31 and CD34 by IHC. The distribution and intensity of staining are less important than the morphologic appearance of capillaries at higher magnification. Crisp linear staining is seen in intact vessels. In the setting of capillary injury, the staining pattern appears frayed and feathered around the capillary circumference (Fig. 14.8). In our experience toggling between C4d/C3d and HLA-DR-stained slides aids in this assessment.

14.3.7 Fibrin

The antibody against fibrin is included in the secondary/optional panel for IF. In severe AMR, endothelial cell injury activates the coagulation

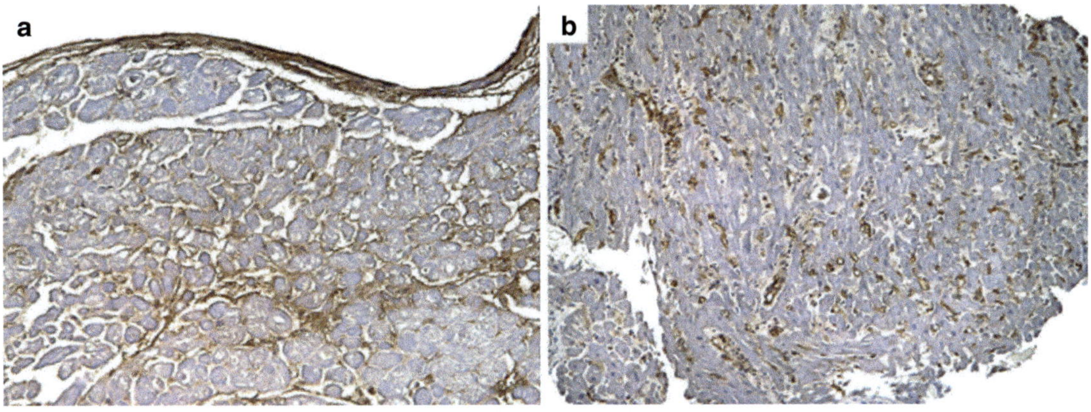

Fig. 14.7 C3d staining profiles by IHC. (Panel **a**) The typical artifactual background staining that is observed on most cases of C3d-stained slides (×200). (Panel **b**) Positive C3d staining showing strong diffuse staining of the interstitial capillaries. C4d was also positive in this case (×125)

system, which leads to the generation of fibrin with or without occlusive thrombi formation. Although fibrin may be observed on H&E slides when there are occlusive microthrombi, the small caliber of capillaries and transient nature of thrombi due to serum plasminogen and other thrombolytic factors complicate the diagnostic assessment. Fibrin staining by IF is technically difficult and challenging to interpret. When convincingly positive, the pattern appears as diffuse flare-like radiations emanating from the capillaries. This likely represents increased capillary permeability and leakage of fibrin into the interstitium. Its presence signifies (and correlates with) more severe AMR episodes, but fibrin staining can also be seen in capillary injury from other causes.

14.3.8 Immunoglobulin Antibodies

The morphological alterations of AMR reflect the interaction of antibodies with endothelial cells, so staining to detect immunoglobulins seems intuitive. However, unlike the covalent linking to endothelial surface molecules that occurs with C4d, immunoglobulin binding to endothelium is weaker and more transient. Routine staining for immunoglobulin heavy and light chains is rarely positive, even when complement fixation can be demonstrated (Rodriguez et al. 2005). Positive immunoglobulin staining may occur in the absence of AMR, such as in perioperative ischemic injury and in patients treated by OKT3 antibody. Nevertheless, staining for IgG and IgM remains part of the routine panel at some institutions. IF staining for immunoglobulin is classified in the secondary/optional panel in the 2013 ISHT WF.

14.3.9 Anticomplement Antibodies C1q/C3c

C1q deposition is a feature of complement activation along the classical pathway. Some studies have evaluated C1q and/or C3c deposition in screening for AMR, but these complement split products, like the immunoglobulin components, are not covalently bound to endothelial cells and are considered not reliable for the IF diagnosis of AMR.

14.4 Pathologic Grading and Reporting of Cardiac AMR

As previously mentioned, the 2013 ISHLT WF states that diagnosis of AMR is rendered by pathologists separately from clinical parameters and DSAs. AMR is reported as "pathologic AMR or pAMR" and graded on the basis of a combina-

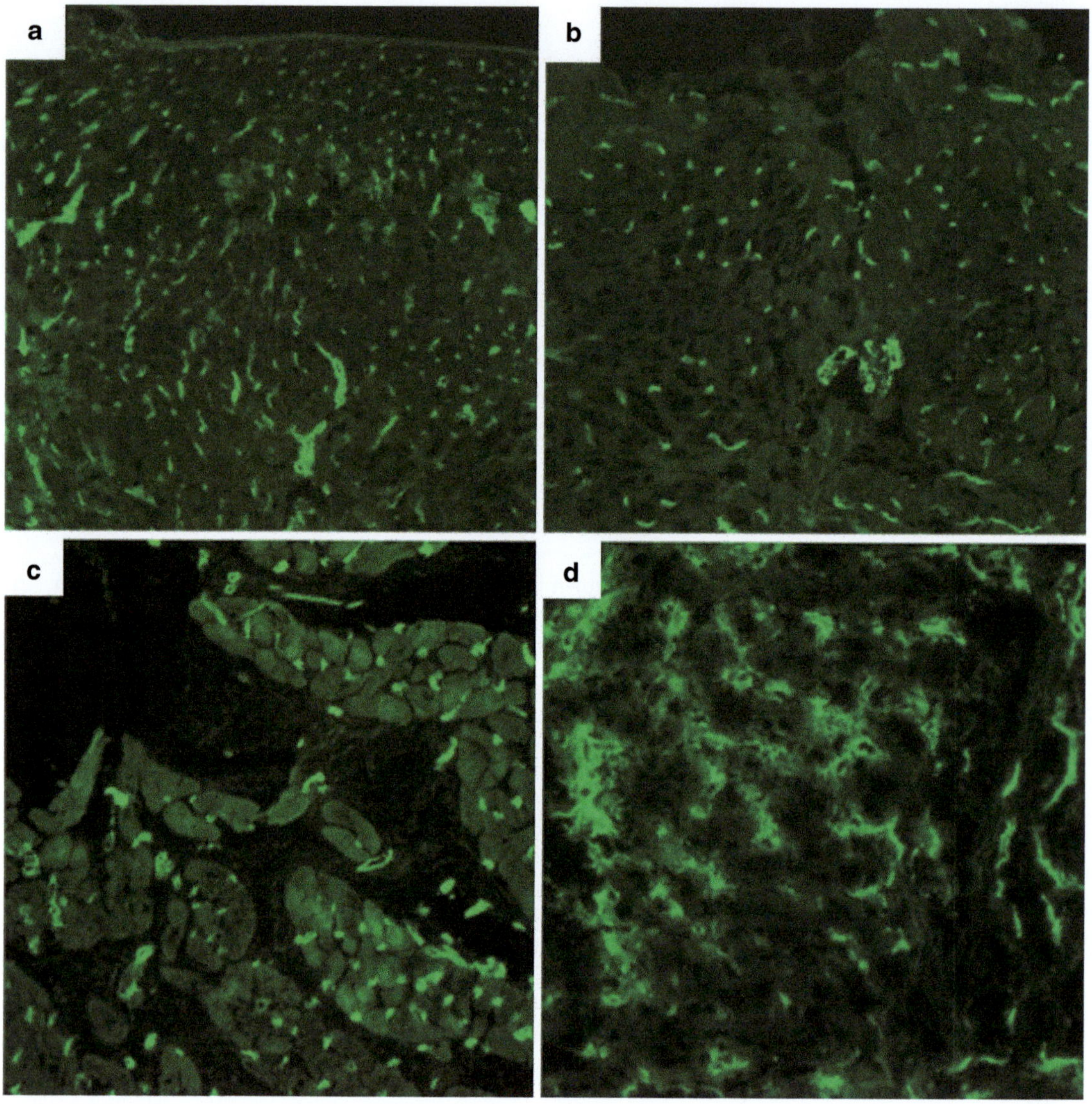

Fig. 14.8 C4d, C3d, and HLA-DR staining profiles by IF. (Panel **a**) Positive C4d staining showing strong diffuse 3+ staining throughout the microvasculature (×200). (Panel **b**) A similar staining pattern for C3d with diffuse 2+ staining intensity (×200). (Panel **c**) The normal staining pattern for HLA-DR showing crisp outlines of the capillaries throughout the biopsy (×200). (Panel **d**) HLA-DR staining displaying frayed, inhomogeneous staining of damaged capillaries following repeated episodes of AMR (×200)

tion of histopathologic and immunopathologic findings as outlined in Table 14.4.

Obviously, pAMR is only one of the factors in the expression of humoral activation, and it should be incorporated in the overall clinical situation (i.e., clinical dysfunction as well as the presence of DSAs) in order to reach therapeutic decisions.

14.5 Controversies and Challenges in Cardiac AMR

The 2013 ISHLT Working Formulation (and its preliminary version in 2011) has now been utilized by cardiac pathologists for a few years. Although one of the recommendations of the

Table 14.4 ISHLT Working Formulation for cardiac antibody-mediated rejection

Grade	Definition	Substrates
pAMR 0	Negative for pathologic AMR	Both histologic and immunopathologic findings negative
pAMR 1: indicative of possible pathologic AMR		
pAMR 1 (H+)	Histopathologic AMR alone	Histologic findings present and immunopathologic findings negative
pAMR 1 (I+)	Immunopathologic AMR alone	Histologic findings negative and immunopathologic findings positive (CD68+ and/or C4d+)
pAMR 2	Pathologic AMR	Both histologic *and* immunopathologic findings present
pAMR 3	Severe pathologic AMR	Interstitial hemorrhage, capillary fragmentation, mixed inflammatory infiltrates, endothelial cell pyknosis and/or karyorrhexis, and marked edema + positive IHC/IF

working group was the request for periodic reassessment of the scheme to examine areas of successful application and deficiencies, it seems prudent to highlight specific areas of controversy and potential difficulty. Some of these reflect technical issues, while others center on interpretative areas and problems that should be evaluated by single-center or multicenter studies. A number of issues have already been addressed in the discussion of individual components of the pathologic evaluation of AMR, but key aspects will be now highlighted.

14.5.1 Mononuclear Cells: What Is Activated? Distinguishing Interstitial from Intravascular Cells

After assessing specimen adequacy, most pathologists proceed to evaluate the endomyocardial biopsy for the presence or absence of ACR. This presumes an appreciation for the "normal" or quiescent myocardium. In adults this is usually straightforward, but pediatric endomyocardial biopsies can be more challenging. The relative size and number of myocyte nuclei imparts a "more cellular" appearance of the myocardium (Fig. 14.9). The interstitium should be carefully assessed at scanning and high-power magnification to evaluate the microvasculature and the presence or absence of increased cellularity. Familiarity with the range of normal changes in the pediatric biopsy is essential to avoid the mistake of overestimating the presence of activated mononuclear cells. Activated mononuclear cells whether they are macrophages and/or swollen endothelial cells produce the appearance of luminal narrowing at high-power magnification.

The primary morphologic finding that should raise consideration for the possibility of AMR is the presence of activated mononuclear cells. As previously discussed, the distinctions of intravascular from interstitial localization and macrophage versus other types of inflammatory cell or endothelial cells can be challenging in some cases. The problem of localization can usually be resolved by IHC. We find that the combination of CD31 (vascular marker), CD68, and a pan-T-cell marker such as CD3 is helpful to distinguish the different cell types. At scanning magnification diffuse mild ACR imparts a "busy" appearance in the myocardial interstitium and can mimic AMR. CD3 can also provide immunophenotypic support for the morphologic impression of mixed diffuse mild ACR and AMR in cases of mixed rejection. Intravascular T-cells are usually sparse or limited to occasional collections. Transformed large lymphocytes and immunoblasts can be difficult to distinguish from macrophages or hyperplastic endothelial cells, and IHC can resolve this problem.

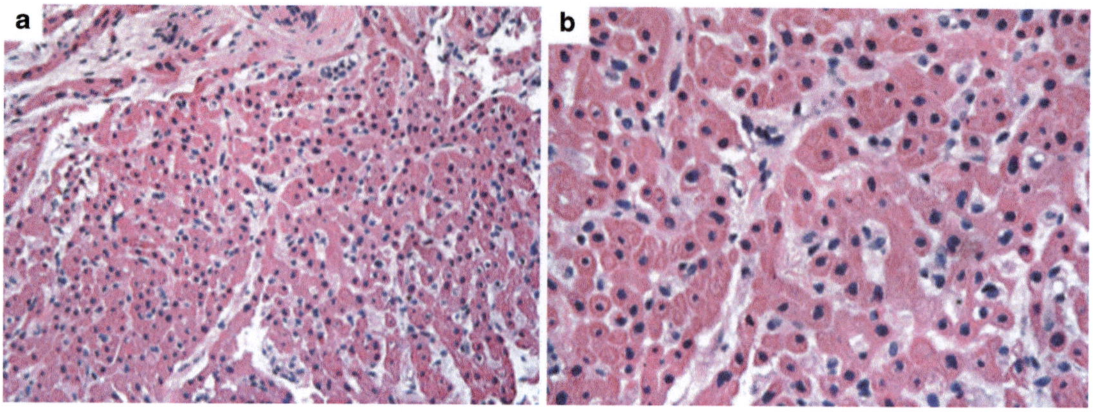

Fig. 14.9 Normal pediatric endomyocardial biopsy. (Panel **a**) Scanning power magnification of a quiescent biopsy in a 3-year-old child after transplant. The biopsy has distinctive features from an adult endomyocardial biopsy (H&E ×200). (Panel **b**) High-power magnification of the same biopsy showing plump myocyte nuclei but indiscernible endothelial cells (H&E ×400)

It should be emphasized that "activated mononuclear cells" can be seen in a variety of settings other than AMR. In general these patterns tend to be focal in distribution rather than the diffuse arrangement of AMR. Ischemic injury, whether found early after transplant on account of ischemic/reperfusion injury or late onset due to TAV, produces focal zones of endothelial swelling, myocyte damage, and limited mixed inflammatory infiltrates. Likewise, the leading edge of a Quilty B lesion can produce reactive changes in the microvasculature. Attention to the focality of the changes, timing of the biopsy, and other findings will resolve the majority of cases; IHC can be useful in the remainder.

A more vexing dilemma for pathologists is the localization of macrophages. The distinction of interstitial from intravascular locales, whether by H&E or CD68 staining, requires an accumulated experience and patience. Careful toggling between the H&E and CD68 stain is very helpful in our experience. The CD68 stain accentuates the intravascular macrophages as linear streaks at scanning magnification. At high-power magnification, expansion of the luminal spaces and the clustering effect of the macrophages provide support for intravascular distribution (Fig. 14.6).

Combined CD31 (or CD34) and CD68 IHC staining may be helpful to identify the intravascular versus extravascular localization of macrophages.

14.5.2 Mixed Cellular and Antibody-Mediated Rejection

Mixed ACR and AMR as defined by the 2013 ISHLT WF requires the presence of mononuclear cell infiltrates of ACR together with the histopathologic and/or immunophenotypic findings of AMR in a biopsy specimen. In our experience concurrent mild ACR (often diffuse mild rejection/Grade 1B in 1990 ISHLT grading scheme) and AMR are not uncommon (Fig. 14.10). Less frequently we encounter moderate or severe ACR and AMR (Fig. 14.11). Each component should be evaluated and graded separately according to ISHLT criteria. We use CD3 staining to confirm the presence of T-cells in the sample but not to screen for or grade the ACR component. Further, the attendant mimics for each type of rejection such as Quilty effect or ischemia should be carefully evaluated before establishing the diagnosis. The clinical significance and treatment aspects of mixed ACR and AMR are not yet fully elucidated. Therapeutic intervention is initiated for the treatable grades of ACR (moderate and severe ACR). In some centers, the decision to treat AMR is reconsidered following the resolution of the

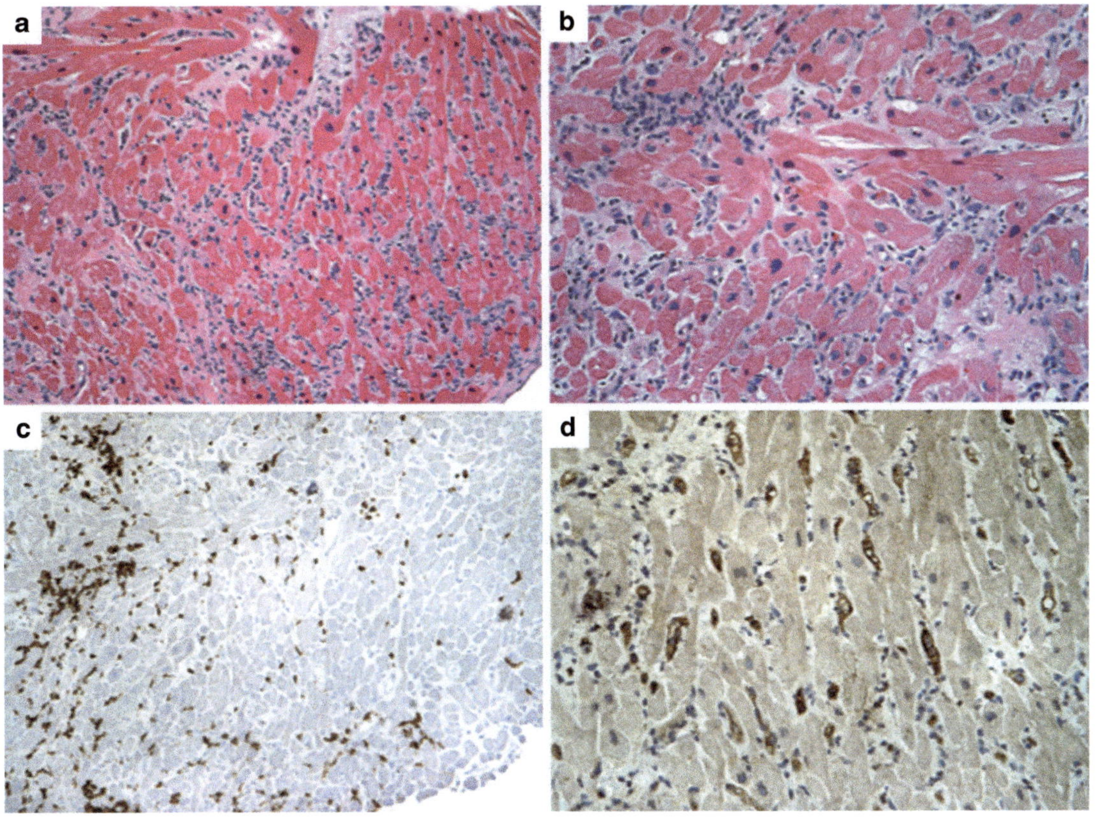

Fig. 14.10 Mixed mild acute cellular rejection and AMR. (Panel **a**) The endomyocardial biopsy shows cellular infiltrates at low-power magnification (H&E ×125). (Panel **b**) At higher magnification both interstitial and activated mononuclear cells are appreciated (H&E ×200). (Panel **c**) CD3 confirms the morphologic impression of mild ACR (×125). (Panel **d**) C4d staining of the same piece shows positive C4d staining (×200)

ACR episode. The prognostic significance of mixed ACR and AMR compared to ACR or AMR alone has not been widely studied. Kfoury and colleagues reported that patients with clinically stable mixed ACR and AMR developed greater cardiovascular mortality such as sudden cardiac death, TAV, heart failure, or cardiogenic shock compared to patients with stable ACR (Kfoury et al. 2009). At this time, the full clinical impact of mixed rejection remains unknown. The diagnostic and prognostic roles of myocardial inflammatory burden and microvascular injury have only recently been addressed (Tavora et al. 2011; Fedrigo et al. 2015). We need to further understand the impact the different cellular constituents and their localization before we can reliably determine if ACR and AMR truly represent separate or intertwined immunologic processes.

This topic is examined in detail in Chap. 15.

14.5.3 C4d: Technical and Interpretative Issues

In the majority of cases, the interpretation of C4d staining is generally straightforward. The presence of weak or strong multifocal or diffuse staining constituents a positive finding, and the staining profile of interstitial capillaries should be "linear endothelial staining producing a "donut" or "elliptical" pattern" (Berry et al. 2013). That said, there are a number of C4d staining results that are encountered that are either mimics of endothelial staining or patterns that are of uncertain significance at this time. These include serum staining that is characterized as

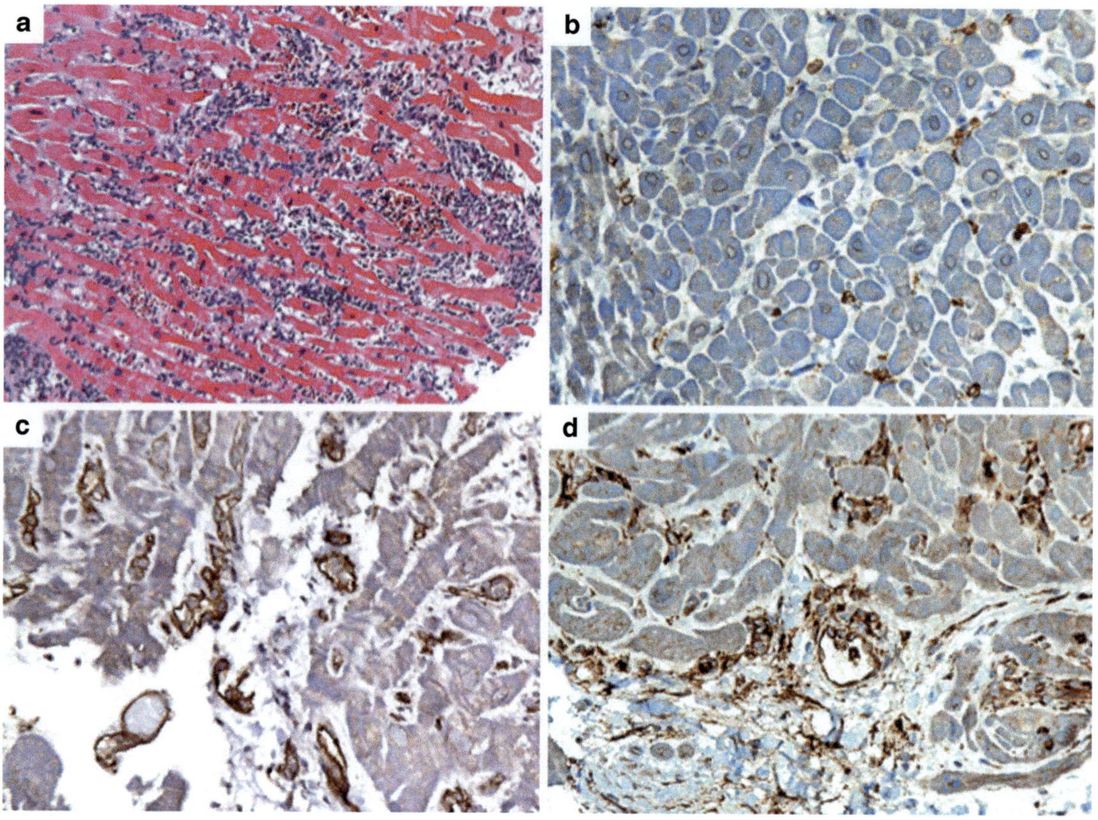

Fig. 14.11 Mixed moderate acute cellular rejection and AMR. (Panel **a**) Dense mononuclear inflammatory cell infiltrates are observed at low-power magnification, and myocyte damage is present suggesting a high-grade ACR (H&E ×200). (Panel **b**) CD3 stains some T-cells in this focus, but the staining was variable in the sample (×400). (Panel **c**) Strong C4d staining of the microvasculature (×400). (Panel **d**) CD68 showing intravascular and interstitial macrophages (×400)

partial or complete luminal aggregates of C4d immunoreactivity or incomplete, granular rather than ringlike endothelial staining of capillaries, venules, or arterioles (Fig. 14.5).

Another pattern that has been described in the IF literature and occasionally encountered in IHC staining is the fine, perimyocytic staining of some or all the myocytes in the biopsy specimen (Fig. 14.12). Following an episode of AMR, it could reflect endothelial injury and seepage of complement from the intravascular to interstitial spaces. The clinical significance in IHC is unknown, and careful attention to the positive and negative controls is recommended to ensure that the antibody titers are accurate. If persistent we recommend both careful clinical evaluation including DSA testing and re-titering of the antibody. Necrotic myocyte fibers will stain strongly against C4d: this artifactual result is observed in ischemic/reperfusion injury early after transplant (Fig. 14.13).

Perhaps the most challenging problem that pathologists encounter in the evaluation of C4d staining is the recognition of diffuse weak endothelial staining. In our experience, this distinction from artifactual serum staining of the microvasculature poses an important decision point: the classification of pAMR 0 versus pAMR 1-I+. Helpful clues include the presence of serum staining and irregular, granular endothelial

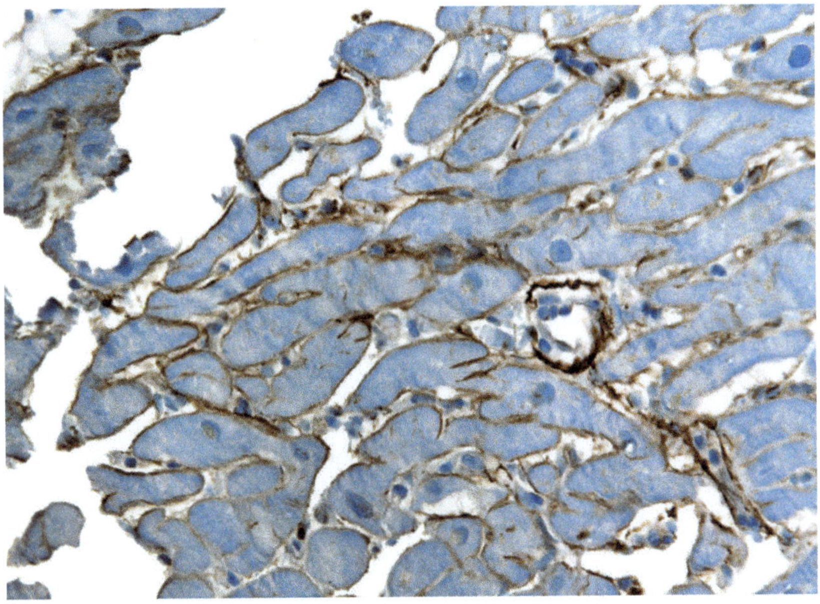

Fig. 14.12 Perimyocytic C4d staining by IHC. The significance of sarcolemmal staining of myocytes by IHC is unknown. Possible explanations are leaking capillaries in the setting of microvascular injury or nonspecific staining artifact (×400)

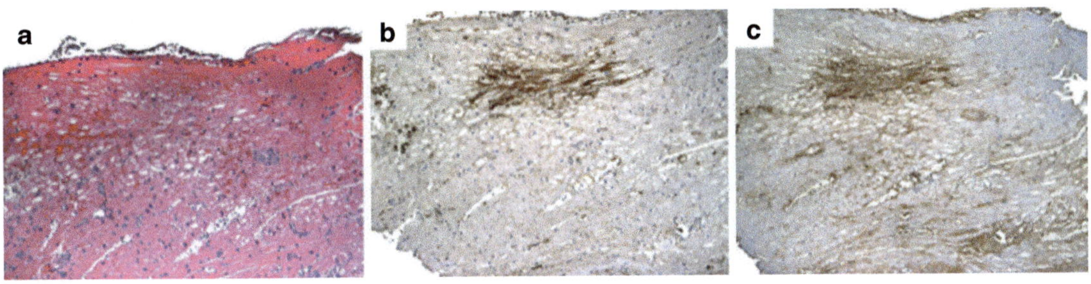

Fig. 14.13 C4d and C3d staining of necrotic myocytes. (Panel **a**) H&E stain showing subendocardial vacuolization and hypereosinophilic necrotic myocytes (H&E ×100). (Panel **b**) C4d stain highlights the necrotic fibers but is of no clinical significance (×100). (Panel **c**) A similar staining profile is observed with C3d (×100)

staining in artifactual C4d staining compared to the linear, uniform staining of C4d in AMR. Attention to both the external control stained slides and internal controls such as C4d staining of larger vessels also helps resolve difficult cases. We report equivocal or unresolvable cases as equivocal in the pathology report and communicate the diagnostic difficulty with our clinical colleagues and classify the pattern as pAMR 0. IHC staining is repeated on the subsequent endomyocardial biopsy.

14.5.4 How Quickly Do C4d and C3d Disappear After Treatment?

The resolution of an AMR episode requires the restitution of normal myocardial morphology and the elimination of antibody deposition and/or intravascular CD68+ macrophages. The recommendation of the 2013 ISHLT WF is to continue immunostaining until this occurs. The challenge lies in determining the pace of resolution. In ACR most episodes of moderate rejection resolve within a few weeks after therapy. In AMR there is limited published data in the IF literature and none in the IHC literature. Tan and colleagues reported that C3d staining was eliminated before C4d and cleared at a pace of 2–4 weeks earlier than C4d (Tan et al. 2009). Anecdotal experience in the IHC realm supports this finding (Fig. 14.14). The rate of C4d clearance can be protracted emphasizing the need to continue immunostaining all positive biopsies until resolution of the AMR episode.

14.5.5 Early- Versus Late-Onset AMR: Are They Different?

As previously discussed the initial AMR experience reported most episodes occurring within the first weeks or months after transplantation, but cases occurring years following transplant are now more frequently recognized. The initiating events in the late cases are often unknown, but episodes of infection and moderate or severe ACR following noncompliance have been associated with aggressive and often poorly responsive forms of AMR in our experience.

There are a number of studies showing the association of late-onset AMR and the development of TAV and other late complications of transplantation (Coutance et al. 2015). The investigation of histopathologic and immunophenotypic differences between early- and late-onset AMR has been recently studied. Fedrigo and colleagues compared the frequency of intravascular macrophages in early AMR (defined as within 1 year of transplant) and late AMR (defined as after 1 year) as a predictor of AMR (Fedrigo et al. 2013). Intravascular macrophages were found more frequently in association with C4d+biopsies in early AMR (70 %) compared to late AMR (30 %) suggesting that their presence is time related. A similar pattern was found for the predictive value of intravascular macrophages for positive DSA in early and late AMR. Intravascular macrophages were also more common in symptomatic AMR patients versus asymptomatic patients within the first year, but this was not observed in the late-onset group. Yerly and colleagues evaluated the prevalence of C4d and CD68 with respect to the pathologic grades of AMR during the first posttransplant year (Yerly et al. 2015). The presence of pAMR2 correlated with both clinical symptoms and positive DSA. Most cases of C4d+CD68+ biopsies occurred within the first 4 months (with highest incidence at 2 weeks) after transplant and then diminished. Further, pAMR1-I+ biopsies also showed a "decrescendo pattern" after 4 months. Additional studies are needed to confirm these sets of observations. The role of molecular analysis and evaluation of other markers of AMR may provide additional insights into the initiation, progression, and cessation of AMR. Immunohistochemical staining of endothelial cell activation by way of mammalian target of rapamycin (mTOR) effector markers, phosphorylated-S6 kinase and S6 ribosomal protein, has been shown to be helpful diagnostic markers of AMR (Li et al. 2015; Tible et al. 2013). Differential microRNA expression has been shown to occur both in serum and in cardiac tissue in patients with allograft rejection (both ACR and AMR). Duong Van Huyen and colleagues found 7 miRNAs expressed in biopsy samples, of which four of the seven demonstrated serologic expression (Duong Van Huyen et al. 2014). Gene expression assessment has been recently shown to be predictive of renal allograft loss in patients with early biopsy-proven AMR in kidney transplant recipients (Loupy et al. 2014). Extension of these techniques to cardiac recipients will hopefully provide similar prognostic information for patient management and surveillance.

14.5.6 Is Pediatric AMR Different from Adult AMR?

Most of our current diagnostic and prognostic information about AMR derives from clinicopathologic studies in adults. There are fewer than ten detailed morphologic studies of pediatric AMR in the published literature, and the majority were published prior to or do not utilize the 2013 WF guidelines (Casarez et al. 2007; Chen et al. 2015; Everitt et al. 2012; Holt et al. 2008; Knecht et al. 2015; Peng et al. 2013; Xu et al. 2013; Zinn et al. 2014). In all but one study, C4d and/or CD68 was applied and IF was used in only one of the studies. In most of the studies,

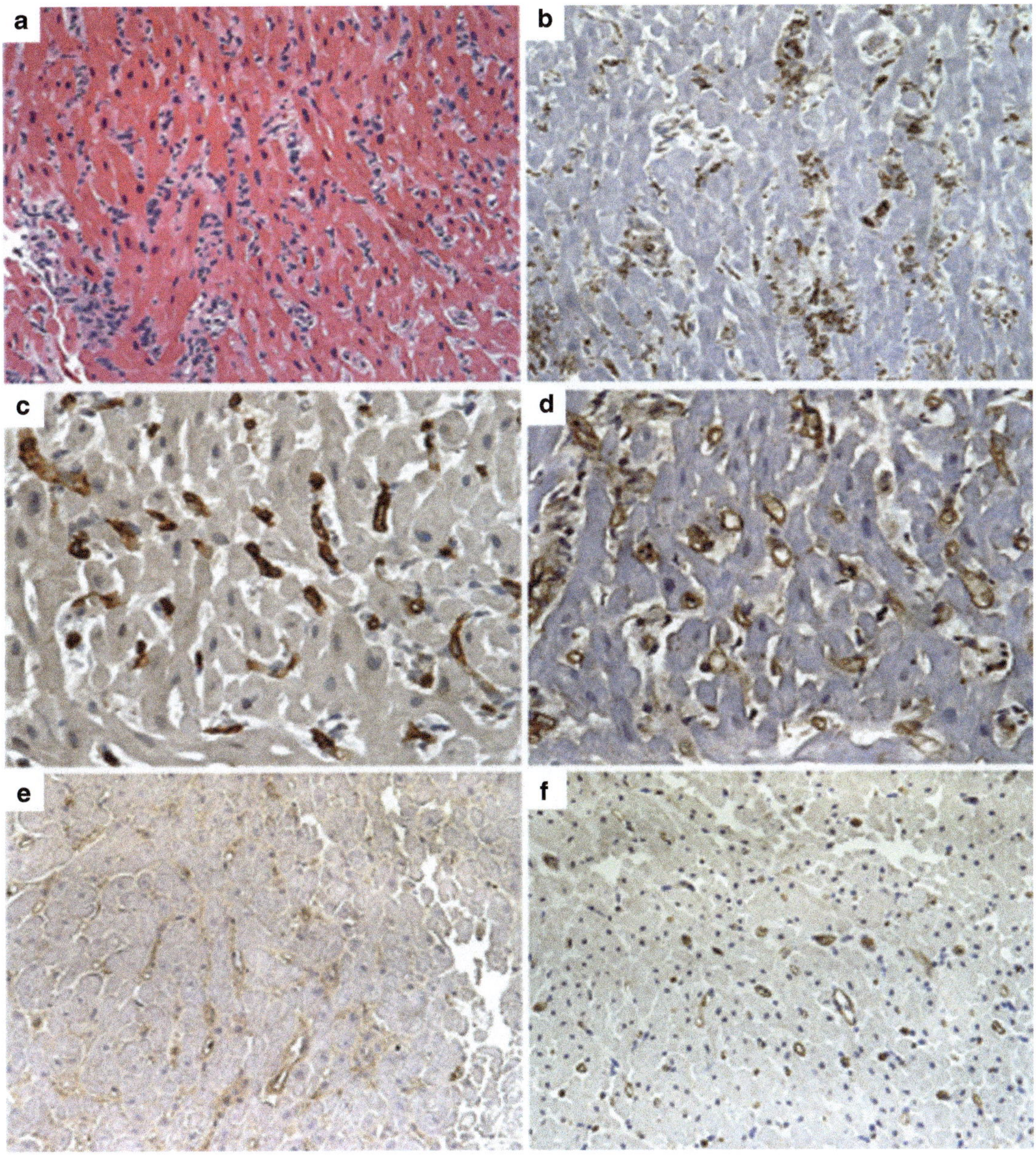

Fig. 14.14 C4d and C3d staining patterns following therapeutic intervention. (Panel **a**) Activated mononuclear cells in an emergent biopsy 1.5 months after transplant in a 12-year-old boy with hemodynamic compromise (H&E ×200). (Panel **b**) Numerous CD68+ intravascular macrophages (×200). (Panel **c**) Strong C4d staining confirming the diagnosis of pAMR 2 (×400). (Panel **d**) C3d also showed strong positivity in the same biopsy sample (×400). (Panel **e**) C3d staining 2 months after therapy showing poorly localized faint staining of the microvasculature (×250). (Panel **f**) The concurrent C4d stain showing persistent strong linear endothelial staining indicating the resolution process is initiated with C3d diminished staining before C4d (×200)

some degree of mixed ACR and AMR was apparent, but the prevalence was variable. Many of the issues presented above also pertain to pediatric AMR such as the incidence and prevalence of AMR; the pace of development and resolution of AMR episodes; the risks for development of accelerated TAV, cardiovascular mortality, and graft loss; and the biologic and prognostic differences between early- and late-onset AMR. As previously discussed, there are inherent differences between the histologic appearance of the myocardium in pediatric compared to adult biopsies in the quiescent state that need to be considered in the morphologic assessment of biopsy findings so as to avoid misinterpreting the histopathologic criteria. As most pediatric centers perform less than 20 transplants annually, additional, large center single- and multicenter studies are needed to resolve these challenges.

14.6 Future Directions

Tremendous progress in our understanding of cardiac AMR has been made over the last 25 years. That said, there remains much to be unraveled, clarified, and expanded. Many of these issues have been enumerated in our discussion of AMR, and others will proceed from newer insights and unresolved questions. The 2013 ISHLT WF attempts to incorporate our current level of understanding into a manageable paradigm for pathologists to apply to endomyocardial biopsy samples in their daily practice. Its utility and reproducibility await further testing and application to clinical practice and multicenter studies. The question of when to initiate therapy is a clinical decision that can only be established by single-center and multi-institutional treatment trials. The role of molecular pathology in the diagnosis and grading of AMR and, in particular, C4d-negative AMR is another unresolved issue. The experience may parallel the renal transplant literature, but detailed studies will need to be performed. The next decade of clinical and basic research will surely prove to be exciting and fruitful.

Key Points

- AMR can occur early, especially in pre-sensitized patients, or late, even year after transplantation.
- A thorough knowledge of the 2013 ISHLT grading scheme for AMR is required.
- AMR is reported as "pathologic AMR or pAMR" and recognizes four grades reflecting the severity of rejection.
- Currently, the diagnosis of AMR is established by pathologists independent of clinical parameters and DSAs.
- Unlike ACR, which is based solely on histopathologic criteria, the pathologic assessment of AMR requires both histopathologic and immunopathologic findings.
- The key histopathologic features are interstitial capillary injury with swollen, enlarged, hyperplastic endothelial cells and intravascular macrophages (*intravascular activated mononuclear cells*)
- The key immunopathologic findings are:
  - IHC: C4d-positive and/or CD68-positive staining results
  - IF: C4d+/-C3d-positive staining results
- Immunopathologic findings together with the histopathologic changes are more sensitive and specific than morphology alone. A low threshold for performing immunophenotypic studies is recommended.
- AMR can coexist with ACR (known as mixed rejection).

References

Berry GJ, et al. The ISHLT working formulation for pathologic diagnosis of antibody-mediated rejection in heart transplantation: evolution and current status(2005-2011). J Heart Lung Transplant. 2011;30(6):601–11.

Berry GJ, et al. The 2013 International Society for Heart and Lung Transplantation Working Formulation for the standardization of nomenclature in the pathologic diagnosis of antibody-mediated rejection in heart

transplantation. J Heart Lung Transplant. 2013;32(12):1147–62.
Billingham ME, et al. A working formulation for the standardization of nomenclature in the diagnosis of heart and lung rejection: Heart Rejection Study Group. The International Society for Heart Transplantation. J Heart Transplant. 1990;9(6):587–93.
Burke M, et al. C4d methodology and interpretation in diagnosis of cardiac antibody-mediated rejection: a European survey from the Association for European Cardiovascular Pathology (ARCVP). J Heart Lung Transplant. 2010;29:S37–8.
Casarez TW, et al. Humoral rejection in pediatric orthotopic heart transplantation. J Heart Lung Transplant. 2007;26:114–9.
Chen CK, et al. Development and impact of de novo anti-HLA antibodies in pediatric heart transplant recipients. Am J Transplant. 2015;20:1–8.
Costanzo-Nordin MR, et al. Role of humoral immunity in acute cardiac allograft dysfunction. J Heart Lung Transplant. 1993;12(2):S143–6.
Coutance G, et al. Late antibody-mediated rejection after heart transplantation: mortality, graft function, and fulminant cardiac allograft vasculopathy. J Heart Lung Transplant. 2015;34(8):1050–7.
Duong Van Huyen J-P, et al. MicroRNAs as non-invasive biomarkers of heart transplant rejection. Eur Heart J. 2014;35:3194–202.
Everitt MD, et al. Biopsy-diagnosed antibody-mediated rejection based on the proposed International Society for Heart and Lung Transplantation working formulation is associated with adverse cardiovascular outcomes after pediatric heart transplant. J Heart Lung Transplant. 2012;31:686–93.
Fedrigo M, et al. Intravascular macrophages in cardiac allograft biopsies for diagnosis of early and late antibody mediated rejection. J Heart Lung Transplant. 2013;32(4):404–9.
Fedrigo M, et al. Inflammatory cell burden and phenotype in endomyocardial biopsies with antibody-mediated rejection (AMR): a multicenter pilot study from the AECVP. Am J Transplant. 2015;15:526–34.
Hammond EH, et al. Vascular (humoral) rejection in heart transplantation: pathologic observations and clinical implications. J Heart Transplant. 1989;8(6):430–43.
Hammond EH, et al. Vascular rejection and its relationship to allograft coronary artery disease. J Heart Lung Transplant. 1992;11:S111–9.
Hammond ME, et al. Utility of histologic parameters in screening for antibody-mediated rejection of the cardiac allograft: a study of 3,170 biopsies. J Heart Lung Transplant. 2005;24(12):2015–21.
Holt DB, et al. Complement fragment C4d and C3d deposition in pediatric heart recipients with a positive crossmatch. J Heart Lung Transplant. 2008;27:1073–8.
Kemnitz J, et al. Hyperacute rejection in heart allografts. Case studies. Pathol Res Pract. 1991;187(1):23–9.
Kfoury AG, et al. Cardiovascular mortality among heart transplant recipients with asymptomatic antibody-mediated or stable mixed cellular and antibody-mediated rejection. J Heart Lung Transplant. 2009;28:781–4.
Knecht KR, et al. Antibody-mediated rejection is associated with impaired graft function in pediatric heart transplant recipients. J Heart Lung Transplant. 2015;34(8):1120–1.
Kobashigawa J, et al. Report from a consensus conference on antibody-mediated rejection in heart transplantation. J Heart Lung Transplant. 2011;30(3):252–69.
Kucirka LM, et al. Survey of North American pathologist practices regarding antibody-mediated rejection in cardiac transplant biopsies. Cardiovasc Pathol. 2011;20(3):132–8.
Li F, et al. Phosphorylated S6 kinase and S6 ribosomal protein are diagnostic markers of antibody-mediated rejection in heart allografts. J Heart Lung Transplant. 2015;34:580–7.
Lones MA, et al. Clinical-pathologic features of humoral rejection in cardiac allografts: a study in 81 consecutive patients. J Heart Lung Transplant. 1995;14:151–62.
Loupy A, et al. Molecular microscope strategy to improve risk stratification in early antibody-mediated kidney allograft rejection. J Am Soc Nephrol. 2014;25:2267–77.
Miller DV, et al. Detection of C4d deposition in cardiac allografts: a comparative study of immunofluorescence and immunoperoxidase methods. Arch Pathol Lab Med. 2010;134:1679–84.
Moseley EL, Atkinson C, Sharples LD, Wallwork J, Goddard MJ. Deposition of C4d and C3d in cardiac transplants: a factor in the development of coronary artery vasculopathy. J Heart Lung Transplant. 2010;29(4):417–23.
Peng DM, et al. Donor-specific antibodies: can they predict C4d deposition in pediatric heart recipients? Pediatr Transplant. 2013;17:429–35.
Ratliff NB, et al. Activation of intravascular macrophages within myocardial small vessels is a feature of acute vascular rejection in human heart transplants. J Heart Lung Transplant. 1995;14:338–45.
Reed EF, et al. Acute antibody-mediated rejection of cardiac transplants. J Heart Lung Transplant. 2006;25:153–9.
Rodriguez ER, et al. Antibody-mediated rejection in human cardiac allografts: evaluation of immunoglobulins and complement activation products C4d and C3d as markers. Am J Transplant. 2005;5:2778–85.
Stewart S, et al. Revision of the 1990 working formulation for the standardization of nomenclature in the diagnosis of heart rejection. J Heart Lung Transplant. 2005;24:1710–20.
Tan CD, et al. Correlation of donor-specific antibodies, complement and its regulators with graft dysfunction in cardiac antibody-mediated rejection. Am J Transplant. 2009;9:2075–84.

Tavora F, et al. Endothelitis in cardiac allograft biopsy specimens: possible relationship to antibody-mediated rejection. J Heart Lung Transplant. 2011;30:435–44.

Tible M, et al. Pathologic classification of antibody-mediated rejection correlates with donor-specific antibodies and endothelial cell activation. J Heart Lung Transplant. 2013;32:769–76.

Xu Y, et al. Utility of C4d immunostaining in the first year after pediatric and young adult heart transplantation. J Heart Lung Transplant. 2013;32:92–7.

Yerly P, et al. Time-dependent specificity of immunopathologic (C4d-CD68) and histologic criteria of antibody-mediated rejection for donor-specific antibodies and allograft dysfunction in heart transplantation. Transplantation. 2015;99:586–93.

Zinn MD, et al. Bortezomib use in a pediatric cardiac transplant center. Pediatr Transplant. 2014;18:469–76.

"Mixed" Rejection in Heart Transplantation

15

Dylan V. Miller and Abdallah G. Kfoury

Contents

D.V. Miller, MD (✉)
Intermountain Central Laboratory,
University of Utah, Salt Lake City, UT, USA
e-mail: Dylan.Miller@imail.org;
Dylan.Miller@imail2.org

A.G. Kfoury, MD
Division of Cardiovascular Disease, Intermountain
Medical Center, Utah Transplant Affiliated Hospitals
(U.T.A.H.) Cardiac Transplant Program,
Murray, UT, USA

15.1 Background

Criteria for T-cell-mediated cellular rejection (CR) as well as antibody-mediated rejection (AMR) are well defined in the working formulations published by the International Society for Heart and Lung Transplantation (ISHLT WF) (Stewart et al. 2005; Berry et al. 2013), and these are a major focus of this book. The mechanisms underlying CR and AMR are distinct but are not necessarily mutually exclusive. In some cardiac allograft biopsies, features of both CR and AMR may be seen concurrently (Fig. 15.1). This has been termed as "mixed" rejection (MR) and has been described in the early case series detailing the features of AMR (Lones et al. 1995; Hammond et al. 1989) and is briefly acknowledged in the 2013 ISHLT WF for AMR (Berry et al. 2013).

Patients may also have variation in patterns of rejection over time, such that one biopsy might show only CR but a subsequent biopsy AMR and vice versa. In this sense, there may also be a "mixed" pattern of rejection for a given patient, even though both processes are not seen simultaneously in the same biopsy tissue. This phenomenon at the patient level raises the question of possibly cross activation of T-cell and B-cell arms of immunity (i.e., one type of rejection occurring first and then initiating events that subsequently lead to the other form of rejection). Data are very sparse on this concept, though there

O. Leone et al. (eds.), *The Pathology of Cardiac Transplantation*,
DOI 10.1007/978-3-319-46386-5_15

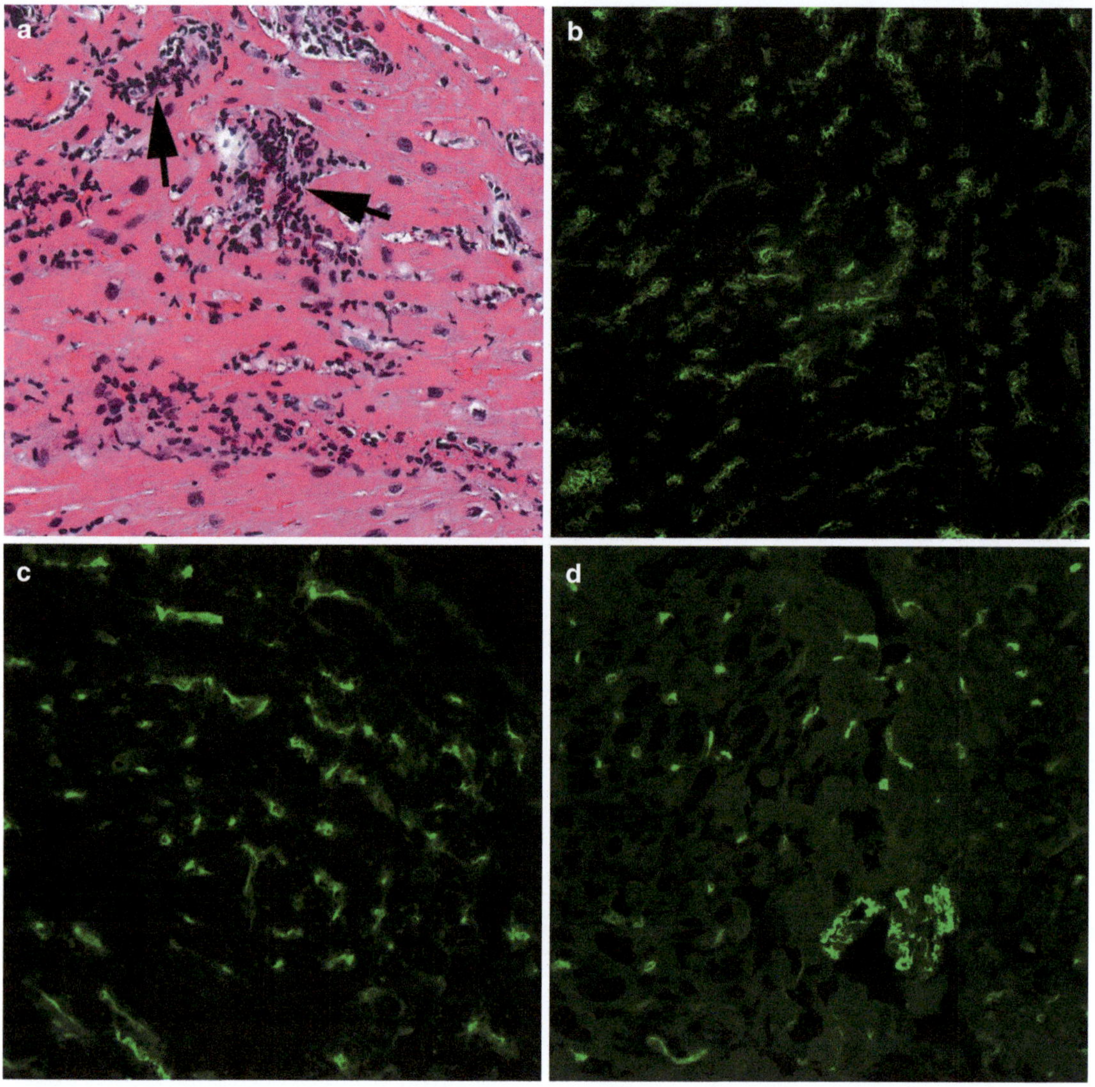

Fig. 15.1 (**a**) Transplant endomyocardial biopsy showing two foci of perivascular lymphocyte inflammation (*arrows*), consistent with cellular rejection. In the background, the capillaries appear congested and show prominent intravascular mononuclear cells [H&E, ×100]. (**b**) Immunofluorescence staining for HLA-DR (expressed on endothelial cells) shows a pattern of capillary injury. Rather than crisp, linear staining the capillaries have a frayed or feathery outline [×100]. (**c**, **d**) Immunofluorescence staining for C4d (**c**) and C3d (**d**) show diffuse positive capillary staining [×200]

are potential mechanisms whereby this could be explained immunologically.

The prospect of such a causal link between the different arms of the immune system is intriguing. If such a link exists, then "mixed rejection" defined at the level of a single biopsy as well as at the level of a patient transitioning between types of rejection may be the same process, just viewed at different points in time. That is, patients whose biopsies show concurrent CR and AMR in the same tissue may have had fortuitous sampling during the window when both are present, and patients whose biopsies show only one pattern in one biopsy and the other pattern in another biopsy may have had tissue sampling on either side of that window.

Alternatively, CR and AMR may not be linked causally at all and may follow separate discrete pathways such that their simultaneous occurrence in a biopsy showing MR may just be coincidental—a random intersection. It is also possible that both of these scenarios occur and that patients may show varying degrees of cross talk between CR and MR. The severity or intensity of the immune response may also impact the extent to which cross activation occurs. Unraveling this complicated conundrum and clarifying the underlying mechanisms at play will be a daunting puzzle.

This chapter focuses on reports of MR in the literature, overlapping morphologic and immunopathologic features between AMR and CR that have relevance for MR and possible mechanisms for cross activation between cellular and humoral immunity that may help conceptually account for MR and serve as possible avenues for further investigation. The available data on clinical implications of MR will also be summarized briefly.

15.2 Review of Other Reports Detailing MR

The phenomenon of MR is mentioned in several reports (Kfoury et al. 2009; Hammond et al. 2005; Taylor et al. 2000) but only reported in detail or as a specific emphasis in a few. Since AMR was not widely recognized until the mid-1990s, there are no reports earlier than this. One of the first reports to detail MR found that 50 % of patients with AMR, defined by the authors using both immunopathologic and histologic criteria, also had mild CR (Lones et al. 1995). Less than 5 % of these patients in their series were said to have severe CR, though these biopsies were not described in further detail. In another review and summary of rejection patterns from published literature, Book et al. described "fulminant" MR as tending to occur early (within 4 months posttransplant) and portending a poor prognosis (Book et al. 2003). More recently, abstracts have been published describing MR (defined as positive C4d and presence of CR) manifesting as mild rejection in 39 % of biopsies and severe in 2 % (Fedrigo et al. 2014). Defining MR more rigidly (as ≥2R CR with positive C3d *and* C4d), Tan et al. reported (Tan et al. 2014) MR in <1 % out of 332 patients.

More recently, Loupy et al. found that explant and biopsy specimens previously classified as moderate ACR at their institution often showed evidence of microvascular inflammation as well. Donor-specific antibody was also present in the serum of these patients more often than expected (Loupy et al. 2011). Tavora et al. also reported "endotheliitis" in up to 10 % of biopsies initially read as ACR. A third of these also had clinical/serologic evidence of AMR (Tavora et al. 2011).

MR is addressed in the ISHLT WF for AMR, where it is defined as the presence of ACR and AMR concurrently in the same biopsy. In the report of the ISHLT Working Group's multicenter digital pathology slide study, it was "not uncommon to find the pattern of both AMR and low-grade ACR" in the same biopsy (Berry et al. 2013). The 2013 ISHLT WF includes a caveat for interpreting immunopathology in possible mixed rejection cases, namely, that C4d and CD68 stains should be "assessed on intact myocardium away from areas of ACR, Quilty lesions, biopsy site scars, and ischemia-related inflammation and necrosis." It also acknowledges that there may be some morphologic overlap between ACR and AMR in some patterns of rejection, particularly the former "1B" type ACR in the 2005 ISHLT scheme (discussed below). Lastly the 2013 ISHLT WF provides a "soft" suggestion that ACR grade ≥2R may be another indication for adding immunopathology (if not done routinely) given the apparent higher incidence of MR in severe rejection episodes (Berry et al. 2013).

15.3 Morphologic and Immunopathologic Overlap Between AMR and CR

The histopathologic manifestations of CR include infiltration by T lymphocytes in clusters that may or may not be associated with myocyte injury. The hallmarks of AMR include accumulation of intravascular mononuclear cells as well as demonstrating evidence of complement activa-

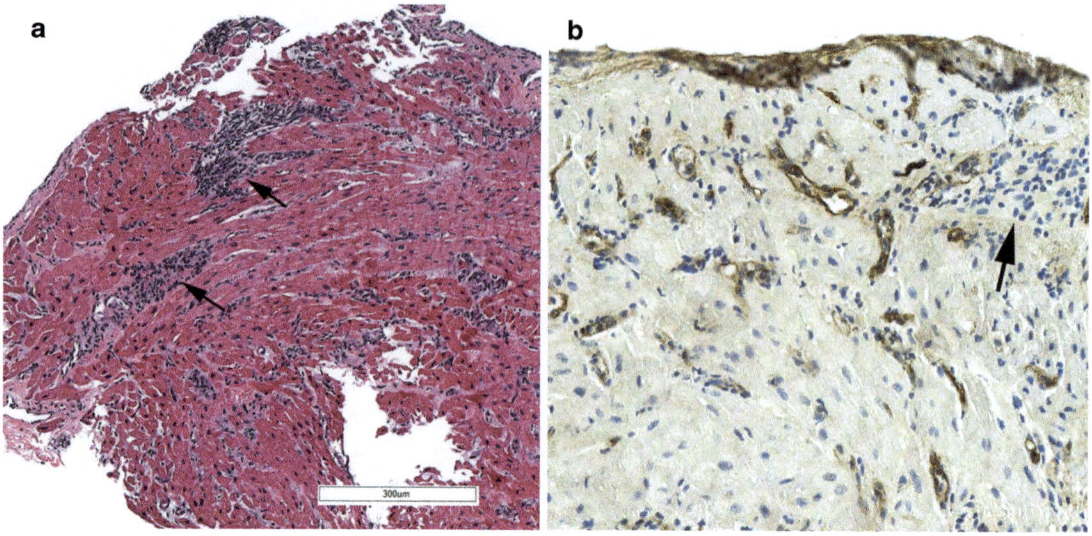

Fig. 15.2 (**a**) Transplant endomyocardial biopsy showing mixed rejection, with areas of cellular rejection (*arrows*) and a "busy" appearance in the surrounding myocardium caused by aggregation of intravascular mononuclear cell [H&E, ×100]. (**b**) Immunoperoxidase staining in this case demonstrated positive capillary staining for C4d. A minor focus of cellular rejection (*arrow*) is also seen at the top right. Swollen endothelial cells and intravascular mononuclear cells can be seen within capillaries as well [×400]

tion or intraluminal macrophages by immunopathologic methods. In general, CR and AMR are relatively easy to separate and in most cases of mild MR give the overall appearance of two separate but overlaid processes (Fig. 15.2). Foci of CR, for example, may be observed in immunohistochemical (Fig. 15.3) or immunofluorescence (Fig. 15.4) stains for complement.

There are cases, however, which present a challenge for pathologic interpretation. While intravascular macrophages are typically associated with AMR and T-cell infiltrates are associated with CR, Fedrigo et al. have demonstrated substantial numbers of T cells in the setting of AMR as well as macrophages in cases of CR (Fedrigo et al. 2015). As described in the 2013 ISHLT WF, some features of severe CR and AMR overlap. Severe AMR is described as showing "Hemorrhage, interstitial edema, myocyte necrosis, capillary fragmentation, [and] mixed inflammatory infiltrates…" (Berry et al. 2013) (Figs. 15.5 and 15.6). The 2005 revised ISHLT WF for CR describes grade 3R rejection as "…a diffuse inflammatory process [with] either predominantly lymphocytes and macrophages or a polymorphous infiltrate…multiple areas of associated myocyte damage…[with] edema, interstitial hemorrhage and vasculitis …" (Stewart et al. 2005). Both descriptions include hemorrhage and myocyte damage, for example.

As mentioned before, the similarities between AMR and CR, when moderate, were recognized by Loupy et al., who observed that "cases previously classified as 3A/2R cellular rejection in the ISHLT consensus actually show evidence for microvascular injury and donor specific antibody, thus suggesting that a substantial part of at least grade 2R rejections may indeed be associated with DSA and may represent mixed rejection" (Loupy et al. 2011).

Neutrophils and eosinophils are more often seen in AMR (Fig. 15.7), especially early in AMR (Berry et al. 2013), but severe CR is also said to show a "polymorphous" infiltrate that may include these cell types. Some of the early reports of severe CR appeared before AMR (so by extension MR) were recognized and must be considered in that context (Billingham et al. 1990; McAllister 1990). Widespread myocyte injury is a fairly constant feature reported in these. When diffuse damage is seen, it can be difficult to separate severe CR from severe AMR

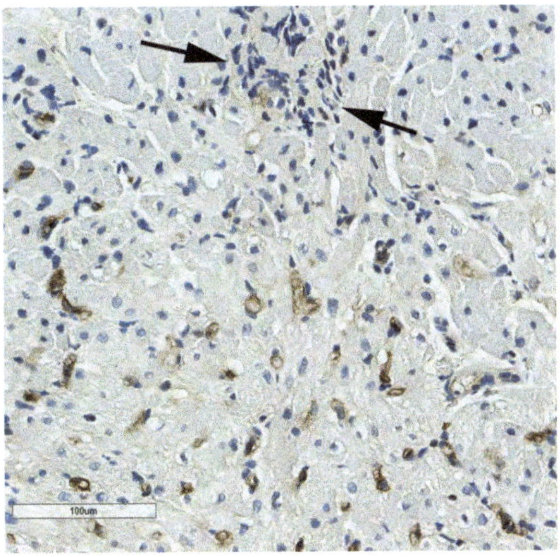

Fig. 15.3 By immunoperoxidase staining, both the histomorphologic features of the biopsy and the expression of complement C4d can be assessed. This photomicrograph shows mixed rejection with an area of cellular rejection (*arrows*) as well as positive C4d staining and intravascular mononuclear cells (ISHLT 2013 1R, pAMR2) [×400]

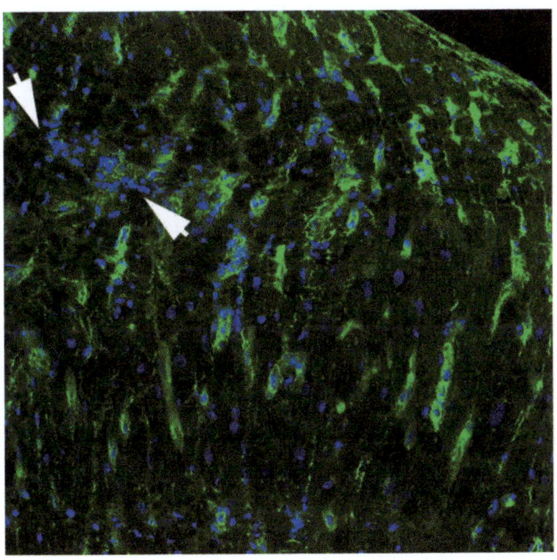

Fig. 15.4 Using DAPI nuclear counterstaining, the features depicted in Fig. 3 can be partly recapitulated by immunofluorescence techniques. This slide showed positive staining for C3d and a collection of nuclei (*arrows*) whose size and morphology suggest lymphocytes in a small focus of cellular rejection. There also appear to be excessive nuclei within positively staining capillaries, consistent with intravascular activated mononuclear cells [×200]

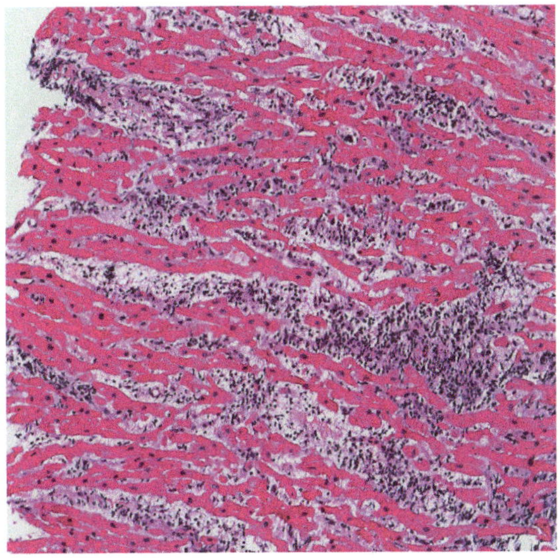

Fig. 15.5 Severe antibody-mediated rejection manifests as widespread diffuse inflammation that is both intravascular and interstitial. It is difficult to appreciate any open lumens of the venules or capillaries, and in fact some of them appear to be overrun, injured, and destroyed. The myocytes also show diffuse injury. This appearance may be complicated by hemorrhage, edema, and neutrophils as well. Positive complement staining is important in establishing a diagnosis of severe AMR (versus severe cellular rejection) [×100]

(or MR). Ultrastructural studies have suggested an important difference however. The injury to myocytes in CR is more often sublethal and reversible, whereas in severe AMR, the cell necrosis is more complete (Myles et al. 1987; Hammond and Yowell 1994).

Complement activation and deposition is almost pathognomonic for AMR and for all intents and purposes does not occur in CR. Complement staining may be seen in and around injured myocytes regardless of etiology (ischemia, CR, or AMR). The myocyte staining pattern, as opposed to capillary pattern, helps avoid confusion and inaccurate stain interpretation. Artifactual complement staining may also cause confusion, especially with paraffin immunohistochemistry, but strict adherence to the ISHLT WF definitions of positive staining (considering both the intensity and distribution of staining) helps reliably AMR from artifactual staining in CR. Alternate mechanisms of complement activation resulting in positive capillary staining (other than AMR) have been

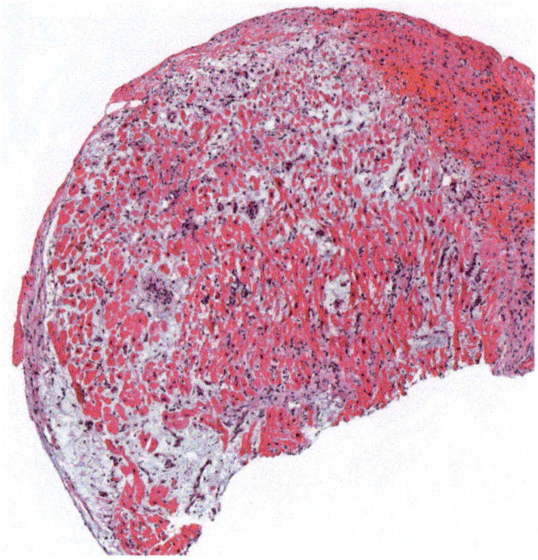

Fig. 15.6 Interstitial edema is prominent in AMR, especially severe episodes. This has also been observed in severe cellular rejection, so is one of the overlapping features that raises the possibility of cross activation or a final common pathway of rejection changes. True edema includes a pale, loose, finely fibrillar extracellular matrix material in the interstices between cells. This helps in distinguishing edema from artifacts of processing and microtomy [×50]

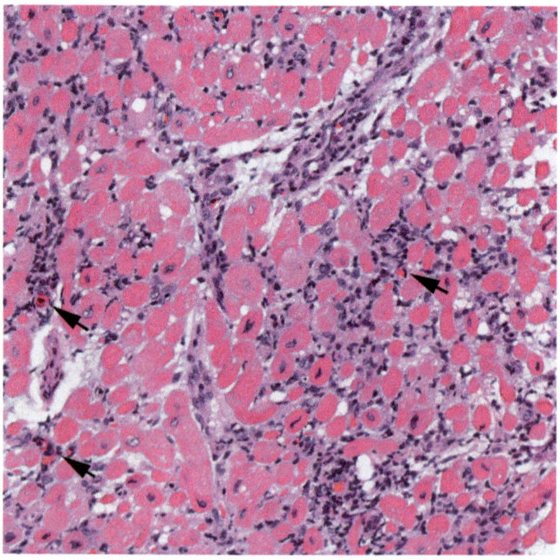

Fig. 15.7 In more severe rejection episodes (whether AMR, cellular, or mixed), there may be prominent eosinophils (*arrows*) as part of the inflammatory infiltrate [×200]

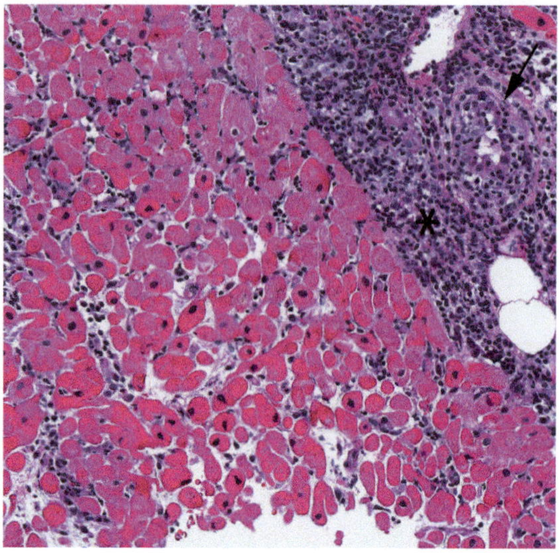

Fig. 15.8 This transplant endomyocardial biopsy shows a mixed pattern of rejection, with prominent intravascular mononuclear cells within myocardial capillaries on the left side and a discrete mass-forming collection of inflammatory cells to the right (*asterisk*). There is an area within the inflammation that appears to be a small branch vessel with transmural inflammation (*arrow*) [×200]

proposed. These include the alternative pathway or mannose-binding lectin pathway in the context of ischemic injury (Loupy et al. 2011).

"Vasculitis" is another feature which has been reported as a feature of both CR and AMR, at the severe end of the spectrum for each (Figs. 15.8 and 15.9). This usually manifests as intimitis or intimal arteritis, but transmural inflammation may also be seen. Since AMR was once synonymous with "vascular" rejection, there is a tendency to assume vasculitis is more specific for AMR. However cases showing clear-cut CR have also demonstrated this feature (Tavora et al. 2011; Johnson et al. 1989; Hammond et al. 1991).

15.4 Mechanisms of Immune Cross Activation in MR

The overlapping features mentioned above may provide insights into common pathways and possible cross activating mechanisms between the cell mediated and humoral arms of the immune

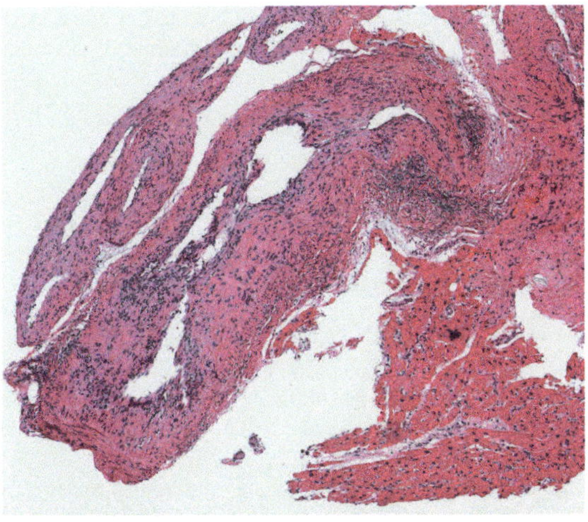

Fig. 15.9 This transplant endomyocardial biopsy included a substantial portion of small muscular artery that is inflamed. There is intimal arteritis and some apparent lymphocytes in the adventitia as well. Curiously, the adjacent myocardium shows only mild equivocal features of AMR. Arterial inflammation has been described in both cellular and antibody-mediated rejection, another overlapping feature raising the possibility of shared or cross activating mechanisms between these two arms of the immune response [×50]

system. These are entirely speculative at this point, but several mechanistic hypotheses exist.

The capillary endothelium is considered the primary point of contact between donor-reactive antibody and the graft in AMR. Capillaries are also affected in CR, since they are the conduit and migration portal for T cells and other leukocytes. It is possible that endothelial activation (usually associated with AMR) may be triggered by capillary level changes in CR, especially in more severe cases.

Several studies have also shown a role for coagulopathy in the potentiation of rejection, especially in AMR. This includes loss of antithrombin III, release of tissue factor, accumulation of fibrin, and aggregation of platelets (Labarrere and Jaeger 2012). Myocyte and vascular injury that occurs in cellular rejection may also result in similar pro-thrombotic events.

Compromise of capillaries and microenvironment ischemia, possibly exacerbated by coagulopathy, may also account cell injury and triggering of immune response in a cyclical feedback loop. The perfusion/reperfusion phenomenon could complicate this mechanism further. These potential mechanisms may have particular relevance to innate immunity (e.g., neutrophils and NK cells). A possible role for activation of T-cell and B-cell pathways via innate immune mechanisms has recently been postulated based on molecular signatures (Hidalgo et al. 2010).

Conclusion

Pathologic observations from several studies seem to lend credence to the concepts of MR as both a coincidental occurrence of CR and AMR as independent processes (in cases of mild MR) and as a non-coincidental "final common pathway" (in moderate/severe MR). The first of those scenarios is much more common, but the second is particularly intriguing and deserves further validation and exploration. Regardless of severity, MR is most often seen following an inflammatory state in a previous biopsy, again suggesting a possible role of cross talk between the different arms of the immune system. Severe MR (like severe CR and severe AMR) portends a significantly worse prognosis.

Much more work is needed to demonstrate the clinical and prognostic import of MR and elucidate potential mechanisms of cross activation that may exist in the coordinated immune response to the cardiac allograft.

Key Points

- It is not uncommon to find features of both AMR (ISHLT pAMR2) and mild CR (ISHLT 1R) occurring in the same biopsy.
- Severe CR (ISHLT 3R) and AMR (ISHLT pAMR3) share overlapping morphologic features including:
  - Edema
  - Polymorphous inflammation
  - Vasculitis

- The mechanisms underlying CR and AMR are distinct but are not necessarily mutually exclusive.
- "Cross talk" between cellular and humoral arms of the immune system may occur via intermediaries such as complement, the coagulation system, innate immune cells, or endothelial activation.

References

Berry GJ, Burke MM, Andersen C, et al. The 2013 International Society for Heart and Lung Transplantation Working Formulation for the standardization of nomenclature in the pathologic diagnosis of antibody-mediated rejection in heart transplantation. J Heart Lung Transplant. 2013;32(12):1147–62.

Billingham ME, Cary NRB, Hammond ME, et al. A working formulation for the standardization of nomenclature in the diagnosis of heart and lung rejection: heart rejection study group. J Heart Transplant. 1990;9:587–92.

Book WM, Kelley L, Gravanis MB. Fulminant mixed humoral and cellular rejection in a cardiac transplant recipient: a review of the histologic findings and literature. J Heart Lung Transplant. 2003;22(5):604–7.

Fedrigo M, Feltrin G, Frigo A, Toscano G, Tona F, et al. Mixed acute cellular rejection and antibody mediated rejection in heart transplantation: a retrospective study in a single transplant center. J Heart Lung Transplant. 2014;33(4S):S113.

Fedrigo M, Leone O, Burke MM, Rice A, Toquet C, et al. Inflammatory cell burden and phenotype in endomyocardial biopsies with antibody-mediated rejection (AMR): a multicenter pilot study from the AECVP. Am J Transplant. 2015;15(2):526–34.

Hammond EH, Yowell RL. Ultrastructural findings in cardiac transplant recipients. Ultrastruct Pathol. 1994;18(1–2):213–20.

Hammond EH, Yowell RL, Nunoda S, et al. Vascular (humoral) rejection in heart transplantation: pathologic observations and clinical implications. J Heart Transplant. 1989;8(6):430–43.

Hammond EH, Ensley RD, Yowell RL, Craven CM, Bristow MR, Renlund DG, O'Connell JB. Vascular rejection of human cardiac allografts and the role of humoral immunity in chronic allograft rejection. Transplant Proc. 1991;23(2 Suppl 2):26–30.

Hammond ME, Stehlik J, Snow G, et al. Utility of histologic parameters in screening for antibody-mediated rejection of the cardiac allograft: a study of 3,170 biopsies. J Heart Lung Transplant. 2005;24(12):2015–21.

Hidalgo LG, Sis B, Sellares J, Campbell PM, et al. NK cell transcripts and NK cells in kidney biopsies from patients with donor-specific antibodies: evidence for NK cell involvement in antibody-mediated rejection. Am J Transplant. 2010;10(8):1812–22.

Johnson DE, Gao SZ, Schroeder JS, DeCampli WM, Billingham ME. The spectrum of coronary artery pathologic findings in human cardiac allografts. J Heart Transplant. 1989;8(5):349–59.

Kfoury AG, Hammond ME, Snow GL, et al. Cardiovascular mortality among heart transplant recipients with asymptomatic antibody-mediated or stable mixed cellular and antibody-mediated rejection. J Heart Lung Transplant. 2009;28(8):781–4.

Labarrere CA, Jaeger BR. Biomarkers of heart transplant rejection: the good, the bad, and the ugly! Transl Res. 2012;159(4):238–51.

Lones MA, Czer LS, Trento A, Harasty D, et al. Clinical-pathologic features of humoral rejection in cardiac allografts: a study of 81 consecutive patients. J Heart Lung Transplant. 1995;14(1):151–62.

Loupy A, Cazes A, Guillemain R, et al. Very late heart transplant rejection is associated with microvascular injury, complement deposition and progression to cardiac allograft vasculopathy. Am J Transplant. 2011;11(7):1478–87.

McAllister Jr HA. Histologic grading of cardiac allograft rejection: a quantitative approach. J Heart Transplant. 1990;9(3 Pt 2):277–82.

Myles JL, Ratliff NB, McMahon JT, Golding LR, Hobbs RE, et al. Reversibility of myocyte injury in moderate and severe acute rejection in cyclosporine-treated cardiac transplant patients. Arch Pathol Lab Med. 1987;111(10):947–52.

Stewart S, Winters GL, Fishbein MC, et al. Revision of the 1990 working formulation for the standardization of nomenclature in the diagnosis of heart rejection. J Heart Lung Transplant. 2005;24(11):1710–20.

Tan CD, Askar M, Rodriguez ER. Mixed rejection is a Low frequency event and not just cellular rejection and C4d deposition in the cardiac allograft. J Heart Lung Transplant. 2014;33(4S):S113.

Tavora F, Munivenkatappa R, Papadimitriou J. Endothelitis in cardiac allograft biopsy specimens: possible relationship to antibody-mediated rejection. J Heart Lung Transplant. 2011;30(4):435–44.

Taylor DO, Yowell RL, Kfoury AG, et al. Allograft coronary artery disease: clinical correlations with circulating anti-HLA antibodies and the immunohistopathologic pattern of vascular rejection. J Heart Lung Transplant. 2000;19(6):518–21.

Pathological Non-rejection Findings in the Endomyocardial Biopsy

16

Helen Doran and Desley A.H. Neil

Contents

H. Doran (✉)
Department of Histopathology, University Hospitals of South Manchester NHS Foundation Trust, Manchester, UK
e-mail: Helen.Doran@uhsm.nhs.uk

D.A.H. Neil
Department of Histopathology, Medical School University Hospitals Birmingham NHS Foundation Trust, Birmingham, UK

16.1 Background

Heart transplant patients undergo scheduled endomyocardial biopsies (EMBs) as part of their routine management. Protocols require frequent biopsies in the early postoperative period followed by a decrease in frequency. EMBs are done for the assessment of rejection, but a range of other pathologies or histological findings may be seen and need to be recognised and distinguished from the changes of cellular and antibody-mediated rejection, as the management is usually different.

These other conditions are related to the time from transplant and to the profile of each patient and are influenced by immunologic and non-immunologic factors. They can manifest with histopathological substrates that need to be differentiated from rejection as most of them share with rejection the key features of inflammation and myocardial damage.

Some of these findings are more common, others are very rare on EMBs, and each of them will be discussed in detail in the chapter.

- Peritransplant injury
- Quilty lesion/effect
- Previous biopsy site
- Subepicardial tissue
- Myocyte calcification
- Intravascular lymphocytes
- Foreign body

O. Leone et al. (eds.), *The Pathology of Cardiac Transplantation*,
DOI 10.1007/978-3-319-46386-5_16

- Tricuspid valve fragments
- Liver fragments
- Late ischaemic damage
- Infection
- Recurrence of primary disease
- Post-transplant lymphoproliferative disorder (PTLD)
- Artefacts (contraction bands, telescopic effects, haemorrhage, clot)

16.2 Peritransplant Injury

There are several causes of myocyte injury before and during the process of transplantation. Myocyte injury often occurs in the donor prior to organ donation, due to effects of hypovolaemia/hypoxia and vasoconstriction related to both inotropic drugs used to support the circulation and catecholamine storm which occur after head injury, particularly sudden onset 'explosive' head injuries and brain death. There may also be coagulation changes and fluctuations in hormone and electrolyte levels which affect blood pressure and organ perfusion generally. Inotropes result in varying degrees of contraction band necrosis and in microinfarcts, when coagulative necrosis occurs and activates complement. This can be detected with anti-complement antibodies, e.g. anti-C4d or anti-C9, before becoming histologically visible as hypereosinophilic myocytes, but in routine practice, it is usually readily identifiable on the haematoxylin–eosin-stained sections. Contraction band necrosis is initially negative with these antibodies; however over the days this starts to become positive (Ferreira et al. 1998).

Mouse studies have shown complement deposition in hearts from brain-dead donors, and this correlates with myocyte changes after transplantation. Studies on the limited number of heart transplant recipients whose donors were not brain dead ('domino' hearts) confirm that these are less prone to early myocyte damage and also less likely to develop acute rejection. Donors may have also suffered other injuries and are likely to be in intensive care units with ventilatory and possibly circulatory support. The hormonal and cardiovascular effects of brain death may vary depending on the speed of onset of brain damage, whether 'explosive' or gradual (Atkinson et al. 2013).

Pre-existing donor-derived coronary atherosclerosis can favour acute ischemic damage in the graft during the agonal period, the organ harvesting and the reperfusion process. This coronary atherosclerosis may have been unrecognised at the time of harvesting and may show accelerated progression during follow-up.

During procurement of the heart, there is a brief period of warm ischaemia before it is chilled by perfusing with cold preservation solution followed by cold storage in the preservation solution on ice and transportation to the site of the recipient. This period is termed the cold ischaemia time and is longer than the initial warm ischaemia time. Here injury can occur due to cold, which results in inactivation of the sodium–potassium pump, the preservation solution per se which may cause some cellular injury and hypoxia. Prior to transplantation the preservation solution is washed out, and there is a second period of warm ischaemia during the transplantation of the heart. After transplantation the heart is perfused by the recipient's warm oxygenated blood, and a paradoxical second phase of injury occurs related to the production of free radicals – the reperfusion injury. Any operative difficulty in restarting the transplanted heart will add to the burden of peritransplant damage to the new organ. In Table 16.1 various peritransplant injury phases are shown.

The changes of peritransplant injury in the endomyocardium are seen early after transplantation within 6 weeks or even up to 3 months after transplant. Pathologic findings of peritransplant injury include myocardial oedema, with fluid separating myocytes and endothelial activation, foci of contraction band necrosis and myocyte fragmentation or coagulative necrosis, associated or not with scant inflammatory infiltrate composed of neutrophils and macrophages, sometimes haemosiderin laden. The main feature which allows the pathologist to differentiate peritransplant damage from rejection is that the degree of myocyte injury, which is usually multifocal throughout the myocardium, tends to be out of proportion to the inflammatory infiltrate compared to that seen in cellular rejection, as the cause of necrosis is ischaemia and the reactive inflammatory infiltrate is suppressed by immunosuppressive treatment (Fig. 16.1). Recently, in routine practice, C4d immunostaining is frequently used to differentiate peritransplant damage from rejection if required in difficult cases, as C4d labels ischemic myocytes (Fig. 16.2). As the injury resolves with time, vascularised loose fibrous tissue replaces the damaged myocardium, often in a subendocardial distribution. Cardiomyocytes in the subendocardium may maintain their integrity, since they are protected by oxygen diffusion from the intracavitary blood. Macrophages can be identified, both in the interstitium and in the areas of loose connective tissue, often containing haemosiderin pigment and so resembling areas of previous biopsy site damage. Table 16.2 summarises the key histologic features helping in distinguishing peritransplant damage from rejection findings.

Table 16.1 Phases of peritransplant injury

1. During agonal events in the donor
2. Short period of warm ischaemia during organ procurement
3. Period of cold storage in hyperosmolar preservation solutions
4. Warm ischaemic period during the transplant procedure
5. Perfusion process
6. Injury related to drugs or hypovolaemia on restarting the heart if any initial poor function occurs

Stages 2–5 are termed ischaemia/reperfusion injury (IRI) or more accurately preservation–reperfusion injury (PRI)

It should be remembered that all EMBs have contraction bands due to the procedure, so that these should be carefully distinguished from the real contraction band necrosis, which may be related to peritransplant injury.

16.3 Quilty Effect

These are the most problematic lesions to differentiate from rejection and are thought to account for the majority of cases called grade 2 rejection in the old ISHLT 1995–2004 grading system. A Quilty lesion is a discrete endocardial-based mononuclear cell infiltrate that may extend into the underlying myocardium and be associated with apparent myocyte damage. Occasionally the Quilty lesion may look like an ‘organoid’ follicle (see below). Quilty lesions do tend to have a denser infiltrate than rejection and can often be seen by macroscopic examination of the slide, unlike rejection. If the biopsy is tangentially cut, it can be difficult or impossible to demonstrate their endocardial origin, even after examination of multiple levels. They are composed predominantly of T lymphocytes, which comprise more than 50% of the infiltrate, with B lymphocytes and macrophages being present in lesser amounts. Sometimes these lesions can be organised in a follicular pattern, which have a central B lymphocyte component with supporting

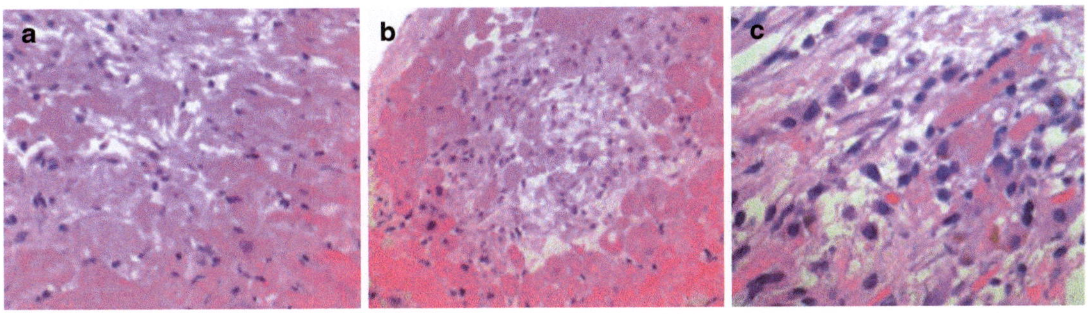

Fig. 16.1 Peritransplant injury. Post-transplant biopsies ranging from 7 to 21 days showing fragmented or hypereosinophilic myocytes, some with coagulation necrosis (**a**, **b**, haematoxylin–eosin, ×200) and scant inflammatory infiltrated (**b**). In (**c**) (haematoxylin–eosin, ×400) a more advanced lesion with necrotic myocytes, mononuclear inflammation and haemosiderin-laden macrophages is shown (Courtesy of Dr. O. Leone)

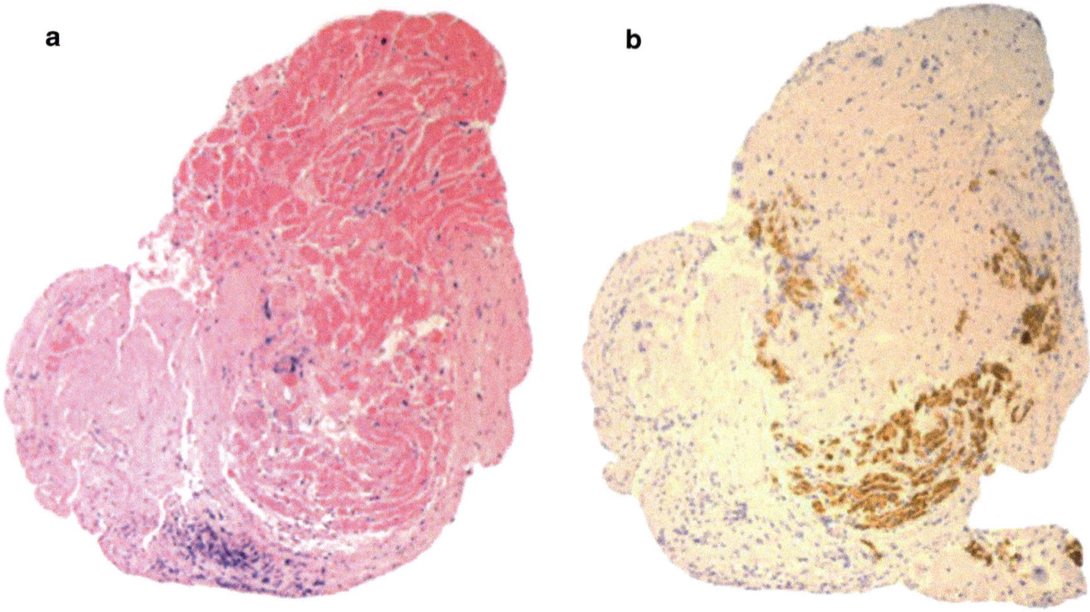

Fig. 16.2 Post-transplant EMB with an extensive area of myocyte necrosis (**a**, haematoxylin–eosin, ×25) highlighted with C4d immunostaining (**b**, ×25)

Table 16.2 Features that help distinguish peritransplant injury from rejection

1. In peritransplant injury the muscle damage is much greater in proportion to the inflammatory infiltrate
2. Hypereosinophilic coagulative necrosis of the myocytes occurs early
3. The inflammatory infiltrate is predominantly macrophages but can consist of neutrophils in the early stages, followed by gradual loss of the myocytes and a macrophage infiltrate
4. The necrotic myocyte stain with C4d or C9

follicular dendritic cells surrounded by T lymphocytes. The follicular dendritic cell framework becomes increasingly extensive in larger lesions (Sattar et al. 2006). Small capillary-sized blood vessels, with high endothelial venule (HEV) features, are frequently present within the lesions. Immunohistochemistry may be helpful in demonstrating the zonation of Quilty lesions with the cellular composition in some areas differing from that of rejection and in identifying the dendritic component of the infiltrating cells (CD21-positive staining) and the rich neovascular net (CD31-/CD34-positive staining). The morphologic similarity of Quilty lesions with the features of a tertiary lymphoid tissue can suggest an attempt to mount a local response to persistent alloantigen stimulation (Di Carlo et al. 2007). This is in contrast to rejection where the same cells are present, but without their organisation into compartments and lacking follicular dendritic cells and a vascular component. In the old 1990 classification, Quilty lesions were described as superficial (Quilty A) and deep (Quilty B): the former lacks myocyte damage, as the infiltrate is less extensive; in the latter inflammatory cells can be massive and infiltrate the underlying myocardium and are often associated with apparent myocyte injury (Fig. 16.3). Staining and evaluation of the intermediate slides in serial sections can help trace the myocardial lesion back to an endocardial origin.

16.4 Previous Biopsy Site

During the first few weeks to months after transplantation, EMBs are likely to be taken on several occasions. The biopsy forceps tend to follow the same path, and often the site of heal-

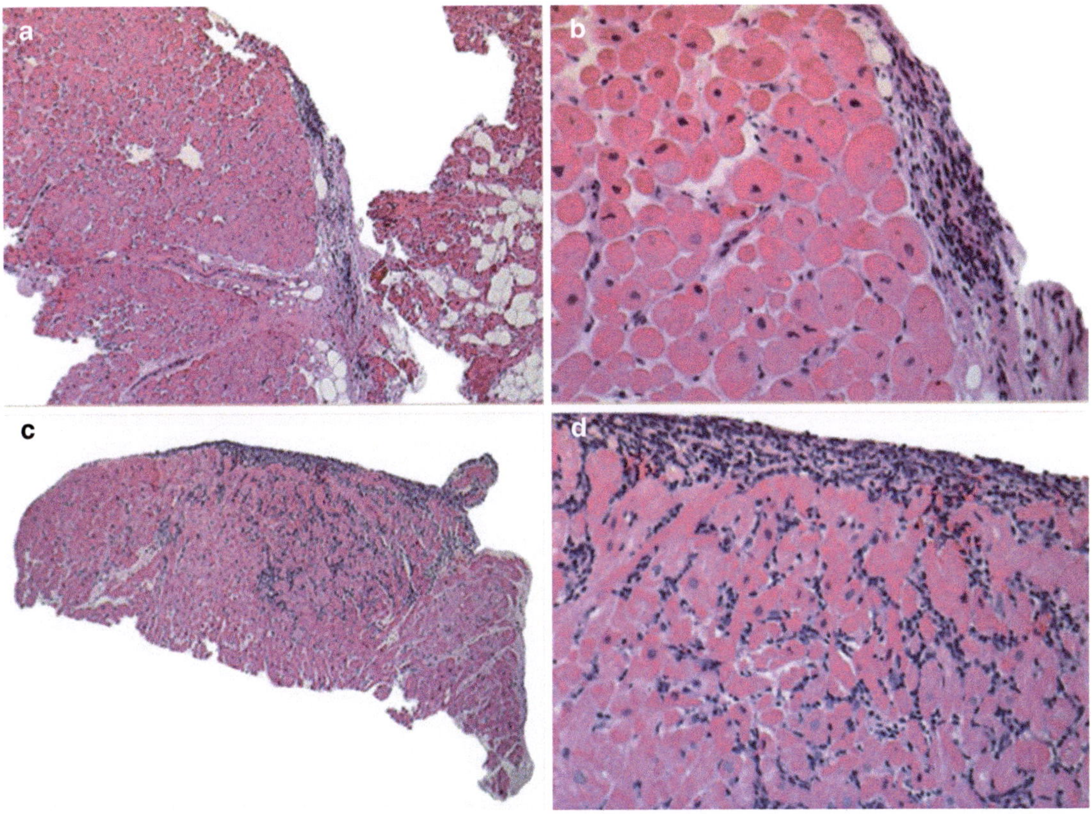

Fig. 16.3 Quilty lesions. (**a**, **b**) Superficial non-encroaching Quilty A lesions (haematoxylin–eosin; **a**, ×25; **b**, ×100) showing location and restriction to the subendocardium. (**c**, **d**) Deep-encroaching Quilty B lesions showing extension of inflammatory infiltrate from the subendocardium to the underlying myocardium and apparent myocyte damage (haematoxylin–eosin, **c**: ×25, **d**: ×100)

ing of a previous biopsy may be included in the samples. Fragments of EMBs which are predominantly previous biopsy sites are excluded by protocol from assessment for rejection grading, as they often include fibrotic reparative tissue/inflammatory granulation tissue or damaged myocytes which should not be mistaken for rejection.

The biopsy forceps cause a traumatic lesion in the myocardium which shows various histologic alterations depending on the time since the traumatic lesion. Recent biopsy sites will have adherent fibrin and blood clots, which organise into granulation tissue and then resolve themselves leaving an area of fibrosis and haemosiderin pigment within macrophages. Altered myocytes (fragmented, vacuolated, hypereosinophilic, coagulated) or necrotic traces of myocytes are scattered within the reparative inflammatory tissue. Moreover, some myocytes, mainly in the border zone between injured and normal myocardium, can be hypertrophic with giant and aberrant nuclei which should not be interpreted as viral cytopathic effect.

The clues to differentiating previous biopsy site from rejection are the subendocardial position, the overlying fibrin if early (assessment of multiple levels may be required to see this feature), the presence of haemosiderin-laden macrophages in intermediate to later lesions and the fact that the myocyte injury is usually disproportionately worse than the infiltrate, unlike rejection where the myocyte injury is

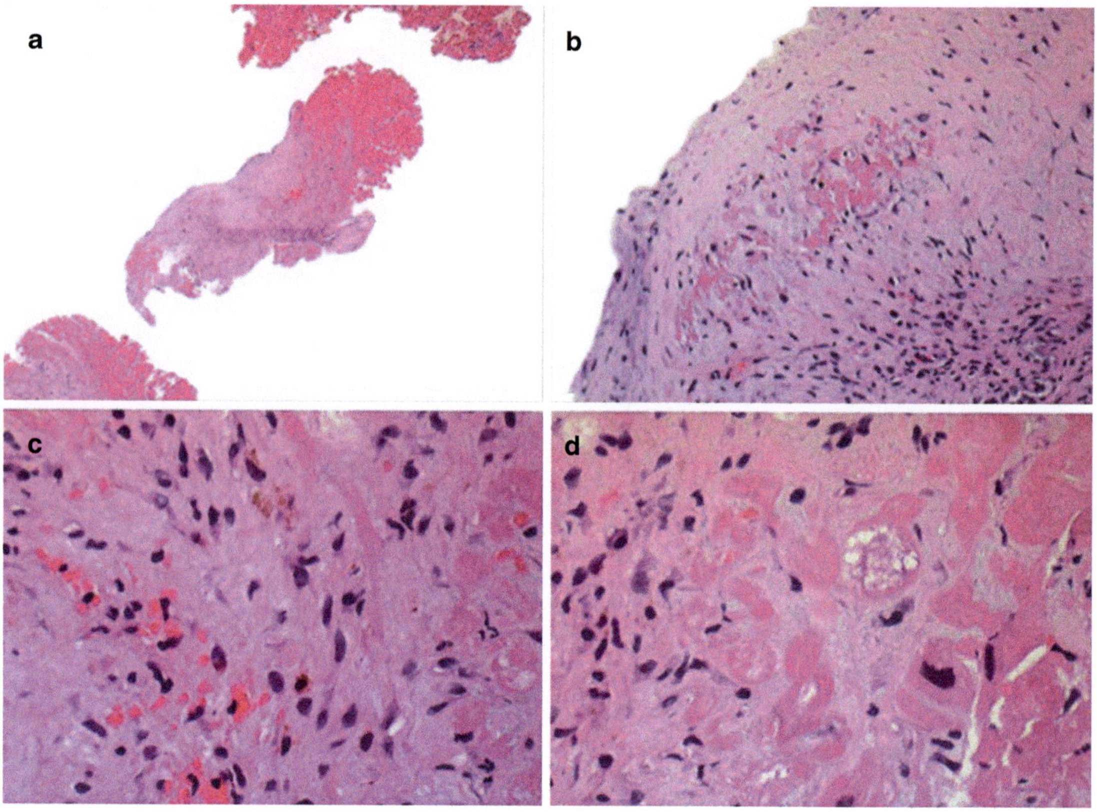

Fig. 16.4 Biopsy site. Routine post-transplant biopsy showing subendocardial location (**a**, haematoxylin–eosin, ×25), wedge shape with organising inflammatory tissue (**b**, haematoxylin–eosin, ×100), pigment in macrophages, fibrin incorporation and damaged myocytes (**c**, **d**: haematoxylin–eosin, ×200)

the consequence of aggressive significant inflammatory infiltrates (Fig. 16.4).

16.5 Subepicardial Tissue

Epicardial adipose tissue is very frequently included in biopsies. In those obtained in the early post-transplant period, fatty tissue may show an inflammatory process related to the postoperative pericarditis: inflammation is usually rich in macrophages and shows reactive multinucleate giant cells and areas of fat necrosis and fibrin (Fig. 16.5). These findings rarely challenge the differential diagnosis of rejection. Subepicardial tissue implies biopsy of the right ventricular free wall, as opposed to the septum, and although a usual finding in EMB, it should be remembered that when it is abundant and includes areas of haemorrhage, a careful assessment for evidence of mesothelium should be undertaken in order to direct clinicians towards possible perforation and check for cardiac tamponade. Later post-transplant perforation is unlikely in transplanted patients, as pericardial adhesions develop with obliteration of the pericardial space.

16.6 Myocyte Calcification

Calcification of myocytes may be seen in EMBs: it is a marker of dead myocytes due to severe mono/paucicellular damage or may be related to

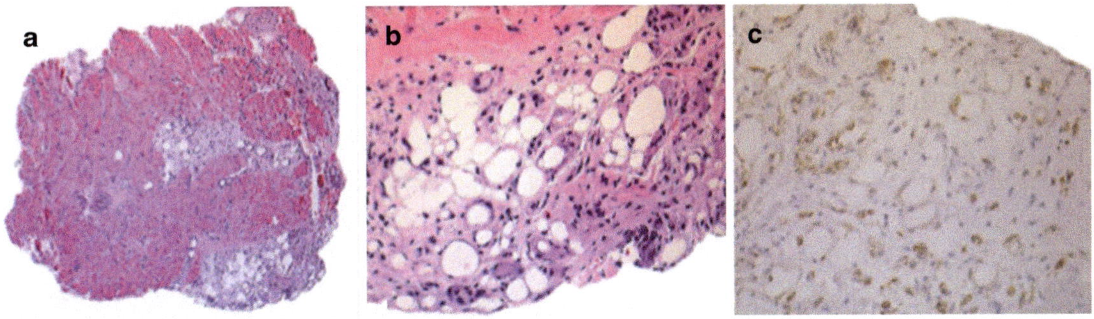

Fig. 16.5 Postoperative pericarditis. Post-transplant EMBs showing steatonecrotic inflammatory process of the subepicardial fat with giant cell reaction and macrophage infiltrate on haematoxylin–eosin (**a**, ×20; **b**, ×200) and on CD68 immunochemistry (**c**: ×200)

clinically significant renal insufficiency. Calcification may appear as blue dots within the cytoplasm and should not be mistaken for bacterial organisms or inclusions (Fig. 16.6): a von Kossa stain can be performed for confirmation if the diagnosis of calcification is not certain.

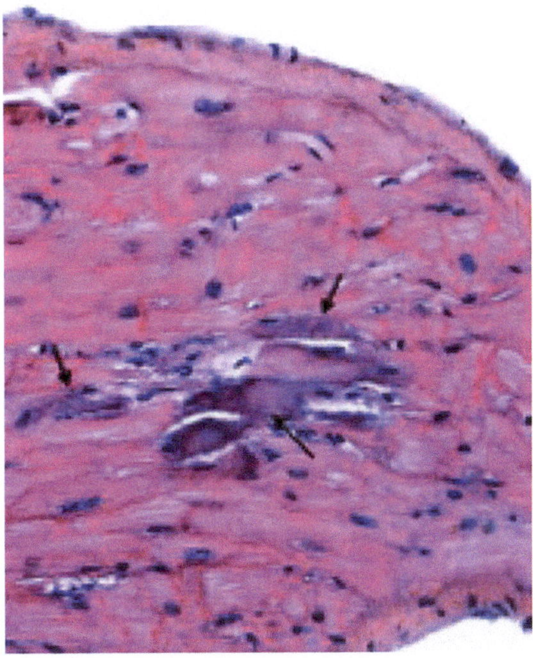

Fig. 16.6 Myocyte calcification. EMB day 8 post-transplant showing myocyte calcification (*arrows*) (haematoxylin–eosin ×200) (Courtesy of Prof A. Angelini)

16.7 Intravascular Lymphocytes

Small lymphatic vessels may show aggregates of lymphocytes within the lumen as a marker of 'lymphatic stasis'. This should not be interpreted as the intravascular activated mononuclear cells of antibody-mediated rejection. The main aspects helping to differentiate this finding from humoral rejection are:

- The focal nature of the lesion
- The packed appearance of the cells
- The absence of any other histologic feature of humoral rejection, especially swelling of the endothelial cells

16.8 Foreign Body

A foreign-body-type reaction with multinucleate giant cells is most often seen in the epicardial adipose tissue as part of postsurgical pericarditis. This finding does not usually determine problems of differential diagnosis with rejection. It should be noted that focal foreign-body-type giant cell reaction may also be found in the subendocardium of the myocardial fragments as a result of the bioptic procedure (due to foreign material adherent to the forceps), and it should not be considered as related to rejection or possible myocarditis.

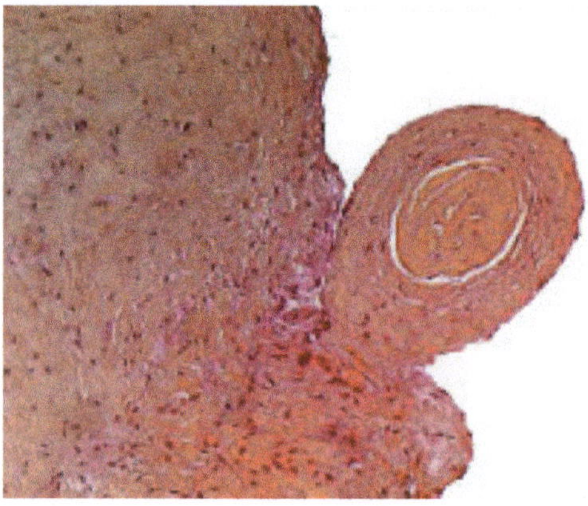

Fig. 16.7 Valve fragments. EMB including a piece of chordae tendineae from the tricuspid valve (haematoxylin–eosin, ×100) (Courtesy of Prof A. Angelini)

16.9 Tricuspid Valve Fragments

Pieces of fibromyxoid connective tissue may be included with the endomyocardial biopsy as the tricuspid valve is biopsied (Fig. 16.7). Clinically significant damage to the valve leading to tricuspid regurgitation is a rare occurrence (Saraiva et al. 2011).

16.10 Liver Fragments

Positioning of the biopsy forceps within the inferior vena cava may lead to a biopsy containing fragments of liver tissue. Fluoroscopic visualisation of the catheter during the procedure reduces the likelihood of malpositioning.

16.11 Late Ischaemic Damage

Late ischaemic damage is characterised by areas of myocytes with sarcoplasmic vacuolisation, scarcely defined contours or actual coagulative necrosis: histologic findings vary with the age of the injury.

There are several possible causes of late ischaemia:

- Cardiac allograft macrovasculopathy
- Cardiac allograft microvasculopathy
- Antibody-mediated rejection
- Native coronary artery atherosclerosis worsening after transplantation

Biopsy findings in the acute phase are similar to those of peritransplant injury (see Table 16.2): myocyte necrosis is typically more prominent than the neutrophilic inflammatory response. Apoptosis of neutrophils follows the initial response, and then macrophages move in as the necrotic myocytes are removed; the dead myocardium is progressively replaced by fibrous tissue.

16.12 Infection

Infections in post-transplant patients are mainly systemic; therefore they are monitored by clinicians using blood tests to evaluate antigenaemia over time and to monitor the therapeutic response to antimicrobiological therapy. However, systemic infections occasionally localise into the cardiac allograft causing an infective myocarditis.

These may occur as a result of one of the following conditions:

- Higher susceptibility to new infections or latent native infection reactivation due to immunosuppressive regimen
- Acquisition of a new infection from the donor when the microorganism is present in the transplanted heart

The incidence of infection is higher in the early post-transplant period, but it may occur at any time.

The principal microorganisms that may be transmitted with the donor organ are viruses, particularly herpesviruses such as cytomegalovirus (CMV) and Epstein–Barr virus (EBV), and intracellular parasites such as toxoplasma and trypanosomes (Chagas' disease).

Myocardial bacteria colonisation is a rare event, and the neutrophil-rich inflammation associated with myocyte necrosis typical of bacterial myocarditis can be easily differentiated from rejection.

Systemic fungal infections are common in transplanted patients, even though rarely localised in the myocardium. Differential diagnosis with rejection is usually not a problem because the inflammatory infiltrates are granulomatous and fungal hyphae can be easily recognised on histologic sections.

The real challenge in histological differential diagnosis with rejection is viral myocarditis, as its histopathological features extensively overlap those associated with rejection, i.e. the presence of lymphocytic inflammatory infiltrates and myocyte damage. However a few hints may facilitate the differential diagnosis. The classic example is CMV infection, where the typical 'owl-eye' intranuclear inclusions within enlarged cells will permit the aetiological diagnosis, which can be easily confirmed by CMV immunostaining. Other viruses, such as herpesvirus, can provoke a peculiar cytopathic effect in infected cells, therefore suggesting a viral aetiology. When suspicion arises it is mandatory to perform molecular tests on cardiac samples (PCR, polymerase chain reaction) for confirmation.

Patients who are antibody negative for CMV pre-transplant are at higher risk of developing the disease post-transplant, especially if the donor is antibody positive. EBV infections may be primary (in patients who were antibody negative before transplant) or reactivations. As well as being a cause of systemic infection, this virus is implicated in 80 % of post-transplant B-cell lymphomas (see below).

In order to reach a correct diagnosis of viral myocarditis, a close interaction between clinicians and pathologists is essential. For instance, an absent response to classical rejection treatment will raise the suspicion of graft infection in the setting of persistence of inflammatory cell infiltrates and myocyte necrosis on EMBs.

Lymphocytic myocarditis may also be the histologic substrate of parasitic infections, such as toxoplasmosis or Chagas' disease, mixed to a variable degree with eosinophils. In toxoplasmosis the diagnosis is based on recognition of the intramyocardial cysts, which appear as a collection of haematoxyphilic 'dots' within the cytoplasm of the myocyte (Fig. 16.8). Chagas' disease is the major cause of cardiac failure in South America where 40 % of transplanted patients experience reactivation of myocarditis in the graft. It is no longer considered a contraindication to transplantation: reactivation causing myocarditis in the new heart is not uncommon but can be treated. In parasitic infections the lymphocytic infiltrates tend to occur away from the infecting organism, so that the inflammatory response may be mistaken for cellular rejection, especially if the biopsy sampling misses the cysts (Fig. 16.9).

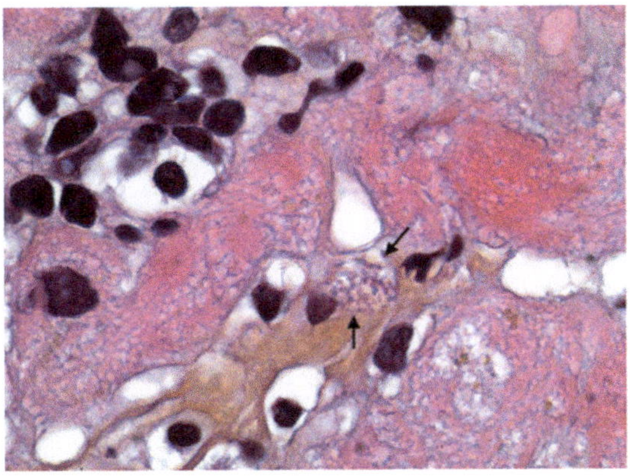

Fig. 16.8 Toxoplasmosis cyst and lymphocytic infiltrate in EMB (haematoxylin–eosin, ×200) (Courtesy of Prof. P. Bruneval)

16.13 Recurrence of Primary Disease

Primary diseases which tend to recur in the cardiac allograft include sarcoid, giant cell myocarditis and amyloid. The pathologist must be informed of the disease of the native heart in order to monitor for possible recurrence.

Giant cell myocarditis is an aggressive inflammatory condition of unknown aetiology which causes rapid onset of cardiac failure and has a high mortality even with aggressive immunosuppressive therapy. Heart transplant often offers the only hope of survival, but recurrence of the disease in the transplanted organ is well recognised and may occur in up to 25 % of cases (Scott et al. 2001). Recurrence has been reported up to 8

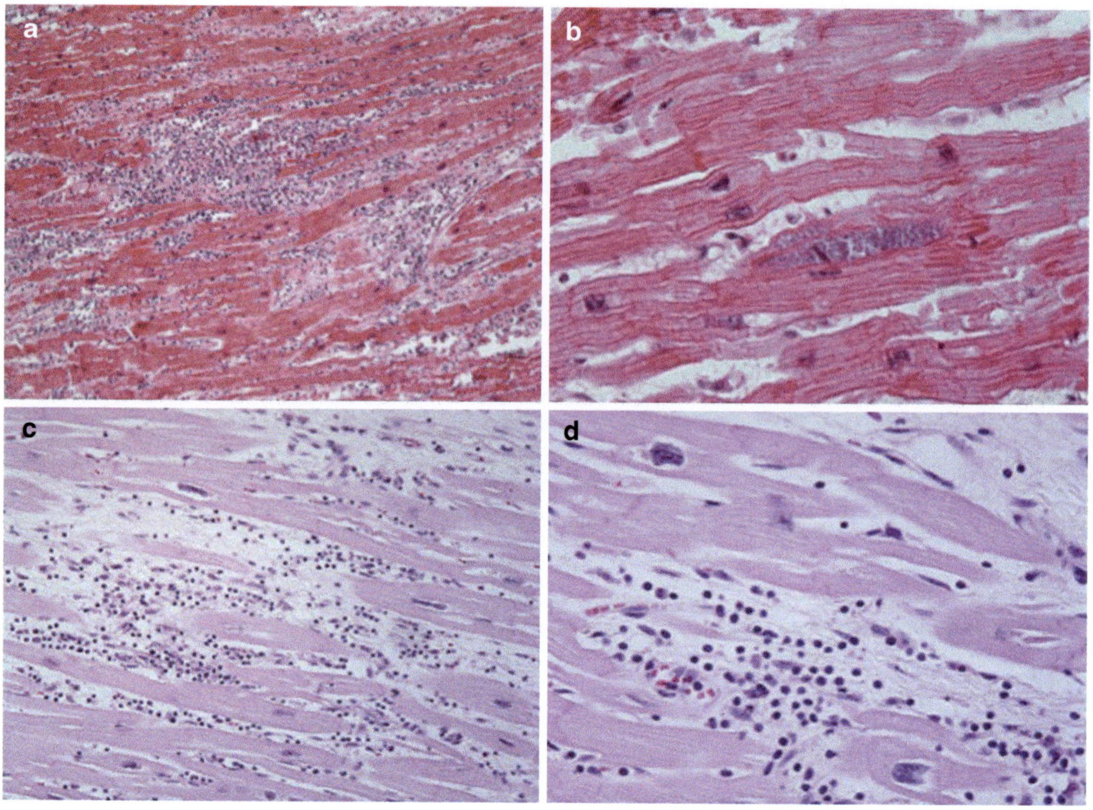

Fig. 16.9 Chagas' disease. EMB showing acute (**a**, **b**: haematoxylin–eosin, ×100, ×200) and chronic (**c**, **d**: ×100, ×200) trypanosomiasis of the myocardium (Courtesy of Prof. G. Berry)

years after transplant (Maleszewski et al. 2015). The diagnosis can be made on endomyocardial biopsy where multinucleate giant cells, extensive myocyte damage and necrosis and a polymorphous inflammatory infiltrate are seen.

Sarcoidosis is a disease with a protean presentation and is frequently diagnosed only on examination of the explanted heart. The granulomatous infiltrate may be asymptomatic for some time and present as the result of extensive fibrosis which can cause restrictive or dilated-type symptomatology, or the presentation may be with arrhythmia. The presence of the typical granulomata in post-transplant EMBs can guide diagnosis, but recurrent disease is rarely of any clinical significance (Banga et al. 2015), and again the immunosuppressive regime post-transplant is likely to suppress the disease systemically and in the cardiac allograft.

A recurrence of amyloidosis can be easily diagnosed at EMB on histological examination; as a noninflammatory process, it does not mimic rejection.

16.14 Post-transplant Lymphoproliferative Disorder (PTLD)

The incidence of PTLD ranges from 2 to 6% in heart transplants, and it is the third leading cause of death in these patients. More than 50% of patients with PTLD present with extra-nodal masses, but involvement of the cardiac allograft or development of lymphoma in the heart is rare: in one meta-analysis, it is reported as 7.3% of heart transplant patients with PTLD (Khemad and Taheri 2011). In those with allograft involvement, the PTLD tends to involve multiple organs and to occur earlier post-transplant with a poorer outcome compared to those with PTLD at another site. There is a higher incidence of PTLD in patients who received higher levels of immunosuppression.

PTLD may present as a polymorphous, polyclonal lymphoplasmacytic proliferation or can be a high-grade lymphoma composed of large poorly differentiated cells. In the former case, it may be difficult to distinguish it in an EMB from Quilty effect or rejection: in the latter immunohistochemistry may be required to distinguish it from other types of poorly differentiated malignancy or from rejection.

The lesions range from lymphocyte hyperplasia to frank lymphomas, and have been divided into four basic histological types in the 2008 WHO classification of tumours of haematopoietic and lymphoid tissues (Table 16.3) (Parker et al. 2010).

In *early lesions* there is preservation of underlying tissue architecture with mixed B and T lymphocytes and plasma cells. Two histological patterns are seen:

1. Plasmacytic hyperplasia
2. Infectious mononucleosis-like

They are usually polyclonal and usually positive for EBV proteins by immunohistochemistry (LMP1) or EBV-encoded RNA (EBERs) by in situ hybridisation.

Polymorphic PTLD is characterised by destruction of underlying tissue architecture and shows a full spectrum of B lymphocytes. Most of these lesions express EBER or LMP1.

Table 16.3 Classification of PTLD

1. Early lesions	Polyclonal, positive for EBV
2. Polymorphic PTLD	Spectrum of B lymphocytes, positive for EBV
3. Monomorphic PTLD	Usually B cell, positive for EBV
4. Classical Hodgkin lymphoma type	Reed–Sternberg cells positive for EBERs

In *monomorphic PTLD* there is architectural and cytological atypia of a degree readily classified as lymphoma on morphological features. It is usually B-cell lineage, but some T-cell and natural killer (NK)-cell lymphomas occur. Most of the B-cell lymphomas are diffuse large B-cell lymphomas, but Burkitt lymphoma, plasma cell myeloma and plasmacytoma-like lesions also occur. The B-cell and NK-cell lymphomas are usually positive for EBV.

In *classical Hodgkin lymphoma type,* the majority of Reed–Sternberg cells are positive for EBERs (Tsao and Hsi 2007). Frequently the inflammatory cell infiltrate is characterised by abundant plasma cells, raising the suspicion of PTLD and triggering further evaluation.

In Western countries 85 % of PTLD is B cell and 80 % of these are EBV driven. Thus it is important to perform EBV in situ hybridisation for detection of EBV viral genome on EMBs if PTLD of B-cell origin is suspected, as well as molecular analysis for monoclonality of B or T cells. It is also important to phenotype the lymphocytes because prognosis and treatment differ for the rarer NK- and T-cell types.

16.15 Artefacts

Contraction bands are routinely seen in EMBs as the fragments of myocardium contract when put into formalin. They are not indicative of myocardial damage.

In addition a blood vessel within or at the edge of the myocardium pulled out by the biopsy forceps may 'telescope' up on fixation so that there appears to be folding of a vessel within the vessel.

Haemorrhage may frequently be seen within the myocardium as a result of trauma during the biopsy. Haemorrhage secondary to the biopsy procedure can be differentiated from haemorrhage seen as part of severe ACR or AMR by the absence of associated oedema or inflammatory infiltrate or other findings of rejection.

Fragments of mural thrombus from the endocardial surface, often showing a degree of organisation, can be sampled instead of the myocardium. These may be difficult to distinguish from the myocardium macroscopically and can lead to inadequate sampling of the myocardium as the clinician mistakes them for myocardial tissue.

Key Points

- Although EMBs are mainly done to assess rejection, a range of other pathologies or histological findings may be found and need to be recognised and distinguished from the changes of cellular- and antibody-mediated rejection.
- Some of these other conditions/findings are easily distinguished from rejection; others share with rejection the key features of inflammation and myocardial damage.
- These findings arise from different situations:
  - The transplant process (peritransplant injury)
  - The immunosuppressive therapy (Quilty effect)
  - Biopsy procedure (previous biopsy site; subepicardial tissue, foreign body, tricuspid valve fragments, liver fragments) or biopsy preparation (artefacts)
  - Events or pathologies/complications occurring post-transplantation (myocyte calcification, intravascular lymphocytes, late ischaemic damage, infection, post-transplant lymphoproliferative disorder, recurrence of primary disease)

Illustrative Case (Fig. 16.10)

A patient was retransplanted for diffuse graft vasculopathy 6.5 years post-heart transplantation for alcoholic cardiomyopathy.

On macroscopic examination the explanted heart had scattered whitish areas in the ventricular myocardium, the most extensive in LV inferior wall (Fig. 16.10a).

Microscopically these consisted of large lymphoid aggregates within the myocardium, associated with infiltration and destruction of the myocardium (Fig. 16.10b). There are prominent vessels with plump endothelium within these nodules (Fig. 16.10c).

The infiltrate consisted of B-cell aggregates (CD20+, CD79a+, Bcl2+, CD5- and CD10-) surrounded by CD3+ T cells with scattered macrophages. There were no CD30-positive blasts. CD21-positive follicular dendritic cells were present within the B-cell areas. There was no evidence of EBV infection with LMP1 and EBERs being negative. Molecular assessment of the B and T cells showed a polyclonal population of cells.

Conclusion: The pattern of lymphoid infiltration is worrying for a PTLD, with morphology suggestive of a follicular lymphoma. The lack of evidence for EBV infection is unusual.

Diagnosis: Suspicion for PTLD (follicular lymphoma).

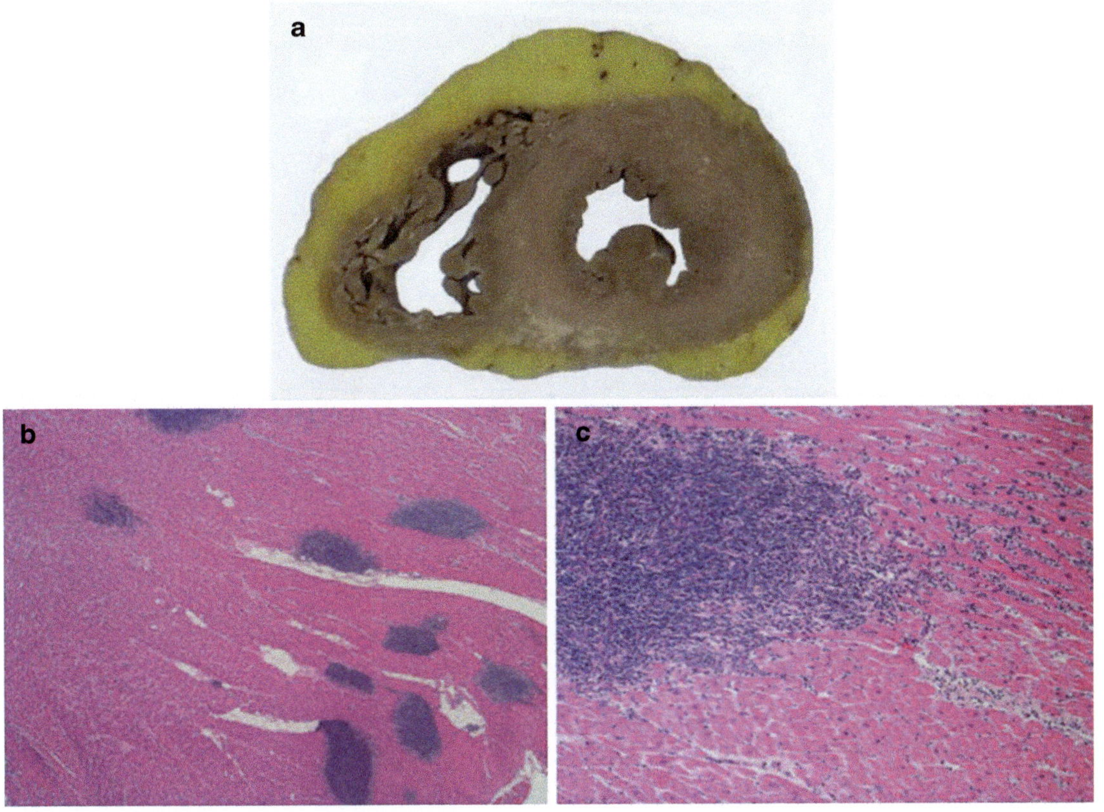

Fig. 16.10 Illustrative case. (**a**) Macroscopic view of a mid-slice of the heart with whitish infiltrate of the left ventricle. (**b**) Histology of the myocardium at low power shows infiltration by lymphoid cells (haematoxylin–eosin, ×100). (**c**) At medium power destruction of the myocardium by lymphoid infiltrate is evident (haematoxylin–eosin, ×200)

References

Atkinson C, Floerchinger B, Qiao F, Casey S, Williamson T, Moseley E, Stoica S, Goddard M, Ge X, Tullius SG, Tomlinson S. Donor brain death exacerbates complement-dependent ischemia/reperfusion injury in transplanted hearts. Circulation. 2013;127:1290–9.

Banga A, Sahoo D, Lane CR, Farver CF, Budev MM. Disease recurrence and acute cellular rejection episodes during the first year after lung transplantation among patients with sarcoidosis. Transplantation. 2015;99(9):1940–5.

Di Carlo E, D'Antuono T, Contento S, Di NM, Ballone E, Sorrentino C. Quilty effect has the features of lymphoid neogenesis and shares CXCL13-CXCR5 pathway with recurrent acute cardiac rejections. Am J Transplant. 2007;7:201–10.

Ferreira MA, Owen HE, Howie AJ. High prevalence of acute myocardial damage in a hospital necropsy series, shown by C9 immunohistology. J Clin Pathol. 1998;51(7):548–51.

Khemad H, Taheri S. Heart allograft involvement by post-transplant lymphoproliferative disorders: report from the PTLD Int survey. Exp Clin Transplant. 2011;9(4):258–64.

Maleszewski JJ, Orellana VM, Hodge DO, Kuhl U, Schultheiss HP, Cooper LT. Long-term risk of recurrence, morbidity and mortality in giant cell myocarditis. Am J Cardiol. 2015;115(12):1733–8.

Parker A, Bowles K, Bradley JA, et al. Diagnosis of post-transplant lymphoproliferative disorder in solid organ transplant recipients – BCSH and BTS guidelines. Br J Haematol. 2010;149:675–92.

Saraiva F, Matos V, Gonçalves L, Antunes M, Providência LA. Complications of endomyocardial biopsy in heart transplant patients: a retrospective study of 2117 consecutive procedures. Transplant Proc. 2011;43(5):1908–12.

Sattar HA, Husain AN, Kim AY, Krausz T. The presence of a CD21+ follicular dendritic cell network distinguishes invasive quilty lesions from cardiac acute cellular rejection. Am J Surg Pathol. 2006;30:1008–13.

Scott RL, Ratliff NB, Starling RC, Young JB. Recurrence of giant cell myocarditis in cardiac allograft. J Heart Lung Transplant. 2001;20(3):375–80.

Tsao L, Hsi ED. The clinicopathologic spectrum of post-transplantation lymphoproliferative disorders. Arch Pathol Lab Med. 2007;131:1209–18.

Noninvasive Tools for Monitoring Acute Cardiac Allograft Rejection: State of the Art

17

Marie-Claude Parent, Brian A. Clarke, and Kiran K. Khush

Contents

M.-C. Parent, MD, MSc, FRCPC
Division of Cardiology, Hôpital du Sacré-Coeur de Montréal, Université de Montréa, Montréal, Québec, Canada
e-mail: drmc.parent@gmail.com

B.A. Clarke
Division of Cardiology, Department of Medicine, Dalhousie University and the QE II Health Science Center, Halifax, NS, Canada

K.K. Khush (✉)
Division of Cardiovascular Medicine, Stanford University School of Medicine, Stanford, CA, USA
e-mail: kiran@stanford.edu

17.1 Background

The diagnosis of acute cardiac allograft rejection in heart transplant patients is challenging because it often presents in the absence of symptoms and is important because it increases the risk of allograft dysfunction, cardiac allograft vasculopathy, and death. Since its introduction in the 1970s, endomyocardial biopsy (EMB) has been the gold standard for routine surveillance and diagnosis of acute rejection. However, significant limitations associated with this invasive technique have spurred clinicians and researchers to develop a noninvasive alternative to endomyocardial biopsy.

Validation of noninvasive markers of heart transplant rejection—one of many obstacles faced in this quest—is inherently challenging for several reasons:

- The limitations of endomyocardial biopsy (Table 17.1)
- The large sample sizes required to prove statistical superiority or equivalence of new monitoring strategies

O. Leone et al. (eds.), *The Pathology of Cardiac Transplantation*,
DOI 10.1007/978-3-319-46386-5_17

- The potentially confounding role of antibody-mediated rejection, a less well-understood and less easily diagnosed process that has been recognized only recently.

Table 17.1 Limitations of endomyocardial biopsy

Patient discomfort
Time and resource intensive
Complications Pneumothorax Tricuspid regurgitation Ventricular perforation, cardiac tamponade Arrhythmias Access site complications
Sampling error (false negative) related to small number of samples and patchy distribution of rejection
"Mimics" of acute rejection (false positive): Quilty B effect, focal ischemic injury
Inter-observer variability (58 % concordance for grade 3 acute cellular rejection (ACR))

Since the majority of clinical studies evaluating novel noninvasive markers of rejection pertain to acute cellular rejection and because of the paucity of data regarding the utility of these makers in the detection of antibody-mediated rejection, the scope of this chapter will focus exclusively on the noninvasive diagnosis of acute cellular rejection (ACR).

17.2 Noninvasive Approaches for Heart Transplant Rejection

17.2.1 Surface and Intramyocardial Electrocardiography

A variety of 12-lead electrocardiographic changes have been observed during acute rejection including atrial premature excitation, atrial fibrillation/flutter, and low QRS amplitude. These observations led to the study of intramyocardial electrocardiography (IMEG) using screw-in epicardial biventricular leads for detection of acute rejection. Although initial studies demonstrated an overall good sensitivity with excellent negative predictive value (NPV), subsequent reports failed to verify the high NPV, thereby limiting widespread adoption of this technique. More recently, an animal model using a small leadless device implanted at the time of transplantation has shown 86 % sensitivity and 100 % specificity for detection of moderate to severe acute cellular rejection (grade ≥2R) (Horai et al. 2009).

17.2.2 Cardiac Imaging

17.2.2.1 Echocardiography

Transthoracic echocardiography is the primary noninvasive imaging modality for heart transplant recipients. It is commonly used to assess left ventricular (LV) systolic function when there is a high suspicion for acute rejection despite negative EMB findings and to subsequently monitor allograft function during confirmed episodes.

Initial echocardiographic studies focused on the increase in LV wall thickness and LV mass, as well as the decrease in systolic function during acute rejection. However, because these changes are not always present and typically occur late in the course of rejection, they were deemed too insensitive for early detection. The presence of a pericardial effusion is also an insensitive marker of acute rejection as it is frequently observed, particularly in the first few months post-transplant, regardless of rejection status.

Another approach has been to evaluate the diastolic function of the transplanted heart with echocardiography. Diastolic dysfunction usually precedes systolic dysfunction in acute rejection and may provide a more sensitive marker. Multiple studies have documented significant differences in Doppler filling parameters between rejecting and non-rejecting allografts and the subsequent normalization to baseline diastolic parameters following rejection treatment (Dandel et al. 2001; Sun et al. 2005). The wide range of accuracy with this method is due to the variability in acute rejection diagnostic criteria, small sample sizes, heterogeneity of the patient populations studied, and the inconsistent definition of diastolic parameters. It is also important to emphasize that modifications in diastolic function may also occur with changes in heart rate and loading conditions, such as is observed with hypertension or allograft vasculopathy, both of which are common in heart transplant recipients. A recent meta-analysis concluded that the inconsistent quality of the studies and the overall low sensitivities do not support the use of traditional diastolic indices by echocardiography as a screening tool for detection of acute rejection after heart transplantation (Mena et al. 2006).

The myocardial performance index (MPI) is a combination of Doppler-derived systolic and diastolic time intervals and has the potential to detect rejection more accurately than traditional Doppler indices. However, the utility of MPI requires further validation (Bader et al. 2011).

Strain and strain rate imaging using tissue Doppler imaging (TDI) or speckle tracking represent relatively new methods in echocardiography that are used to demonstrate quantitatively the changes in dimension of a specific segment of the myocardium (Saleh et al. 2011). These methods have demonstrated promising results in recent studies for early detection of acute cardiac rejection (Kato et al. 2010), but have not yet been tested extensively. The evaluation of LV systolic torsion (LV-Tor) derived from two-dimensional speckle-tracking echocardiography could also be of clinical value for noninvasive monitoring of acute rejection in the near future (Sato et al. 2011).

In summary, clinical studies have demonstrated that no single echocardiographic feature has enough sensitivity or specificity to detect acute rejection. Future studies focusing on combinatorial methods, incorporating both diastolic and systolic parameters, in addition to newer modalities such as strain imaging, may plausibly lead to the development and validation of an "echo rejection score" (Roshanali et al. 2010). Large multicenter studies will be necessary to evaluate the utility of echocardiography for detection of acute rejection as well as to set cutoff values for newly developed echocardiographic indices (Kato et al. 2013).

17.2.2.2 Cardiac Magnetic Resonance Imaging

Cardiac magnetic resonance (CMR) imaging is a potentially attractive screening modality for detection of acute rejection. Its lack of ionizing radiation and its ability to assess multiple aspects of myocardial injury in a single examination make it a promising imaging modality. CMR imaging is also able to survey the entire myocardium, thereby possibly decreasing the likelihood of false-negative results secondary to sampling error, as is seen in endomyocardial biopsy.

T2-weighted imaging has been the most widely studied sequence in the setting of acute rejection. T2 values are known to be prolonged in tissues with high water content, which appears during tissue injury process, subsequent inflammation, and edema, as is seen in acute myocardial infraction, myocarditis, and acute rejection. In the largest human study using T2-weighted imaging, T2 relaxation times were higher in patients with moderate to severe rejection at biopsy (grades 2 and 3, ISHLT 1990 grading system) than in those without rejection (60 ± 7 ms vs. 51 ± 6 ms, $p = 0.0001$) (Marie et al. 2001). A T2 value ≥ 2 standard deviations (SD) of normal (i.e., ≥ 56 ms) was the best cutoff value to separate patients with and without grade ≥ 2 rejection with a sensitivity of 89 % and specificity of 70 %. This criterion was associated with a high NPV of 97 %, but with a much lower PPV of 35 %. These results need to be interpreted with caution as this study primarily recruited patients suspected of having acute rejection, thus introducing a potential sample bias. More recently, T2 mapping without contrast has also been tested with sensitivity and specificity of 86 % and 95 %, respectively, using T2 time cutoff of 56.4 ms (Usman et al. 2012). The results also suggested that T2 mapping may be useful for assessing the response to acute rejection therapy as resolution of elevated T2 relaxation times indicates that the treatment for acute rejection was successful, whereas T2 values that remain elevated may indicate ongoing rejection.

Currently, the utility of late gadolinium enhancement (LGE) imaging in the transplant population is unclear as most investigations were not performed on patients with acute rejection (Steen et al. 2008). The sensitivity of LGE is likely insufficient to detect the microscopic and diffuse nature of myocyte necrosis that occurs during acute rejection episodes; however, cumulative insults may result in patchy myocardial fibrosis more easily revealed with LGE (Miller et al. 2013). Only limited reports of LGE in the presence of acute cardiac rejection have been described in the literature, and further studies on a larger cohort of patients with acute rejection will be needed to adequately validate this approach (Estep et al. 2009). However, the presence of *early* gadolinium enhancement has been described in the setting of acute rejection due to regional hyperemia, vasodilatation, and capillary leakage associated with inflammation. A recent study found a positive association between rejection and early relative myocardial enhancement with 82 % sensitivity and 79 % specificity (Taylor et al. 2010). When rejection was defined as an increase in early contrast enhancement *or* myocardial edema on T2-weighted imaging (STIR), the sensitivity improved to 100 %, with a minimal reduction in specificity to 73 % (Taylor et al. 2010).

In the near future, investigational contrast agents such as ultrasmall superparamagnetic iron oxide (USPIO) particles may improve the sensitivity of CMR in detecting areas of inflammation (Wu et al. 2009). When injected intravenously, these particles are ingested by circulating macrophages. The labeled macrophages migrate into the rejecting graft, and in situ macrophage accumulation can be detected as hypointense regions on T2-weighted CMR. Although current USPIO preparations are safe for human administration, there have been no human studies applying USPIO-enhanced CMRI for detection of acute cardiac rejection to date.

Finally, novel sequences using contrast-free T1-mapping and T2-mapping techniques have opened a new frontier for the quantitative exploration of tissue characteristics using CMR imaging. More studies with contemporary CMR imaging platforms and sequences are needed to evaluate the sensitivity and specificity for acute rejection diagnosis. A systematic rejection scoring system with CMR may provide a more standardized assessment of rejection (Butler et al. 2009).

17.2.2.3 Nuclear Imaging

Radionuclide imaging techniques have also been studied for the noninvasive detection of acute rejection. Many cellular components have been targeted, including ^{111}indium-labeled antibodies targeted to myosin, which is released in the setting of inflammation with disruption of cellular membranes (Hesse et al. 1995); ^{99m}technetium-labeled annexin-V, a marker of apoptotic cell death (Narula et al. 2001; Kown et al. 2001); and ^{111}indium-labeled lymphocytes and ^{99m}technetium-labeled oligonucleotides complementary to mRNA of interleukin-2, which is overexpressed during acute rejection (Rubin et al. 1996; Gierthmuehlen et al. 2010). However, the clinical utility of these imaging techniques has not been proven thus far, and the radiation burden associated with repeated tests is possibly deleterious.

PET imaging was tested recently in a well-established murine cardiac rejection model. PET imaging with [18F]FDG was able to detect heart transplant rejection and to monitor the evolution of rejection (Daly KP et al. 2015). More recent systems combining CT imaging with either single-photon emission computed tomography (SPECT) or positron emission tomography (PET) have led to improve image quantification. PET/CT imaging of monocyte/macrophage infiltration in a murine heart transplant model using phagocytosable nanoparticles with the long-lived PET isotope copper-64 may offer a quantitative and noninvasive alternative to EMB (Ueno et al. 2013).

17.3 Breath Testing

Allograft rejection is accompanied by oxidative stress resulting from increased production of reactive oxygen species (ROS) in the myocardium. These ROS subsequently degrade cellular membranes by lipid peroxidation generating alkanes that are excreted in the breath as volatile organic compounds (VOCs). Theoretically, these VOCs could provide markers of the intensity of rejection. A study published by Phillips et al.

(2004) demonstrated that breath testing has a high negative predictive value to identify grade 3 rejection (1990 ISHLT grading scheme) and could potentially reduce the number of endomyocardial biopsies performed. A multicenter study to validate these findings is ongoing (http://clinicaltrials.gov).

17.4 Biomarkers

17.4.1 Brain Natriuretic Peptide (BNP) and N-Terminal Pro-brain Natriuretic Peptide (NT Pro-BNP)

Studies correlating absolute BNP or NT pro-BNP levels with episodes of allograft rejection have been sparse and conflicting. However, more recent analysis showed that serial BNP monitoring may be effective for clinical and functional allograft surveillance if combined with clinical examination and/or echocardiography, once routine endomyocardial biopsies have been discontinued. The main advantage of serial BNP monitoring is its wide availability, rapid turnaround time, low cost, and excellent negative predictive value of 95–97 % (Kittleson et al. 2009; Garrido et al. 2009; Damodaran et al. 2012).

17.4.2 Serum Troponin (TnT, TnI) and High-Sensitivity Troponin (hs-TnT, hs-TnI)

Since acute rejection is characterized by myocardial cell destruction, the use of cardiac troponin (troponin T and troponin I) has been examined as a marker of acute rejection. However, most studies have documented poor sensitivity and inadequate negative predictive value for clinical use.

New high-sensitivity (hs) troponin assays are approximately tenfold more sensitive than assays evaluated in these previous studies (Mohammed and Januzzi 2010; Morrow 2009). The performance of the hs-cTnI assay for rejection using a cut point of 15 ng/L demonstrated a sensitivity of 94 %, specificity of 60 %, positive predictive value of 18 %, and negative predictive value of 99 % (Patel et al. 2014). Based on these results, the measurement of hs-TnI could be a useful surveillance method to rule out acute rejection, especially in low-risk subjects. Another study using hs-TnT suggested that concentrations <17 ng/L may rule out acute rejection with a sensitivity and negative predictive value (NPV) of 100 % (Méndez et al. 2014). This noninvasive test may be particularly useful in patients with contraindications to EMB and in those with insufficient material for histopathologic analysis.

Finally, a multimarker approach using a combination of biomarkers, such as change in BNP or NT pro-BNP with hs-TnI/T, may improve on the test performance of each assay alone (Dyer et al. 2012).

17.4.3 Immunologic Biomarkers

The usefulness of a noninvasive biomarker resides in its ability to detect early signs of acute rejection, as opposed to confirmation of the process once it is well underway. As such, markers of myocyte death may be inadequate, as they reflect late tissue degradation. Growing attention has been focused on chemokines, a family of powerful small chemotactic peptides that play a pivotal role in the control of leukocyte trafficking during acute rejection and other inflammatory conditions. In particular, CXCL10 constitutes a potential biomarker of acute rejection as it initiates and amplifies the host alloresponse (Crescioli et al. 2009). A recently described and innovative method utilizes integrated RNA data-driven proteomics (IRDDP) to discover candidate proteomic biomarkers of allograft rejection (Chen et al. 2010). Using this method, three candidate biomarkers were found to be significantly upregulated in patients undergoing acute cellular rejection: PECAM 1 (CD31 antigen), CXCL9 (MIG, chemokine ligand 9), and CD44 (hyaluronic acid receptor). The integration of gene expression microarray measurements from disease samples with publicly available data sets could be a powerful, fast, and cost-effective strategy for discovering diagnostic serum protein biomarkers.

17.5 Genomic Markers

17.5.1 Gene Expression Profiling (GEP)

Recent studies have investigated the value of genomic markers of acute rejection using the gene expression profile of peripheral blood leukocytes. In the multicenter Cardiac Allograft Rejection Gene Expression Observation (CARGO) study, a multigene algorithm based on the differential expression of 20 genes (11 informative, 9 control) in peripheral blood mononuclear cells was developed and validated to discriminate between a quiescent state (grade 0) and moderate/severe rejection (grade ≥2R) in cardiac transplant recipients (Deng et al. 2006). A scoring system based on the differential gene expression profile identified patients at low risk for moderate/severe rejection (84 % agreement with biopsy results) and an NPV of 99.6 % in patients with a score <30 beyond the first year post-transplant. This gene expression profiling (GEP) technology is now commercially available (AlloMap®) and is used at many US transplant centers and has become available in Europe in the late 2015. Patients who are either more than 2 months post-transplant with an AlloMap® score <20, more than 6 months post-transplant with an AlloMap® score <30, or greater than 1 year post-transplant with an AlloMap® score <34 have a very low risk of acute cellular rejection and therefore may not require endomyocardial biopsy (Fig. 17.1) (Starling et al. 2006).

The IMAGE study was a multicenter, nonblinded, randomized clinical trial that compared a noninvasive rejection surveillance strategy using gene expression profiling (GEP) with AlloMap®, to an invasive endomyocardial biopsy-based strategy (Pham et al. 2010). Over 600 patients between 6 months and 5 years post-transplant were randomized. The IMAGE study results suggest that GEP with AlloMap® is non-inferior to the standard EMB protocols in surveillance for cellular rejection in low-risk patients who are more than 6 months post-transplant, utilizing a threshold AlloMap® value of 34, and resulted in the performance of significantly fewer biopsies. Furthermore, a low GEP score was associated with a low future risk of rejection, suggesting that the test may be useful in identifying low-risk patients. It is important not to extrapolate these findings to patients felt to be at high risk of acute rejection, such as those with recurrent or persistent rejection, with recent changes to their immunosuppressive drug regimens, or with high-risk demographic profiles (e.g., multiparous women, blacks, and highly sensitized patients), and on its value in excluding antibody-mediated rejection (AMR Mehra and Parameshwar 2010; Patel et al. 2011).

The preliminary results of Early IMAGE (EIMAGE) study, a randomized trial of AlloMap® vs. EMB, were published recently (Kobashigawa et al. 2013). This trial recruited 60 patients in their first year post-transplant, beginning 2 months after transplant. A biopsy was performed if AlloMap® score was >30 in the first 6 months or >34 in the second 6 months. The primary endpoint was a composite of death or re-transplant, hemodynamic compromise with rejection, or graft dysfunction. There was no significant difference in the primary endpoint between AlloMap® and EAMB groups ($p = 0.45$), and left ventricular ejection fraction was also similar. Patient satisfaction score was higher in AlloMap® group vs. EMB group ($p = 0.003$). IVUS data that could confirm the safety of this approach are still pending.

The variability of GEP test scores within a single patient over time may be used to predict risk of future clinical events, including allograft dysfunction and death. For example, a recipient predicted to be at low risk for future events may become a candidate for further minimization of immunosuppressive maintenance regimen. Conversely, an individual predicted to be at higher risk for future events may receive further evaluation to detect possible underlying causes of the variability such as overlooked infections or noncompliance to medications (Deng et al. 2014). Similarly, the results of CARGO 2 study showed that after 12 months, GEP score instability ($p = 0.001$) and GEP ≥34 ($p = 0.06$) may predict future events (Crespo-Leiro et al. 2012, 2013).

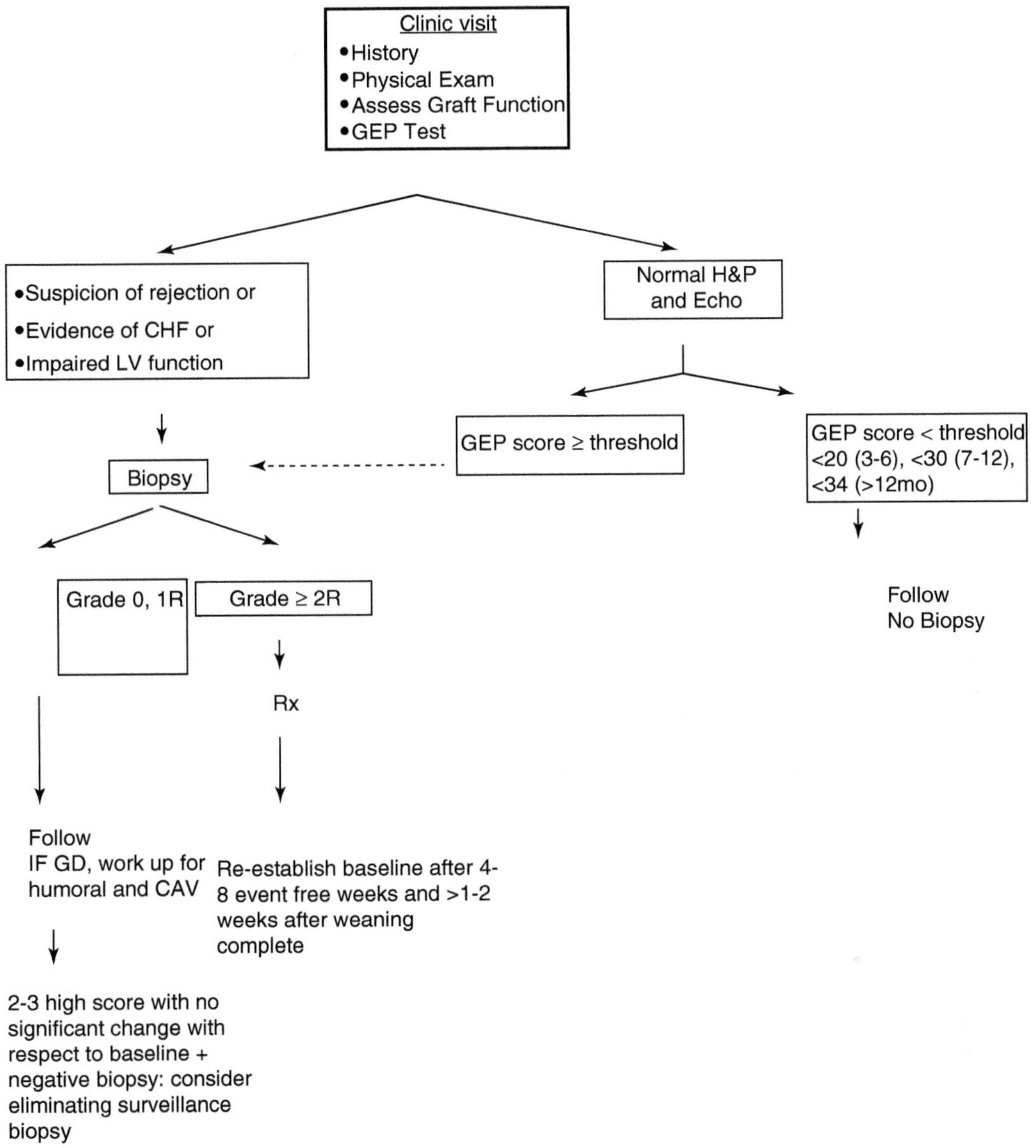

Fig. 17.1 Proposed rejection surveillance using gene expression profiling (*GEP*) in stable heart transplant recipients (From: Starling et al. 2006)

A study by McManus et al. evaluated the whole blood samples from cardiac transplant recipients and identified 12 candidate genes that correlated well with acute cellular rejection (sensitivity 83 %, specificity 75 %) (Lin et al. 2009; Hollander et al. 2010). Of note, none of the 12 genes in the panel were identified in CARGO. This discrepancy may possibly be due to the difference between the whole blood versus peripheral blood monocyte samples and to the use of different microarrays. There is a prospective Canadian trial underway testing this biomarker panel in multiple independent settings.

Interestingly, there seems to be a common immunological mechanism for acute rejection across different solid organ transplants. Serum proteins highly increased in acute renal transplant rejection were also increased during cardiac and liver acute rejection (Khatri et al. 2013). Recently, ten genes associated with renal allograft rejection in blood were tested in the diagnosis and prediction of cardiac allograft rejection (Li et al. 2013). The original ten-gene panel was then narrowed to a smaller set of five genes (DUSP1, FNGR1, MAPK9, PBEF1, and RYBP) that were not confounded by clinical variables, such as transplant recipient age and sex, time post-transplant, or innate immune activation. The five-gene panel discriminated acute rejection from concomitant CMV infection with 87 % sensitivity, 90 % specificity, 94 % PPV, and 80 % NPV. The high specificity and PPV—features unique to the five-gene panel—could help clinicians *rule in* the presence of rejection in contrast to AlloMap® testing which can *rule out* the presence of rejection by virtue of its high NPV. Further studies are required to evaluate the usefulness of this gene set as a means to titrate immunosuppression in heart transplantation, while reducing the need for frequent protocol biopsies.

17.5.2 Genome Transplant Dynamics

Current investigational efforts have focused on the detection and quantification of donor-derived cell-free DNA (dd-cfDNA) in the peripheral blood of heart transplant recipients (Fig. 17.2). Instead of monitoring the recipient immune response, an assay that directly measures the amount of dd-cfDNA, as a marker of graft injury, has been developed (Tong and Lo 2006). The theory underlying this approach lies in the observation that cellular rejection results in myocyte lysis and apoptosis, causing the release of donor DNA into the recipient circulation. Past research in solid organ transplantation attempted to identify cell-free DNA in sex-mismatched female recipients of male donor organs, where chromosome Y served as the donor genetic signature, but these studies disagreed on whether any donor-specific signature was detectable in the recipient plasma (Lo et al. 1998; Lui et al. 2003). This approach was also limited to the case of women who receive male organs, which precluded its use for most transplant procedures. The new genome transplant dynamics (GTD) approach uses high-throughput shotgun sequencing techniques to identify single nucleotide polymorphism (SNP) differences between donor and recipient. It is therefore possible to identify and quantify dd-cfDNA, regardless of donor and recipient sex. Preliminary studies in heart transplantation demonstrated that dd-cfDNA levels increase in the recipient plasma during episodes of significant cellular rejection (grade ≥2R) (Synder et al. 2011). Moreover, it was demonstrated that GTD is able to detect rises in donor DNA levels prior to a biopsy-proven rejection event.

Recently, a prospective cohort study that evaluated the performance of dd-cfDNA to detect acute rejection after heart transplantation was reported (De Vlaminck et al. 2014). A total of 565 plasma samples were collected longitudinally from 65 adult and pediatric heart transplant recipients. The genomes of the transplant donors and recipients were characterized using SNP genotyping. The SNP genotyping information obtained before transplant was used to discriminate donor- and recipient-derived sequences. SNPs were selected from single-base alleles that were distinct between donor and recipient and homozygous within each individual. The enrolled patients had a total of 356 endomyocardial biopsies during the study period. Levels of dd-cfDNA were significantly lower in stable transplant recipients without evidence of rejection (biopsy grade 0) than for recipients diagnosed with mild ACR (grades ≥1R/1A and <2R/3A) and recipients diagnosed with moderate or severe ACR (grade ≥2R/3A) or AMR. The dd-cfDNA levels were significantly higher for heart transplant recipients during acute rejection and correlated with the severity of the rejection episode as determined by biopsy (comparing biopsy grades 0 and 1R/1A and biopsy grades 0 and ≥2R/3A or AMR). The data furthermore indicate the potential for early diagnosis of acute rejection, up to 5 months before detection by biopsy. Early diagnosis, before the appearance of graft damage on biopsy, may prevent severe rejection events and allograft dysfunction.

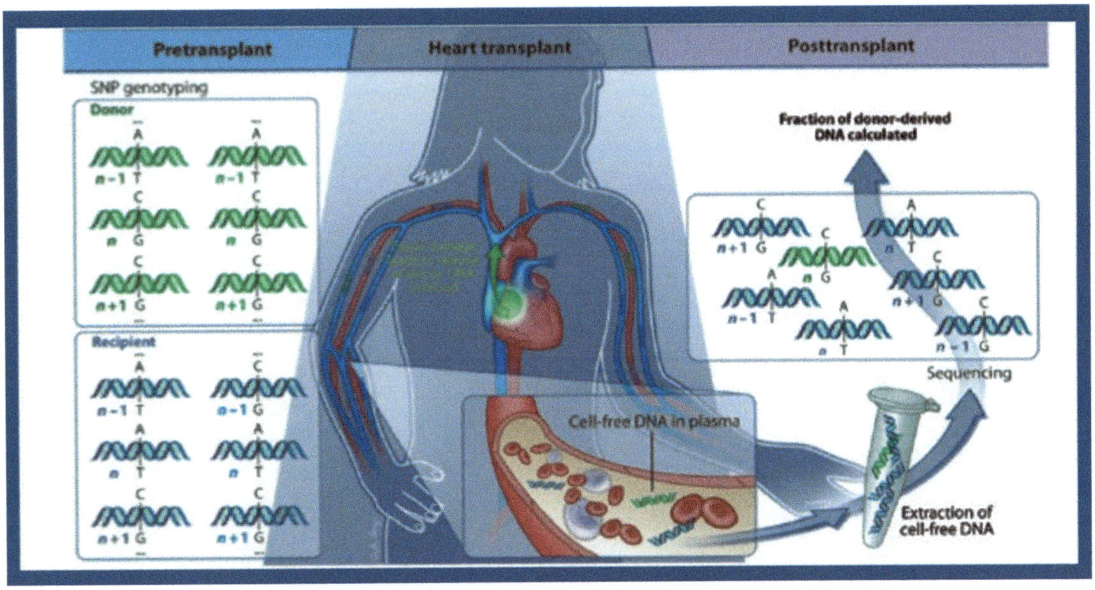

Fig. 17.2 Cell-free donor DNA is detectable in greater amount in the plasma of the transplant recipients during episodes of significant cellular rejection. Cell-free DNA collected in plasma contains a majority of molecules from the recipient (in *blue*) but may also include some from the transplanted organ (*green*). Due to the increased cell death in the organ during a rejection episode, more donor molecules are expected to be present in the blood at these times. Shotgun sequencing of the purified DNA allows for quantification of recipient versus donor molecules by looking at single nucleotide polymorphisms (SNPs) that vary between donor and recipient. Significant increases in the percentage of donor-derived cell-free DNA may indicate the onset of rejection (From: De Vlaminck et al. 2014)

In summary, these findings indicate that dd-cfDNA measurements have the potential to replace the endomyocardial biopsy and that these measurements may even be used for other aspects of patient management, such as prediction of rejection events and management of immunosuppressant dosing. Donor-derived DNA is therefore a promising biomarker for acute rejection; however, clinical utility studies are required before widespread adoption of this approach.

Conclusion

The search for easily measureable and cost-effective biomarkers for allograft rejection continues. An improved understanding of the physiologic and molecular mechanisms of acute rejection has led to the discovery of several promising noninvasive alternatives to EMB in rejection surveillance, which may significantly reduce the number of biopsies performed and increase patient satisfaction.

Several important questions remain. The appropriate criteria for selection of candidates for noninvasive monitoring need to be determined; rejection history and other post-transplant complications must be considered. Inclusion of screening strategies able to detect both antibody-mediated and cellular rejection must also be considered. Currently, graft injury after AMR may only be detected with dd-cfDNA measurements, but the test is not able to distinguish graft damage from AMR versus ACR, which have different therapeutic consequences and outcomes. Hence, this strategy may require follow-up testing, such as biopsy or measurement of donor-specific antihuman leukocyte antigen antibodies, if rejection is determined. Also, differentiating AMR from a state of accommodation (development of donor-specific anti-HLA antibodies without graft injury) will be essential to this end.

There are likely to be several equivalent noninvasive rejection surveillance strategies that will depend on patients' clinical history and comorbidities during the first year post-transplant. An integrated assessment with non-genomic and genomic biomarkers, echocardiography, and/or functional imaging could provide a more effective, but potentially more costly, noninvasive screening modality. Alternatively, intraindividual longitudinal follow-up of biomarkers such as BNP, combined with less frequent echocardiography, may be the most cost-effective approach. Currently, biomarker-based strategies may be best employed starting several months post-transplant to allow host-graft adaptation with respect to hemodynamic, metabolic, and biomarker stabilization.

In conclusion, several major limitations in the evaluation of noninvasive modalities of rejection surveillance remain to be addressed. These include the systematic exclusion of AMR in the majority of the studies, the inherent limitations of EMB as the gold standard, and, more importantly, the lack of appropriately powered and randomized clinical trials in this field. Finally, while most recent studies are looking for a noninvasive substitute for biopsies, the more clinically relevant objective could be the prediction of future rejection that would permit the customization of immunosuppressive therapy for individual patients before rejection occurs. However, the study designs and statistical methods suitable to develop such predictive models are substantially more complex than those suitable for the development of biomarkers for acute rejection (Hollander et al. 2013).

Key Points

- Endomyocardial biopsy is still regarded as the standard tool for the diagnosis of acute myocardial rejection, although several methodological limitations have been identified since its introduction.
- Imaging techniques may be used to diagnose graft dysfunction, which can largely be related to acute rejection. Cardiac ultrasound is routinely used in clinical practice, although no single echocardiographic feature has enough sensitivity or specificity to detect acute rejection, and studies investigating combinatorial methods, incorporating both diastolic and systolic parameters, are needed. Cardiac MRI has the greatest potential to develop as a standard imaging technique for the diagnosis of rejection.
- Cardiac biomarkers provide controversial information: the pro is that they are easily accessible and noninvasive; the con is that they often have low specificity.
- Molecular biomarkers, including gene expression profiling and donor-derived cell-free DNA, are the noninvasive tests with the highest evidence available supporting a substitution of routine biopsy surveillance in clinical practice. The cost and need of multicenter reproducibility, respectively, are the main obstacles to their widespread adoption.
- Future prospective studies aiming to validate noninvasive tools for the diagnosis of rejection will have to focus on clinical outcomes instead of trying to replicate the result of the biopsy. Histology and immunohistochemistry will remain precious tools to finalize the diagnosis but could be supplanted for routine patient monitoring.

References

Bader FM, Islam N, Mehta NA, et al. Noninvasive diagnosis of cardiac allograft rejection using echocardiography indices of systolic and diastolic function. Transplant Proc. 2011;43:3877–81.

Butler CR, Thompson R, Haykowsky M, Toma M, Paterson I. Cardiovascular magnetic resonance in the diagnosis of acute heart transplant rejection: a review. J Cardiovasc Magn Reson. 2009;11:7.

Chen R, Sigdel TK, Li L, et al. Differentially expressed RNA from public microarray data identifies serum protein biomarkers for cross-organ transplant rejection and other conditions. PLoS Comput Biol. 2010;6(9):1–12.

Crescioli C, Buonamano A, Scolletta S, Sottili M, Francalanci M, Giomarelli P, Biagioli B, Lisi G, Pradella F, Serio M, Romagnani P, Maccherini M. Predictive role of pretransplant serum CXCL10 for cardiac acute rejection. Transplantation. 2009;87(2):249–55.

Crespo-Leiro MG, Schulz U, Zuckermann A, et al. Prediction of allograft clinical outcomes and risk of acute cellular rejection with a non-invasive gene expression profiling test (AlloMap): results from the CARGO 2 European-Based Multicenter Trial. J Heart Lung Transplant. 2012;31:S113.

Crespo-Leiro MG, Stypmann J, Zuckermann A, et al. Utility of gene expression profiling test (GEP) score instability to predict future clinical outcomes in heart transplant: results from the CARGO 2 European-based multicenter trial. J Heart Lung Transplant. 2013;32:S113.

Daly KP, Dearling JL, Seto T et al. Use of [18F] FDG Positron Emission Tomography to Monitor the Development of Cardiac Allograft Rejection. Transplantation. 2015;99(9):e132–9.

Damodaran A, Dardas T, Wu AH, Dyke DB, Hummel SL, Cowger JA, Koelling TM. Changes in serial B-type natriuretic peptide level independently predict cardiac allograft rejection. J Heart Lung Transplant. 2012;31(7):708–14.

Dandel M, Hummel M, Muller J, Wellnhofer E, Meyer R, Solowjowa N, et al. Reliability of tissue Doppler wall motion monitoring after heart transplantation for replacement of invasive routine screenings by optimally timed cardiac biopsies and catheterizations. Circulation. 2001;104(12 Suppl 1):I184–91.

Deng MC, Eisen HJ, Mehra MR, et al. Noninvasive discrimination of rejection in cardiac allograft recipients using gene expression profiling. Am J Transplant. 2006;6:150–60.

Deng MC, Elashoff B, Pham MX, Teuteberg JJ, Kfoury AG, Starling RC, Cappola TP, Kao A, Anderson AS, Cotts WG, Ewald GA, Baran DA, Bogaev RC, Shahzad K, Hiller D, Yee J, Valantine HA, IMAGE Study Group. Utility of gene expression profiling score variability to predict clinical events in heart transplant recipients. Transplantation. 2014;97(6):708–14.

Dyer AK, Barnes AP, Fixler DE, Shah TK, Sutcliffe DL, Hashim I, Drazner MH, de Lemos JA. Use of a highly sensitive assay for cardiac troponin T and N-terminal pro-brain natriuretic peptide to diagnose acute rejection in pediatric cardiac transplant recipients. Am Heart J. 2012;163:595–600.

De Vlaminck I, Valantine HA, Snyder TM, Strehl C, Cohen G, Luikart H, Neff NF, Okamoto J, Bernstein D, Weisshaar D, Quake SR, Khush KK. Circulating cell-free DNA enables noninvasive diagnosis of heart transplant rejection. Sci Transl Med. 2014;6(241):241ra77.

Estep JD, Shah DJ, Nagueh SF, Mahmarian JJ, Torre-Amione G, Zoghbi WA. The role of multimodality cardiac imaging in the transplanted heart. JACC Cardiovasc Imaging. 2009;2:1126–40.

Garrido IP, Pascual-Figal DA, Nicolas F, et al. Usefulness of serial monitoring of b-type natriuretic peptide for the detection of acute rejection after heart transplantation. Am J Cardiol. 2009;15(103):1149–53.

Gierthmuehlen M, Sommer P, Zuhayra M, et al. Imaging of acute heart-transplant rejection using 99m-technetium labelled oligonucleotides against interleukin-2 mrna in rats. Eur J Cardiothorac Surg. 2010;37:1111–6.

Hesse B, Mortensen SA, Folke M, et al. Ability of antimyosin scintigraphy monitoring to exclude acute rejection during the first year after heart transplantation. J Heart Lung Transplant. 1995;14:23–31.

Hollander Z, Lin D, Chen V, Ng R, Wilson-McManus J, Ignaszewski A, Cohen Freue G, Balshaw R, Mui A, McMaster R, Keown PA, McManus BM; NCE CECR PROOF Centre of Excellence. Whole blood biomarkers of acute cardiac allograft rejection: double-crossing the biopsy. Transplantation. 2010;90(12):1388–93.

Hollander Z, Chen V, Sidhu K, Lin D, Ng RT, Balshaw R, Cohen-Freue GV, Ignaszewski A, Imai C, Kaan A, Tebbutt SJ, Wilson-McManus JE, McMaster RW, Keown PA, McManus BM; NCE CECR PROOF Centre of Excellence. Predicting acute cardiac rejection from donor heart and pre-transplant recipient blood gene expression. J Heart Lung Transplant. 2013;32(2):259–65.

Horai T, Fumoto H, Saeed D, et al. Novel implantable device to detect cardiac allograft rejection. Circulation. 2009;120:S185–90.

http://clinicaltrials.gov/show/NCT01397812.

Kato K, Oda N, Hashimura K, et al. Strain rate imaging would predict sub-clinical acute rejection in heart transplant recipients. Eur J Cardiothorac Surg. 2010;37:1104–10.

Kato TS, Homma S, Mancini D. Novel echocardiographic strategies for rejection diagnosis. Curr Opin Organ Transplant. 2013;18:573–80.

Khatri P, Roedder S, Kimura N, De Vusser K, Morgan AA, Gong Y, Fischbein MP, Robbins RC, Naesens M,

Butte AJ, Sarwal MM. A common rejection module (CRM) for acute rejection across multiple organs identifies novel therapeutics for organ transplantation. J Exp Med. 2013;210(11):2205–21.

Kittleson MM, Skojec DV, Wittstein IS, et al. The change in B-type natriuretic peptide levels over time predicts significant rejection in cardiac transplant recipients. J Heart Lung Transplant. 2009;28:704–9.

Kobashigawa J, Patel J, Kittleson M, et al. Results of a randomized trial of Allomap vs heart biopsy in the 1st year after heart transplant: early invasive monitoring attenuation through gene expression trial. J Heart Lung Transplant. 2013;32:S203.

Kown MH, Strauss HW, Blankenberg FG, et al. In vivo imaging of acute cardiac rejection in human patients using (99m)technetium labeled annexin v. Am J Transplant. 2001;1:270–7.

Li L, Khush K, Hsieh SC, Ying L, Luikart H, Sigdel T, Roedder S, Yang A, Valantine H, Sarwal MM. Identification of common blood gene signatures for the diagnosis of renal and cardiac acute allograft rejection. PLoS One. 2013;8(12):e82153.

Lin D, Hollander Z, Ng RT, et al. Whole blood genomic biomarkers of acute cardiac allograft rejection. J Heart Lung Transplant. 2009;28:927–35.

Lo YM, Tein MS, Pang CC, Yeung CK, Tong KL, Hjelm NM. Presence of donor-specific DNA in plasma of kidney and liver-transplant recipients. Lancet. 1998;351:1329–30.

Lui YY, Woo KS, Wang AY, et al. Origin of plasma cell-free DNA after solid organ transplantation. Clin Chem. 2003;49(3):495–6.

Marie PY, Angioi M, Carteaux JP, Escanye JM, Mattei S, Tzvetanov K, Claudon O, Hassan N, Danchin N, Karcher G, Bertrand A, Walker PM, Villemot JP. Detection and prediction of acute heart transplant rejection with the myocardial T2 determination provided by a black-blood magnetic resonance imaging sequence. J Am Coll Cardiol. 2001;37:825–31.

Mehra MR, Parameshwar J. Gene expression profiling and cardiac allograft rejection monitoring: is IMAGE just a mirage? J Heart Lung Transplant. 2010;29(6):599–602.

Mena C, Wencker D, Krumholz HM, McNamara RL. Detection of heart transplant rejection in adults by echocardiographic diastolic indices: a systematic review of the literature. J Am Soc Echocardiogr. 2006;19:1295–300.

Méndez AB, Cardona M, Ordóñez-Llanos J, Mirabet S, Perez-Villa F, Roig E. Predictive value of high-sensitive troponin T to rule out acute rejection after heart transplantation. Rev Esp Cardiol (Engl Ed). 2014;67(9):775–6.

Miller CA, Fildes JE, Ray SG, Doran H, Yonan N, Williams SG, Schmitt M. Non-invasive approaches for the diagnosis of acute cardiac allograft rejection. Heart. 2013;99(7):445–53.

Mohammed AA, Januzzi Jr JL. Clinical applications of highly sensitive troponin assays. Cardiol Rev. 2010;18:12–9.

Morrow DA. Clinical application of sensitive troponin assays. N Engl J Med. 2009;361:913–5.

Narula J, Acio ER, Narula N, et al. Annexin-v imaging for noninvasive detection of cardiac allograft rejection. Nat Med. 2001;7:1347–52.

Patel JK, Kittleson M, Kobashigawa JA. Cardiac allograft rejection. Surgeon. 2011;9:160–7.

Patel PC, Hill DA, Ayers CR, Lavingia B, Kaiser P, Dyer AK, Barnes AP, Thibodeau JT, Mishkin JD, Mammen PP, Markham DW, Stastny P, Ring WS, de Lemos JA, Drazner MH. High-sensitivity cardiac troponin I assay to screen for acute rejection in patients with heart transplant. Circ Heart Fail. 2014;7(3):463–9.

Pham MX, Teuteberg JJ, Kfoury AG, et al. Gene-expression profiling for rejection surveillance after cardiac transplantation. New Engl J Med. 2010;362:1890–900.

Phillips M, Boehmer JP, Cataneo RN, Cheema T, Eisen HJ, Fallon JT, Fisher PE, Gass A, Greenberg J, Kobashigawa J, Mancini D, Rayburn B, Zucker MJ. Heart allograft rejection: detection with breath alkanes in low levels (the HARDBALL study). J Heart Lung Transplant. 2004;23(6):701–8.

Roshanali F, Mandegar MH, Bagheri J, et al. Echo rejection score: new echocardiographic approach to diagnosis of heart transplant rejection. Eur J Cardiothorac Surg. 2010;38:176–80.

Rubin PJ, Hartman JJ, Hasapes JP, et al. Detection of cardiac transplant rejection with 111in-labeled lymphocytes and gamma scintigraphy. Circulation. 1996;94:II298–303.

Saleh HK, Villarraga HR, Kane GC, et al. Normal left ventricular mechanical function and synchrony values by speckle-tracking echocardiography in the transplanted heart with normal ejection fraction. J Heart Lung Transplant. 2011;30:652–8.

Sato T, Kato TS, Kamamura K, et al. Utility of left ventricular systolic torsion derived from 2-dimensional speckle-tracking echocardiography in monitoring acute cellular rejection in heart transplant recipients. J Heart Lung Transplant. 2011;30:536–43.

Synder TM, Khush KK, Valantine HA, Quake SR. Universal noninvasive detection of solid organ transplant rejection. Proc Natl Acad Sci U S A. 2011;108:6229–34.

Starling RC, Pham M, Valantine H, et al. Molecular testing in the management of cardiac transplant recipients: initial clinical experience. J Heart Lung Transplant. 2006;25:1389–95.

Steen H, Merten C, Refle S, et al. Prevalence of different gadolinium enhancement patterns in patients after heart transplantation. J Am Coll Cardiol. 2008;52:1160–7.

Sun JP, Abdalla IA, Asher CR, Greenberg NL, Popovic ZB, Taylor DO, et al. Non-invasive evaluation of orthotopic heart transplant rejection by echocardiography. J Heart Lung Transplant. 2005;24(2):160–5.

Taylor AJ, Vaddadi G, Pfluger H, et al. Diagnostic performance of multisequential cardiac magnetic resonance imaging in acute cardiac allograft rejection. Eur J Heart Fail. 2010;12:45–51.

Tong YK, Lo YM. Diagnostic developments involving cell-free (circulating) nucleic acids. Clin Chim Acta. 2006;363:187–96.

Ueno T, Dutta P, Keliher E, Leuschner F, Majmudar M, Marinelli B, Iwamoto Y, Figueiredo JL, Christen T, Swirski FK, Libby P, Weissleder R, Nahrendorf M. Nanoparticle PET-CT detects rejection and immunomodulation in cardiac allografts. Circ Cardiovasc Imaging. 2013;6(4):568–73.

Usman AA, Taimen K, Wasielewski M, McDonald J, Shah S, Giri S, Cotts W, McGee E, Gordon R, Collins JD, Markl M, Carr JC. Cardiac magnetic resonance T2 mapping in the monitoring and follow-up of acute cardiac transplant rejection: a pilot study. Circ Cardiovasc Imaging. 2012;5:782–90.

Wu YL, Ye Q, Sato K, et al. Noninvasive evaluation of cardiac allograft rejection by cellular and functional cardiac magnetic resonance. JACC Cardiovasc Imaging. 2009;2:731–41.

Cardiac Allograft Vasculopathy 18

Marny Fedrigo, Jorge Pombo Otero,
Francesco Tona, Carlo Dal Lin,
Marisa Crespo Leiro, and Patrick Bruneval

Contents

18.1 Background

Cardiac allograft vasculopathy (CAV) is the complex phenomenon that frequently develops in the vasculature of grafted hearts in both adult and pediatric cardiac transplantations, leading to progressive stenosing of cardiac vessels. Since

M. Fedrigo
Cardiovascular Pathology Unit, Department of Cardiac, Thoracic and Vascular Sciences, Azienda Ospedaliera Padua, Padua, Italy
e-mail: marny.fedrigo@unipd.it

J. Pombo Otero
Cardiac Pathology Department, Complejo Hospitalario Universitario A Coruña, A Coruña, Spain
e-mail: jorge.pombo.otero@sergas.es

F. Tona • C. Dal Lin
Cardiology Unit, Department of Cardiac, Thoracic and Vascular Sciences, University of Padua, Padua, Italy
e-mail: francesco.tona@unipd.it; griska3@yahoo.it

M. Crespo Leiro
Unidad de Insuficiencia Cardiaca Avanzada y Trasplante Cardiaco, Servicio de Cardiología, Complexo Hospitalario Universitario A Coruña e Instituto de Investigación Biomédica (INIBIC) A Coruña, A Coruña, Spain
e-mail: marisa.crespo.leiro@sergas.es

P. Bruneval (✉)
Department of Pathology, Hopital Europeen Georges Pompidou, 20 rue Leblanc, 75015 Paris, France
e-mail: patrick.bruneval@egp.aphp.fr

O. Leone et al. (eds.), *The Pathology of Cardiac Transplantation*,
DOI 10.1007/978-3-319-46386-5_18

the early days of cardiac transplantation it has been recognized in patients surviving beyond 1 month (Bieber et al. 1970; Milam et al. 1970).

Over the years, many synonyms have been used by both clinicians and pathologists to identify this pathologic vascular process: chronic rejection, allograft vasculopathy, transplant vasculopathy, accelerated atherosclerosis, transplant coronary artery disease, allograft arteriopathy, cardiac transplant arteriosclerosis, and transplant atherosclerosis (Angelini et al. 2014).

Although the posttransplantation interval for CAV onset varies, ranging from months to years, CAV was always considered a chronic process, and the most common term was chronic rejection (Bieber et al. 1970; Milam et al. 1970). The term CAV is now preferred to chronic rejection for two main reasons: (1) a number of nonimmune factors contribute significantly to the pathogenesis, and (2) the alloimmune responses contributing to the disease are basically acute rejection processes, namely, acute cellular rejection and antibody-mediated rejection. Moreover given that these two types of rejection often fluctuate, and are ongoing or recurrent, the concepts of acute and chronic processes are no longer adequate to explain the phenomenology and pathophysiology of immunologic aspects of the various forms of rejection as well as the development of CAV.

In this chapter, we will present the clinical background of CAV, its imaging, and its pathology with controversial aspects and some pathophysiologic aspects of the disease.

18.2 Risk Factors Influencing the Development of Cardiac Allograft Vasculopathy

Despite the abundant literature, not a lot is known about the risk factors that determine CAV development. These factors are both immunologic and non-immunologic:

1. *Immunologic risk factors*. HLA mismatching, humoral immune response against graft antigens, and increased T-helper activity are recognized immune risk factors for CAV development. These may activate immune inflammation, which in turn activates fibroproliferative processes.

   The role of the cumulative effects of recurrent rejection episodes is still under debate. There is a long-standing controversy as to the role of acute cellular rejection in CAV. An association between CAV and acute cellular rejection had already been reported (Stoica et al. 2006; Mehra et al. 1997; Jimenez et al. 2001; Raichlin et al. 2009; Alexander et al. 2005), and the most recent paper on this topic supports the role of episodes of acute cellular rejection $\geq$ ISHLT grade 2 in CAV (Sato et al. 2016). Stovin et al. on the other hand found no association between CAV and acute cellular rejection (Stovin et al. 1993).

   Current thinking considers antibody-mediated rejection to be more significant than acute cellular rejection, and several recent studies support this association (Loupy et al. 2015; Kfoury et al. 2012; Wu et al. 2009; Frank et al. 2014): in many cases CAV even developed in the presence of subclinical antibody-mediated rejection. Antibody-mediated rejection seems to act as a subtle fluctuating phenomenon, which over time produces CAV. In support of this, a retrospective study was made of a group of patients retransplanted for CAV; their previous endomyocardial biopsies were found to show markers of antibody-mediated rejection (C4d deposition, presence of intravascular activated mononuclear cells within the microcirculation, and/or intravascular CD68-positive cells) (Loupy et al. 2015). Recently, Coutance et al. (Coutance et al. 2015) reported cases of severe, rapidly progressing CAV, in patients with de novo immunization and late episodes of antibody-mediated rejection after 1 year posttransplantation, despite aggressive treatment for rejection.
2. *Non-immunologic risk factors*. Besides the major contribution of immune risk factors to CAV development, the following are also involved in varying degrees (Rahmani et al. 2006):
   - The usual atherosclerosis risk factors (hyperlipidemia, diabetes mellitus, hypertension,

smoking) (Kapadia et al. 2001; Wenke et al. 1997).

- Infection which can be linked to onset and progression of the disease. Among various infectious agents, *Cytomegalovirus* is the most important in CAV development and progression. Several studies found a deleterious effect of CMV infection in vascular cells and/or an association with CAV (Delgado et al. 2015; Graham et al. 2009; Potena et al. 2006), although the matter is still controversial (Sambiase et al. 2000; Gulizia et al. 1995).
- C-reactive protein as indicator of an inflammatory condition.
- Ischemia-reperfusion injury related to harvesting and preservation of the graft as central factor in endothelial damage and dysfunction (Gaudin et al. 1994).
- Brain death which acts as dramatic central injury with its hemodynamic, metabolic, and neurohormonal consequences and the potential damage to the graft, especially vascular injury (Mehra et al. 2004).
- Transmission of donor-related coronary artery disease which, although controversial, can progress independently of CAV or may accelerate CAV, thus contributing to vessel remodeling (Rahmani et al. 2006).

18.3 Clinical Presentation

Though its incidence and mortality have fallen somewhat in recent years, CAV remains a major cause of late graft failure and death after heart transplantation (Lund et al. 2014). It affects 8 %, 30 %, and 50 % of patients still alive 1, 5 and 10 years, respectively, after heart transplantation, and after 1 year is the main indication for retransplantation (Lund et al. 2014). Clinically, it commonly presents only in its later stages, as progressive heart failure, arrhythmia, or sudden death (Hamon et al. 2014; Chantranuwat et al. 2004). Though myocardial infarction is also common, it is generally silent, the cardiac denervation consequent upon heart transplantation preventing premonitory angina pectoris. Any symptoms are thus nonspecific: effort-related chest pain, dyspnea, diaphoresis, gastrointestinal distress, pre-syncope, and syncope. Signs suggestive of CAV can appear in echocardiograms (mainly left ventricular systolic dysfunction) (Bolad et al. 2006) and on ECGs (both atrial and ventricular arrhythmias, but particularly ventricular extrasystoles and conduction disorders), but its diagnosis requires appropriate imaging studies supplemented by hemodynamic data (see below).

18.4 Imaging

18.4.1 Invasive Techniques

- *Coronary angiography* enables detection of coronary luminal narrowing and assessment of flow velocity. In coronary angiograms, CAV is typically visualized as luminal irregularity or concentric stenosis. Table 18.1 and Fig. 18.1 present the types of lesions of an early classification of CAV by Gao et al. (1988). A minor limitation of coronary angiography for detection of CAV is that the lesions can be mimicked by vasospasm; however, the two conditions can easily be distinguished by intracoronary administration of nitroglycerine. A

Table 18.1 Angiographic description of cardiac allograft vasculopathy

Type of anatomic abnormality	Description
Type A lesion	Discrete or tubular stenosis and multiple stenosis in the proximal, middle, or distal segment branches
Type B1 lesion	Proximal vessel maintaining normal diameter with abrupt onset of distal concentric narrowing and obliterations
Type B2 lesion	Gradual transition from the normal proximal vessel with tapering, concentric narrowing progressively increasing in severity distally
Type C lesion	Diseased vessel, diffusely irregular which has lost small branches with terminations, often non-tapered, squared off, and ending abruptly

From Gao et al. (1988)

more basic limitation is that the often diffuse and concentric stenosis of early CAV is generally accompanied by vascular remodeling, including vasodilation, with the result that angiograms, which of course are luminograms, appear normal. Nevertheless, the 2010 ISHLT working formulation of a standardized nomenclature for CAV (Mehra et al. 2010) is based on coronary angiography, partly because of its universal availability and partly because coronarograms are in any case necessary for planning revascularization procedures. Except for the inclusion of hemodynamic considerations (evaluated by echocardiography or catheterization), the staging criteria of the working formulation, displayed in Table 18.2, are very similar to those of the earlier classification of Costanzo et al. (Costanzo et al. 1998) (Table 18.3), which was adopted in large part because, unlike the classification of Gao et al. (1988), it had shown prognostic value: 50 % of patients with CAV classified as severe by the Costanzo system died or underwent retransplantation within 5 years. Baseline coronarography is commonly performed 4–6 weeks after transplantation to rule out donor-transmitted coronary lesions (unless the donor underwent catheterization during pre-transplant evaluation of the potential graft). After that, it is generally performed at 1-year follow-up and then every 2–5 years. CAV classified at 1 year post-heart transplantation as moderate or severe according to the Table 18.2 classification has been reported as associated with subsequent major adverse cardiac events (Prada-Delgado et al. 2012).

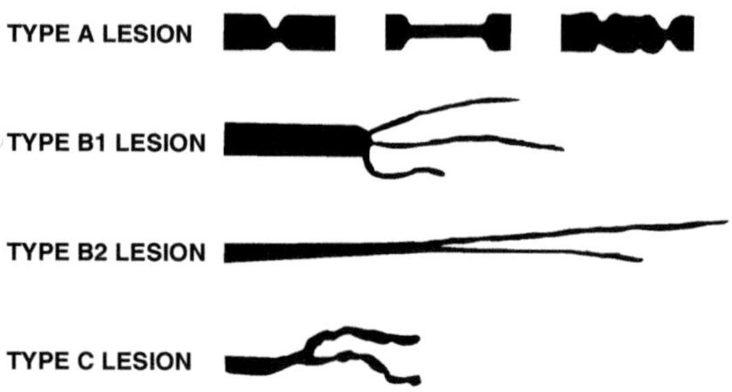

Fig. 18.1 Types of anatomic abnormality in cardiac allograft vasculopathy (From Gao et al. 1988)

Table 18.2 International Society for Heart and Lung Transplantation (ISHLT) recommended cardiac allograft vasculopathy (CAV) 2010 nomenclature

Nomenclature	Definition
ISHLT CAV0 (not significant)	No detectable angiographic lesion
ISHLT CAV1 (mild)	Angiographic left main (LM) <50 %, or primary vessel with maximum lesion of <70 %, or any branch stenosis <70 % (including diffuse narrowing) without allograft dysfunction
ISHLT CAV2 (moderate)	Angiographic LM <50 %, a single primary vessel ≥70 %, or isolated branch stenosis ≥70 % in branches of two systems, without allograft dysfunction
ISHLT CAV3 (severe)	Angiographic LM ≥50 %, or two or more primary vessels ≥70 % stenosis, or isolated branch stenosis ≥70 % in all three systems or ISHLT CAV1 or CAV2 with allograft dysfunction (defined as LVEF ≤45 % usually in the presence of regional wall motion abnormalities) or evidence of significant restrictive physiology (which is common but not specific; see text for definitions)

Definitions:

(a) A "primary vessel" denotes the proximal and middle 33 % of the left anterior descending

(b) Artery, the left circumflex, the ramus and the dominant or codominant right coronary artery with the posterior descending, and posterolateral branches

(c) A "secondary branch vessel" includes the distal 33 % of the primary vessels or any segment within a large septal perforator, diagonals and obtuse marginal branches, or any portion of a nondominant right coronary artery

(d) "Restrictive cardiac allograft physiology" is defined as symptomatic heart failure with echocardiographic E to A velocity ratio > 2 (>1.5 in children), shortened isovolumetric relaxation time (<60 ms), shortened deceleration time (<150 ms), or restrictive hemodynamic values (right atrial pressure >12 mmHg, pulmonary capillary wedge pressure >25 mmHg, cardiac index <2 l/min/m^2)

From Mehra et al. (2010)

Table 18.3 Cardiac allograft vasculopathy (CAV) categories according to the Cardiac Transplant Research Database (CRTD)

	Description
Normal	No lesions
Mild CAV	Left main (LM) < 50 %, or primary vessel with maximum lesion < 70 %, or isolated single-branch stenosis > 70 %, or any branch
Moderate CAV	LM 50–69 %, or a single primary vessel > 70 %, or isolated branch stenosis > 70 % in branches of 2 systems
Severe CAV	LM > 70 %, or ≥ primary vessels > 70 %, or isolated branch stenosis > 70 % in all 3 systems.
Definitions	
"*Primary vessels*": the proximal or middle 33 % of the left anterior descending, left circumflex, and dominant or codominant right coronary artery	
"*Branch vessels*": the diagonal branches, obtuse marginal branches, or the distal 33 % of a primary vessel or any part of a nondominant right coronary artery	

From Costanzo et al. (1998)

- *Intravascular ultrasound (IVUS) imaging* uses 10–40 MHz ultrasound emitted by a miniature transducer at the end of a flexible catheter to visualize the walls of coronary arteries (Topilsky et al. 2012) (Fig. 18.2) The normal coronary artery appears as three zones: a bright echo from the intima, a dark zone due to the media, and multiple bright echoes from the adventitia. Abnormal thickening of the intima and the morphology and distribution of plaques show up very well. IVUS-measurable parameters that have been used to evaluate coronary arteries in relation to CAV include intimal thickness, maximal intimal thickness, intimal index (intimal area/[intimal area + luminal area]), change in the maximal intimal index at a reference point, and atheroma volume expressed as a percentage of the volume within the external elastic membrane (PAV). A drawback of IVUS is that each artery must be explored separately; the greater number of arteries explored, the greater the likelihood of detecting intimal thickening. In clinical trials, the left anterior descending artery was explored first, followed by the right coronary artery and the circumflex when possible, using automated pullback to ensure consistent sampling and facilitate identification of the branch vessels used as landmarks. At 1-year follow-up, IVUS detects intimal thickening in more than 80 % of heart transplantation patients (Tuzcu et al. 1995), and thickening exceeding 0.5 mm at this time has been reported as predicting angiographic CAV, myocardial infarction, and mortality within 4 years (Tuzcu et al. 2005). However, these findings have not been confirmed, and IVUS is still largely used experimentally to evaluate the outcome of therapy.
- *Optical coherence tomography* and other advanced intravascular imaging methods are similarly of limited availability. Although their high-resolution images allow early detection of morphological changes in the arterial wall, their predictive value remains to be determined.

18.4.2 Noninvasive Imaging

- *Conventional ECG stress testing* is of limited value for detection of CAV because basal ECG abnormalities are frequent and prevent interpretation of ECG changes. However, *dobutamine stress echocardiography* has been reported to have a sensitivity of 85 % for CAV, with a high negative predictive value, and deterioration of dobutamine stress results in serial studies is associated with increased risk of adverse events (Spes et al. 1999). *Stress technetium-99m tetrofosmin myocardial perfusion imaging* has been reported to predict cardiac death (Elhendy et al. 2002), and *gated single-photon emission computed tomography (gated SPECT)* may be useful for screening for myocardial ischemia (Manrique et al. 2010), but neither of these techniques is as sensitive as coronary angiography for CAV detection.
- *Coronary computed tomography angiography (CCTA)*, which is not only noninvasive, but also less costly than conventional angiography, is attractive as a potential screening tool,

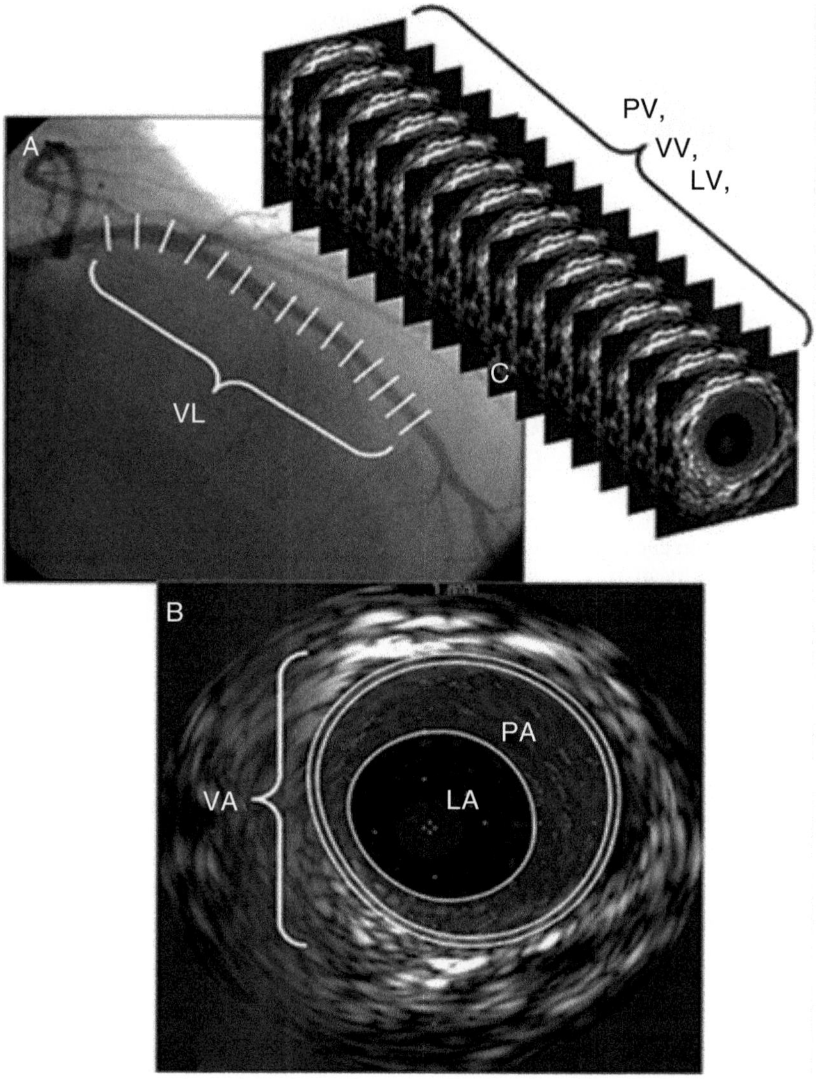

Fig. 18.2 Methods for conducting three-dimensional intravascular ultrasound (IVUS) examinations and definitions of IVUS measurements (From Topilsky et al. 2012). IVUS is performed during coronary angiography with mechanical pullback (0.5 mm/s) usually from the mid-to-distal left anterior descending coronary artery to the left main coronary artery. Parameters and definitions: *VL* vessel length, *LA* lumen area, *VA* vessel area (media adventitia interface), *PA* plaque area (difference between VA and LA for each two-dimensional image), *VV* vessel volume, *LV* lumen volume, *PV* plaque volume, *PI* plaque index (PV/VV) × 100 %

having achieved mean-weighted sensitivities of 97 % for any trace of CAV and 94 % for significant CAV (stenosis ≥ 50 %) in a recent meta-analysis of 30 studies; the respective specificities were 81 and 92 %, the negative predictive values 97 and 99 %, the positive predictive values 78 and 67 %, and the diagnostic accuracy 88 and 94 % (Wever-Pinzon et al. 2014).

As in the case of other noninvasive techniques, a major limitation of CCTA is that it does not reliably detect early or limited disease, particularly in the small coronary arteries, although it does appear capable of excluding significant CAV in arteries susceptible to stenting or surgical revascularization. Also, though noninvasive, it shares drawbacks with coronary angiography in that its use of iodinated dye increases the risk of renal failure, while repeated radiation increases the risk of malignancy. Accordingly, current ISHLT guidelines do not recommend CCTA for monitoring CAV.

18.5 Recommendations

In summary, the five consensus recommendations achieved in the current ISHLT guidelines (Mehra et al. 2010) were as follows: (1) Coronary angiography coupled with assessment of allograft function maintains the highest level of evidence for CAV nomenclature. The advantages of angiography are that it is universally available for both adult and pediatric patients, clinically accepted and applicable at any time in the posttransplantation process (favorable for longitudinal and snapshot assessments); (2) IVUS-detected maximal intimal thickness may be most useful for its negative predictive value at any time after transplant. A role for routine IVUS surveillance was not identified. (3) IVUS-detected first-year change in maximal intimal thickening (6 weeks to 1 year) is a putative surrogate marker for prognosis, but evaluation as a robust marker for reliable late outcomes is uncertain and at present should be considered investigational. (4) Noninvasive computed tomography-based angiography should not be used in a manner equivalent to invasive coronary angiography for the assessment of CAV. There is lack of adequate branch vessel assessment; accuracy, sensitivity, and specificity still remain uncertain in heart transplantation and concerns for excess radiation in this vulnerable population exist. Furthermore, data providing prognostic outcomes are lacking. (5) Endomyocardial biopsy findings, immune-based markers, gene-based and protein-based biomarkers, microvascular function test, and stress-based imaging were not recommended for inclusion in the nomenclature algorithm as markers to define CAV severity. This decision was reached due to lack of specificity for diagnosis and issues of inherent broad reproducibility.

For practical implementation of this nomenclature, it is recommended:

1. Using a combination of visual angiographic vessel descriptors in concert with measures of allograft function.
2. Each angiographic report must include a description of the maximum stenosis at the level of the left main artery, primary vessels, and secondary vessels.
3. For optimal assessment, resting vasospasm in the coronary vessels must be excluded.
4. Allograft dysfunction must be defined by allograft imaging: left ventricular ejection fraction coupled with hemodynamic assessment (restrictive physiology), as described in Table 18.2.

18.6 Pathology

CAV is a pathological disease of cardiac vessels leading to a progressive intimal thickening which causes narrowing of the vessel lumen until occlusion.

The disease typically involves epicardial coronary arteries and intramyocardial vessels with diameter greater than 500 μm (macrovasculopathy) and/or small intramyocardial vessels (diameter <500 μm) (microvasculopathy). Veins and venules may also be affected.

Although CAV has long been considered a graft arteriopathy, it is now recognized that veins and venules may be affected.

Pathologic features are heterogeneous and include three main types of lesion (Angelini et al. 2014; Loupy et al. 2015; Lu et al. 2011; Seki and Fishbein 2014; Huibers et al. 2014):

1. Proliferative/hyperplastic intimal lesions
2. Vasculitis/perivascular inflammation
3. Conventional atherosclerotic lesions

It should be noted that even in CAV nonculprit and culprit (lesions complicated by thrombosis or hemorrhages), lesions may be found.

Although pathologic features of CAV and native atherosclerosis may overlap and features typical of classical atherosclerosis may be found, they are two distinctive diseases in relation to onset, to progression, and of course to pathologic findings. CAV is often concentric and diffusely distributed in the vascular tree.

As de novo proliferative fibrocellular lesions and remodeling of the vessel wall due to already existing or superimposed atherosclerotic lesions can coexist, it is difficult to give a systematic pathologic categorization of CAV lesions or explain their origins. So it is time that pathologists worked on a standardized pathological classification of this important disease in order to avoid varying and confusing terminology among transplant centers.

18.6.1 Macrovasculopathy

1. *Proliferative/hyperplastic intimal lesions* are made up by a mixture of fibroblasts, myofibroblasts, smooth muscle cells mainly migrating from the media, and various components of extracellular matrix. These lesions are typically concentric and may show areas of both loose and dense tissue, in keeping with the ongoing nature of the disease. The medial layer is usually preserved, although it may be thinner or show replacement of fibrous tissue similar to healed arteritis; the internal elastic lamina frequently remains intact or is duplicated (Figs. 18.3 and 18.4). Fibrocellular lesions are present in two-thirds of CAV cases in the first year after transplantation, but their incidence drops markedly in the long term, when the fibrolipid plaques are more frequently found (Angelini et al. 2014). The origin of the migrated smooth muscle cells infiltrating the intima and producing extracellular matrix is controversial: either of host origin (Atkinson et al. 2004; Shimizu et al. 2001; Minami et al. 2005) or of donor origin (Pober et al. 2014), the latter hypothesis now being the more probable.
2. *Vasculitis/perivascular inflammation*. Inflammation is a significant component of CAV. It is frequently seen and ranges from focal involvement of the intima (endothelialitis) to transmural spreading of inflammatory infiltrates to the media and adventitia: the degree varies from mild to severe, the latter being more frequently associated with rapid progression of the disease (Fig. 18.5). Inflammatory infiltrates are usually chronic and made up by macrophages and T lymphocytes. Adventitial inflammation is frequently organized in a follicular-like pattern (Seki and Fishbein 2014).
   Several studies have emphasized that atherosclerosis plaques associated with CAV are more inflamed than those in native atherosclerosis (Lu et al. 2011; Castellani et al. 2014); the cell types however do not differ and macrophages are the major component (Fig. 18.6) (Angelini et al. 2014).
   In spite of this greater inflammation in grafted hearts, the prevalence of atherosclerosis in CAV does not correlate with the general vascular inflammatory burden within the

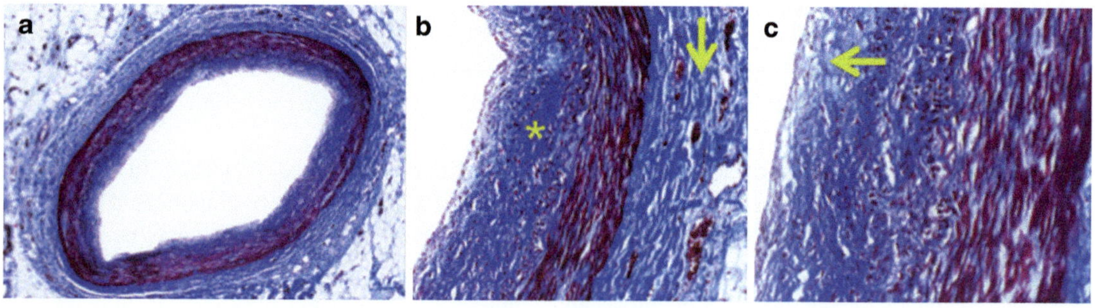

Fig. 18.3 Macrovasculopathy: early proliferative/hyperplastic intimal lesions. Left anterior descending coronary artery with an early hyperplastic intimal proliferative lesion. (**a**) Cross section showing the concentric intimal lesion, the preserved tunica media, and the fibrotic adventitia. (Azan Mallory trichrome, original magnification 25×). (**b**) High-power view showing the neo-angiogenesis in the adventitia with increased fibrosis (*arrow*) and the abundant extracellular collagen (*asterisk*) in the intima. (Azan Mallory trichrome, original magnification 100×). (**c**) High-power view showing the two-layer stratification of the hyperplastic lesion with loose collagen in the outer layer (*arrow*) (Azan Mallory trichrome, original magnification 200×)

vasculature of the grafted heart, i.e., endotheliitis, media inflammation, and microvascular inflammation (Loupy et al. 2015).

3. *Conventional atherosclerotic lesions* are seen in CAV, especially in the advanced disease. They are found as individual lesions or combined

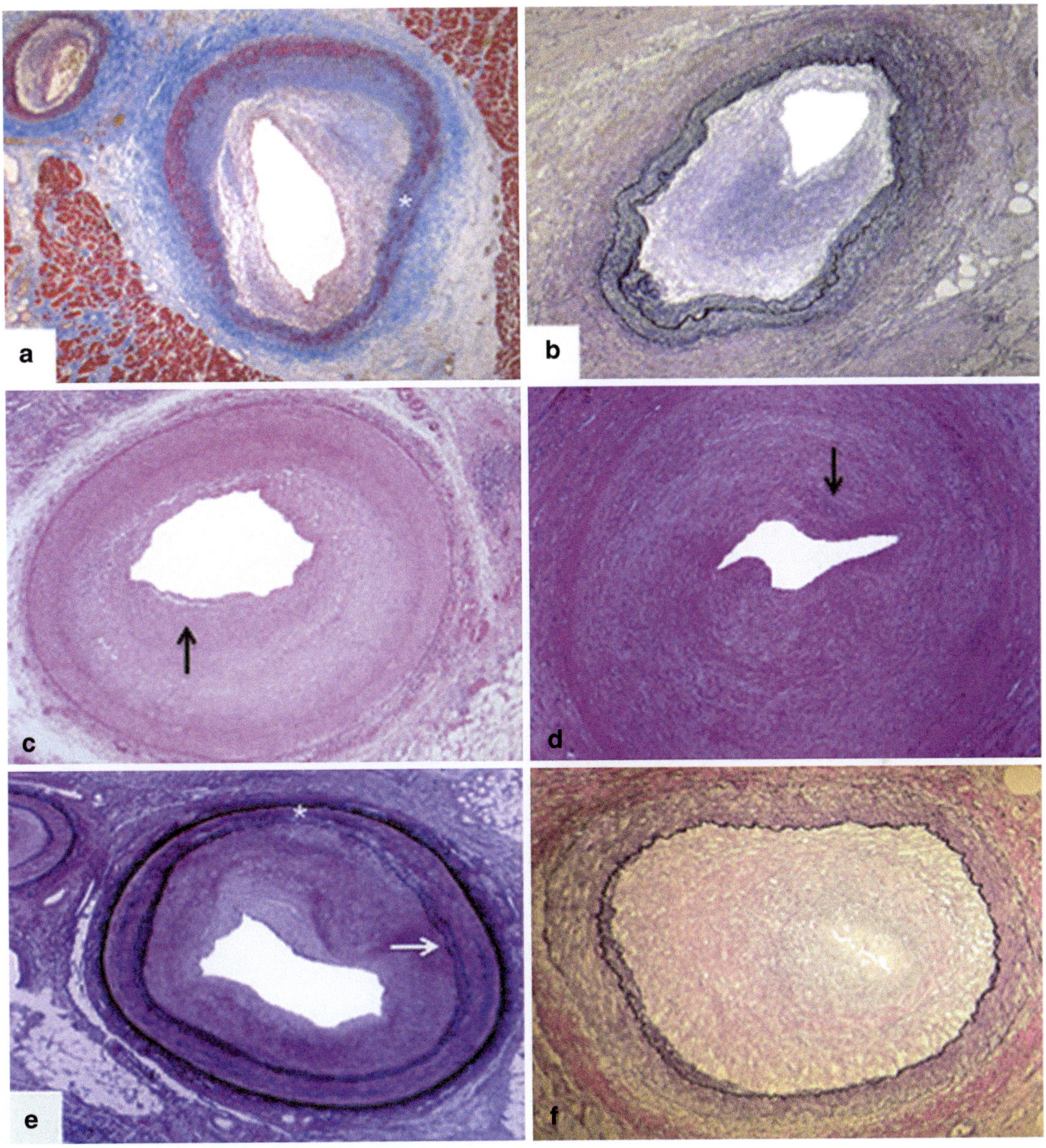

Fig. 18.4 Macrovasculopathy: more advanced proliferative/hyperplastic intimal lesions. Intimal thickening is made up of a mixture of smooth muscle cells mainly migrating from the media and various components of extracellular matrix. The lesions are concentric and made up of fibroblasts, myofibroblasts, smooth muscle cells, collagen, and other components of extracellular matrix leading to a loose mesenchymal tissue (**a**, **b**) or to a more dense tissue (**c**, **d**). Endothelialitis (**c**) or some chronic inflammation (*arrows*) is also present. The medial layer is preserved or shows focal fibrosis (**a**, *asterisk*) or thinning (**e**, *asterisk*). The internal elastic lamina is intact or duplicated (**e**, *arrow*). Azan Mallory trichrome (**a**), Weigert van Gieson (**b**, **e**, **f**), hematoxylin-eosin (**c**, **d**), original magnification 25×. **a**, **b**, **f** (Courtesy of Dr. Leone, Bologna, Italy)

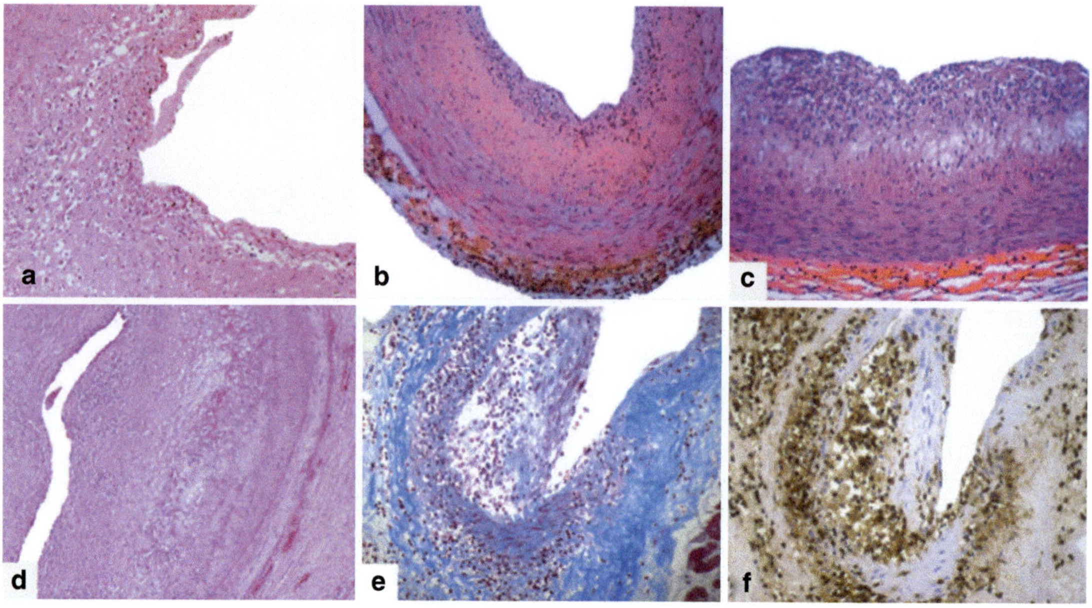

Fig. 18.5 Inflammation of CAV lesions may, to varying extent, involve the intima layer of fibrocellular lesions (endothelialitis) (**a**, **b** hematoxylin-eosin, 200×; 100×), the intima layer of the lesions with both intimal proliferation and lipid deposits (**c**, hematoxylin-eosin 200×), or the superficial layer of a conventional fibrolipid plaque (**d**, hematoxylin-eosin 50×). It may also spread to the entire wall and extend to the periadventitial tissue (**e**, **f**, 200×, Azan Mallory trichrome, immunostaining for CD45). **e**, **f** (Courtesy of Dr. Leone, Bologna, Italy)

Fig. 18.6 Many macrophages in a fibrolipid plaque of an epicardial coronary artery. CD163 immunohistochemical staining for macrophages. Original magnification 100×

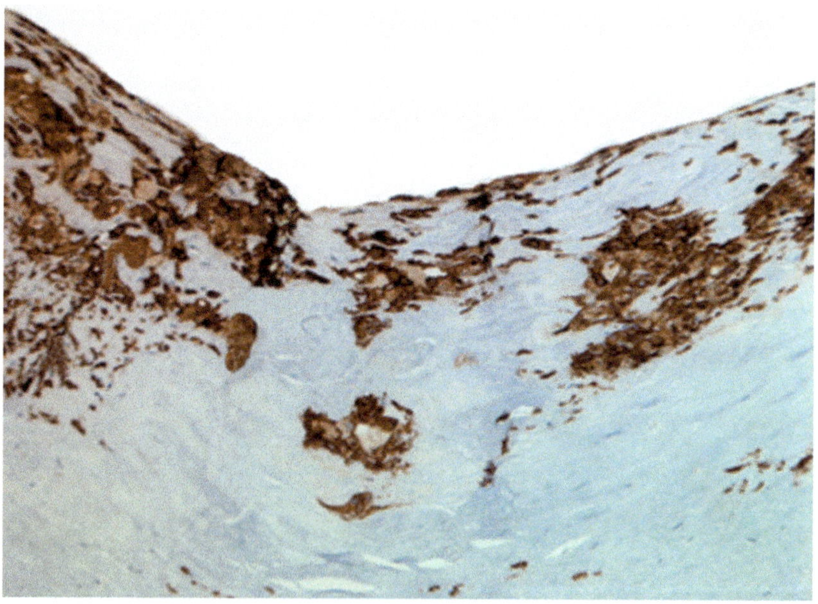

with the typical fibrocellular intimal lesions, both in the same coronary artery or even in the same section (Fig. 18.7) (Lu et al. 2011). Besides the possible presence of macrophage aggregates and lipid deposits within the proliferative CAV lesions, atherosclerotic lesions are usually eccentric fibrolipid plaques similar to those observed in native atherosclerosis and cause variable lumen stenosis. Occlusive thrombosis, hemorrhage, and calcifications

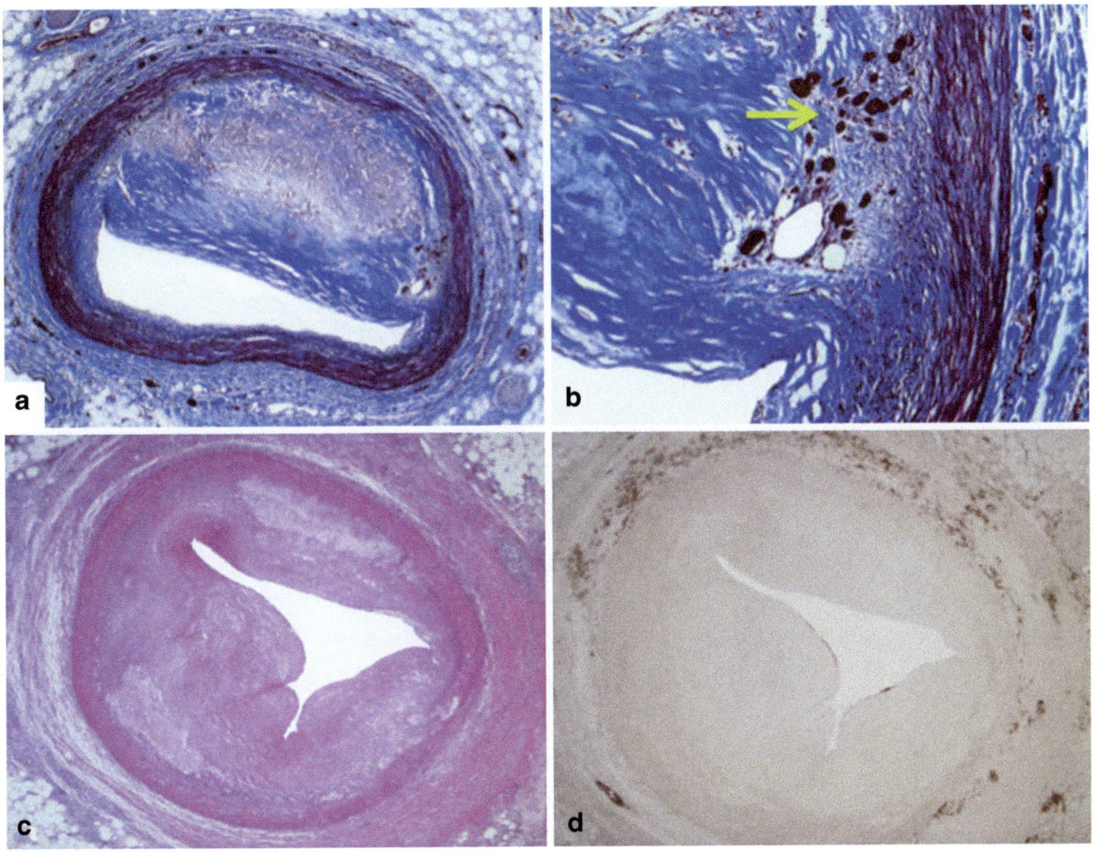

Fig. 18.7 (**a**) Cross section of a right coronary artery with an isolated eccentric atherosclerotic plaque, with the typical lipid core rich in cholesterol cleft and a thick fibrous cup (Azan Mallory trichrome, original magnification 25×). (**b**) High-power view showing neo-angiogenesis at the shoulder of the plaque (*arrow*) (Azan Mallory trichrome, original magnification 200×). (**c**) Cross section of a right coronary artery showing a combined concentric plaque, mainly fibrous with a necrotic core (hematoxylin-eosin, original magnification 25×). (**d**) The concentric plaque stained with glycophorin to identify hemorrhagic component (original magnification 25×)

may complicate both proliferative and atherosclerotic lesions, frequently leading to acute coronary syndromes (Fig. 18.8).

Nevertheless, atherosclerosis in CAV may exhibit some peculiar features such as concentric fibrolipid plaques, spreading of plaques into intramyocardial arteries, frequent mural thrombosis, and lipid-rich or foamy macrophage-rich plaques (Fig. 18.9). Recently another plaque complication, the intraplaque hemorrhage (Fig. 18.10), has been highlighted in CAV, thanks to an original study comparing plaques in paired hearts, i.e., native hearts and autopsied grafted hearts from the same patient (Castellani et al. 2014). The authors showed the increased incidence of intraplaque hemorrhage in plaques from CAV: of the 35 plaques analyzed, 60% were in grafted hearts and 22.9% in native hearts. Since intraplaque hemorrhage is associated with sudden plaque progression, its high incidence in CAV coronary arteries could support the hypothesis of an accelerated atherosclerosis process. The pathophysiology of the intraplaque hemorrhage involves neo-angiogenesis with leaky microvessels within the plaque (Castellani et al. 2014) (Fig. 18.10).

18.6.1.1 Some Remarks on the Relationship Between Primary CAV and Native Atherosclerosis Lesions

Observing atherosclerosis in the epicardial coronary arteries of a grafted heart, whether using vascular imaging in live hearts or pathology in autopsy

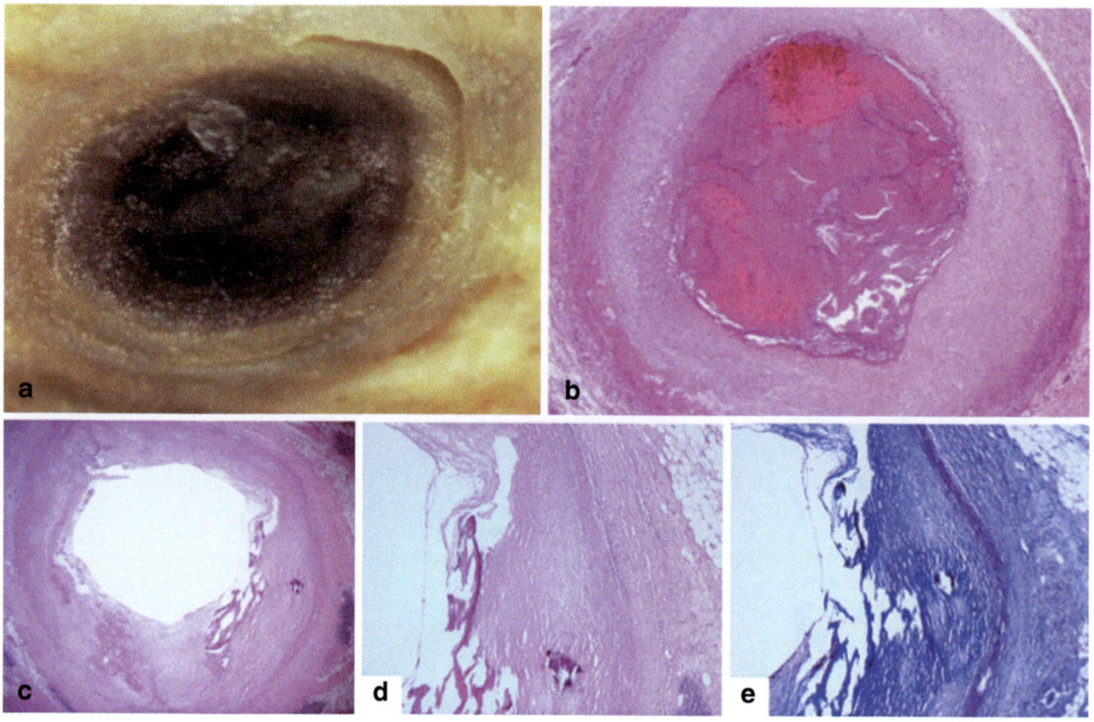

Fig. 18.8 (**a**) Cross section stereomicroscopic view of occlusive thrombosis in a fibrous plaque. (**b**) Histology of the occlusive thrombosis: focal attenuation of the tunica media and significant fibrosis of the adventitia are evident (hematoxylin-eosin, original magnification 125×). (**c**) Calcifications may complicate atherosclerotic lesions (hematoxylin-eosin, original magnification 125×). (**d, e**) High-power view of the calcified plaque (**d**, hematoxylin-eosin; **e**, Azan Mallory trichrome, original magnification ×200)

or explanted hearts, raises the question of whether it is a condition acquired during transplantation or a lesion transmitted from the donor heart. An IVUS analysis of the coronary arteries, performed very early after cardiac transplantation, found donor lesions in 30% of the hearts with more lesions in older patients (Li et al. 2006). As average donor age has risen and continue to rise, the incidence and severity of coronary atherosclerosis in donor hearts is expected to increase (Lund et al. 2015; Schumer et al. 2015). A study using echocardiography and stress echocardiography showed a high prevalence of atherosclerosis in marginal donor hearts (11 out of 18 candidates had abnormal tests) (Leone et al. 2009). Another study using IVUS of a cohort of young donors (31.4 ± 11 years) found atherosclerosis (defined as intimal thickness ≥ 0.5 mm) in as many as 48.5%, with incidence increasing with donor age (Kim et al. 2013). Techniques to differentiate donor-transmitted atherosclerosis from CAV in live grafted hearts are under development: they are based on modern in vivo coronary artery imaging techniques like optical coherence tomography that shows a double intimal layer pattern in donor-transmitted atherosclerosis (Imamura et al. 2014) and three-dimensional IVUS (Yamasaki et al. 2011). That donor-transmitted atherosclerosis could be a determinant of plaque progression during the first year posttransplantation is controversial, with pros (Yamasaki et al. 2011) and contras (Li et al. 2006).

18.6.2 Microvasculopathy

The involvement of small intramyocardial vessels is peculiar to CAV, since it is not usually observed in native coronary artery atherosclerosis, and has long been known to be an immune injury (Salomon et al. 1991).

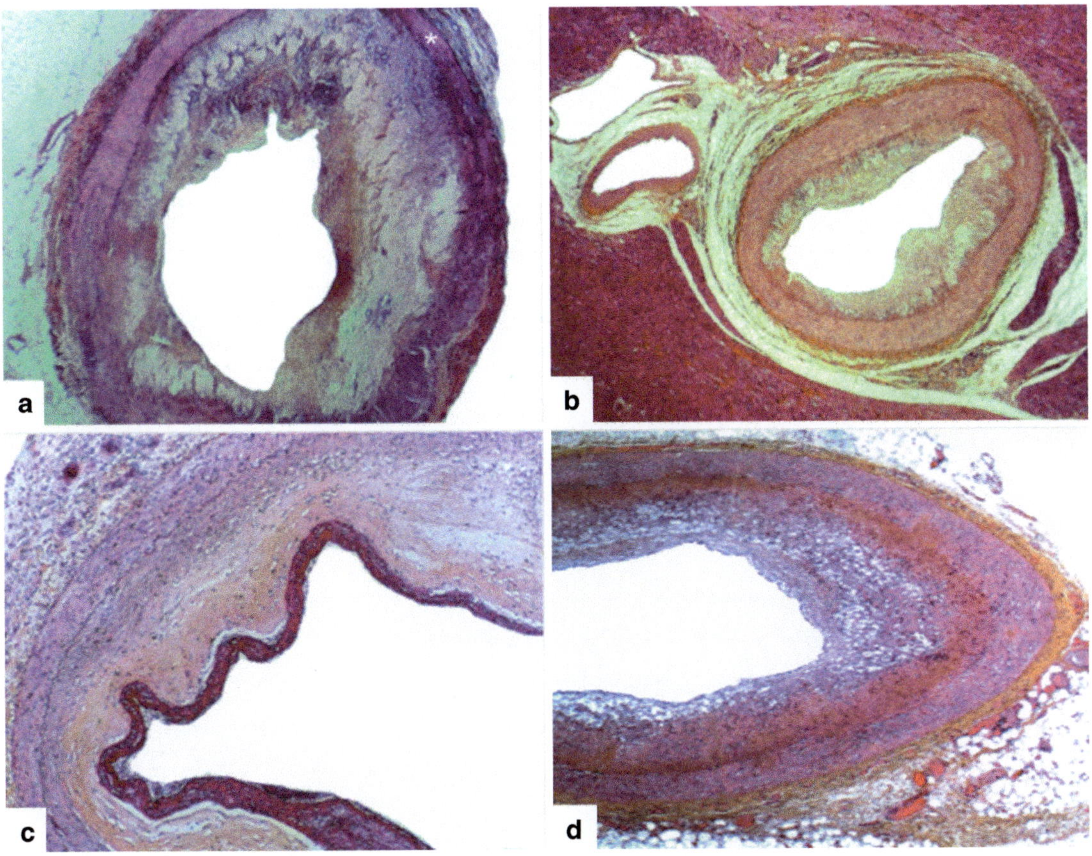

Fig. 18.9 (**a**) Epicardial coronary artery in an explanted cardiac graft obtained at retransplantation for CAV. Note the concentric pattern of the fibrolipid plaque, with multifocal disruption of the internal elastic lamina and atrophy of the media (*asterisk*) (hematoxylin-eosin, original magnification 25×). (**b**) Intramyocardial coronary artery branch showing fibrolipid plaque and well-preserved tunica media (hematoxylin-eosin, original magnification 25×). (**c**) Mural thrombosis stratified on a fibrous atherosclerotic plaque in an epicardial coronary artery (hematoxylin-eosin, original magnification 50×). (**d**) Non-stenotic atherosclerotic plaque containing many foam cells and a few inflammatory cells in an epicardial coronary artery, with a well-preserved tunica media (hematoxylin-eosin, original magnification 25×)

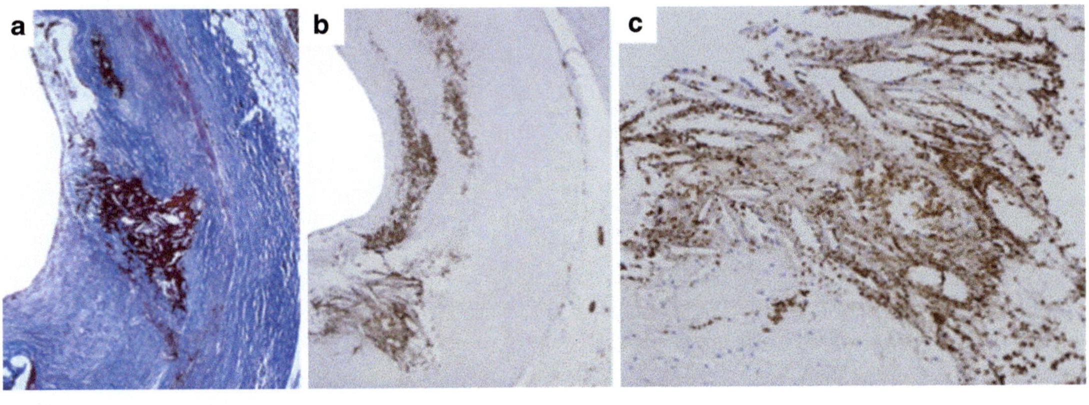

Fig. 18.10 (**a**) Hemorrhage in a fibrolipid plaque (Azan Mallory trichrome, original magnification 100×). (**b, c**) Glycophorin immunostaining shows red blood cells or remnants of the red cell membranes within the lipidic core close to the cholesterol clefts and in the fibrotic component (original magnification **b**, 100×; **c**, 200×)

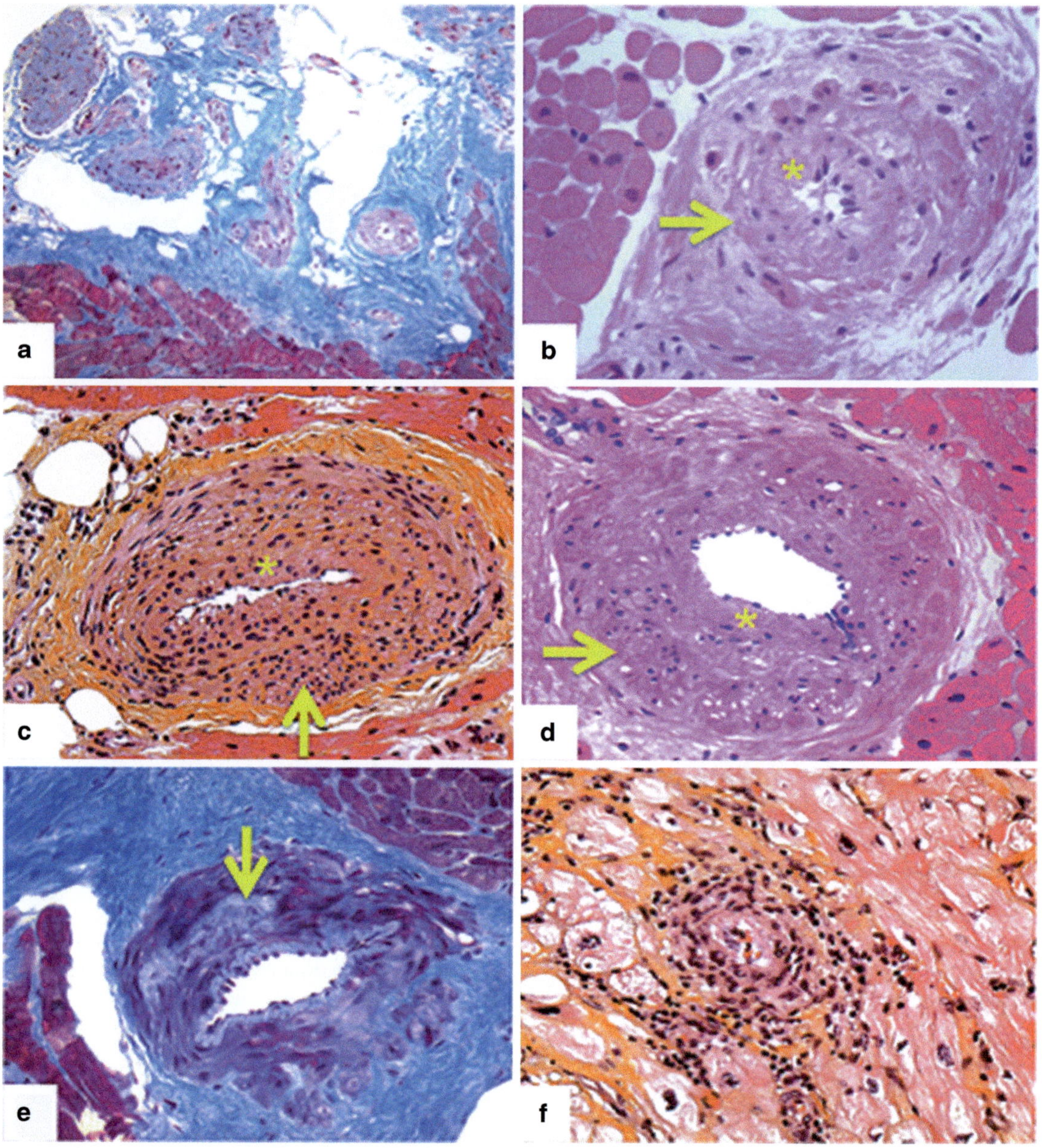

Fig. 18.11 Pathology of microvasculopathy in small-sized intramyocardial coronary artery branch at endomyocardial biopsy. (**a**) Prevalent intimal disease with fibrocellular proliferation (Azan Mallory trichrome, 200×), (**b–d**) mixed intimal (*asterisks*) and medial (*arrows*) disease (hematoxylin-eosin, 400×). (e) Medial disease with hypertrophy and fibrosis (*arrow*) (Azan Mallory trichrome, 400×). (**f**) Thickening of an arteriola in keeping with the structural changes associated with microangiopathy or vasculitis (hematoxylin-eosin, 400×)

Microvasculopathy is characterized by concentric intimal thickening made up of migrated vascular smooth muscle cells embedded in extracellular matrix and covered by a lining of endothelial cells (Mitchell 2004; Jansen et al. 2015). It is often called immune arteriosclerosis, a term borrowed from atherosclerosis nomenclature (Salomon et al. 1991).

Pathologic changes consist of (Fig. 18.11):

- Myointimal proliferative lesions (fibrocellular intimal proliferation and/or fibrous intimal thickening)

- Medial disease with hypertrophy/hyperplasia of smooth muscle cells and/or fibrosis
- Endothelialitis/vasculitis

These lesions may be independently present or coexist with one prevailing. The media of the intramyocardial arteries is frequently normal or mildly fibrous and in some instances may show a pattern of atrophy with complete loss of vascular smooth muscle cells, resulting in acellular fibrous media (Loupy et al. 2015; Lu et al. 2011). This media pattern reflects vascular smooth muscle cell apoptotic death in the context of alloimmunization, mainly due to antibodies against histocompatibility antigens (Thaunat et al. 2006).

The pathology of the microcirculation in grafted hearts, whether with or without involvement of epicardial branches, has not yet been definitively characterized, and discordant data exist.

Armstrong et al. found no stenosis or intimal thickening of arterioles in myocardial biopsies obtained in 36 months posttransplant (Armstrong et al. 1996), while Hiemann et al. (Hiemann et al. 2007) found stenotic microvasculopathy in 43 % of patients in biopsies as early as 1 year posttransplantation, implying decreased survival independently of epicardial coronary artery lesions. In the latter study, the stenotic arteriolar lesions included media thickening associated with inconstant endothelial thickening, but a subjective grading system was used. Other researchers also found a high incidence of microvascular changes and no correlation with CAV (Abu-Qaoud et al. 2012).

18.6.3 Pathogenesis of CAV Proliferative Lesions

Inflammatory cells found in the thickened intima of epicardial and intramyocardial arteries have a crucial function in the pathogenesis, since they are the signature of an immune/inflammatory process in the arterial wall that triggers the endothelial cells and the smooth muscle cells (Mitchell 2004; van Loosdregt et al. 2006). The cell population present is, in descending order, CD3-positive T lymphocytes (twice more CD4 than CD8), CD68-positive macrophages, and CD20-positive B lymphocytes (van Loosdregt et al. 2006). Host T lymphocytes represent cellular immunity within the intima and are activated by HLA antigens present on donor endothelial cells. Activated T cells produce interferon-γ and TGF-β and in turn stimulate vascular smooth muscle cells to proliferate and produce extracellular matrix (Pober et al. 2014). Innate immunity acting through NK cells and macrophages is also a source of cytokines including interferon-γ. Humoral rejection is now recognized as a major factor in CAV; donor-specific antibodies target the smooth muscle cells (Thaunat et al. 2006; Zhang et al. 2012) and the endothelial cells via complement-dependent and independent mechanisms (Zhang and Reed 2009; Jane-Wit et al. 2013).

B lymphocytes and plasma cells have been detected in the epicardial arteries with CAV either in adventitia with lymphoid nodules or a diffuse pattern or within intimal hyperplasia (Wehner et al. 2010). The lymphoid nodules, resembling tertiary lymphoid nodules, may be a local immune response; the cells in the intima or diffusely distributed in the adventitia may simply be a scarring process (Wehner et al. 2010).

18.6.4 Myocardial Lesions in CAV

Data on pathology of the myocardium comes from autopsy and analysis of failing grafted hearts removed during retransplantation for severe CAV.

In the presence of a culprit lesion, the most frequent substrate is acute myocardial infarction or focal/multifocal acute ischemic/subischemic damage with non-infarction distribution (Fig. 18.12).

In cases of sudden death or cardiac failure, as well as in retransplanted patients, acute lesions can be absent and the pathologic substrate can show chronic myocyte changes (cytoplasmic vacuolization – especially subendocardial, hypertrophy, attenuation, irregular and hyperchromic nuclei, architectural disarrangement) and varying degrees of patchy interstitial fibrosis.

In a series of 64 hearts retransplanted for CAV, Lu et al. (Lu et al. 2011) found cardiomegaly, rarely, gross scarring, indicative of previous infarction, despite severe CAV, and frequently multifocal/diffuse fibrosis (Fig. 18.13). In addition, in these failing grafts, the myocardium quite often displayed features of rejection, mainly antibody-mediated type (Loupy et al. 2015).

Identifying CAV requires repeated coronary angiograms, although this invasive procedure is not frequently performed during patient follow-up. Given that protocol endomyocardial biopsies are mainly performed to detect rejection, an ancillary goal of the analysis of these biopsies is to assess myocardial fibrosis, considering that fibrosis could be an indirect myocardial marker of CAV. Yamani et al. (Yamani et al. 2002) found an increased semiquantitative score of myocardial fibrosis associated with CAV. However, in transplanted hearts, myocardial fibrosis may be the final reparative process of many different noxae. Morphometric quantification of myocardial fibrosis in transplanted patients monitored by endomyocardial biopsy showed that fibrosis increases slowly in long-term survivors without any correlation with CAV (Armstrong et al. 2000). Furthermore in a morphometric study on sequential biopsies, fibrosis has been found to vary from biopsy to biopsy in a given patient and did not correlate with the highest grade of cellular rejection or CAV (Fornes et al. 1996). These data prove that fibrosis found in endomyocardial

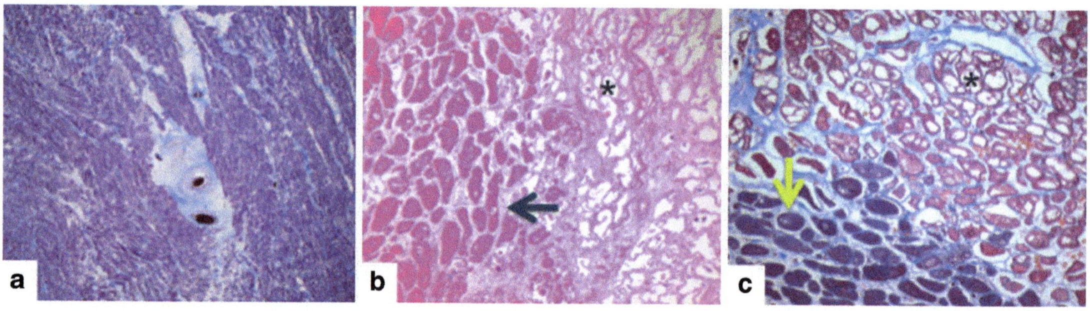

Fig. 18.12 Acute/chronic myocardial ischemic lesions due to CAV. (**a**) Acute myocardial infarct with coagulative necrosis and waviness of myofibers. Note the interstitial fibrosis as sign of previous ischemic damage and the microvasculopathy of small intramyocardial arteries and veins (Azan Mallory trichrome, original magnification 100×). (**b, c**) Coagulative necrosis (*arrows*) associated with cytoplasmic vacuolization (i.e., coagulative myocytolysis) (*asterisks*). (**b**) Hematoxylin-eosin, original magnification 200×; (**c**) Azan Mallory trichrome, original magnification 200×)

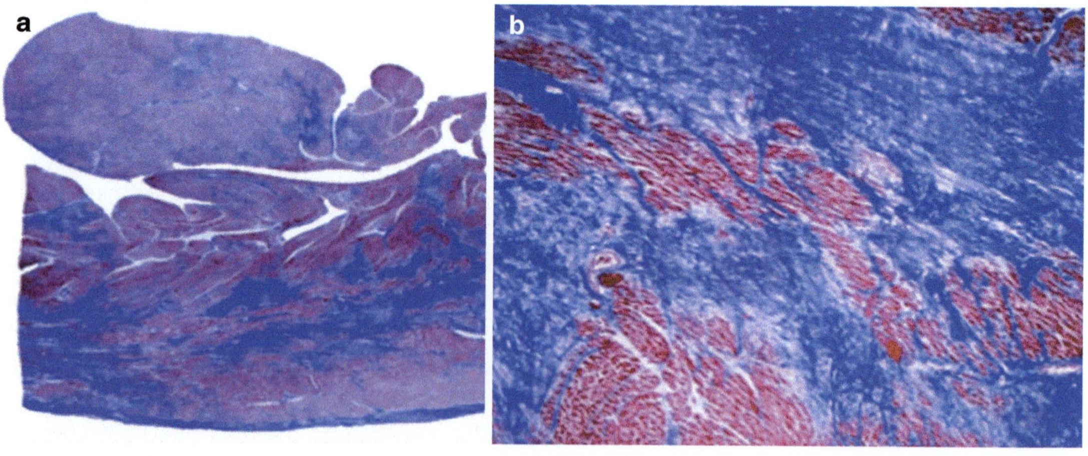

Fig. 18.13 Chronic myocardial ischemic lesions due to CAV. (**a**) Panoramic view of the left ventricle wall with diffuse myocardial fibrosis (Azan Mallory trichrome, original magnification 25×). (**b**) High-power view of A (Azan Mallory trichrome, original magnification 200×)

biopsies cannot be used as a surrogate marker of CAV, but is the result of many pathologic processes built up over time, which all contribute to the restrictive hemodynamics typical of the grafted heart (Kobashigawa et al. 2013; Law et al. 2006).

18.7 Pathophysiology of Microvasculopathy

Functional tests analyzing the coronary circulation are able to distinguish abnormal epicardial coronary function from coronary microvascular dysfunction. Several studies have emphasized the dysfunction of coronary microcirculation in transplanted hearts (Tona et al. 2006, 2015; Haddad et al. 2012), and interestingly this dysfunction has been correlated with the onset of CAV (Tona et al. 2015). This data raises the hypothesis of a common pathophysiologic pathway linking CAV and microcirculation dysfunction with a common target, the endothelial cell (Deng et al. 1995).

Coronary circulation, from a physiological point of view, can be divided into three areas arranged in series, although, anatomically, the boundaries of each compartment are not so clearly defined (Dal Lin et al. 2015; Herrmann et al. 2012; Chilian 1997) (Fig. 18.14). The proximal compart-

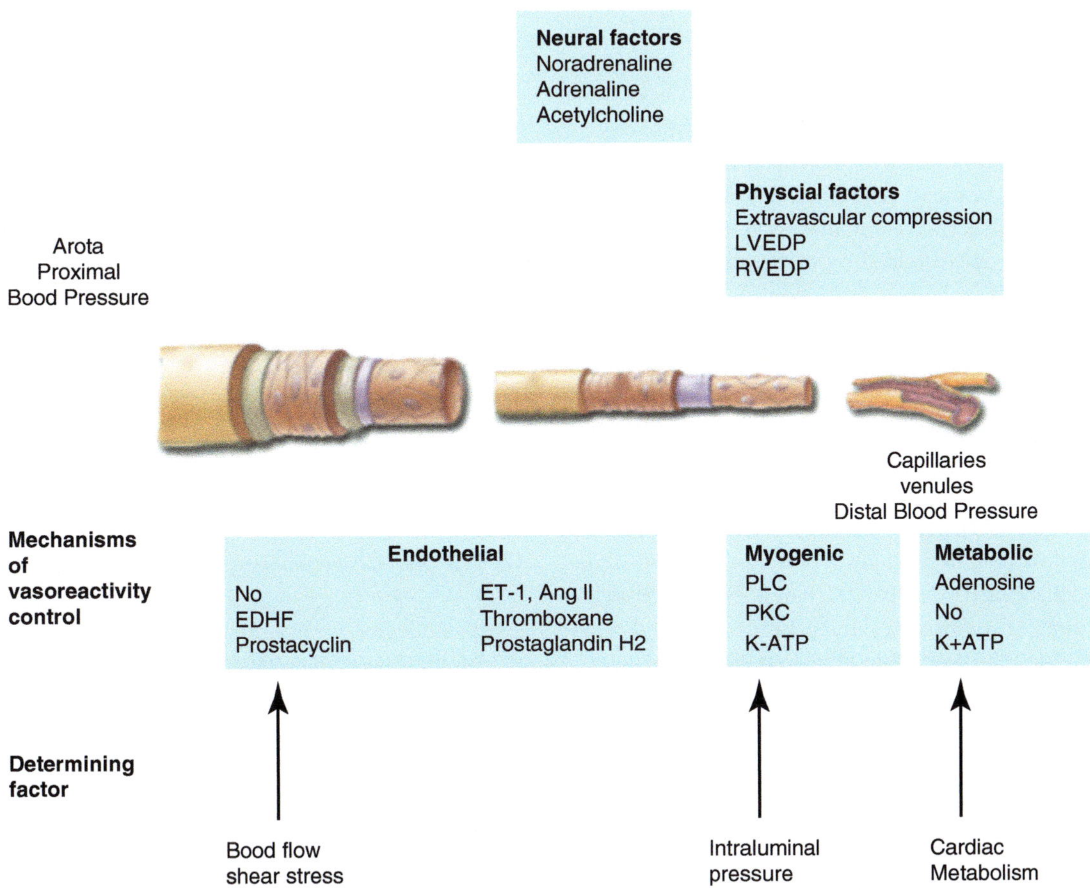

Fig. 18.14 Physiology of coronary circulation (From Dal Lin et al. 2015). The coronary blood flow is driven by the pressure difference between the aorta and the capillary bed and is further modulated by various physical and neural factors influencing the microcirculation. Thus, the coronary circulation adjusts the blood flow to myocardial oxygen requirement, harmonizing the resistances of the various compartments of the microcirculation, each regulated by a separate mechanism

ment consists of the conductance epicardial arteries (diameter 500 μm to 2–5 mm), which offer little resistance to blood flow. They are regulated by the sympathetic system but also possess an inherent tendency to maintain a given level of shear stress through endothelial vasodilation. The intermediate compartment consists of arterioles, characterized by a drop in pressure along their course. Their diameter varies from 100 to 500 μm, and their function is to maintain constant coronary perfusion, regulating blood flow and pressure within the coronary vasculature. The tone of the arterioles depends on intravascular pressure (myogenic autoregulation), local or circulating vasoactive substances, and neurogenic stimuli, but not on the metabolic activity of cardiomyocytes. The distal compartment consists of the intramural arterioles whose diameter is less than 100 μ and which are characterized by a considerable decrease of internal pressure. Their function is to coordinate the requirement for blood with myocardial oxygen consumption. They are responsible for about 55 % of total coronary resistance and are regulated by local vasoactive circulating or neurogenic factors; they are also affected by myocardial cell metabolites (metabolic autoregulation).

Four main factors influence vascular resistance: (1) anatomical (left ventricular wall thickness and the presence of collateral circulation), (2) mechanical (flow systemic vascular resistance, systolic compression, myogenic reflex, blood viscosity or hemolysis, and platelet aggregation), (3) neuro-immune (through alpha- and beta-2 receptors, vagal action), and (4) endocrine-metabolic (pO2, pH, K, adenosine, prostaglandins, thromboxane, hyperlipidemia, and nitric oxide (NO)) (Camici and Crea 2007).

Therefore, the mechanisms underlying the regulation of coronary blood flow are metabolic and myogenic autoregulation, nervous system regulation, and humoral control.

18.7.1 Coronary Self-Regulation

Coronary self-regulation or autoregulation means the intrinsic ability of the heart to maintain blood flow relatively constant, despite changes in perfusion pressure (within the limits of pressure from 60 to 180 mmHg, provided that the level of oxygen incorporation remains constant). These mechanisms predominate in the microcirculation where they mostly impact on total coronary resistance.

(a) *Metabolic autoregulation.* Metabolic action, adjusting the flow to tissue metabolic demand, is mainly mediated by adenosine, although this is not the only factor involved. Adenosine is released from the myocardial cells in the interstitial space (Rubio and Berne 1975) in various conditions, both physiological and pathophysiological: when the metabolic demand increases, adenosine triphosphate (ATP) hydrolysis takes place and adenosine is released into the interstitium causing vasodilation and, therefore, increases blood flow.
(b) *Myogenic autoregulation.* The mechanism by which vascular wall tone changes as a result of endovascular pressure changes, and, therefore, wall tension is regulated according to the "stretch stress," in order to maintain a stable flow within a certain range of perfusion pressure variation. It is more evident in the subepicardial than in subendocardial layer and can also be adjusted by NO and interferes with metabolic vasodilation (Jones et al. 1993).

18.7.2 Autonomic Regulation

Sympathetic and parasympathetic autonomic control of microvascular resistance has two effects, one direct and one indirect. Through activation of β1 receptors, sympathetic tone increases oxygen consumption and metabolic active vasodilation. As a direct effect on receptors α, we get vasoconstriction, which can lead to an increase up to 20–30 % of resistances at the subepicardial level with the purpose of limiting metabolic vasodilation and ensuring a more homogeneous distribution of the transmural flow. Cholinergic activation has the indirect effect of myocardial oxygen consumption (bradycardia) and extravascular compression (negative inotropy) reduction. The direct effect is endothelium dependent: it has been shown that inhibiting the endothelial NO synthesis eliminates cholinergic reflected vasodilation (Hodgson and Marshall 1989).

18.7.3 Humoral Regulation

The substances involved in the humoral control of coronary microvascular resistance consist of circulating, non-circulating, and endothelium-derived factors. The circulating ones are primarily catecholamines, vasopressin, angiotensin II with a vasoconstrictor effect, and the atrial natriuretic factor with a vasodilator effect. Among the non-circulating, there are arachidonic acid derivatives such as prostacyclin (vasodilator) and thromboxane A2 with vasoconstrictor effect. Among the factors of endothelial origin, NO and endothelium-derived relaxing factors (EDRF) are vasodilators, and endothelin is a vasoconstrictor (Dal Lin et al. 2015).

Moreover, there is a constant production of NO in basal conditions as a result of physical or neurohumoral factors (Kelm and Schrader 1990) which is an important control factor for endothelial coronary microvascular tone. Endothelial control directs both the myogenic self-regulation processes and the effects of autonomic stimulation. The inhibition of NO production leads to an increase in coronary vascular resistance, thus confirming a basic NO-dependent vasodilator tone (Kuo et al. 1992).

18.8 Coronary Flow Reserve

18.8.1 Definition

The functional status of coronary circulation can be clinically assessed by measuring the coronary flow reserve (CFR), defined as the ratio between the speed of the hyperemic diastolic flow ceiling and the diastolic baseline. The value of the CFR is, therefore, the ability of both the vascular coronary components (i.e., vascular resistance at the epicardial and microvascular levels), responding to a hyperemizing stimulus to obtain a maximal coronary flow. Thus, thanks to its self-regulating coronary mechanism, the heart, in rest conditions, can maintain coronary blood flow constant along a wide range of pressures at the expense of a coronary vasodilation. However, when the vasodilation becomes maximal, the pressure-flow relationship becomes linear. The difference between the coronary flow ceiling and the self-regulated flow represents the coronary flow reserve (Fig. 18.15), which indicates the proportion of "additional" flow (expressed in ml/min/g) which can be obtained at a given pressure when the vessels have reached maximum vasodilatation.

18.8.2 Factors Affecting the Coronary Reserve

The CFR is affected by vascular resistance, by myocardial extravascular resistance, and by rheological components (Dal Lin et al. 2015). Since CFR is expressed by a ratio, it may fall as a result of an increase in coronary blood flow at rest, secondary to the increased metabolic demands (due to tachycardia, pathological myocardial hypertrophy, hypoxemia, anemia, vasodilators and vasoconstrictors, increased myocardial contractility), or as a result of a reduction in the flow's hyperemic ceiling as in the case of microcirculatory dysfunction, epicardial stenosis, blood hyperviscosity, and abnormal cardiovascular function (as in the case of elevated diastolic pressure of the left ventricle or aortic mean pressure reduction) (Dal Lin et al. 2015). In other words, the CFR can be reduced by structural or functional causes. It is proved that in the presence of single-vessel stenosis and normal ventricular function, the flow at baseline remains constant with increasing severity of the stenosis, while the maximal flow decreases in a gradual manner (not linear) (Uren et al. 1994); vasodilator capacity is diminished because the coronary reserve is already recruited in basal conditions due to the presence of the stricture (Fig. 18.16). Among the structural causes of reduced CFR, we must consider vasculitis, microvascular alterations in systemic inflammatory diseases, posttransplant

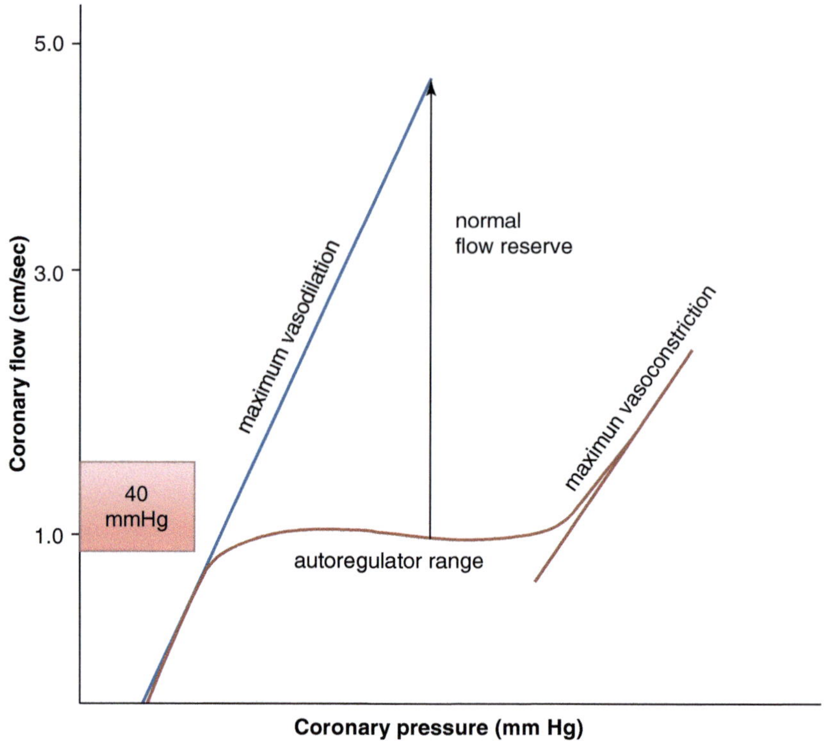

Fig. 18.15 Relationship between perfusion pressure and coronary flow

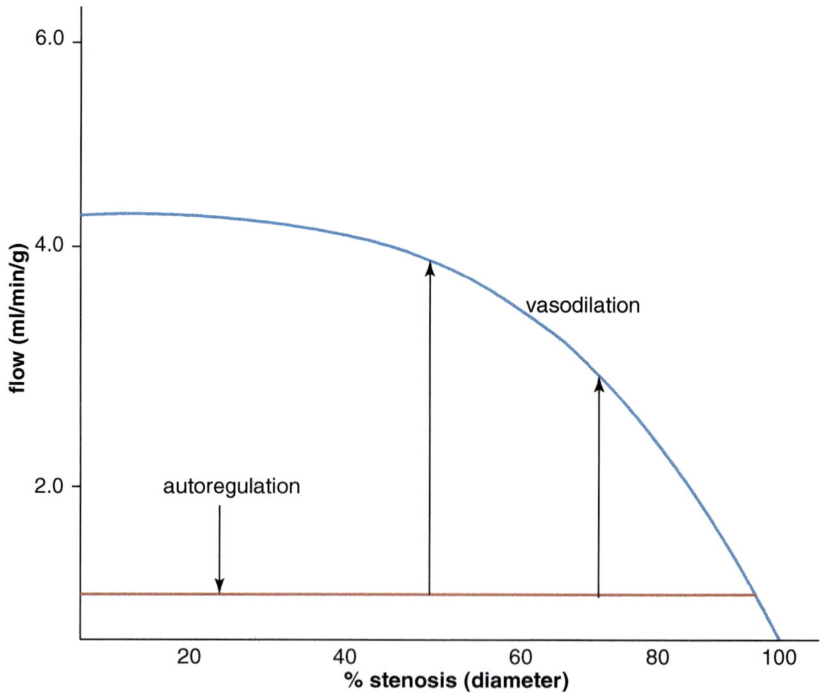

Fig. 18.16 Schematic representation of reduction of the CFR with progression of stenosis. With stenosis less than 40 %, CFR remains normal

vasculopathy (Hiemann et al. 2007), diabetic microangiopathy, or arterial remodeling with intimal and media thickening as in hypertrophic cardiomyopathy (Cecchi et al. 2003). Finally, Buus et al. have shown that in healthy subjects, myocardial hyperemia induced by adenosine is partially dependent on the normal endogenous production of NO, suggesting that adenosine-induced vasodilation is partially endothelium dependent (Buus et al. 2001); other studies (van den Heuvel et al. 2000; Osto et al. 2012) confirm a decrease in coronary reserve caused by coronary endothelial dysfunction. In conclusion, the CFR is a global parameter of coronary flow, which is immediately altered in the presence of microvascular dysfunction or stenosis of epicardial coronary arteries. It has been shown that, in the absence of the latter, CFR value is a good marker of microcirculatory function. Its normal value is greater than 2.5 (Dal Lin et al. 2015). Camici and Crea (Crea et al. 2014) proposed a classification of coronary microvascular dysfunction (CMVD) into four types:

1. Coronary microvascular dysfunction in the absence of coronary artery disease or myocardial disease: it is the counterpart of traditional coronary risk factors such as smoking, hypertension, hyperlipidemia, diabetes, and the state of insulin resistance. It is a microcirculatory dysfunction at least partially reversible.
2. Coronary microvascular dysfunction in the presence of a myocardial pathology (secondary heart disease and primary cardiomyopathies): it is represented by remodeling of the intramural coronary arterioles. It could have a role in inducing myocardial ischemia.
3. Coronary microvascular dysfunction in the presence of obstructive coronary artery disease: it can be identified in the context of stable coronary disease or acute coronary syndrome with or without ST-segment elevation.
4. Iatrogenic coronary microvascular dysfunction: after revascularization, CMVD may be caused either by vasoconstriction or by distal embolization (Camici and Crea 2007). The alterations of the tunica media have an independent negative effect on prognosis (Hiemann et al. 2007).

Microcirculatory dysfunction, defined as reduced coronary flow reserve and/or coronary endothelial dysfunction, is associated with 2.5 % of major annual adverse events, including death, nonfatal myocardial infarction, nonfatal stroke, and congestive heart failure (Dal Lin et al. 2015). It is the mechanism responsible for the onset of ischemic phenomena in the absence of critical angiographically visible atherosclerotic lesions in epicardial vessels.

The integrity of the endothelial cells is critical for endothelial homeostatic response. Endothelial cells are in a strategic anatomical position, placed between the bloodstream and the vessel wall; they regulate the function and structure of the vessel and release vasoconstrictors and vasodilating agents (Cosentino and Luscher 1995).

In physiological conditions, the synergistic action of endothelial factors allows maintenance of normal vascular tone and blood fluidity while limiting inflammatory damage to the vessel and the proliferation of smooth muscle cells. Among substances with a vasodilating effect, the most important is NO, which is produced by the catabolism of L-arginine by the enzyme NO synthetase and expressed constitutively by endothelial cells. NO is released as a result of different stimuli, both mechanical (shear wall stress) and biochemical (acetylcholine, bradykinin, serotonin, etc.), and acts on both the smooth muscle cells of the vessel and on the corpuscular elements of blood (monocytes, platelets), so mediating the expression of adhesion molecules through guanylate cyclase activation (Dal Lin et al. 2015). Due to its powerful anti-inflammatory effects, NO derived from the endothelium can be considered the most important endogenous antiatherogenic molecule.

In pathological conditions, however, the endothelium changes and becomes susceptible to damage and, even worse, promotes inflammation and thrombosis. It also loses its active vascular control on permeability so causing vasoconstriction and circulating leukocyte adhesion, which in turn give rise to formation and progression of atherosclerotic plaque (Luscher and Barton 1997). In the presence of disease or cardiovascular risk factors, which alter endothelial physiology, endothelial cells decrease their ability to release vasodilating substances, which allows the predominance of vasoconstrictive products (Behrendt and Ganz 2002). Risk factors that damage the endothelium are divided into modifiable (hypertension, diabetes, smoking, high cholesterol, obesity, sedentary lifestyle associated with unbalanced diet) and non-modifiable (old age and male gender). Chronic inflammation and infections have recently been suggested as risk factors for endothelial dysfunction (Dal Lin et al. 2015).

The vasoconstrictive mediators are prostanoids: thromboxane A2, vasoconstrictive prostaglandins, and free radicals which, in addition to directly causing vasoconstriction, reduce the bioavailability of NO by destroying it. Endothelin 1 and angiotensin II are vasoconstrictors and also induce cell growth by modifying the vascular structure (Osto et al. 2010).

Generally, therefore, the bioavailability of NO indicates the state of health and functionality of the vessel. As described by Osto et al. (2012): "the increased production of reactive oxygen species (ROS) is considered a major determinant of the reduction in the levels of NO. The loss of NO, due to increased oxidative stress in the vessel wall, can be considered the central mediator of all the different aspects related to endothelial dysfunction, contributing to the destabilization of the atherosclerotic plaque. The loss of NO produced by the endothelium leads to an increase in gene transcription of pro-inflammatory nuclear factor kappa B (NF-KB), resulting in the increased expression of adhesion molecules and the production of cytokines and chemokines. These actions promote the migration of monocytes and vascular smooth muscle cells in the intima of the vessels and in the transformation of macrophages in foam cells, phenomena that are characteristic of early morphological changes of atherosclerosis." So, altered bioavailability of NO, leading to endothelial dysfunction, is a key pathological condition that is associated with most if not all cardiovascular risk factors (Dal Lin et al. 2015).

18.9 Endothelial Function After Heart Transplant

After heart transplant, the restoration of endothelial function is neither immediate nor complete, although the coronary endothelium is replaced by a presumably healthier one, and hemodynamics improve along with endothelial shear stress. After transplantation, the coronary endothelium is characterized by chimerism, with donor- and recipient-derived endothelial cells (Minami et al. 2005; Angelini et al. 2007). Studies of sex-mismatched heart-transplanted patients have shown that as early as 1 month after transplantation, up to 22 % of endothelial cells in the coronary arteries are of recipient origin (Minami et al. 2005). Chimerism continues over time, with recipient origin endothelial cells increasing by about 0.43+−0.77 % per month following transplantation (Angelini et al. 2007), in both pediatric and adult patients.

Probably the high prevalence of coronary endothelial dysfunction described shortly after heart transplant is due to the persistence of atherosclerosis risk factors, inflammation, and the use of immunosuppressive drugs (such as cyclosporine) that decrease NO and increase levels of endothelin and ROS production (Fig. 18.17).

Coronary endothelial dysfunction in early posttransplant patients has been correlated with a higher risk of developing cardiac allograft vasculopathy (Tona et al. 2006).

Key Points

- Cardiac allograft vasculopathy (CAV) is the complex phenomenon which frequently affects the vasculature of grafted hearts in both adult and pediatric cardiac transplantations, leading to progressive stenosing of cardiac vessels.
- CAV remains a major cause of late graft failure and death after heart transplantation.
- Over the years, many synonyms have been used for CAV: chronic rejection, allograft vasculopathy, transplant vasculopathy, accelerated atherosclerosis, transplant coronary artery disease, allograft arteriopathy, cardiac transplant arteriosclerosis, and transplant atherosclerosis.
- CAV risk factors are both immunologic and non-immunologic.
- Clinically, CAV presents as progressive heart failure, arrhythmia, or sudden death in the later stages. Myocardial infarction is also common but is generally silent due to cardiac denervation.
- Coronary angiography coupled with assessment of allograft function offers the highest level of evidence for CAV identification and nomenclature.
- Pathologically, cardiac vessels progressively develop an intimal thickening,

which causes narrowing of the vessel lumen until occlusion.

- The disease typically involves epicardial coronary arteries and intramyocardial vessels with diameter greater than 500 μm (macrovasculopathy) and/or small intramyocardial vessels (<500 μm) (microvasculopathy). Veins and venules may also be affected.
- Pathologic changes of *macrovasculopathy* consist of:
  - Proliferative/hyperplastic intimal lesions
  - Vasculitis/perivascular inflammation
  - Conventional atherosclerotic lesions
- Pathologic changes of *microvasculopathy* consist of:
  - Myointimal proliferative lesions (fibrocellular intimal proliferation and/or fibrous intimal thickening)
  - Medial disease with hypertrophy/hyperplasia of smooth muscle cells and/or fibrosis
  - Endothelialitis/vasculitis
- *Myocardial lesions*. In the presence of a culprit lesion, the most frequent substrate is acute myocardial infarction; in cases of sudden death or cardiac failure, the most frequent pathologic substrate includes chronic myocyte changes and varying degrees of patchy interstitial fibrosis.
- Dysfunction of the coronary microcirculation in transplanted hearts has been correlated with the onset of CAV, thus raising the hypothesis of a common pathophysiologic pathway linking CAV and microcirculation.

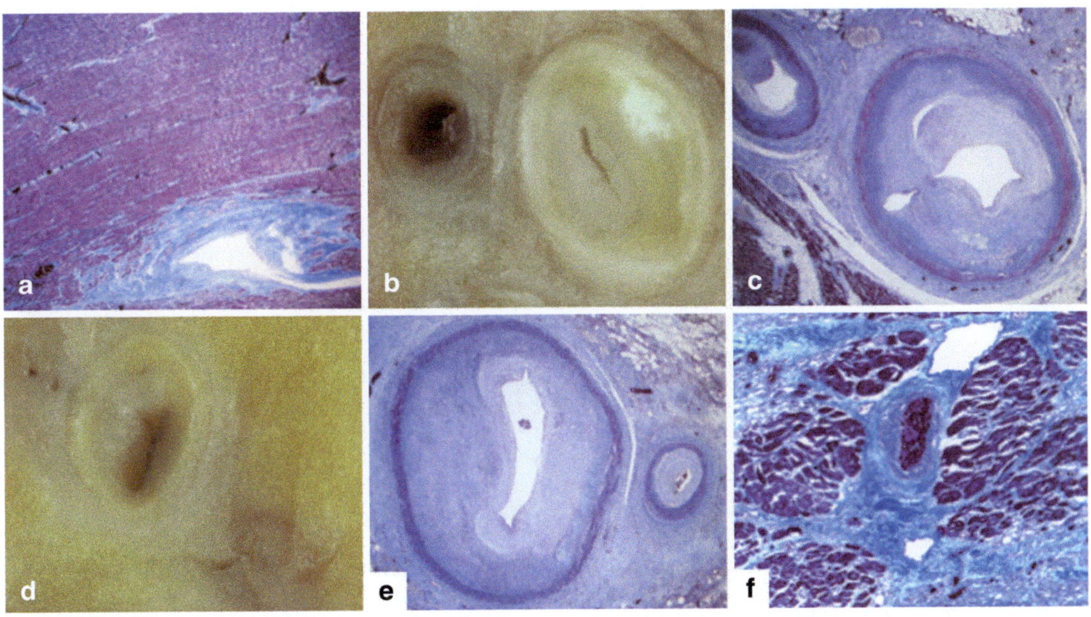

Fig. 18.17 Illustrative case. A 40-year-old male, transplanted in 2004 for Ebstein's anomaly, died suddenly of severe coronary allograft vasculopathy after 10 years. The myocardium showed severe multifocal areas of fibrosis but no sign of acute myocardial infarction (**a**, Azan Mallory trichrome, original magnification 100×). The left anterior descending coronary artery (**b**, stereomicroscopic view; **c**, histologic section; Azan Mallory trichrome, original magnification 125×) and the right coronary artery (**d**, stereomicroscopic view; **e**, histologic section; Azan Mallory trichrome, original magnification 125×) showed severe diffuse concentric hyperplastic proliferative lesions, with well-preserved tunica media and enlarged fibrotic adventitia. Intramyocardial small vessels were also involved (**f**, Azan Mallory trichrome, original magnification 200×)

References

Abu-Qaoud MS, Stoletniy LN, Chen D, Kerstetter J, Kuhn M, Pai RG. Lack of relationship between microvascular and macrovascular disease in heart transplant recipients. Transplantation. 2012;94:965–70.

Alexander RT, Lathrop S, Vollmer R, Blue L, Russell SD, Steenbergen C. Graft vascular disease after cardiac transplantation and its relationship to mean acute rejection score. Arch Pathol Lab Med. 2005;129:1283–7.

Angelini A, Castellani C, Tona F, Gambino A, Caforio AP, Feltrin G, Della Barbera M, Valente M, Gerosa G, Thiene G. Continuous engraftment and differentiation of male recipient Y-chromosome-positive cardiomyocytes in donor female human heart transplants. J Heart Lung Transplant. 2007;26(11):1110–8.

Angelini A, Castellani C, Fedrigo M, de Boer OJ, Meijer-Jorna LB, Li X, Valente M, Thiene G, van der Wal AC. Coronary cardiac allograft vasculopathy versus native atherosclerosis: difficulties in classification. Virchows Arch. 2014;464:627–35.

Armstrong AT, Strauch AR, Kardan A, Starling RC. Morphometric and immunocytochemical analysis of coronary arterioles in human transplanted hearts. J Heart Lung Transplant. 1996;15:818–26.

Armstrong AT, Binkley PF, Baker PB, Leier CV. Histologic comparison of allograft myocardium between short- and long-term survivors of human cardiac transplantation. Am J Cardiol. 2000;86:1148–51. A1149.

Atkinson C, Horsley J, Rhind-Tutt S, Charman S, Phillpotts CJ, Wallwork J, Goddard MJ. Neointimal smooth muscle cells in human cardiac allograft coronary artery vasculopathy are of donor origin. J Heart Lung Transplant. 2004;23:427–35.

Behrendt D, Ganz P. Endothelial function. From vascular biology to clinical applications. Am J Cardiol. 2002; 90:40L–8.

Bieber CP, Stinson EB, Shumway NE, Payne R, Kosek J. Cardiac transplantation in man. VII. Cardiac allograft pathology. Circulation. 1970;41:753–72.

Bolad IA, Robinson DR, Webb C, Hamour I, Burke MM, Banner NR. Impaired left ventricular systolic function early after heart transplantation is associated with cardiac allograft vasculopathy. Am J Transplant. 2006;6: 161–8.

Buus NH, Bottcher M, Hermansen F, Sander M, Nielsen TT, Mulvany MJ. Influence of nitric oxide synthase and adrenergic inhibition on adenosine-induced myocardial hyperemia. Circulation. 2001;104:2305–10.

Camici PG, Crea F. Coronary microvascular dysfunction. N Engl J Med. 2007;356:830–40.

Castellani C, Angelini A, de Boer OJ, van der Loos CM, Fedrigo M, Frigo AC, Meijer-Jorna LB, Li X, Ploegmakers HJ, Tona F, Feltrin G, Gerosa G, Valente M, Thiene G, van der Wal AC. Intraplaque hemorrhage in cardiac allograft vasculopathy. Am J Transplant. 2014;14:184–92.

Cecchi F, Olivotto I, Gistri R, Lorenzoni R, Chiriatti G, Camici PG. Coronary microvascular dysfunction and prognosis in hypertrophic cardiomyopathy. N Engl J Med. 2003;349:1027–35.

Chantranuwat C, Blakey JD, Kobashigawa JA, Moriguchi JD, Laks H, Vassilakis ME, Fishbein MC. Sudden, unexpected death in cardiac transplant recipients: an autopsy study. J Heart Lung Transplant. 2004;23: 683–9.

Chilian WM. Coronary microcirculation in health and disease. Summary of an NHLBI workshop. Circulation. 1997;95:522–8.

Cosentino F, Luscher TF. Maintenance of vascular integrity: role of nitric oxide and other bradykinin mediators. Eur Heart J. 1995;16(Suppl K):4–12.

Costanzo MR, Naftel DC, Pritzker MR, Heilman 3rd JK, Boehmer JP, Brozena SC, Dec GW, Ventura HO, Kirklin JK, Bourge RC, Miller LW. Heart transplant coronary artery disease detected by coronary angiography: a multiinstitutional study of preoperative donor and recipient risk factors. Cardiac Transplant Research Database. J Heart Lung Transplant. 1998;17:744–53.

Coutance G, Ouldamar S, Rouvier P, Saheb S, Suberbielle C, Brechot N, Hariri S, Lebreton G, Leprince P, Varnous S. Late antibody-mediated rejection after heart transplantation: Mortality, graft function, and fulminant cardiac allograft vasculopathy. J Heart Lung Transplant. 2015;34:1050–7.

Crea F, Camici PG, Bairey Merz CN. Coronary microvascular dysfunction: an update. Eur Heart J. 2014;35: 1101–11.

Dal Lin C, Tona F, Osto E. Coronary microvascular function and beyond: the crosstalk between hormones, cytokines, and neurotransmitters. Int J Endocrinol. 2015;31:28–48.

Delgado JF, Reyne AG, de Dios S, Lopez-Medrano F, Jurado A, Juan RS, Ruiz-Cano MJ, Dolores Folgueira M, Gomez-Sanchez MA, Aguado JM, Lumbreras C. Influence of cytomegalovirus infection in the development of cardiac allograft vasculopathy after heart transplantation. J Heart Lung Transplant. 2015;34:1112–9.

Deng MC, Bell S, Huie P, Pinto F, Hunt SA, Stinson EB, Sibley R, Hall BM, Valantine HA. Cardiac allograft vascular disease. Relationship to microvascular cell surface markers and inflammatory cell phenotypes on endomyocardial biopsy. Circulation. 1995;91:1647–54.

Elhendy A, van Domburg RT, Vantrimpont P, Poldermans D, Bax JJ, van Gelder T, Baan CC, Schinkel A, Roelandt JR, Balk AH. Prediction of mortality in heart transplant recipients by stress technetium-99m tetrofosmin myocardial perfusion imaging. Am J Cardiol. 2002;89:964–8.

Fornes P, Heudes D, Simon D, Guillemain R, Amrein C, Bruneval P. Influence of acute or chronic rejection on myocardial collagen density in serial endomyocardial biopsy specimens from cardiac allografts. J Heart Lung Transplant. 1996;15:796–803.

Frank R, Molina MR, Goldberg LR, Wald JW, Kamoun M, Lal P. Circulating donor-specific anti-human leukocyte antigen antibodies and complement C4d deposition are associated with the development of cardiac allograft vasculopathy. Am J Clin Pathol. 2014;142:809–15.

Gao SZ, Alderman EL, Schroeder JS, Silverman JF, Hunt SA. Accelerated coronary vascular disease in the heart transplant patient: coronary arteriographic findings. J Am Coll Cardiol. 1988;12:334–40.

Gaudin PB, Rayburn BK, Hutchins GM, Kasper EK, Baughman KL, Goodman SN, Lecks LE, Baumgartner WA, Hruban RH. Peritransplant injury to the myocardium associated with the development of accelerated arteriosclerosis in heart transplant recipients. Am J Surg Pathol. 1994;18:338–46.

Graham JA, Wilkinson RA, Hirohashi T, Chase CM, Colvin RB, Madsen JC, Fishman JA, Russell PS. Viral infection induces de novo lesions of coronary allograft vasculopathy through a natural killer cell-dependent pathway. Am J Transplant. 2009;9:2479–84.

Gulizia JM, Kandolf R, Kendall TJ, Thieszen SL, Wilson JE, Radio SJ, Costanzo MR, Winters GL, Miller LL, McManus BM. Infrequency of cytomegalovirus genome in coronary arteriopathy of human heart allografts. Am J Pathol. 1995;147:461–75.

Haddad F, Khazanie P, Deuse T, Weisshaar D, Zhou J, Nam CW, Vu TA, Gomari FA, Skhiri M, Simos A, Schnittger I, Vrotvec B, Hunt SA, Fearon WF. Clinical and functional correlates of early microvascular dysfunction after heart transplantation. Circ Heart Fail. 2012;5:759–68.

Hamon D, Taleski J, Vaseghi M, Shivkumar K, Boyle NG. Arrhythmias in the heart transplant patient. Arrhythm Electrophysiol Rev. 2014;3:149–55.

Herrmann J, Kaski JC, Lerman A. Coronary microvascular dysfunction in the clinical setting: from mystery to reality. Eur Heart J. 2012;33:2771–2782b.

Hiemann NE, Wellnhofer E, Knosalla C, Lehmkuhl HB, Stein J, Hetzer R, Meyer R. Prognostic impact of microvasculopathy on survival after heart transplantation: evidence from 9713 endomyocardial biopsies. Circulation. 2007;116:1274–82.

Hodgson JM, Marshall JJ. Direct vasoconstriction and endothelium-dependent vasodilation. Mechanisms of acetylcholine effects on coronary flow and arterial diameter in patients with nonstenotic coronary arteries. Circulation. 1989;79:1043–51.

Huibers MMH, Vink A, Kaldeway J, Huisman A, Timmermans K, Leenders M, Shipper MEI, Laphor JR, Kirkels HJH, Klöpping C, de Jonge N, de Weger RA. Distinct phenotypes of cardiac allograft vasculopathy after heart transplantation: a histopathological study. Atherosclerosis. 2014;236:353–9.

Imamura T, Kinugawa K, Murasawa T, Kagami Y, Endo M, Muraoka H, Fujino T, Inaba T, Maki H, Hatano M, Kinoshita O, Nawata K, Kyo S, Komuro I, Ono M. Cardiac allograft vasculopathy can be distinguished from donor-transmitted coronary atherosclerosis by optical coherence tomography imaging in a heart transplantation recipient: double layered intimal thickness. Int Heart J. 2014;55:178–80.

Jane-Wit D, Manes TD, Yi T, Qin L, Clark P, Kirkiles-Smith NC, Abrahimi P, Devalliere J, Moeckel G, Kulkarni S, Tellides G, Pober JS. Alloantibody and complement promote T cell-mediated cardiac allograft vasculopathy through noncanonical nuclear factor-kappaB signaling in endothelial cells. Circulation. 2013;128:2504–16.

Jansen MA, Otten HG, de Weger RA, Huibers MM. Immunological and Fibrotic Mechanisms in Cardiac Allograft Vasculopathy. Transplantation. 2015;99:2467–75.

Jimenez J, Kapadia SR, Yamani MH, Platt L, Hobbs RE, Rincon G, Botts-Silverman C, Starling RC, Young JB, Nissen SE, Tuzcu M, Ratliff NB. Cellular rejection and rate of progression of transplant vasculopathy: a 3-year serial intravascular ultrasound study. J Heart Lung Transplant. 2001;20:393–8.

Jones CJ, Kuo L, Davis MJ, Chilian WM. Myogenic and flow-dependent control mechanisms in the coronary microcirculation. Basic Res Cardiol. 1993;88:2–10.

Kapadia SR, Nissen SE, Ziada KM, Rincon G, Crowe TD, Boparai N, Young JB, Tuzcu EM. Impact of lipid abnormalities in development and progression of transplant coronary disease: a serial intravascular ultrasound study. J Am Coll Cardiol. 2001;38:206–13.

Kelm M, Schrader J. Control of coronary vascular tone by nitric oxide. Circ Res. 1990;66:1561–75.

Kobashigawa JA, Itagaki BK, Razi RR, Patel JK, Chai W, Kawano MA, Goldstein Z, Kittleson MM, Fishbein MC. Correlation between myocardial fibrosis and restrictive cardiac physiology in patients undergoing retransplantation. Clin Transplant. 2013;27:E679–84.

Kfoury AG, Snow GL, Budge D, Alharethi RA, Stehlik J, Everitt MD, Miller DV, Drakos SG, Reid BB, Revelo MP, Gilbert EM, Selzman CH, Bader FM, Connelly JJ, Hammond ME. A longitudinal study of the course of asymptomatic antibody-mediated rejection in heart transplantation. J Heart Lung Transplant. 2012;31:46–51.

Kim MS, Kang SJ, Lee CW, Han S, Park DW, Lee SW, Kim YH, Park SW, Park SJ, Kim JJ. Prevalence of coronary atherosclerosis in asymptomatic healthy subjects: an intravascular ultrasound study of donor hearts. J Atheroscler Thromb. 2013;20:465–71.

Kuo L, Davis MJ, Cannon MS, Chilian WM. Pathophysiological consequences of atherosclerosis extend into the coronary microcirculation. Restoration of endothelium-dependent responses by L-arginine. Circ Res. 1992;70:465–76.

Law Y, Boyle G, Miller S, Clendaniel J, Ettedgui J, Beerman L, Counihan P, Webber S. Restrictive hemodynamics are present at the time of diagnosis of allograft coronary artery disease in children. Pediatr Transplant. 2006;10:948–52.

Leone O, Gherardi S, Targa L, Pasanisi E, Mikus P, Tanganelli P, Maccherini M, Arpesella G, Picano E, Bombardini T. Stress echocardiography as a gatekeeper to donation in aged marginal donor hearts: anatomic and pathologic correlations of abnormal stress echocardiography results. J Heart Lung Transplant. 2009;28:1141–9.

Li H, Tanaka K, Anzai H, Oeser B, Lai D, Kobashigawa JA, Tobis JM. Influence of pre-existing donor atherosclerosis on the development of cardiac allograft vasculopathy and outcomes in heart transplant recipients. J Am Coll Cardiol. 2006;47:2470–6.

Loupy A, Toquet C, Rouvier P, Beuscart T, Bories MC, Varnous S, Guillemain R, Pattier S, Suberbielle C, Leprince P, Lefaucheur C, Jouven X, Bruneval P, Duong Van Huyen JP. Late failing heart allografts: pathology of cardiac allograft vasculopathy and association with antibody-mediated rejection. Am J Transplant. 2015;16:111–20.

Lu WH, Palatnik K, Fishbein GA, Lai C, Levi DS, Perens G, Alejos J, Kobashigawa J, Fishbein MC. Diverse morphologic manifestations of cardiac allograft vasculopathy: a pathologic study of 64 allograft hearts. J Heart Lung Transplant. 2011;30:1044–50.

Lund LH, Edwards LB, Kucheryavaya AY, Benden C, Dipchand AI, Goldfarb S, Levvey BJ, Meiser B, Rossano JW, Yusen RD, Stehlik J. The Registry of the International Society for Heart and Lung Transplantation: Thirty-second Official Adult Heart Transplantation Report--2015; Focus Theme: early graft failure. J Heart Lung Transplant. 2015;34:1244–54.

Lund LH, Edwards LB, Kucheryavaya AY, Benden C, Christie JD, Dipchand AI, Dobbels F, Goldfarb SB, Levvey BJ, Meiser B, Yusen RD, Stehlik J. The registry of the International Society for Heart and Lung Transplantation: thirty-first official adult heart transplant report--2014; focus theme: retransplantation. J Heart Lung Transplant. 2014;33:996–1008.

Luscher TF, Barton M. Biology of the endothelium. Clin Cardiol. 1997;20:II-3-10.

Manrique A, Bernard M, Hitzel A, Bubenheim M, Tron C, Agostini D, Cribier A, Vera P, Bessou JP, Redonnet M. Diagnostic and prognostic value of myocardial perfusion gated SPECT in orthotopic heart transplant recipients. J Nucl Cardiol. 2010;17:197–206.

Mehra MR, Ventura HO, Chambers RB, Ramireddy K, Smart FW, Stapleton DD. The prognostic impact of immunosuppression and cellular rejection on cardiac allograft vasculopathy: time for a reappraisal. J Heart Lung Transplant. 1997;16:743–51.

Mehra MR, Uber PA, Ventura HO, Scott RL, Park MH. The impact of mode of donor brain death on cardiac allograft vasculopathy: an intravascular ultrasound study. J Am Coll Cardiol. 2004;43:806–10.

Mehra MR, Crespo-Leiro MG, Dipchand A, Ensminger SM, Hiemann NE, Kobashigawa JA, Madsen J, Parameshwar J, Starling RC, Uber PA. International Society for Heart and Lung Transplantation working formulation of a standardized nomenclature for cardiac allograft vasculopathy-2010. J Heart Lung Transplant. 2010;29:717–27.

Milam JD, Shipkey Jr FH, Lind Jr CJ, Nora JJ, Leachman RD, Rochelle DG, Bloodwell RD, Hallman GL, Cooley DA. Morphologic findings in human cardiac allografts. Circulation. 1970;41:519–35.

Minami E, Laflamme MA, Saffitz JE, Murry CE. Extracardiac progenitor cells repopulate most major cell types in the transplanted human heart. Circulation. 2005;112:2951–8.

Mitchell RN. Allograft arteriopathy: pathogenesis update. Cardiovasc Pathol. 2004;13:33–40.

Osto E, Tona F, De Bon E, Iliceto S, Cella G. Endothelial dysfunction in cardiac allograft vasculopathy: potential pharmacological interventions. Curr Vasc Pharmacol. 2010;8:169–88.

Osto E, Fallo F, Pelizzo MR, Maddalozzo A, Sorgato N, Corbetti F, Montisci R, Famoso G, Bellu R, Luscher TF, Iliceto S, Tona F. Coronary microvascular dysfunction induced by primary hyperparathyroidism is restored after parathyroidectomy. Circulation. 2012; 126:1031–9.

Pober JS, Jane-wit D, Qin L, Tellides G. Interacting mechanisms in the pathogenesis of cardiac allograft vasculopathy. Arterioscler Thromb Vasc Biol. 2014;34:1609–14.

Potena L, Holweg CT, Chin C, Luikart H, Weisshaar D, Narasimhan B, Fearon WF, Lewis DB, Cooke JP, Mocarski ES, Valantine HA. Acute rejection and cardiac allograft vascular disease is reduced by suppression of subclinical cytomegalovirus infection. Transplantation. 2006;82:398–405.

Prada-Delgado O, Estevez-Loureiro R, Paniagua-Martin MJ, Lopez-Sainz A, Crespo-Leiro MG. Prevalence and prognostic value of cardiac allograft vasculopathy 1 year after heart transplantation according to the ISHLT recommended nomenclature. J Heart Lung Transplant. 2012;31:332–3.

Rahmani M, Cruz RP, Granville DJ, McManus BM. Allograft vasculopathy versus atherosclerosis. Circ Res. 2006;99:801–15.

Raichlin E, Edwards BS, Kremers WK, Clavell AL, Rodeheffer RJ, Frantz RP, Pereira NL, Daly RC, McGregor CG, Lerman A, Kushwaha SS. Acute cellular rejection and the subsequent development of allograft vasculopathy after cardiac transplantation. J Heart Lung Transplant. 2009;28:320–7.

Rubio R, Berne RM. Regulation of coronary blood flow. Prog Cardiovasc Dis. 1975;18:105–22.

Salomon RN, Hughes CC, Schoen FJ, Payne DD, Pober JS, Libby P. Human coronary transplantation-associated arteriosclerosis. Evidence for a chronic immune reaction to activated graft endothelial cells. Am J Pathol. 1991;138:791–8.

Sambiase NV, Higuchi ML, Nuovo G, Gutierrez PS, Fiorelli AI, Uip DE, Ramires JA. CMV and transplant-related coronary atherosclerosis: an immunohistochemical, in situ hybridization, and polymerase chain reaction in situ study. Mod Pathol. 2000;13:173–9.

Sato T, Seguchi O, Ishibashi-Ueda H, Yanase M, Okada N, Kuroda K, Hisamatsu E, Sunami H, Watanabe T, Nakajima S, Wada K, Hata H, Fujita T, Fukushima N, Kobayashi J, Nakatani T. Risk stratification for cardiac allograft vasculopathy in heart transplant recipients-annual intravascular ultrasound evaluation. Circ J. 2016;80:395–403.

Schumer EM, Ising MS, Trivedi JR, Slaughter MS, Cheng A. Early outcomes with marginal donor hearts compared with left ventricular assist device support in patients with advanced heart failure. Ann Thorac Surg. 2015;100:522–7.

Seki A, Fishbein MC. Predicting the development of cardiac allograft vasculopathy. Cardiovascular Phatol. 2014;23:253–60.

Shimizu K, Sugiyama S, Aikawa M, Fukumoto Y, Rabkin E, Libby P, Mitchell RN. Host bone-marrow cells are a source of donor intimal smooth- muscle-like cells in murine aortic transplant arteriopathy. Nat Med. 2001;7:738–41.

Spes CH, Klauss V, Mudra H, Schnaack SD, Tammen AR, Rieber J, Siebert U, Henneke KH, Uberfuhr P, Reichart B, Theisen K, Angermann CE. Diagnostic and prognostic value of serial dobutamine stress echocardiography for noninvasive assessment of cardiac allograft vasculopathy: a comparison with coronary angiography and intravascular ultrasound. Circulation. 1999;100:509–15.

Stoica SC, Cafferty F, Pauriah M, Taylor CJ, Sharples LD, Wallwork J, Large SR, Parameshwar J. The cumulative effect of acute rejection on development of cardiac allograft vasculopathy. J Heart Lung Transplant. 2006;25:420–5.

Stovin PG, Sharples LD, Schofield PM, Cary NR, Mullins PA, English TA, Wallwork J, Large SR. Lack of association between endomyocardial evidence of rejection in the first six months and the later development of transplant-related coronary artery disease. J Heart Lung Transplant. 1993;12:110–6.

Thaunat O, Louedec L, Dai J, Bellier F, Groyer E, Delignat S, Gaston AT, Caligiuri G, Joly E, Plissonnier D, Michel JB, Nicoletti A. Direct and indirect effects of alloantibodies link neointimal and medial remodeling in graft arteriosclerosis. Arterioscler Thromb Vasc Biol. 2006;26:2359–65.

Tona F, Caforio AL, Montisci R, Angelini A, Ruscazio M, Gambino A, Ramondo A, Thiene G, Gerosa G, Iliceto S. Coronary flow reserve by contrast-enhanced echocardiography: a new noninvasive diagnostic tool for cardiac allograft vasculopathy. Am J Transplant. 2006;6:998–1003.

Tona F, Osto E, Famoso G, Previato M, Fedrigo M, Vecchiati A, Perazzolo Marra M, Tellatin S, Bellu R, Tarantini G, Feltrin G, Angelini A, Thiene G, Gerosa G, Iliceto S. Coronary microvascular dysfunction correlates with the new onset of cardiac allograft vasculopathy in heart transplant patients with normal coronary angiography. Am J Transplant. 2015;15:1400–6.

Topilsky Y, Hasin T, Raichlin E, Boilson BA, Schirger JA, Pereira NL, Edwards BS, Clavell AL, Rodeheffer RJ, Frantz RP, Maltais S, Park SJ, Daly RC, Lerman A, Kushwaha SS. Sirolimus as primary immunosuppression attenuates allograft vasculopathy with improved late survival and decreased cardiac events after cardiac transplantation. Circulation. 2012;125:708–20.

Tuzcu EM, Hobbs RE, Rincon G, Bott-Silverman C, De Franco AC, Robinson K, McCarthy PM, Stewart RW, Guyer S, Nissen SE. Occult and frequent transmission of atherosclerotic coronary disease with cardiac transplantation. Insights from intravascular ultrasound. Circulation. 1995;91:1706–13.

Tuzcu EM, Kapadia SR, Sachar R, Ziada KM, Crowe TD, Feng J, Magyar WA, Hobbs RE, Starling RC, Young JB, McCarthy P, Nissen SE. Intravascular ultrasound evidence of angiographically silent progression in coronary atherosclerosis predicts long-term morbidity and mortality after cardiac transplantation. J Am Coll Cardiol. 2005;45:1538–42.

Uren NG, Melin JA, De Bruyne B, Wijns W, Baudhuin T, Camici PG. Relation between myocardial blood flow and the severity of coronary-artery stenosis. N Engl J Med. 1994;330:1782–8.

van den Heuvel AF, van Veldhuisen DJ, van der Wall EE, Blanksma PK, Siebelink HM, Vaalburg WM, van Gilst WH, Crijns HJ. Regional myocardial blood flow reserve impairment and metabolic changes suggesting myocardial ischemia in patients with idiopathic dilated cardiomyopathy. J Am Coll Cardiol. 2000;35:19–28.

van Loosdregt J, van Oosterhout MF, Bruggink AH, van Wichen DF, van Kuik J, de Koning E, Baan CC, de Jonge N, Gmelig-Meyling FH, de Weger RA. The chemokine and chemokine receptor profile of infiltrating cells in the wall of arteries with cardiac allograft vasculopathy is indicative of a memory T-helper 1 response. Circulation. 2006;114:1599–607.

Wehner JR, Fox-Talbot K, Halushka MK, Ellis C, Zachary AA, Baldwin 3rd WM. B cells and plasma cells in coronaries of chronically rejected cardiac transplants. Transplantation. 2010;89:1141–8.

Wenke K, Meiser B, Thiery J, Nagel D, von Scheidt W, Steinbeck G, Seidel D, Reichart B. Simvastatin reduces graft vessel disease and mortality after heart transplantation: a four-year randomized trial. Circulation. 1997; 96:1398–402.

Wever-Pinzon O, Romero J, Kelesidis I, Wever-Pinzon J, Manrique C, Budge D, Drakos SG, Pina IL, Kfoury AG, Garcia MJ, Stehlik J. Coronary computed tomography angiography for the detection of cardiac allograft vasculopathy: a meta-analysis of prospective trials. J Am Coll Cardiol. 2014;63:1992–2004.

Wu GW, Kobashigawa JA, Fishbein MC, Patel JK, Kittleson MM, Reed EF, Kiyosaki KK, Ardehali A. Asymptomatic antibody-mediated rejection after heart transplantation predicts poor outcomes. J Heart Lung Transplant. 2009;28:417–22.

Yamani MH, Haji SA, Starling RC, Tuzcu EM, Ratliff NB, Cook DJ, Abdo A, Crowe T, Secic M, McCarthy P, Young JB. Myocardial ischemic-fibrotic injury after human heart transplantation is associated with increased progression of vasculopathy, decreased cellular rejection and poor long-term outcome. J Am Coll Cardiol. 2002;39:970–7.

Yamasaki M, Sakurai R, Hirohata A, Honda Y, Bonneau HN, Luikart H, Yock PG, Fitzgerald PJ, Yeung AC, Valantine HA, Fearon WF. Impact of donor-transmitted atherosclerosis on early cardiac allograft vasculopathy: new findings by three-dimensional intravascular ultrasound analysis. Transplantation. 2011;91:1406–11.

Zhang X, Reed EF. Effect of antibodies on endothelium. Am J Transplant. 2009;9:2459–65.

Zhang X, Valenzuela NM, Reed EF. HLA class I antibody-mediated endothelial and smooth muscle cell activation. Curr Opin Organ Transplant. 2012;17:446–51.

Part V

Post-cardiac Transplantation: Complications Other than Rejection

Infections

19

David Lebeaux, Julien Coussement, Sylvain Poiree, and Olivier Lortholary

Contents

D. Lebeaux • O. Lortholary (✉)
Université Paris Descartes, Sorbonne Paris Cité, AP-HP, Hôpital Necker Enfants Malades, Centre d'Infectiologie Necker-Pasteur and Institut Imagine, Paris, France
e-mail: olivier.lortholary@wanadoo.fr

J. Coussement
Division of Infectious Diseases, CUB-Erasme, Université Libre de Bruxelles, Brussels, Belgium

S. Poiree
Service de Radiologie Adulte, Hôpital Necker-Enfants Malades, Assistance Publique-Hôpitaux de Paris, Paris, France

19.1 Background

Heart transplantation has revolutionized the outcome of patients with terminal chronic heart failure. Worldwide, about 5,000 heart transplantations are performed annually (Stehlik et al. 2011). Survival after heart transplant is continuously increasing due to advances in drug-induced immunosuppression, improvement of surgical procedures, optimal pretransplant risk assessment, and close patient monitoring (Stehlik et al. 2011; Gavalda et al. 2014a).

Soon after the first heart transplantations were performed in the late 1960s, infection appeared to be a major complication and a significant cause of mortality. Indeed, infectious events are responsible for 30 % of deaths, with a significant weight between 30 days and 1 year posttransplant (Stehlik et al. 2011). Beyond morbidity

O. Leone et al. (eds.), *The Pathology of Cardiac Transplantation*,
DOI 10.1007/978-3-319-46386-5_19

and mortality, infectious complications are also associated with a high economic burden due to higher length of hospital stay, increased graft losses, and costs related to indirect effects such as virus-induced malignancies (Gavalda et al. 2014a; Menzin et al. 2011). Beyond this direct burden, microorganisms are also involved in indirect transplant-related complications. For instance, it has been repeatedly shown that the "microbially determined immune modulation (MDIM)" could increase the risk of allograft injury or rejection, atherogenesis, malignancies (such as PTLD), and other opportunistic pathogens (Gavalda et al. 2014a). Therefore, preventive measures are cornerstone for the management of heart-transplanted patients (Fishman 2014).

There are many challenges in the management of infectious diseases after heart transplantation. First, infectious processes may originate from a wide range of sources (hospital environment, recipient community, reactivation of a latent process, transmission by the donor organ) (Fishman 2014; Wright and Fishman 2014). Therefore, a high number of bacterial, viral, fungal, and parasitic agents may be causative in heart transplant recipients. Second, the use of immunosuppressive agents may modify the clinical presentations associated with infectious events (Fishman 2014). Finally, drug toxicities and interactions are frequent and hamper antimicrobial treatment once the infectious diagnosis is made in such patients (Fishman 2014).

For all these reasons, diagnosis, prevention, and treatment of infectious complications appear as a cornerstone aspect of the management of heart-transplanted patients.

19.2 Clinics and Management

After solid organ transplantation, infectious risk may be stratified according to two axes: time posttransplantation and source of the infection.

Follow-up after heart transplantation can be divided into three time periods: less than 4 weeks after SOT (phase 1), between 1 and 6 months (phase 2), and more than 6 months after SOT (phase 3) (Fig. 19.1) (Fishman 2014; Wright and Fishman 2014). Besides that transplantation timeline, four distinct infection sources should be distinguished: the hospital environment, community exposure, donor (or graft) derived, and reactivation of an infection from the recipient (Fishman 2014; Wright and Fishman 2014). Taken together, these elements lead to distinct microbiological hypothesis.

- In the early phase after heart transplantation, most of infections are related to surgery and/or postoperative supportive care. Among these infections should be included surgical site and wound infections and catheter-related or urinary tract infections. The frequent use of antibiotics before or after surgery increases the risk of *C. difficile*-associated diarrhea (Fishman 2014). Lastly, donor-derived infections can be revealed early after heart transplantation if donor had an active viral, bacterial, or fungal infection or in case of graft contamination (Fishman 2014; Wright and Fishman 2014).
- Between 1 and 6 months, co-trimoxazole prophylaxis significantly reduces the risk of major opportunistic infections such as *P. jirovecii* pneumonia, *T. gondii* encephalitis, or listeriosis and may also reduce the risk of urinary tract infections. Most of febrile episodes are caused by viruses and graft rejection at that time (Fishman 2014). Depending on the level of immunosuppression, a broad spectrum of pathogens can occur such as *Aspergillus* spp., *Cryptococcus* spp., or *Nocardia* spp.
- More than 6 months after transplantation, drug-induced immunosuppression is tapered for most of patients. Thus, opportunistic pathogens are less common (Fishman 2014). However, opportunistic infections might occur late after transplantation, especially if immunosuppression has been beforehand intensified due to allograft rejection (Fishman 2014). The risk of CMV late-onset infection should be considered if an antiviral prophylaxis has been used and stopped. Besides, transplanted patients can experience more severe complications from community-acquired infections.

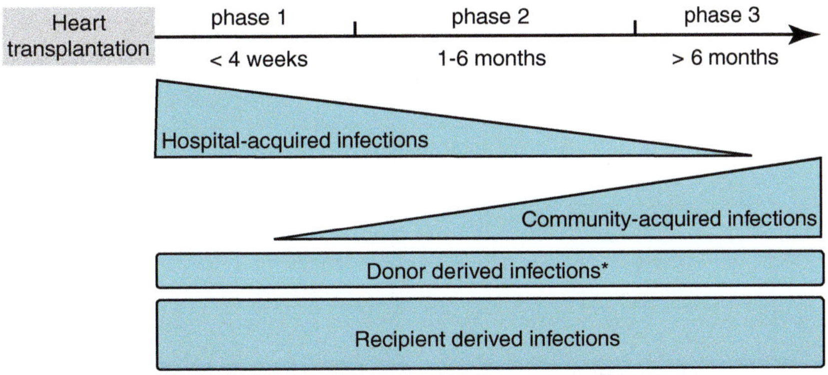

Fig. 19.1 Infectious timeline after heart transplantation and most frequent sources of infections. To note, even if donor-derived or recipient-derived infections are always possible, different pathogens can be involved, depending on the delay after transplantation (Adapted from Fishman 2014). *Of note, after 6 months, donor-derived infections are rare, with the notable exception of CMV disease

Even if infection is usually suspected because of fever, the first diagnostic step is to perform a complete clinical examination in order to identify a focus of infection.

19.2.1 Lung Infections

In case of respiratory symptoms (e.g., cough, dyspnea, chest pain), lung infection should be suspected, and a radiological work-up is mandatory. Even if chest radiography is still an important first-line exam, computed tomodensitometry (CT) scan is now considered cornerstone in order to obtain a clearer view of the type and extension of the lung lesions (Gavalda et al. 2014b). Indeed, depending on the type of radiological aspect, oriented diagnostics should be suspected (Fig. 19.2). In case of radiological abnormalities, a microbiological work-up is mandatory in order to increase the likelihood of pathogen identification.

In case of pneumonia occurring early after transplantation (phase 1), a ventilator-associated pneumonia should be suspected. In that case, a distal sample is mandatory, due to the broad spectrum of possible pathogens and the high frequency of resistant bacteria. In that case, bronchoscopy is mandatory and allows performing bronchoalveolar lavage (BAL), distal protected specimen with a plugged telescoping catheter or a brush. If the patient is ventilated, bronchoscopy is not mandatory and a blinded protected telescoping catheter sampling is feasible.

If pneumonia occurs in phase 2 or 3, community-acquired or opportunistic pathogens are responsible for most cases of infections. In that case, chest CT scan is important as microbiological diagnosis can be suspected based on the radiological picture (Fig. 19.2).

In any case, noninvasive diagnostic procedures are cornerstone such as sputum analysis (for Gram staining, bacterial cultures, fungal and mycobacterial examinations), urine antigen assays (for *S. pneumonia* and *L. pneumophila*), and blood cultures.

However, due to the broad spectrum of responsible pathogens, an invasive procedure is frequently required and relies on the BAL. Usually, BAL is required in case of nodular or interstitial pneumonia or in case of lung consolidation without clinical improvement after a 3-day course of antibiotics. Lastly, bronchoscopy and BAL should be proposed in case of relapsing infection, despite a complete course of antibiotics. This procedure will allow obtaining specimen for bacterial, mycobacterial, and viral examinations (Tables 19.1 and 19.2). Fungal examination is also important and should include the identification of *P. jirovecii* with Grocott–Gomori methenamine silver (GMS) staining, immunofluorescence ± quantitative PCR-based assay. Furthermore, indirect tests can be proposed in the blood and in

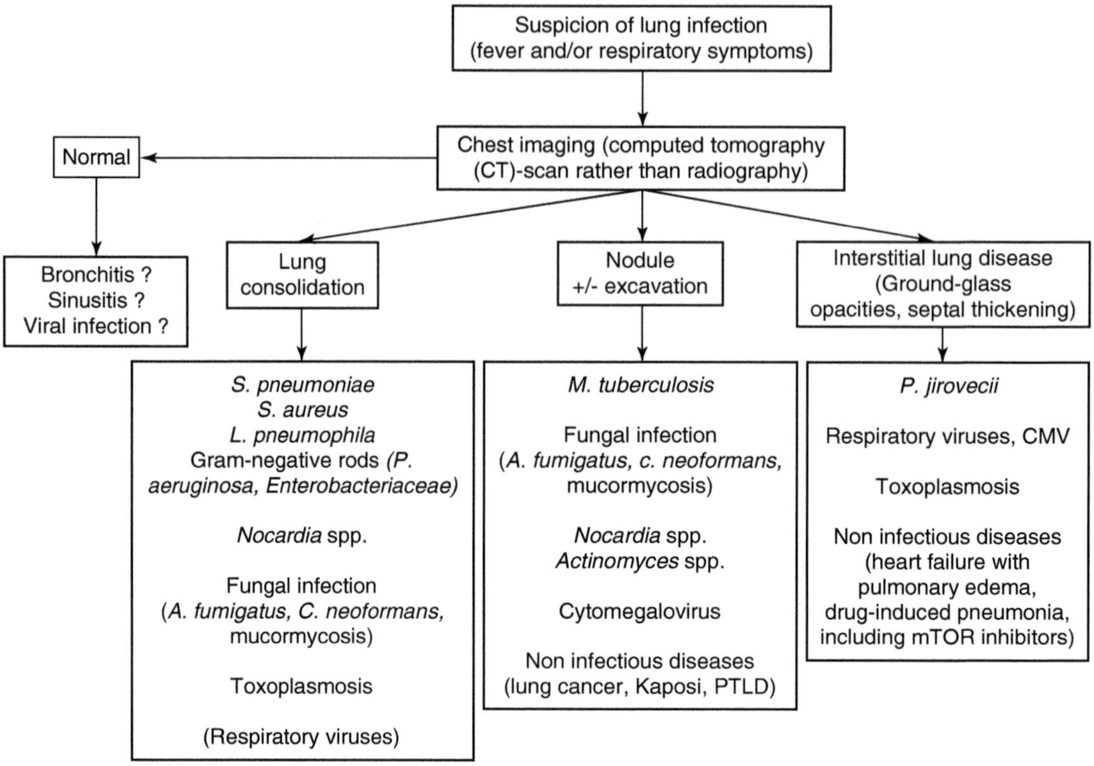

Fig. 19.2 Microbial etiologies as a function of radiological findings during pneumonia, in heart transplant recipients

the BAL, depending on the radiological aspects such as galactomannan antigen (for the identification of *Aspergillus* spp.), *Cryptococcus* spp. antigen, or β-D-glucan.

In case of nodular pneumonia and if BAL is negative, a lung biopsy should be proposed for microbial identification but also to rule out a noninfectious diagnosis (PTLD, cancer). In that case, a complete microbiological work-up is also mandatory (Table 19.1).

19.2.2 Neurological Symptoms

Between 10 and 85 % of SOT recipients experience central nervous system (CNS) symptoms (Wright and Fishman 2014). Among them, infections are one of the most severe etiologies. However, due to the use of drug-induced immunosuppression, clinical signs and symptoms may be reduced. Of note, noninfectious causes such as metabolic disorders, drug-induced side effects, and primary brain lymphoma should be considered. Early CNS infections (during phase 1) are rare, unless the patient experiences a massive microbial exposure or exhibits an anatomic underlying factor (Wright and Fishman 2014). Furthermore, donor-derived infections may occur in this time period, such as lymphocytic choriomeningitis, West Nile virus or herpes simplex virus (HSV) encephalitis, or, in case of graft contamination, cryptococcosis, even if the latter case is rare. CNS opportunistic infections mainly occur during phases 2 and 3. Fungal infections (*Aspergillus*, *C. neoformans*, *Histoplasma*, *Coccidioides*), nocardiosis, toxoplasmosis (if the chosen prophylaxis is not active against *T. gondii*), and tuberculosis should be considered (Wright and Fishman 2014; Lebeaux et al. 2014a). Viral infections are also possible at that phase (such as HSV or VZV encephalitis). After 6 months, even if the patient may experience infection caused by community-acquired pathogens (*S. pneumoniae*), the risk of opportunistic

Table 19.1 Microbiological work-up in heart-transplanted patients according to different clinical sample

	Bronchoalveolar lavage	Lumbar puncture	Stools	Biopsy
Bacteria: Gram staining + bacterial culture + culture for *Nocardia* (4w)	Yes	Yes	No Gram staining but detection of *Salmonella, Shigella, Yersinia,* specific groups of *E. coli*, and *Campylobacter*	Yes + molecular testing (16S)
Mycobacteria: Ziehl staining + long-term cultures (6–8w)	Yes	Yes + molecular testing (GeneXpert *M. tuberculosis*)	No	Yes + molecular testing (*M. tuberculosis*)
Mycology: PAS, GMS stainings + cultures	Yes + *P. jirovecii* IF and/or PCR	Yes	No	Yes
Parasites	No (with the exception of *T. gondii*)	Yes + PCR (*T. gondii*)	Yes + microsporidia, cryptosporidia, *Strongyloides*	No
Virology IF and/or PCR	IF or PCR (CARVs)	PCR (EBV, HSV, VZV, CMV)	PCR (*Norovirus*, *Enterovirus*, *Rotavirus*, adenovirus)	No
Indirect tests	Galactomannan antigen, *Cryptococcus* spp. antigen (BAL+serum)	*Cryptococcus* spp. antigen and β-D-glucan (CSF+serum)	Detection of *C. difficile* toxin (PCR based)	
Other	*Legionella* antigen in urine	Biochemical (proteins and differential glucose level) + CSF opening pressure measurement for *Cryptococcus*		Gram, PAS, GMS stainings on histology

CARVs community-acquired respiratory viruses (see Table 19.3), CSF cerebrospinal fluid, EBV Epstein–Barr virus, HSV herpes simplex virus, IF immunofluorescence, GMS Grocott–Gomori methenamine silver, PAS periodic acid–Schiff, PCR polymerase chain reaction, VZV varicella-zoster virus

Table 19.2 Seasonal predominance and management of CARVs

Virus	Seasonal predominance	Etiologic therapy
Respiratory syncytial virus (RSV)	Autumn and winter	Discuss ribavirin ± antibody-based treatment ± steroids
Human metapneumovirus	Winter	Discuss ribavirin
Influenza	Winter	Neuraminidase inhibitor
Parainfluenza viruses (types 1–4)	Throughout the year	Discuss ribavirin
Rhinoviruses	Throughout the year	None
Coronaviruses	Winter	None

pathogens can be increased as prophylaxis is usually interrupted at that stage: herpesviruses, nocardiosis, invasive molds, tuberculosis, and cryptococcosis can be encountered.

If CNS infection is suspected, two cornerstone elements are mandatory: lumbar puncture and brain imaging (CT scan or, ideally, magnetic resonance imaging, MRI). Indeed, MRI has been shown to be superior, especially in the case of invasive fungal infections (Gavalda et al. 2014b). Lumbar puncture should be performed first in case of meningeal syndrome. However, brain

Table 19.3 Management of CMV in heart transplant recipients according to donor and recipient serostatus (Kotton et al. 2013)

Donor serology (D)	Recipient serology (R)	Risk of CMV disease	Role of CMV prevention
D+	R−	High	Prophylaxis is often considered to be the best option (duration: at least 6 months) Consider the risk of late-onset CMV disease after discontinuing prophylaxis, in which case a hybrid strategy (i.e., using a preemptive strategy after the cessation of prophylaxis) should be helpful
D+	R+	Intermediate	Prophylaxis or preemptive strategy should be used. As there is no strong published data to decide whether one of these two strategies is best, physicians should decide according to local possibilities. Particular attention should be made for patients with additional risk factors (e.g., use of antilymphocyte therapy or treatment of acute rejection episode)
D−	R+		
D−	R−	Low	The use of prophylaxis against CMV is not recommended. Consider prophylaxis against other herpes infections

imaging should be performed before LP in case of localizing neurological signs, seizure, or reduced vigilance. Indeed, these clinical signs might be suggestive of intracranial hypertension. In that case, LP increases the risk of brain herniation (Duffy 1969). If lumbar puncture is performed, several microbiological tests should be performed (Table 19.1). If *Cryptococcus* infection is suspected or diagnosed, CSF opening pressure should be measured (see below). Based on the results of brain MRI and LP, different pathogens are possible (Fig. 19.3).

Furthermore, the presence of extra-neurological symptoms can be cornerstone for the microbial diagnosis. For instance, concomitant skin lesions can suggest disseminated nocardiosis and mycobacterial or fungal infections (Wright and Fishman 2014; Lebeaux et al. 2014a). In that case, a skin biopsy should be performed. In this regard, lung infection, heart murmur, and sinusitis should also be investigated.

Lifestyle is also important to assess neurological symptoms, and an extensive travel history should be made for these patients. For instance, a recent travel in tropical zone should prompt malaria testing. Even if the travel occurred years ago, the diagnosis of endemic fungus should be investigated (e.g., *Coccidioides immitis*, *Histoplasma*)

If LP and the abovementioned extensive extra-neurological work-up did not lead to a microbial diagnosis, neurosurgery should be considered for biopsy or debridement, in case of brain abscess (Wright and Fishman 2014).

19.2.3 Skin and Soft Tissue Infections

Most of skin and soft tissue infections occurring during phase 1 are related to the surgical procedure. In that case, the most worrisome diagnosis should be mediastinitis. Indeed,

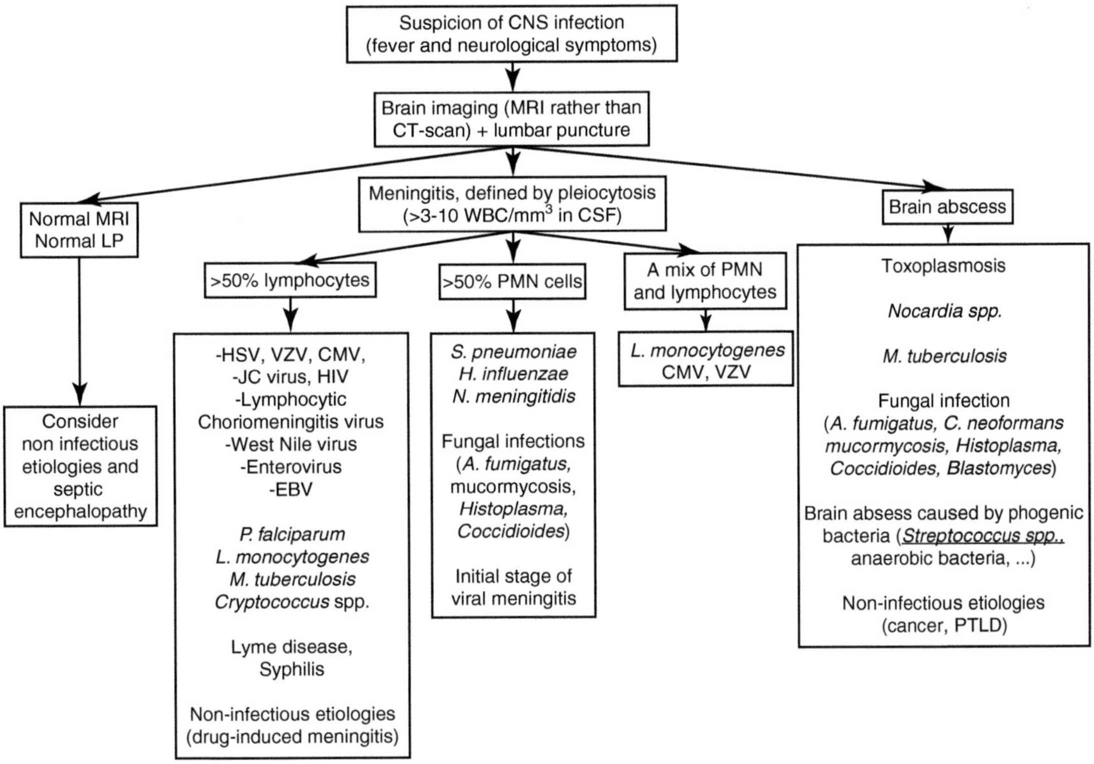

Fig. 19.3 Microbial etiologies in case of neurological signs, based on the results of brain imaging and lumbar puncture. *At the initial stage of viral meningitis, PMN cells can prevail. *CSF* cerebrospinal fluid, *CT* computed tomography, *EBV* Epstein–Barr virus, *HSV* herpes simplex virus, *LP* lumbar puncture, *MRI* magnetic resonance imaging, *PMN* polymorphonuclear, *PTLD* posttransplant lymphoproliferative disorder, *VZV* varicella-zoster virus, *WBC* white blood cells

heart transplant recipients have an increased risk of surgical wound infections, as compared with patients undergoing conventional heart surgeries (Zuckermann and Barten 2011). After heart transplantation, surgical wound infections are observed in 8–15 % of patients with some groups reporting incidence of mediastinitis up to 40 % (Zuckermann and Barten 2011). The diagnosis of surgical wound infection may be difficult as fever, erythema, and purulent discharge are sometimes absent (Zuckermann and Barten 2011). Therefore, chest CT scan and needle aspiration are cornerstone for the diagnosis of posttransplant mediastinitis.

Due to prophylaxis with aciclovir or valaciclovir, viral recurrences caused by HSV or VZV are rare but can be severe with more extensive zona or herpes lesions. Without prophylaxis, reactivation of HSV or VZV can occur in more than 35 % of cases (Ulrich et al. 2008).

During phases 2 and 3, other cutaneous findings may be related to community-acquired infections caused by group A *Streptococcus* or *S. aureus*. Strikingly, Gram-negative rods can be responsible for skin and soft tissue infections in immunocompromised patients. Opportunistic pathogens can also be causative, especially in case of nodular skin lesions or relapse after an antibiotic course. In that case, main diagnosis includes bacteria (*Nocardia* spp.), mycobacteria, and fungus (*Cryptococcus*, invasive dermatophytosis, *Aspergillus* spp.) (Lebeaux et al. 2014a; Ulrich et al. 2008). Skin lesions may be secondary to direct skin inoculation (after telluric or soil trauma, for instance) or because of a disseminated disease (in which a hematogenous spread is observed). Therefore, skin lesions should always be considered after heart transplantation, and skin biopsy performed when possible.

During phase 3, *human herpesvirus 8* (HHV8) can be responsible for Kaposi sarcoma, human papilloma viruses (HPV) can cause warts, and mucocutaneous candidiasis are frequent (Ulrich et al. 2008).

Lastly, heart-transplanted patients have an increased risk of skin cancer. Thus, a yearly dermatological examination is mandatory.

19.2.4 Digestive Tract Infections

During phase 1, most of the digestive tract infections are caused by *C. difficile*. This infection is related to nosocomial exposure and frequent antibiotic prescription. During the second and the third phases, community-acquired as well as opportunistic pathogens can be found. In case of diarrhea after heart transplantation, an exhaustive microbiological work-up is mandatory (Table 19.1). In this setting, viruses can be responsible for long-term aqueous diarrhea. Of note, if the patient has been exposed to *Strongyloides*, even decades ago, initiation of corticosteroids and/or immunosuppressive drugs can be responsible for hyperinfection syndrome (see below).

19.2.5 Isolated Fever

Lastly, infection can be suspected in heart-transplanted patients only because of an isolated fever. If none of the abovementioned symptoms are present, a minimal work-up is mandatory and should include at least blood and urine cultures and chest radiography. If uninformative, chest and abdominal CT scan, cryptococcal antigen, serum PCR for CMV, and toxoplasmosis should be performed. Cardiac echocardiography can also be performed to investigate infective endocarditis. Lastly, noninfectious etiologies must be considered such as PTLD.

19.3 Viral Diseases

19.3.1 *Cytomegalovirus*

Cytomegalovirus (CMV) is the major viral agent after heart transplantation, increasing both morbidity and mortality. CMV may cause direct effects (ranging from benign viral syndrome to life-threatening tissue-invasive disease) as well as indirect effects such as allograft rejection, coronary vasculopathy, accelerated atherosclerosis, new-onset diabetes mellitus after transplantation, and opportunistic infections. International consensus guidelines on the management of CMV after solid organ transplantation have recently been published (Kotton et al. 2013).

"CMV infection" usually applies to the evidence of CMV replication without any signs of disease. When attributable symptoms are associated with this viral replication, the process is called "CMV disease." CMV disease is divided into "viral syndrome" (fever, malaise, hematological cytopenia) and "tissue-invasive disease," a process that may, for example, affect the digestive tract, the eyes, the central nervous system, the pancreas, or the liver and the lungs. Therefore, complete physical examination and adapted work-up should be conducted when a CMV infection is suspected.

Risk stratification is of great importance to prevent CMV after transplantation. A CMV IgG screening test should be performed for both donor (D) and recipient (R) before transplantation to allow for risk stratification of CMV disease. Beyond serostatus, some specific cell-mediated immunity tests such as QuantiFERON-CMV and ELISpot have been developed to better predict the risk of CMV disease (Manuel et al. 2013a). Due to the strong impact of CMV infection on clinical outcomes, a preventive strategy should be used for both CMV-positive recipients (R+) and CMV-negative recipients with a positive donor (D+/R-). Two preventive strategies are currently available: universal prophylaxis (i.e., administration of antiviral therapy in the first months after transplantation) and preemptive therapy (i.e., repeated realizations of laboratory assays such as (ideally) quantitative nucleic acid amplification testing or pp65 antigenemia ± administration of antiviral therapy once an early viral replication has been diagnosed). Their roles are summarized in Table 19.3. If universal prophylaxis is selected, routine viral load monitoring should not be encouraged in asymptomatic patients as this strategy is not cost-benefit. For CMV prophylaxis, oral valganciclovir (900 mg once daily) and intravenous ganciclovir (5 mg/kg once daily) have proven their efficacy. Both valganciclovir and ganciclovir dosages should be adjusted to renal function. Limited data suggest that the preventive use of CMV hyperimmune globulin may decrease the cardiac consequences of CMV infection after heart transplantation (Valantine et al. 2001).

While serological tools have no role after transplantation, both CMV pp65 antigenemia and PCR assays are highly useful tools for the diagnosis of CMV infection. Of note, sensitivity of pp65 antigenemia decreases significantly in neutropenic recipients, defined as less than 1000 polymorphonuclear cells/mm^3. Mainly because of poor interhospital correlation of PCR assays until the recent creation of an international World Health Organization (WHO) standard, no consensual cutoff value has been determined to initiate antiviral therapy in patients with isolated replication without identified disease. While a low threshold should most likely be used in D+/R- couples to initiate antiviral therapy and prevent direct and indirect effects of CMV infection, it is unclear when to initiate therapy in CMV seropositive heart transplant recipients. Kinetics of DNAemia may offer additional information. The role of CMV detection by PCR in bronchoalveolar lavage is still a matter of debate. Last, physicians should be aware of the possibility of a compartimentalized CMV disease. A common illustration is that of digestive CMV disease which may be seen with undetectable or low viral load values in blood samples.

Curative treatment of CMV infection in heart transplant recipients does not differ from other solid organ transplant recipients. Briefly, oral valganciclovir as well as intravenous ganciclovir could be used for nonlife-threatening CMV disease, with the notable exception of gastrointestinal tract infections. In that case, oral valganciclovir should be avoided. Treatment dose should be adapted with great attention according to the estimated glomerular filtration rate. Duration of treatment is based on the monitoring of CMV DNAemia. A minimum length of treatment of 2 weeks should be used, at the condition of obtaining one or more negative CMV tests (i.e., pp65 antigenemia or PCR). Antiviral drug resistance is a cause of persisting infection despite antiviral treatment at an adapted dose. Testing for mutations of viral UL97 kinase and/or UL54 DNA polymerase should be conducted in such cases.

19.3.2 Herpes Simplex and Varicella-Zoster Viruses

Like CMV, other *Herpesviridae* viruses are able to cause infection in transplant recipients. Among them, herpes simplex virus (HSV) and varicella-zoster virus (VZV) are of importance. Due to the impaired cell-mediated immunity observed after transplantation, both these agents may progress from latency in sensory nerve ganglia to reactivation. HSV and VZV may also be transmitted via the graft from an infected donor.

HSV type 1 (HSV-1) and type 2 (HSV-2) are generally transmitted by direct contact with a subject actively infected. While primary HSV-1 infection usually occurs during childhood via oral secretions, HSV-2 is sexually transmitted. In the absence of antiviral prophylaxis, HSV replicates in the first weeks after transplantation and symptoms ranging from mucocutaneous viral reactivation to lethal multiple visceral organ involvement may be observed. Atypical presentations require adapted specimen collection and laboratory confirmation. In case of benign mucocutaneous lesions due to HSV, aciclovir (400 mg PO three times daily) and valaciclovir (1 g PO twice daily) are effective agents when started early after the onset of symptoms. In case of severe disease such as meningoencephalitis or disseminated disease, aciclovir should be used intravenously at a dose of 10 mg/kg every 8 h.

More than 90% of adults are infected by VZV. Serological testing should be conducted before transplantation to identify VZV-naïve patients as the occurrence of primary infection after transplantation may lead to severe dermatologic lesions and visceral involvement (e.g., pneumonitis) in such subjects. In seropositive transplant patients, herpes zoster (also known as shingles or zona) may present as dermatomal herpes zoster or as varicella-like skin lesions. In most cases, a clinical diagnosis can be made. Contact with infected subjects may be a clue to diagnosis. Unlike CMV, asymptomatic replication is not observed after solid organ transplantation. As a consequence, identification of VZV (e.g., by PCR) from lesions or plasma is a highly valuable tool. Aggressive therapy is needed once the diagnosis of VZV disease has been made in an immunocompromised patient. Intravenous aciclovir should be used at a dose of 10 mg/kg every 8 h. Dosing adjustments with renal impairment is required. Localized shingles may be treated orally with valaciclovir (1 g three times daily). Of note, aciclovir-resistant VZV isolates have been described.

Preventive strategies play a significant role for both HSV and VZV. Prophylaxis against HSV should be used for 1–3 months after solid organ transplantation. Aciclovir (400–800 mg per os twice daily) and valaciclovir (500 mg per os twice daily) are effective to prevent HSV infections in transplant recipients. Of note, ganciclovir and valganciclovir (the most widely used anti-CMV drugs) also offer protection against HSV and VZV. Patients who are seronegative pretransplant for VZV should receive vaccination before transplantation. Indeed, the use of this live virus vaccine is not recommended after transplantation.

19.3.3 Epstein–Barr Virus

More than 90% of the world population is infected with Epstein–Barr virus (EBV). Such as other *Herpesviridae* viruses described supra, it persists lifelong. After transplantation, the use of immunosuppressive agents imbalance the relation established between EBV-infected B-cells and the host's cytotoxic T lymphocyte response. As a consequence, it may lead to a wide range of presentations ranging from asymptomatic viremia to posttransplantation lymphoproliferative disorder (PTLD). EBV serological testing should be realized for risk stratification before transplant for both donor and recipient. EBV-negative recipients of EBV-positive heart transplants (D+/R-) have the highest risk of PTLD. In this high-risk population, EBV-positive PTLD typically occurs within 1 year after transplantation. Because increased EBV viral load is linked to aberrant EBV-induced B-cell proliferation, the question of viral load monitoring is of interest. However, such strategies of monitoring are imperfectly correlated with the risk of developing EBV-positive PTLD, especially due to a low-positive predictive value. Moreover, this tool has no utility for predicting EBV-negative PTLD. In patients who are at high risk for PTLD (such as EBV D+/R− patients and/or recipients with chronic EBV viremia), preemptive reduction in immune suppression appears to be an effective first-line strategy. The role of adjunctive therapies such as rituximab is an ongoing debate in solid organ transplant recipients. Apart from PTLD, uncommon events such as infections of the central nervous system and aplastic anemia have been associated with EBV in transplant recipients.

19.3.4 Influenza and Other Community-Acquired Respiratory Viruses

In immunocompromised subjects such as heart transplant recipients, community-acquired respiratory viruses (CARVs) have been shown to be responsible for severe respiratory diseases (Table 19.2) (Manuel et al. 2013b). Progression from upper to lower respiratory infection is common. Clinical symptoms are poor tools to distinguish one CARV from one other. Infections with

CARVs should be suspected in all solid organ transplant recipients with symptoms of upper or lower respiratory tract infection. Specimens should be taken as soon as possible from the site of clinical involvement. In case of upper respiratory tract symptoms, pooled nasopharyngeal and throat swabs are recommended. In case of lower respiratory tract infection, BAL should be made when possible, in order to exclude other infectious diseases. Laboratory diagnostic methods mainly include antigen detection assays, virus isolation by cell culture, and nucleic acid amplification testing. When available, the latter is a rapid and highly sensitive tool for clinicians. Prevention is a major tool to prevent infection by CARVs in solid organ transplant recipients. Inactivated vaccination is highly recommended to prevent influenza in solid organ transplant recipients, even if conflicting results have been published concerning its immunogenicity in heart transplant recipients. Meanwhile, vaccination of household contacts and health-care workers attending transplanted patients should be done annually. To prevent infections with CARVs in transplant recipients, general preventive measures are also mandatory (including contact avoidance with individuals suffering from respiratory tract infection and young children, hand hygiene, and adapted isolation of infected patients). Promising results have been published concerning the use of prophylaxis by neuraminidase inhibitors in solid organ transplant recipients during influenza season (Ison et al. 2012). Curative treatment options are presented in Table 19.2. Antiviral therapy using neuraminidase inhibitors should be administered in all heart transplant recipients with suspected influenza infection, even if symptoms started several days earlier. In severe cases, reduction of immune suppression should be considered.

19.3.5 West Nile Virus

West Nile virus (WNV) is an arthropod-born agent. WNV is mainly acquired via *Culex* that are infected by wild birds. While this disease has been first described in the West Nile district of Uganda in 1937, many countries are currently concerned all over the world. Notably, a worrisome outbreak is observed in North America since 1999. Transmission has also occurred through blood transfusion and transplantation with an infected organ. While 80 % of WNV infections are asymptomatic in immunocompetent subjects, symptomatic forms range from West Nile fever (a self-limiting febrile illness) to neuroinvasive diseases (meningitis, encephalitis, or acute flaccid paralysis) and myocarditis. Solid organ transplant recipients are at higher risk for severe disease (Singh et al. 2013). Incubation varies from 3 to 14 days. The diagnosis of WNV depends on a high index of suspicion. Serum and cerebrospinal fluid analysis should include WNV serological assays and nucleic acid testing. WNV treatment is mainly supportive and may include reduction of immunosuppression, use of interferon or passive immunization using anti-WNV antibodies. In the absence of an available vaccine, protection against mosquito bites should be recommended in the concerned areas.

19.4 Nonviral Diseases

19.4.1 Management of Fungal and Parasitic Infections

Candidiasis *Candida* is the most frequent agent of invasive fungal infection (IFI) after SOT, accounting for more than half of the cases (Gavalda et al. 2014b). Most cases occur during phase 1 and originate from the gut and an indwelling device (such as intravenous catheter) or can be caused by a graft contamination (even if this latter event is more frequently associated with kidney transplantation). Invasive candidiasis is associated with a high mortality (≈30–40 %) (Gavalda et al. 2014b). Even if blood cultures are cornerstone, it has been repeatedly shown that their sensitivity for invasive candidiasis was 50–75 %, therefore leading scientific societies to propose other diagnostic options such as the detection of β-D-glucan in the serum that can be useful for its negative predictive value (Gavalda et al. 2014b). Initial treatment of

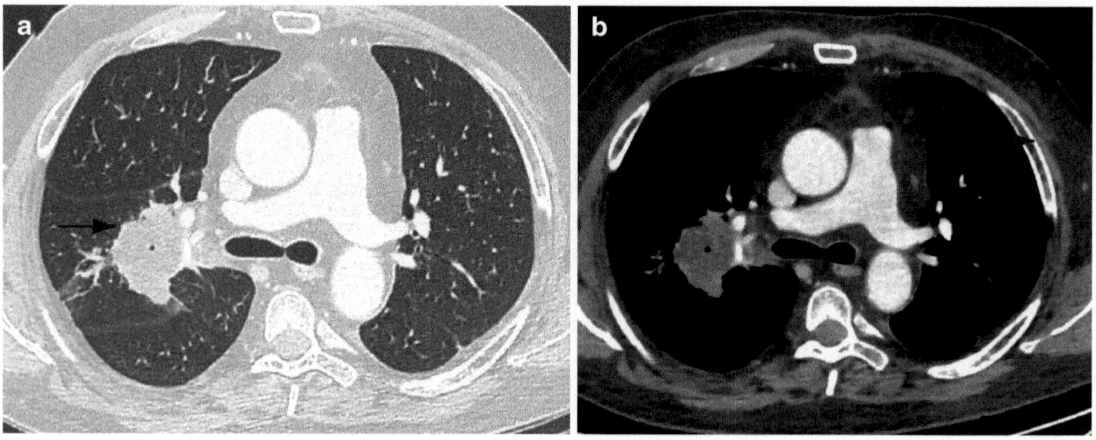

Fig. 19.4 Invasive aspergillosis after transplantation. Axial non-enhanced computed tomography (NECT) of a transplanted patient with invasive aspergillosis shows a right hilar mass (**a**, *black arrow*) with central low attenuation and intrinsic air (**b**), consistent with tissue necrosis and early cavitation

candidemia should rely on intravenous echinocandins. All central venous catheters should be removed, except in specific and complex situations, and venous ultrasonography, cardiac echocardiography, and funduscopy should be performed. Antifungal treatment should be prescribed for 14 days after the first negative blood culture (Gavalda et al. 2014b). Asymptomatic candiduria, a common phenomenon, should not be treated unless the patient is neutropenic or is about to have a urological procedure. However, symptomatic candiduric patients must be treated, and urinary catheters should be removed or replaced.

Aspergillosis *Aspergillus* is the second most frequent fungal pathogen after SOT, and heart- and lung-transplanted patients are at higher risk. Most of cases are invasive aspergillosis (IA) with an acute pulmonary (Fig. 19.4) or neurological infection that is associated with a high mortality (up to 80 %) (Gavalda et al. 2014b). IA can be considered proven if specific diagnostic criteria are met (Table 19.4) (De Pauw et al. 2008). In other cases, IA is considered probable or possible (Table 19.5). To note, even if the detection of galactomannan antigen in the serum is not recommended in SOT recipients due to its low sensitivity, it can be performed in BAL or CSF (Gavalda et al. 2014b). β-D-Glucan can be used for the diagnosis of IA even if false-positive or false-negative results have been reported.

No universal antifungal prophylaxis is proposed, but some groups propose an itraconazole-based prevention only to patients at high risk of IFI (acute rejection, hemodialysis, reexploration after transplantation, CMV disease, or excessive *Aspergillus* spp. in the air of the center) (Gavalda et al. 2014b).

Antifungal therapy should be initiated early in case of suspicion of IA, and immunosuppression should be reduced. First-line treatment should rely on voriconazole, and therapeutic drug monitoring is mandatory with a trough concentration target between 2 and 4 mg/l. Drug-to-drug interactions and liver and skin toxicities (including squamous cell carcinoma, in case of long-term therapy) should be closely monitored. Treatment duration is difficult to standardize but usually lasts for 6–12 weeks. Surgery should be proposed in case of hemoptysis, endocarditis, sinus disease, pericardium, or large vessels involvement (Gavalda et al. 2014b).

Cryptococcosis The third most frequent fungal pathogen is *Cryptococcus*, especially in patients receiving high doses of corticosteroids, monoclonal antibodies, alemtuzumab, or infliximab. Most of cases occur lately after transplantation

Table 19.4 Criteria for the diagnostic classification of proven invasive fungal infection

Specimen and type of analysis	Molds	Yeasts
Microscopic analysis: sterile material	Histopathologic, cytopathologic, or direct microscopic examination of a specimen obtained by biopsy in which fungus are seen and associated with evidence of tissue damage	Histopathologic, cytopathologic, or direct microscopic examination of a specimen obtained by biopsy from a normally sterile site (other than mucous membranes) showing yeast cells
Culture		
Sterile material	Recovery of a fungus by culture of a specimen obtained by a sterile procedure from a normally sterile and clinically or radiologically abnormal site consistent with an infectious disease process, excluding bronchoalveolar lavage fluid, a cranial sinus cavity specimen, and urine	Recovery of a yeast by culture of a sample obtained by a sterile procedure (including a freshly placed [<24 h ago] drain) from a normally sterile site showing a clinical or radiological abnormality consistent with an infectious disease process
Blood	Blood culture that yields a mold (e.g., *Fusarium* species) in the context of a compatible infectious disease process	Blood culture that yields yeast (e.g., *Cryptococcus* or *Candida* species) or yeast-like fungi (e.g., *Trichosporon* species)
Serological analysis: CSF	Not applicable	Cryptococcal antigen in CSF indicates cryptococcal meningitis

Adapted from De Pauw et al. (2008)

(16–21 months), and mortality may reach 25 % (Gavalda et al. 2014b). Cryptococcosis can be revealed by CNS or lung infection (Fig. 19.5), associated or not with fungemia and skin lesions. Besides blood, urine, and skin culture (in case of skin lesions), diagnostic relies on the detection of cryptococcal antigen in CSF and blood (Gavalda et al. 2014b). For meningoencephalitis, disseminated disease, and severe pneumonia, first-line treatment is liposomal amphotericin B (3–4 mg/kg/day) or amphotericin B lipid complex + flucytosine (25 mg/kg x4/j) for 2 weeks (induction therapy) (Gavalda et al. 2014b). Then if CSF culture is sterile, consolidation with fluconazole 400–800 mg/j for 8 weeks. Lastly, maintenance therapy with fluconazole 200 mg/j is prescribed for 6–12 months. In case of elevated intracranial pressure, large volume taps are required to reduce the intracranial pressure < 20 cmHg. Even if a reduction of immunosuppressant drugs should be proposed, immune reconstitution inflammatory syndrome (IRIS) can occur in 5–11 % of cases (Gavalda et al. 2014b). For focal pulmonary infections, fluconazole can be used first at 400 mg/day (6 mg/kg/day) for 6–12 months.

Pneumocystosis Pneumocystis pneumonia (PcP) is a fungal infection responsible for an asymptomatic or mild disease in the normal host but severe interstitial lung infection (PcP) in immunocompromised patients. Despite intense controversies, it is now considered that infection originates from recent acquisition of *Pneumocystis jirovecii* rather than reactivation of a latent infection. After transplantation, the risk of PcP is high, especially in the first year posttransplant. As the use of prophylaxis with trimethoprim–sulfamethoxazole significantly decreases this risk, most of cases occur after cessation of this preventive agent (Wang et al. 2012). Thus, several groups propose a lifelong prophylaxis. Atovaquone or pentamidine can also be proposed as prophylaxis. The diagnosis of PcP can be difficult as PCR-based assays are highly sensitive and can reveal only colonization. β-D-Glucan has been demonstrated to have a high negative predictive value in this setting.

Toxoplasmosis This life-threatening opportunistic infection is caused by *T. gondii*, a parasite able to encyst in several organs, such as the heart.

Table 19.5 Host, clinical, and mycologic criteria used for the definition of probable or possible invasive fungal infections

Host factors
Recent history of neutropenia (<500 neutrophils/mm3 for >10 days) temporally related to the onset of fungal disease
Receipt of an allogeneic stem cell transplant
Prolonged use of corticosteroids at a mean minimum dose of 0.3 mg/kg/day of prednisone equivalent for >3 weeks
Treatment with other recognized T cell immunosuppressants, such as cyclosporine, TNF-a blockers, specific monoclonal antibodies (such as alemtuzumab), or nucleoside analogues during the past 90 days
Inherited severe immunodeficiency (such as chronic granulomatous disease or severe combined immunodeficiency)
Clinical criteria
Lower respiratory tract fungal disease
The presence of one of the following three signs on CT: dense, well-circumscribed lesion(s) with or without a halo sign, air-crescent sign, cavity
Tracheobronchitis
Tracheobronchial ulceration, nodule, pseudomembrane, plaque, or eschar seen on bronchoscopic analysis
Sinonasal infection
Imaging showing sinusitis plus at least one of the following three signs: acute localized pain (including pain radiating to the eye), nasal ulcer with black eschar, extension from the paranasal sinus across bony barriers, including into the orbit
CNS infection
One of the following two signs: focal lesions on imaging, meningeal enhancement on MRI or CT
Disseminated candidiasis
At least one of the following two entities after an episode of candidemia within the previous 2 weeks: small, target-like abscesses (bull's-eye lesions) in liver or spleen, progressive retinal exudates on ophthalmologic examination
Mycological criteria
Direct test (cytology, direct microscopy, or culture)
Mold in sputum, bronchoalveolar lavage fluid, bronchial brush, or sinus aspirate samples, indicated by one of the following: the presence of fungal elements indicating a mold, recovery by culture of a mold (e.g., *Aspergillus, Fusarium, Zygomycetes*, or *Scedosporium* species)
Indirect tests (detection of antigen or cell-wall constituents)
Aspergillosis: galactomannan antigen detected in plasma, serum, bronchoalveolar lavage fluid, or CSF
Invasive fungal disease other mucormycoses: b-d-glucan detected in serum

Adapted from De Pauw et al. (2008)
Probable IFI requires that a host factor, clinical features, and mycological evidence are present; in possible IFI, mycological evidence is lacking

In transplant recipients, toxoplasmosis can result from the transmission of the parasite with the graft (D+) to a seronegative recipient (R-) or from a reactivation of a pretransplant latent infection in a seropositive recipient (R+) (Derouin et al. 2008). In the first case, clinical signs usually occur in the first 3 months after heart transplantation (sometimes earlier, within 2 weeks) with febrile myocarditis, encephalitis, or pneumonia. Without prophylaxis, incidence of disseminated toxoplasmosis in case of mismatch (D+/R-) may reach 75 %, but trimethoprim–sulfamethoxazole prophylaxis efficiently prevents this complication. The second option (reactivation of a latent infection R+ patient) is less frequent. Even if serological reactivation (defined by a rise in IgG antibody titers, with a high avidity index) occurs in ≈5 % of R+ patients, a clinical toxoplasmosis is exceptional (Derouin et al. 2008). The diagnosis of disseminated toxoplasmosis relies on the identification of the parasite or its DNA (through PCR testing) in any involved organ or in the blood. Serologic diagnostic might be useful but does not have enough sensitivity or specificity. Even if trimethoprim–sulfamethoxazole is highly effective in preventing toxoplasmosis, the risk might appear after cessation of the drug or if it is replaced by aerosolized pentamidine prophylaxis

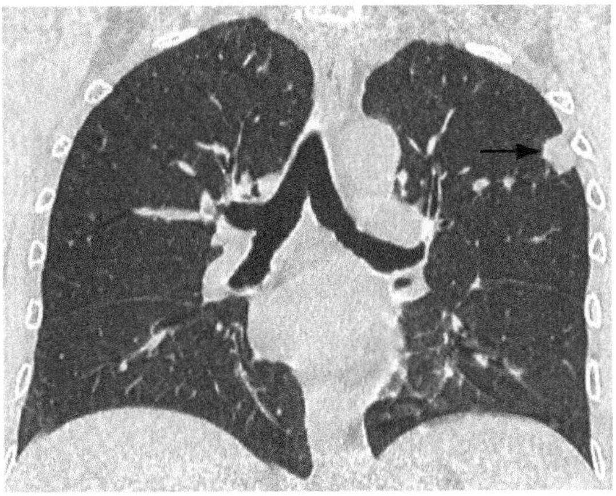

Fig. 19.5 Coronal non-enhanced computed tomography of a transplanted patient with pulmonary cryptococcosis demonstrates a subpleural left upper lobe solid nodule (*black arrow*)

against PcP. Beside trimethoprim–sulfamethoxazole, pyrimethamine alone or atovaquone can also be used as prophylaxis.

Strongyloidiasis Strongyloides stercoralis is a parasite that is present in tropical and subtropical regions. *Strongyloides* can complete an entire life cycle through an autoinfection pattern, allowing a prolonged survival within the host, up to several decades (Roxby et al. 2009). The immunodepression induced after transplantation may lead to hyperinfection, through a massive increase in the reproductive cycle of the larvae (Roxby et al. 2009). After a proliferation step in the duodenum, larvae may reach the bloodstream, the lungs, and then the gut. Thus, hyperinfection syndrome usually associates respiratory symptoms leading to acute respiratory distress syndrome, gastrointestinal symptoms (from abdominal pain to gastrointestinal bleedings or occlusion), and neurological involvement. A frequent complication is the occurrence of a bloodstream coinfection or meningitis cause by Gram-negative enteric bacteria. Due to its severity, hyperinfection syndrome should be prevented in patients awaiting heart transplantation who lived or stayed in area of endemicity (South America, Africa, Southeast Asia), even decades ago. The prevention relies on the treatment of chronic intestinal strongyloidosis with ivermectin before starting chemical immunosuppression (Roxby et al. 2009).

Chagas disease

This vector-borne (reduviid bug) parasitic infection caused by *Trypanosoma cruzi* is widespread in Latin America where seven to eight million people are chronically infected (Andrade et al. 2014). Human disease can be separated in two different phases: acute and chronic infection (Lattes and Lasala 2014). In most of adult cases, acute infection is spontaneously cleared and frequently asymptomatic. However, without any specific treatment, infection can evolve to the chronic phase. This chronic infection can be asymptomatic but can lead in 30 % of patients to irreversible damages of the following organs: the heart, esophagus, colon, and peripheral nervous system. During acute infection, diagnosis can be made through direct parasitologic examination of the whole blood (with and without concentration) or serologic tests. The later methods only can be used for the diagnosis of the chronic phase. More recently, PCR-based methods performed on the blood, body fluid, or tissues emerged as sensitive tools for the diagnosis of chronic Chagas disease with low parasite burden or in case of reactivation.

Two connections between Chagas disease and transplantation are described: reactivation and graft-transmitted disease.

In the first case, chronic Chagas was not known before transplantation. For instance, the patient can suffer from end-stage heart dysfunction requiring transplantation because of chronic Chagas disease. After heart transplantation, immunosuppressant drugs are responsible for parasitic reactivation with parasitemia, meningoencephalitis, panniculitis, or erythema nodosum-like lesions and myocarditis. In case of heart transplantation, mortality may reach 100 %.

In the other scenario, the organ donor was suffering from an unknown chronic Chagas disease. Kidney and liver transplantation are associated with a risk of graft-transmitted disease of 19 and 29 %, respectively, but heart transplantation is contraindicated if the donor had a chronic Chagas disease (Andrade et al. 2014).

Because of these two scenarios, serologic screening for chronic Chagas disease is mandatory for donors and recipients originating from or who lived in endemic areas. In this regard, increased traveling and migrations are leading to difficulties regarding organ transplantation and blood donation systems.

19.4.2 Management of Mycobacterial Infections

- Active tuberculosis (TB) is a severe disease after SOT with mortality ranging between 9.5 and 17 % (Meije et al. 2014). Most cases occur within the first year after transplantation. Strikingly, extrapulmonary or disseminated TB is more frequent than in the general population. As a consequence, all transplant candidates and living donors should ideally be screened for latent tuberculosis with a tuberculin skin test (lecture at 48–72 h, positive if induration ≥5 mm). However, due to a reduced sensitivity and false positiveness of tuberculin skin test after vaccination, interferon gamma release assay (IGRA) should be done when possible, independently of the tuberculin skin test result (Meije et al. 2014). In case of positive tuberculin skin test or IGRA test, active TB should be investigated.
  Active TB can be confirmed only by culturing *M. tuberculosis* or detecting nucleic acid sequence from a clinical specimen. In case of lung infection, if sputum is negative, BAL, transbronchial biopsy, or mediastinoscopy should be considered. For extrapulmonary TB, any involved site might be sampled (Table 19.1). If active TB is not present, treatment of latent TB is recommended for patients awaiting heart transplantation in any of the following cases: (i) positive TST or IGRA test, (ii) history of untreated TB, or (iii) history of contact with a subject with active TB. In that case, treatment relies on isoniazid (300 mg/day) + vitamin B6 for 9 months, associated with a close monitoring of liver tests and signs of neuropathy (Meije et al. 2014).
  For the treatment of active TB, rifamycins (rifampicin or rifabutin) can be avoided in case of localized and non-severe infections. In that case, maintenance therapy should last for 12–18 months. However, for severe or disseminated TB, a regimen containing rifampicin or rifabutin is mandatory, with a close monitoring of calcineurin or mTOR inhibitors and corticosteroid levels (Meije et al. 2014). In that case, maintenance therapy should last for 9 months. IRIS during the treatment of active TB is possible.
- Nontuberculous mycobacteria are ubiquitous and found in a wide range of environments. Even if their incidence is low, it is much higher after SOT than in the general population and may reach 0.24–2.8 % after heart transplantation (Meije et al. 2014). Most cases develop cutaneous lesions of the extremities, tenosynovitis, or arthritis (Meije et al. 2014). The diagnosis is confirmed by the isolation of NTM from a normally sterile body site. Even if lung infection is rare (beside lung recipients), its diagnosis is more complex and requires compatible clinical and radiological presentation (Fig. 19.6), exclusion of other diagnosis, and identification of NTM in BAL or two consecutive sputa or pulmonary tissue. Treatment of NTM requires antimicrobial therapy, surgical excision, or drainage and reduction of immunosuppressant drugs. Association of two or three drugs will be chosen, based on the initial severity and the identification of the bacterial species (Meije et al. 2014).

19.4.3 Management of Opportunistic Bacterial Infections

Nocardia. Nocardiosis is a rare opportunistic infection caused by *Nocardia* spp., an ubiquitous aerobic actinomycete that is commonly found in a wide range of environments such as decaying vegetation, soil, and water. In recent reports, incidence after heart transplantation ranges between 0.65 and 2.5 % (Lebeaux et al. 2014a). Nocardiosis during the first month after SOT is uncommon and about 2/3 of cases occur during the first year after transplantation. Main risk factors are high-dose corticosteroids, cytomegalovirus (CMV) disease in the preceding 6 months,

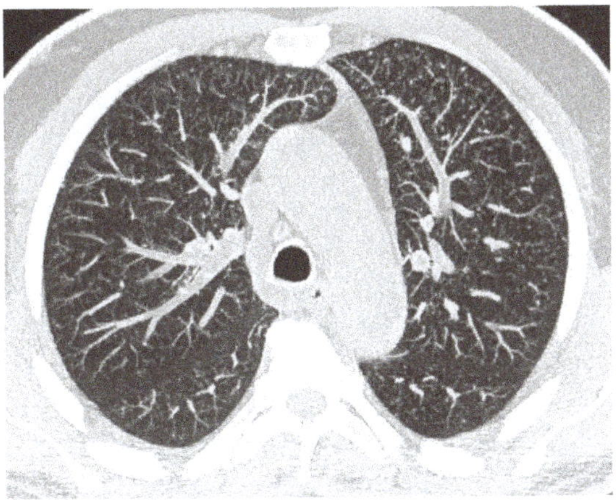

Fig. 19.6 Transplanted patient with pulmonary *Mycobacterium bovis* infection. Axial non-enhanced computed tomography (Maximal intensity projection images) shows multiple scattered centrilobular nodules

and a high median calcineurin inhibitor serum level in the preceding 30 days. Invasive nocardiosis accounts for 80–90 % of cases and is caused by bacterial inhalation, therefore leading to pneumonia in most cases. CT scan discloses lung infiltrates with consolidation (Fig. 19.7), nodules, excavations, or pleural effusion. Bacteria may then reach the bloodstream and disseminate to all organs: the CNS (with brain abscess), skin, soft tissue, eyes, liver, bone, heart valve, joint, muscle, and testis (Fig. 19.7). Overall mortality is ≈30 % but may reach 50 % in case of brain abscess. Strikingly, coinfections are possible with viral, bacterial, or fungal pathogens and are associated with a worst outcome. Primary cutaneous or subcutaneous nocardiosis is also possible in case of direct bacterial inoculation

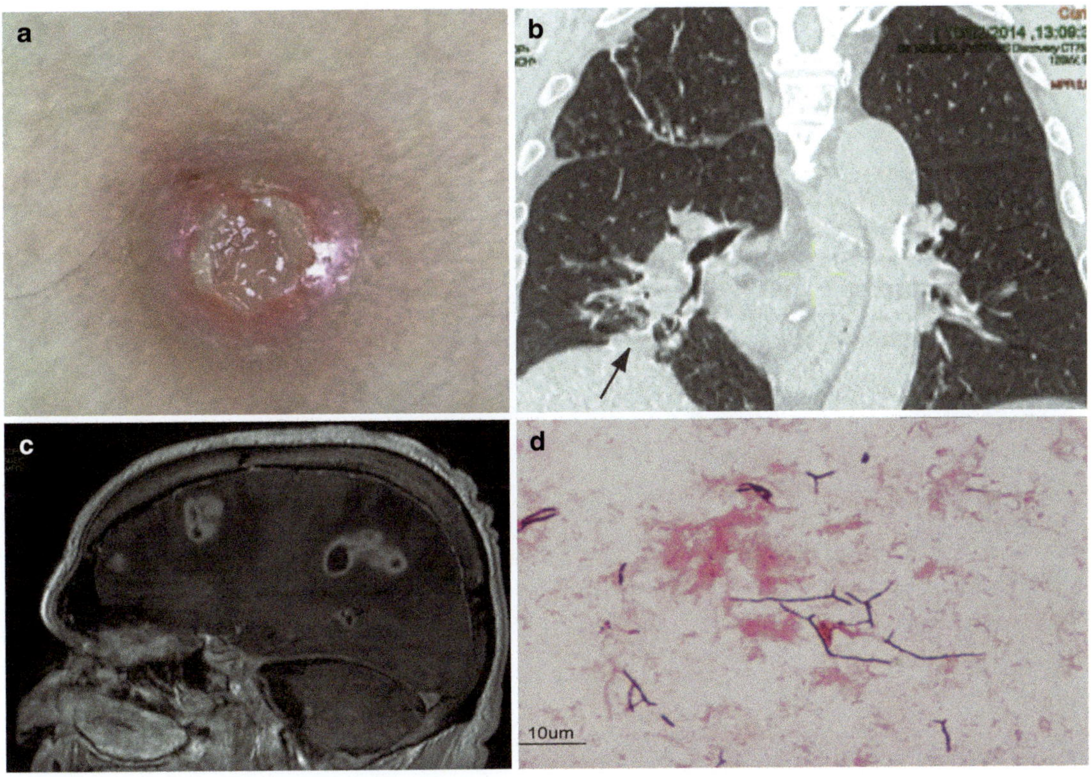

Fig. 19.7 Disseminated nocardiosis in a transplanted patient. (**a**) Nodular skin lesion of the right leg, (**b**) lung consolidation (coronal non-enhanced computed tomography, *black arrow*), (**c**) postcontrast sagittal T1-weighted magnetic resonance image showing multiple rim-enhancing brain lesions with a central hypointensity and peripheral edema, (**d**) Gram staining of the skin biopsy reveals filamentous and branching Gram-positive rods. Figure previously published in (Lebeaux et al. 2014b)

after a penetrating skin trauma. First-line treatment relies on trimethoprim–sulfamethoxazole, amikacin, third-generation cephalosporin, imipenem, or linezolid, depending on initial severity and dissemination (Lebeaux et al. 2014a). To reduce the risk of relapse, treatment is usually administered for 6 months in case of lung infection or 12 months in case of brain abscess.

Listeriosis *Listeria monocytogenes* is a Gram-positive bacillus that is transmitted to humans through contaminated foods such as milk and cheese or undercooked meat. It is responsible for bloodstream infection and meningoencephalitis in immunocompromised patients, including SOT recipients.

Conclusion

Even if heart transplantation dramatically changed the care of patients with terminal chronic heart disease, several challenges remain. Among them infections put the emphasis on the importance of mixing several medical skills including surgeon, infectious diseases specialist, radiologist, and microbiologist, among many.

Furthermore, there is still a lot to do regarding the challenges of donor-derived infection, in the context of a severe lack of grafts.

Key Points

- Infection, a major complication which increases mortality after heart transplantation, should be suspected early in this population.
- Due to the important number of causative pathogens, advances in molecular diagnostic tools, new therapeutic options, and interactions between antimicrobial agents and immunosuppressive drugs, a close collaboration between infectious diseases specialists and heart transplantation teams is mandatory.
- Pretransplant evaluation of the heart transplant candidate should assess the risk of posttransplant infections with agents such as *Herpesviridae*, tuberculosis, and *Strongyloides*. Needed vaccinations should also be initiated during pretransplant care.
- Preventive strategies (prophylaxis and preemptive therapy) increase the survival of heart transplant recipients. Main agents to consider are *Herpesviridae* (such as CMV, HSV, and VZV), influenzae, hepatitis viruses, *Pneumocystis jirovecii*, *Toxoplasma gondii*, and *Mycobacterium tuberculosis*.
- Depending on factors such as donor specificities, pretransplant colonizations, drug-induced immunosuppression used, time post heart transplantation, local specificities, prophylactic regimen used, and clinical presentation, likely pathogens should be considered and guide first-line diagnostic investigations once an infection is suspected.
- A wide range of viral, bacterial, fungal, and parasitic agents may cause infection after heart transplantation. An extensive clinical and radiological work-up is mandatory due to diagnostic pitfalls in these patients.
- Early infections (within 4 weeks) after heart transplantation suggest surgical site and wound infections or graft-transmitted disease.
- Clinical and radiological aspects have low predictive values to predict the causative microbial pathogen involved. Bronchoalveolar lavage and biopsy of any involved organ play an important role due to the broad spectrum of causative pathogens.
- Antimicrobial resistance is a matter of concern in heart transplant recipients. Useless antimicrobial therapies should be avoided, and catheters and other devices should be removed when no longer essential. Antimicrobial therapies should be targeted against identified pathogen(s).

References

Andrade DV, Gollob KJ, Dutra WO. Acute chagas disease: new global challenges for an old neglected disease. PLoS Neglect Tropical Dis. 2014;8, e3010.

De Pauw B, Walsh TJ, Donnelly JP, Stevens DA, Edwards JE, Calandra T, Pappas PG, Maertens J, Lortholary O, Kauffman CA, Denning DW, Patterson TF, Maschmeyer G, Bille J, Dismukes WE, Herbrecht R, Hope WW, Kibbler CC, Kullberg BJ, Marr KA, Munoz P, Odds FC, Perfect JR, Restrepo A, Ruhnke M, Segal BH, Sobel JD, Sorrell TC, Viscoli C, Wingard JR, Zaoutis T, Bennett JE,; European Organization for R; Treatment of Cancer/Invasive Fungal Infections Cooperative G; National Institute of A; Infectious Diseases Mycoses Study Group Consensus G. Revised definitions of invasive fungal disease from the European Organization for Research and Treatment of Cancer/Invasive Fungal Infections Cooperative Group and the National Institute of Allergy and Infectious Diseases Mycoses Study Group (EORTC/MSG) Consensus Group. Clin Infect Dis. 2008;46:1813–21.

Derouin F, Pelloux H, Parasitology ESGoC. Prevention of toxoplasmosis in transplant patients. Clin Microbiol Infect. 2008;14:1089–101.

Duffy GP. Lumbar puncture in the presence of raised intracranial pressure. Br Med J. 1969;1:407–9.

Fishman JA. From the classic concepts to modern practice. Clin Microbiol Infect 2014;20(Suppl 7):4–9.

Gavalda J, Aguado JM, Manuel O, Grossi P, Hirsch HH, Hosts ESGoIiC. A special issue on infections in solid organ transplant recipients. Clin Microbiol Infect. 2014;20(Suppl 7):1-3.

Gavalda J, Meije Y, Fortun J, Roilides E, Saliba F, Lortholary O, Munoz P, Grossi P, Cuenca-Estrella M, Hosts ESGfIiC. Invasive fungal infections in solid organ transplant recipients. Clin Microbiol Infect. 2014;20(Suppl 7):27–48.

Ison MG, Szakaly P, Shapira MY, Krivan G, Nist A, Dutkowski R. Efficacy and safety of oral oseltamivir for influenza prophylaxis in transplant recipients. Antivir Ther. 2012;17:955–64.

Kotton CN, Kumar D, Caliendo AM, Asberg A, Chou S, Danziger-Isakov L, Humar A, Transplantation Society International CMVCG. Updated international consensus guidelines on the management of cytomegalovirus in solid-organ transplantation. Transplantation. 2013; 96:333–60.

Lattes R, Lasala MB. Chagas disease in the immunosuppressed patient. Clin Microbiol Infect. 2014;20:300–9.

Lebeaux D, Morelon E, Suarez F, Lanternier F, Scemla A, Frange P, Mainardi JL, Lecuit M, Lortholary O. Nocardiosis in transplant recipients. Eur J Clin Microbiol Infect Dis. 2014a;33:689–702.

Lebeaux D, Rodriguez-Nava V, Laurent F, Mainardi JL, Meynard JL, Toro A, Boiron P, Lecuit M, Lortholary O. Diagnosis and treatment of nocardiosis. Lettre de l'Infectiologue. 2014. XXIX:20–5.

Manuel O, Husain S, Kumar D, Zayas C, Mawhorter S, Levi ME, Kalpoe J, Lisboa L, Ely L, Kaul DR, Schwartz BS, Morris MI, Ison MG, Yen-Lieberman B, Sebastian A, Assi M, Humar A. Assessment of cytomegalovirus-specific cell-mediated immunity for the prediction of cytomegalovirus disease in high-risk solid-organ transplant recipients: a multicenter cohort study. Clin Infect Dis. 2013;56:817–24.

Manuel O, Estabrook M, Practice ASTIDCo. RNA respiratory viruses in solid organ transplantation. Am J Transplant. 2013;13(Suppl 4):212–9.

Meije Y, Piersimoni C, Torre-Cisneros J, Dilektasli AG, Aguado JM, Hosts ESGoIiC. Mycobacterial infections in solid organ transplant recipients. Clin Microbiol Infect. 2014;20(Suppl 7):89–101.

Menzin J, Meyers JL, Friedman M, Korn JR, Perfect JR, Langston AA, Danna RP, Papadopoulos G. The economic costs to United States hospitals of invasive fungal infections in transplant patients. Am J Infect Control. 2011;39:e15–20.

Roxby AC, Gottlieb GS, Limaye AP. Strongyloidiasis in transplant patients. Clin Infect Dis. 2009;49:1411–23.

Singh N, Levi ME, Practice ASTIDCo. Arenavirus and West Nile virus in solid organ transplantation. Am J Transplant. 2013;13(Suppl 4):361–71.

Stehlik J, Edwards LB, Kucheryavaya AY, Benden C, Christie JD, Dobbels F, Kirk R, Rahmel AO, Hertz MI. The Registry of the International Society for Heart and Lung Transplantation: Twenty-eighth Adult Heart Transplant Report--2011. J Heart Lung Transplant. 2011;30:1078–94.

Ulrich C, Hackethal M, Meyer T, Geusau A, Nindl I, Ulrich M, Forschner T, Sterry W, Stockfleth E. Skin infections in organ transplant recipients. J German Soc Dermatol. 2008;6:98–105.

Valantine HA, Luikart H, Doyle R, Theodore J, Hunt S, Oyer P, Robbins R, Berry G, Reitz B. Impact of cytomegalovirus hyperimmune globulin on outcome after cardiothoracic transplantation: a comparative study of combined prophylaxis with CMV hyperimmune globulin plus ganciclovir versus ganciclovir alone. Transplantation. 2001;72:1647–52.

Wang EH, Partovi N, Levy RD, Shapiro RJ, Yoshida EM, Greanya ED. Pneumocystis pneumonia in solid organ transplant recipients: not yet an infection of the past. Transplant Infect Dis. 2012;14:519–25.

Wright AJ, Fishman JA. Central nervous system syndromes in solid organ transplant recipients. Clin Infect Dis. 2014;59:1001–11.

Zuckermann A, Barten MJ. Surgical wound complications after heart transplantation. Transplant Int. 2011;24:627–36.

Malignancies After Heart Transplantation

20

Valentina Agostini, Heike Goebel, Luciano Potena, Gerald J. Berry, and Ornella Leone

Contents

V. Agostini, MD • O. Leone, MD (✉)
Cardiovascular and Cardiac Transplant Pathology Program, Department of Pathology, Sant'Orsola-Malpighi University Hospital, Bologna, Italy
e-mail: ornella.leone@aosp.bo.it

H. Goebel, MD
Institute of Pathology, University of Cologne, Köln, Germany

L. Potena, MD, PhD
Heart Failure and Heart Transplant Program, Cardiology Unit, Sant'Orsola-Malpighi University Hospital, Bologna, Italy

G.J. Berry, MD
Department of Pathology, Stanford Medical Center, Stanford, CA, USA

20.1 Background

Since the introduction of cyclosporin A, solid organ transplantation is an acknowledged treatment option in end-stage organ failure. Over time many new potent immunosuppressant agents and multidrug immunosuppressive regimens have been introduced into clinical practice. Different management strategies have also been designed for the various transplant organs and can now be further refined to meet individual patient needs. With a greater proportion of patients now surviving for more than a decade, continuous immunosuppression is prolonged and creates new problems such as drug toxicity and secondary malignancies with their attendant treatment challenges (Nair et al. 2014; Collett et al. 2010; Jiang et al. 2010; Krynitz et al. 2013).

For many years the primary objective of heart transplant patient management was necessarily the control of acute cellular rejection. Today it remains a major cause of death in the first 1–3 years after transplantation (around 10 %, according to the 2015 International Society for Heart and Lung Transplantion (ISHLT) Adult Heart Transplantation Statistics). More recently efforts have been increasingly focused on the study of cardiac allograft vasculopathy (at present 13.3 % of patients die 10–15 years after transplantation and 11.7 % after 15 years) to permit early detection and follow-up of the disease with the goal of reduced morbidity and mortality.

O. Leone et al. (eds.), *The Pathology of Cardiac Transplantation*,
DOI 10.1007/978-3-319-46386-5_20

Now is probably the time for a closer look at malignancies, although the balance between under- and over-immunosuppression is complex.

While the malignancies commonly observed in the general population (e.g. lung, prostate, colo-rectal and breast cancer) occur at the same or slightly greater rates in heart transplant recipients, some that are rare in the general population are quite common in transplanted patients. For example, lympho-proliferative disorder, ano-genital squamous cell carcinoma and Kaposi sarcoma develop in this patient population on account of dysregulation of the immune system and/or viral infections (Nair et al. 2014).

This chapter examines risk factors for tumour initiation and development, the main groups of tumour encountered in heart-transplanted patients and therapeutic strategies.

20.2 Risk Factors for Tumour Development

Solid organ and haematopoietic stem cell transplant (HSCT) recipients have an increased risk of developing malignancies. There is variation in the types and frequencies of malignancies in the different transplant groups, e.g. non-melanoma skin cancers are the most common in solid organ recipients and B-cell lymphomas the most common in HSCT patients. Moreover, within the solid organ group, heart and combined heart-lung recipients have higher incidence than renal transplant patients. Previous studies have shown that lymphomas and visceral malignancies are four and six times, respectively, more common in cardiac transplantation compared to renal transplantation (Engels et al. 2011; Sampaio et al. 2012; Jiang et al. 2010).

Immunosuppressive therapy is the major risk factor in the development of malignancies, although various aspects of immunosuppressive regimens should be considered: type, intensity and duration. Each of these can also vary according to recipient potential for developing acute rejection, such as pre-transplant panel-reactive antibody titres, donor-specific crossmatches and the number of rejection episodes after transplantation. The direct toxic/oncogenic effects of some immunosuppressive agents as well as the increased risk of oncovirus activation (e.g. Epstein-Barr virus -EBV, human papillomavirus -HPV, and human herpesvirus-8 -HHV8) and/or reactivation are important related issues. Moreover current knowledge of the relationship between different immunosuppressant drugs, their duration and intensity and subsequent malignancy risk is still limited, as is the efficacy (and safety) of lower immunosuppression regimens.

Additional risk factors for post-transplant malignancies have been enumerated: older patients, recipient tumour history, genetic predisposition for certain tumours and common risk factors such as smoking or high sun exposure (AlBugami and Kiberd 2014; Kuijken and Bouwes Bavinck 2000; Epailly et al. 2011).

In addition, many patients have multiple documented risk factors that further augment the overall predisposition for neoplasia.

Although a rare occurrence, there are published case reports of malignancies developing following the transfer of malignant cells from the donor, via the transplanted organ. One should always keep this possibility in mind since the recipient immune system will be diminished by the immunosuppression, and cells with a different genetic background will escape the normal host defence mechanisms (Pandanaboyana et al. 2016; Buell et al. 2001).

20.2.1 Risks Related to Immunosuppressive Drugs

20.2.1.1 Induction Immunosuppression

- *Antithymocyte globulin* (*ATG*)
  These polyclonal antibodies derived from rabbit or equine sources belong to the group of lymphocyte-depleting agents. They are effective, potent therapeutic drugs that promptly reduce circulating T-cells, and

B-cells. They are often used in induction protocols prior to transplantation in selective patient groups, e.g. presensitized patients, to reduce perioperative rejections and also after transplant in severe hemodynamic compromise or refractory acute cellular rejection episodes. In heart transplantation there are only a few published studies demonstrating the usefulness of ATG as induction therapy or rejection treatment, and they show a benefit in reducing acute cellular rejection episodes. Unfortunately, they are associated with an increased risk in late-onset cytomegalovirus (CMV) infections, but this is avoided by instituting antiviral prophylaxis at the time of administration. There is an association with post-transplant malignancies, especially lymphomas, skin cancer and lung cancer when ATG is used repeatedly in high doses (Ducloux et al. 2004; Gharekhani et al. 2013).

- *OKT3*
  This murine antibody targets T-cells by binding to the T-cell receptor complex in the CD3 region of the T-cell and inhibiting its function. T-cell depletion enhances susceptibility to a variety of viral infections. Repeated intravenous bolus injections or prolonged high doses precipitate an increase in post-transplant lymphoproliferative disorders. Other viral-associated neoplasms such as ano-genital squamous cancers due to HPV and Kaposi sarcoma associated with HHV8 have been reported (Swinnen et al. 1990; Kobashigawa and Patel 2006). The drug was withdrawn from clinical utilization in 2009 due to reduced clinical demand.
- *Anti-CD52 antibodies*
  Anti-CD52 antibodies such as alemtuzumab target T-cells, natural killer (NK) cells, monocytes, macrophages and B-cells act by binding to the glycoprotein CD52. They are used primarily for induction therapy although it has been initiated as rescue therapy in some solid organ transplant recipients. Leukopenia, delayed T-cell cell recovery, cytokine release syndrome and autoimmune disorders such as haemolytic anaemia and thyroiditis are reported complications, but there are no reports of increased viral infections or malignancy. That said only a few clinical trials with small numbers of patients have been published to date so that information of the drug's neoplastic potential is scarce (Söderlund and Rådegran 2015).
- *Interleukin-2 (IL-2) receptor antagonists*
  This group of non-lymphocyte-depleting biologics are directed at the alpha chain of the IL-2 receptor of T-cells and act to inhibit T-cell differentiation and proliferation. Neither basiliximab nor daclizumab has been associated with increased risk for infection or malignancy.

20.2.1.2 Maintenance Immunosuppression

- *Cyclosporin A (CyA)*
  This agent uses calcineurin inhibition to prevent T-cell proliferation and differentiation. Apart from its recognized nephrotoxicity, gingival hyperplasia is a prominent side effect (Ho et al. 2010). These are often indications to consider switching to other calcineurin inhibitors or reducing the dosage used for patients. One mechanism is up-regulation of the plasminogen activator inhibitor-1 pathway that promotes the accumulation of extracellular matrix seen in gingival hyperplasia. Furthermore, CyA appears to increase the development of basal cell carcinoma and squamous cell carcinoma, possibly due to its influence on the p53-pathway and its role in DNA repair after ultraviolet-light exposure (Krynitz et al. 2016). Therefore, typical precautions with respect to sunlight are essential for patients after transplant (Kuijken and Bouwes Bavinck 2000).
- *Azathioprine (AZA)*
  This antimetabolite drug inhibits purine nucleotide synthesis in the cell cycle of both T- and B-cells. It was one of the first immunosuppressive drugs and has been largely replaced by mycophenolate mofetil as

the anti-proliferative agent of choice in most centres (Keogh et al. 2004; David et al. 2005; Eisen et al. 2005). AZA appears to be associated with increased incidence of post-transplant malignancies (Kobashigawa et al. 1998), especially lymphoproliferative disorders and acute myeloid leukaemia, as it impairs DNA repair (Swann et al. 1996; O'Donovan et al. 2005). Acute myeloid leukaemia is considered a separate form, but, on account of its rarity, it is difficult to estimate the contribution of AZA as a risk factor (Rashidi and Fisher 2014).

- *Mycophenolate mofetil (MMF)*
  Like AZA, it inhibits the cell cycle of both T- and B-lymphocytes by reversibly blocking the enzyme that is critical to guanosine synthesis, type 2-inosine-monophosphate-dehydrogenase (IMPDH). Its primary adverse effects are gastro-intestinal and, less commonly, pulmonary (Keogh et al. 2004; David et al. 2005). It is not associated with increased risk for malignancy, but there is a potential interaction with antiviral drugs like acyclovir and ganciclovir.
- *Proliferation signal inhibitors (PSI) (mammalian target of rapamycin – mTOR – inhibitors)*
  This recent class of immunosuppressive drugs, which includes sirolimus and everolimus, inhibits the proliferation and differentiation of both T-cells and B-cells by binding to the tacrolimus binding protein (FKBP12). Principle among their reported side effects is impaired wound healing and lung and renal toxicity. Interestingly, these compounds also appear to have antineoplastic properties (Geissler 2008; 2015; Valantine 2007), as they have antiproliferative effects and can also interfere with several pro-oncogenic pathways of malignancy development (Dantal and Pohanka 2007). Indeed mTOR inhibitors are currently registered for the treatment of some breast cancers and renal clear cell carcinoma – although at higher dosages than are used for transplant immunosuppression.

20.3 Malignancies Occurring in Heart-Transplanted Patients

20.3.1 Post-transplant Lymphoproliferative Disorders

Post-transplant lymphoproliferative disorders (PTLDs) are defined as lymphoid or plasmacytic proliferations that develop as a consequence of immunosuppression following solid organ or haematopoietic cell transplantation (Swerdlow et al. 2008).

Four general types of PTLDs are described in the fourth edition of the WHO classification of haematopoietic and lymphoid tissue:

- Early lesions
- Polymorphic PTLD
- Monomorphic PTLD
- Classical Hodgkin lymphoma PTLD

Indolent small B-cell lymphomas such as follicular lymphoma and EBV-negative extranodal marginal zone lymphoma arising in transplant patients are currently not considered PTLD. There are rare exceptions such as EBV+ mucosa-associated neoplasms (MALT lymphoma).

An updated PTLD classification is forthcoming, although it is likely that the current scheme will not be substantially altered.

PTLD risk and incidence depends on the intensity and type of immunosuppressive regimen and the type of organ transplanted: recent data describe an incidence of PTLDs between 3 and 9 % in heart and lung transplantation compared with 1.4–2.9 % in renal transplantation and 0.9–2.6 % in liver transplantation. A recent study in cardiac recipients reported an incidence of 5.4 % in a population of 763 patients transplanted between 1984 and 2010 (Kumarasinghe et al. 2015).

The most important risk factor for PTLD is EBV serum negativity at the time of transplantation, thus explaining the high rate in children and young adults (Caillard et al. 2006; Webber 1999).

Up to 30 % of PTLDs are EBV negative (even more in some studies) (Leblond et al. 1998; Nelson et al. 2000): these are more likely to be of monomorphic type and tend to occur later than EBV-positive cases, on average 4–5 years later (Nelson et al. 2000; Leblond et al. 1998).

CMV negativity at the time of transplantation may also be associated with increased incidence of PTLDs, and the effects of EBV and CMV may be synergic (Jaffe 2011).

Most PTLDs present within 1 year of transplantation and the clinical presentation is often non-specific. Allograft involvement makes the differential diagnosis between lymphoma and rejection challenging, but cardiac localization by PTLD is rare (2.4 % according to Kumarasinghe G. et al.) (Fig. 20.2). General features that support the diagnosis of lymphoma are the presence of a mass-forming lesion, a B-cell-rich infiltrate, lymphoid cytologic atypia and extensive necrosis. Paraffin section immunohistochemistry and EBV in situ hybridization are useful tools to distinguish rejection from PTLD, as are flow cytometry, clonality studies and mutational analysis. Lymphomas involving the heart allograft are more likely to be disseminated, and aggressive neoplasms develop in a significantly shorter time from transplantation (Khedmat and Taheri 2011).

Early lesions These are lymphoplasmacytic proliferations characterized by architectural preservation and admixture of polyclonal T-cells, B-cells and/or plasma cells. The term "early" implies a pathogenetic rather than a temporal focus, as many cases arise years after transplantation. They are classified as plasmacytic hyperplasia or infectious mononucleosis-like lesions (IM-like); the distinction depends on the number of transformed cells (immunoblasts). Some authors recognize florid follicular hyperplasia as a third type of early lesion. These occur at a younger age than other PTLDs and are often seen in extranodal sites such as tonsils and adenoids in patients with no prior EBV infection. They can regress spontaneously with the reduction of immunosuppression or precede polymorphic or monomorphic PTLDs in some cases. Most of these proliferations are EBV positive, although the positivity may be variable. There are no clear criteria to distinguish these early lesions from the other reactive lymphoplasmacytic proliferations, and diagnosis rests on clinical correlations and presence of increased numbers of EBV+ cells compared to immunocompetent patients. Small monoclonal or oligoclonal populations may be demonstrated with Southern blot, but their significance is unknown.

Polymorphic PTLDs (P-PTLDs) These are lymphoplasmacytic proliferations that efface the architecture of underlying tissue or form destructive masses but do not fulfil the criteria for any of the recognized types of lymphoma. P-PTLDs are defined as an admixture of the full range of B-cell maturation (immunoblasts, plasma cells, small- or intermediate-sized lymphoid cells and scattered large bizarre cells that resemble Reed-Stenberg cells) with a variable proportion of heterogeneous T-cells.

P-PTLDs and monomorphic PTLDs of B-cell origin form a morphologic spectrum, so clonally rearranged immunoglobulin genes are not infrequent in P-PTLDs, but the clones are less dominant than in monomorphic PTLDs; T-cell clones are not expected. Most P-PTLDs contain numerous EBV-positive cells.

Monomorphic PTLDs (M-PTLDs) These are lymphoid or plasmacytic proliferations that fulfil the criteria for one of the non-Hodgkin lymphomas or plasma cell neoplasms that arise in the immunocompetent host. They are categorized according to the WHO classification and should be designated as M-PTLDs in the diagnostic report. The major types are diffuse large B-cell lymphoma, Burkitt lymphoma and plasma cell myeloma/plasmacytoma. In North

America and Western Europe, peripheral T-cell and T/NK cell neoplasms account for less than 15 % of PTLDs. Mucosa-associated lymphoid tissue lymphomas and other small B-cell lymphomas are not considered PTLDs. Clonal immunoglobulin gene or T-cell receptor gene rearrangement is characteristic of M-PTLDs. EBV positivity is more variable than other categories.

Classical Hodgkin lymphoma PTLD (CHL-PTLD) It fulfils the criteria for classical Hodgkin lymphoma in the immunocompetent host and is the least common major form of PTLD. CHL-PTLD often resembles mixed cellularity classical Hodgkin lymphoma. Reed-Stenberg cells should be both CD15 and CD30 positive and weak PAX5 positive, in order to distinguish a CHL-PTLD from a Hodgkin-like polymorphic lesion, such as ALK+ anaplastic lymphoma. In differential diagnosis detecting EBV in small- and medium-sized lymphoid cells is a useful tool.

PTLD mortality rates have been historically high and vary widely (32 % 5-year overall survival in the American Registry and 20 % in the Spanish study group). More recent studies have suggested improved survival with anti-CD20 monoclonal antibody therapy like rituximab and other therapeutic strategies, but there are limited large series for comparison.

The first-line management is reduction of immunosuppression, as it may reverse the lymphoproliferative process in some cases, particularly the "early" lesions and a subset of polymorphous-PTLD. Unfortunately this is not always feasible because of the increased risk of acute rejection (Tsai et al. 2001).

Other potential treatments include antiviral therapy, monoclonal antibodies such as anti-CD20 monoclonal antibody and conventional chemotherapy in cases of therapeutic failure with rituximab. Surgery or radiation may be considered for selected patients with localized lesions. Surgery may be necessary in the setting of organ perforation or obstruction (Choquet et al. 2006).

An uncommon manifestation of EBV+ proliferations is in the form of smooth muscle neoplasms (Deyrup et al. 2006; Jonigka et al. 2012). The morphologic spectrum ranges from benign leiomyomas to leiomyosarcoma, and the cells are immunoreactive for smooth muscle markers like desmin and caldesmon. In situ hybridization for EBV-encoded RNA (EBER) shows strong nuclear staining.

At the end of the chapter, a wide selection of illustrative cases of PTLD from different solid organ transplant and HSCT patients is provided.

20.3.2 Skin Neoplasms

The skin is the most common site for malignancy in Caucasian organ recipients, with one patient in two developing at least one cutaneous neoplasm during their follow-up (Euvrad et al. 2003).

These tumours, especially non-melanocytic tumours, seem to be more frequent in heart recipients than in liver and renal transplantations, but this is not confirmed in all cohort studies (Euvrad et al. 2006; Jensen et al. 1999).

Cumulative risk of development of a skin neoplasm such as squamous cell carcinoma, basal cell carcinoma and Merkel cell carcinoma increases with time, intensity and duration of immunosuppression, sun exposure history, geographic location and skin type according to the Fitzpatrick scale (Euvrad et al. 2003). The impact of specific immunosuppressant drugs on the development of skin cancer is still debated, but mTOR inhibitors may reduce the risk for non-melanoma skin neoplasms, while MMF seems to increase the risk (Campbell et al. 2012; Euvrad et al. 2003).

The pathways that lead to an elevated risk for cutaneous malignancies in transplanted patients are complex, and proposed mechanisms include reduced immune surveillance, direct carcinogenic effects of immunosuppressive drugs and proliferation of oncogenic viruses (e.g. HPV and Merkel cell polyomavirus).

Squamous cell carcinoma (SCC) is the predominant skin neoplasm in this group, constituting 90 % of the lesions, followed by basal cell carcinoma (BCC), Merkel cell carcinoma (MCC) and Kaposi sarcoma (KS). Solid organ transplantation is associated with a slightly increased risk for melanoma (it is higher in HSCT recipients), but this neoplasm remains rare in heart recipients compared to other skin tumours.

Clinical presentation and morphologic appearance of SCC and BCC in transplant recipients are similar in the general population; these neoplasms are more frequent in older males and most often develop in sun-exposed areas.

The prognostic value of the seventh edition American Joint Committee on Cancer (AJCC) staging system has been substantiated in a retrospective study including heart transplant patients (Metchnikoff et al. 2012). High-risk factors should be highlighted in the pathology report (i.e. >4 mm depth, perineural and lymphovascular invasion, primary site on the ear or lip, poorly differentiated histology) (Leboit et al. 2006).

In immunocompromised patients SCCs and BCCs are often multiple and tend to be more aggressive, with high tumour burden and frequent local recurrence (Brewer et al. 2009). In a multicentre collaborative study by Martinez and colleagues, 5–8 % of transplant recipients developed metastases from non-melanoma skin cancer (Martinez et al. 2003) with its attendant poor prognosis. A study performed in Australia reported a 42 % mortality rate in cardiac transplant patients with non-melanoma skin cancer, but this rate seems to be much lower in other countries and is closely linked to early management and geographic considerations (Veness et al. 1999). Even in organ graft recipients, death due to SCC and BCC is preventable in most cases with early detection and aggressive clinical management.

Merkel cell carcinoma arising in transplant patients tends to have an aggressive course with approximately 70 % of patients developing lymph node involvement. At 2 years, the mortality rate is 56 % (Bajetta et al. 2007).

The management of SCC, BCC and MCC in heart recipients is based on surgical excision with adequate margins and usually parallels the management in immune-competent patients. In the metastatic setting, conventional chemotherapy should be considered, but data on its efficacy and safety for this group are limited.

Kaposi sarcoma is the most frequent skin neoplasm in African-American transplant recipients and, unlike other cutaneous malignancies, often develops in the first 2 years after organ transplantation. The clinical presentation resembles that of classic KS, manifesting as angiomatous lesions predominantly affecting the legs. Visceral involvement is especially common in heart recipients as it develops in 50 % of KS cases, twice as frequently as in renal recipients (Euvrad et al. 2003). HHV-8 is demonstrated in the neoplastic cells of KS, frequently with serologic evidence of infection.

The primary therapy for KS in transplant patients is a reduction in immunosuppression. Complete tumour regression of cutaneous lesions has been reported after switching from cyclosporine to sirolimus (Stallone et al. 2005).

20.3.3 Other Tumours

In recent years survival of heart transplanted patients has improved, and the overall rate of malignancy has decreased. However, as cardiac transplant patients live longer, the risk of developing other neoplasms not unique to this group remains high, at least as high as for the general population (Collett et al. 2010; Higgins et al. 2014). The ISHLT registry 2010 report gave the combined incidence of non-skin, non-lymphoproliferative malignancies as 1 %, 7 %, 15 % and 22 % at 1, 5, 10 and 14 years after transplant (Stehlick et al. 2010).

In most studies greater age, male gender and frequent episodes of treated allograft rejection are related to an increased incidence of solid neoplasms (Collett et al. 2010; Stehlick et al. 2010; Crespo-Leiro et al. 2010).

Another important factor for tumour development in the transplant era is that the probability of neoplasm has decreased in recent years compared to the early 90s (Higgins et al. 2014; Stehlick et al. 2010).

A recent study by Higgins and colleagues compared the malignancy rate in the Cardiac Transplant Research Database with that in the Surveillance Epidemiology and End Results (SEER) Cancer Statistics Review: after correction for age, gender and race, they found that the aggregate malignancy rate for transplanted patients in the modern era does not significantly differ from that of the non-transplanted population.

In recent years, while some cancers have declined in incidence, others such as lung cancer have remained high. Lung cancer occurs more frequently in heart recipients than in the general population, with an actual/expected ratio of 1.86 (Higgins et al. 2014). Most of these pulmonary neoplasms are carcinomas, but mesothelioma and carcinoid tumours have also been reported. Patients transplanted at 55–65 years are at highest risk for lung cancer (Rinaldi et al. 2001; Strecker et al. 2013).

In male recipients the second most frequent solid neoplasm is prostate cancer and in females breast cancer, mirroring the incidence in the non-transplanted population (Higgins et al. 2014). Standard therapeutic interventions such as surgery, radiation therapy and chemotherapy are used depending on the tumour type and stage. In general the prognosis is similar to that of the general population.

20.4 Management of Recipients

Management of heart transplant patients, with their higher risk of developing malignancies, is a complex process and should involve a multidisciplinary approach.

It starts before transplantation with an individualized assessment of recipient risk factors (individual and familial history of malignancy and general risk factors, such as smoking, sun exposure, oncovirus infections, etc.) and proceeds to careful pre-transplant screening for tumours or premalignant lesions and for biological markers of tumour risk.

After transplantation, early diagnosis of neoplasms and premalignant conditions is essential: these patients should be more frequently screened than the general population, using the usual tests for tumour prevention (Nägele et al. 1999), as clearly underlined by current ISHLT guidelines for the care of heart transplant recipients (Costanzo et al. 2010).

All patients - and paediatric recipients - in particular should have frequent monitoring of peripheral blood EBV loads to identify patients at higher risk for PTLD.

The last step is modulating immunosuppressive therapy when malignancies occur. There are no randomized studies exploring this issue and practice varies from centre to centre. Recently, a group of transplant cardiologists, surgeons and oncologists, relying on both published and personal experience, have attempted to establish clinical guidelines for cardiac recipient patients with malignancy, with the specific aim of reducing the immunosuppression burden (Fig. 20.1). In this guide the authors emphasize the importance of a multidisciplinary approach with collaboration between the various clinical and laboratory specialists (Epailly et al. 2011).

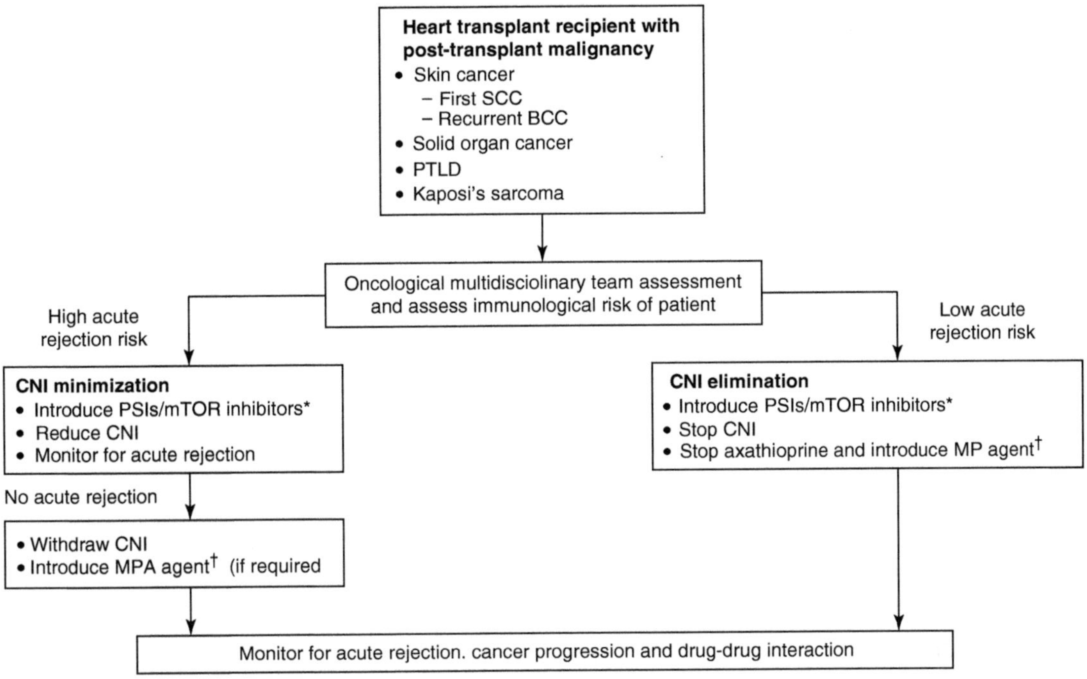

BCC, basal cell carcinoma; inhibitor; MPA, mycophenolic acid; PSIs/mTOR inhibitors, proliferation signal inhibitor/mammalian target of rapamycin inhibitor: PTLD, post-transplant lymphoproliferative disorder: SSC, squamous cell carcinoma (recommended trough levels: 3–8 ng/mL for everolimus and 5–15 ng/mL for sirolimus).

*If the patient is to receive surgery for cancer, delay the initiation of PSIs/m TOR inhibitors until the risk of wound healing has subsidied. †Decreases MPA dose if converting from CsA and using in combination with everolimus or sirolimus.

Fig. 20.1 Proposed algorithm for management of post-transplant malignancies with proliferation signal inhibitors (From Epailly et al. 2011)

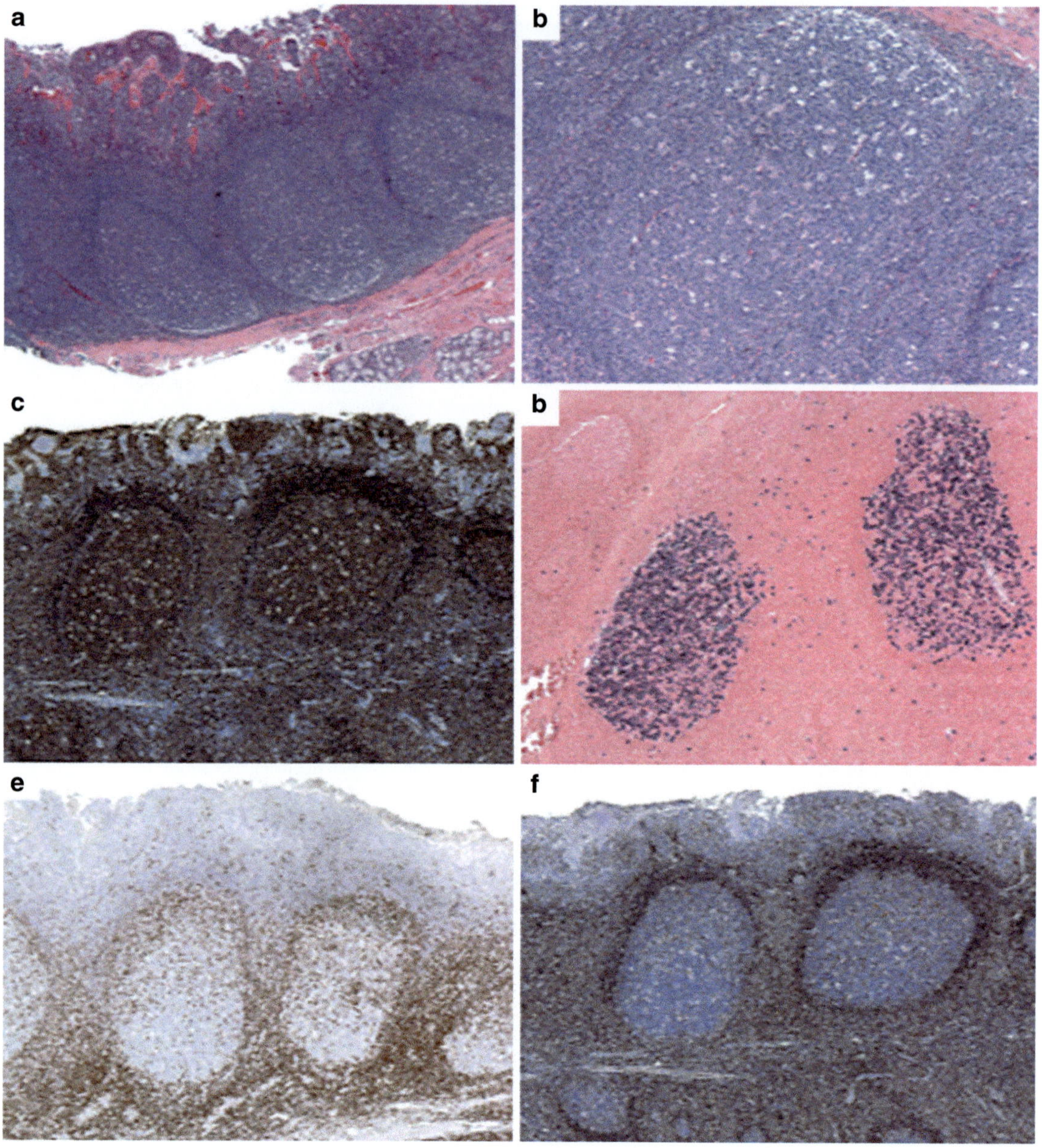

Fig. 20.2 (**a**) The tonsils and adenoids showed early lesion PTLD with florid reactive follicular hyperplasia (Haematoxylin-eosin, ×40). (**b**) High power showing prominent reactive germinal centre within the tonsillar tissue (Haematoxylin-eosin, ×200). (**c**) CD20 immunohistochemical staining highlights B-cells within the germinal centres (×50). Kappa and lambda light chain staining demonstrated a polytypic pattern (not shown). (**d**) In situ hybridization for EBV RNA shows marked increase in EBV in many of the germinal centres (×60). (**e**) CD3+ highlights the T-cells in the interfollicular regions (×50). (**f**) BCL2 shows a normal staining pattern (×50)

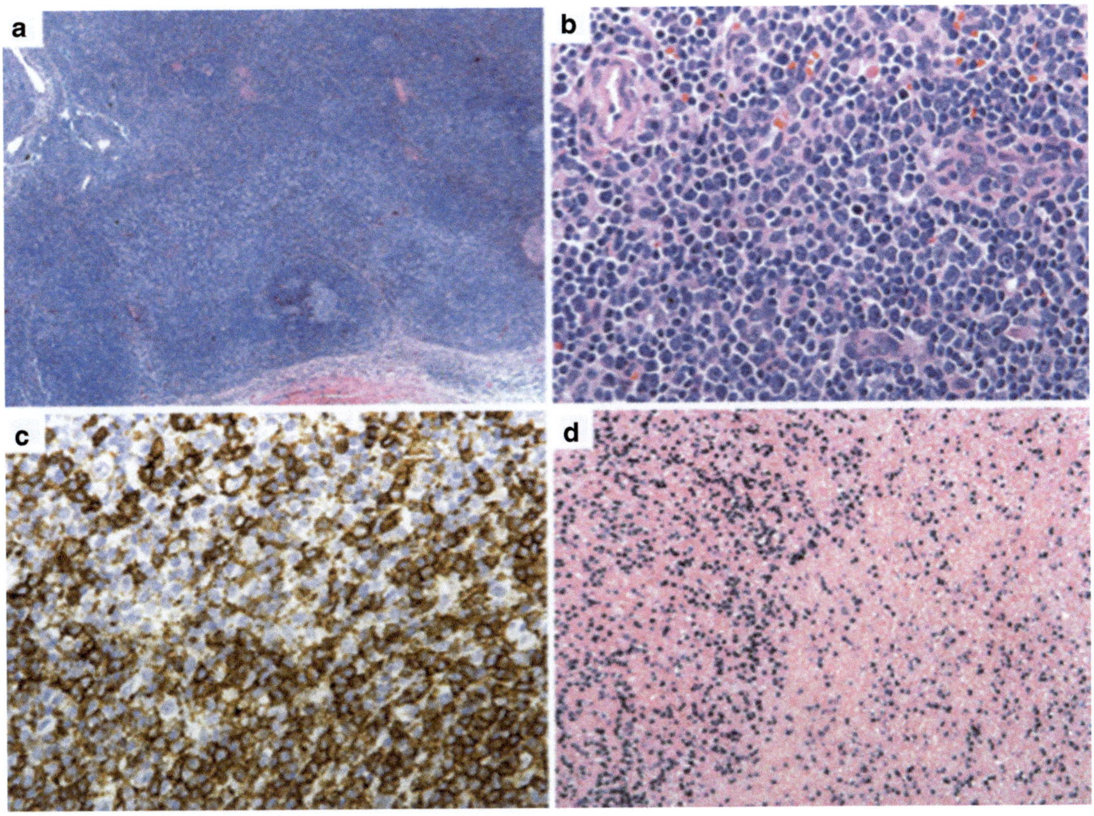

Fig. 20.3 (**a**) Partial effacement of the nodal architecture with expansion of the paracortical regions by a mixed infiltrate (Haematoxylin-eosin, ×40). (**b**) High-power magnification of the paracortical region showing a polymorphous collection of small lymphocytes, plasmacytoid lymphocytes and immunoblasts (Haematoxylin-eosin, ×400). (**c**) Both the small and large cells are immunoreactive against the B-cell marker-CD20 (×400). Flow cytometry on the lymph node showed a heterogeneous population of lymphocytes, including mostly T-cells and fewer B-cells and NK-cells. The B-cells showed polytypic light chain expression (not shown). (**d**) Strong EBV positivity mirroring the CD20 B-cell staining in the paracortical regions (×100)

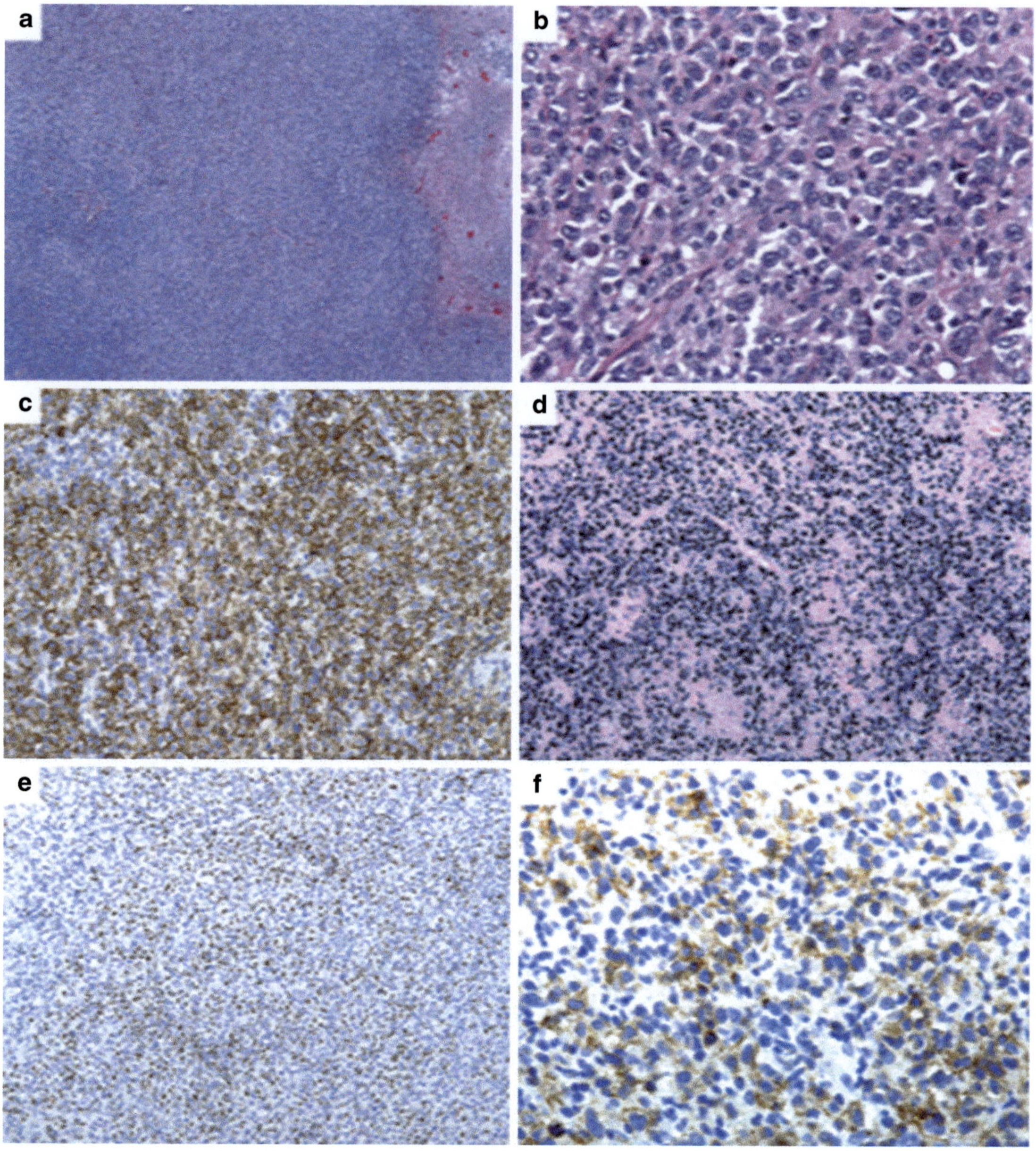

Fig. 20.4 (**a**) Complete effacement of nodal architecture with foci of necrosis (Haematoxylin-eosin, ×40). (**b**) High-power magnification showing sheets of monotonous atypical large lymphoid cells (Haematoxylin-eosin, ×400). (**c**) Strong diffuse staining of neoplastic cells with the B-cell marker, CD20 (×200). (**d**) Diffuse staining for EBER by EBV in situ hybridization (×100). (**e**) High proliferation rate of 50–60 % by Ki-67 immunostaining (×100). (**f**) Positive CD30 staining of 50 % (×400)

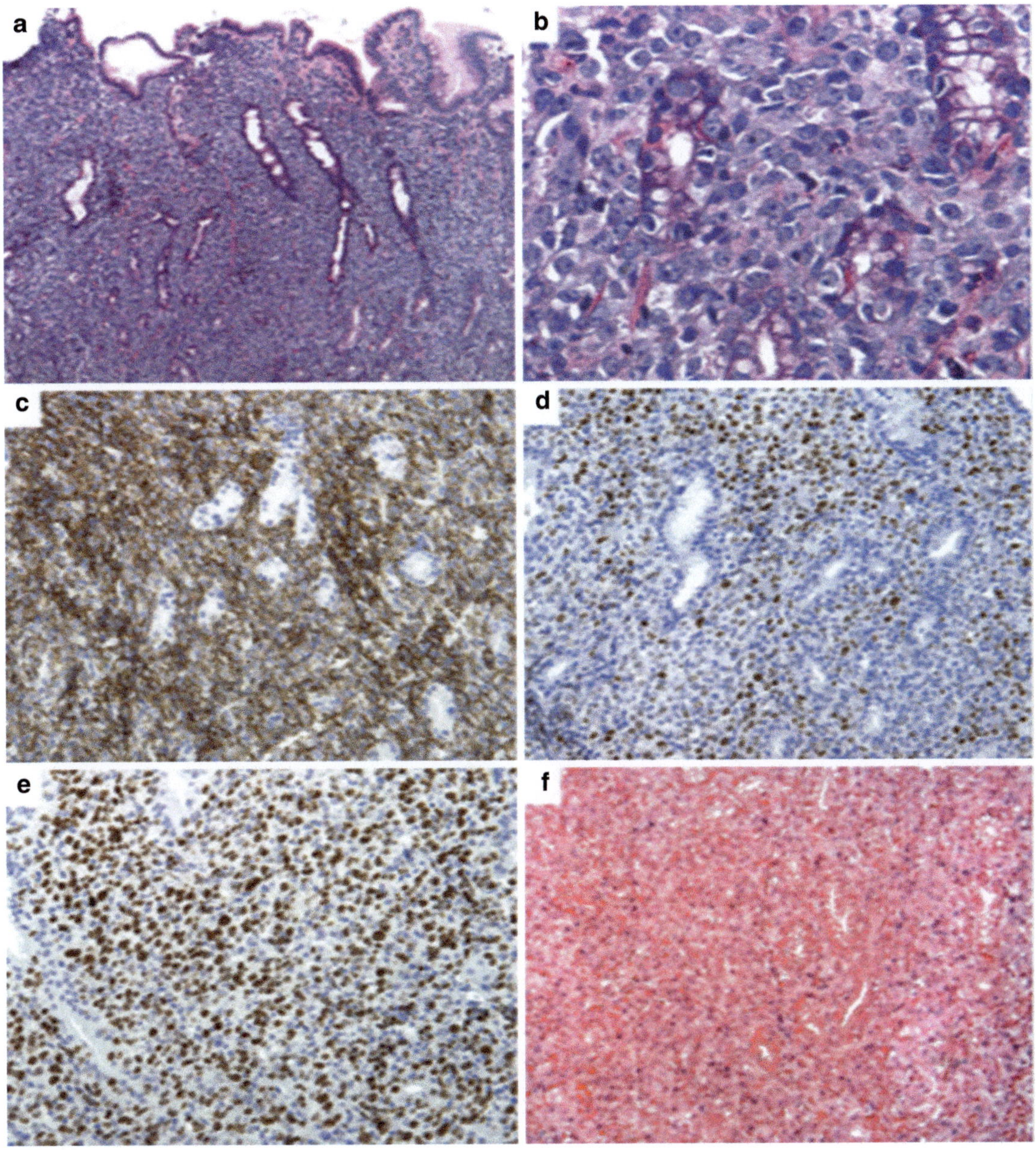

Fig. 20.5 (**a**) Gastric antrum showing extensive infiltration by an atypical lymphoid infiltrate (Haematoxylin-eosin, ×100). (**b**) High-power magnification showing a monotonous population of large lymphoid cells with intraepithelial intrusion (Haematoxylin-eosin, ×600). (**c**) Diffuse CD20 immunoreactivity indicating diffuse large B-cell lymphoma (×200). (**d**) Myeloma-associated oncogene (MUM1, IRF4) showing nuclear positive staining supporting non-germinal centre origin (×200). (**e**) High proliferation rate of 80 % shown by Ki67 staining (×200). (**f**) EBV in situ hybridization for EBER is negative (×200)

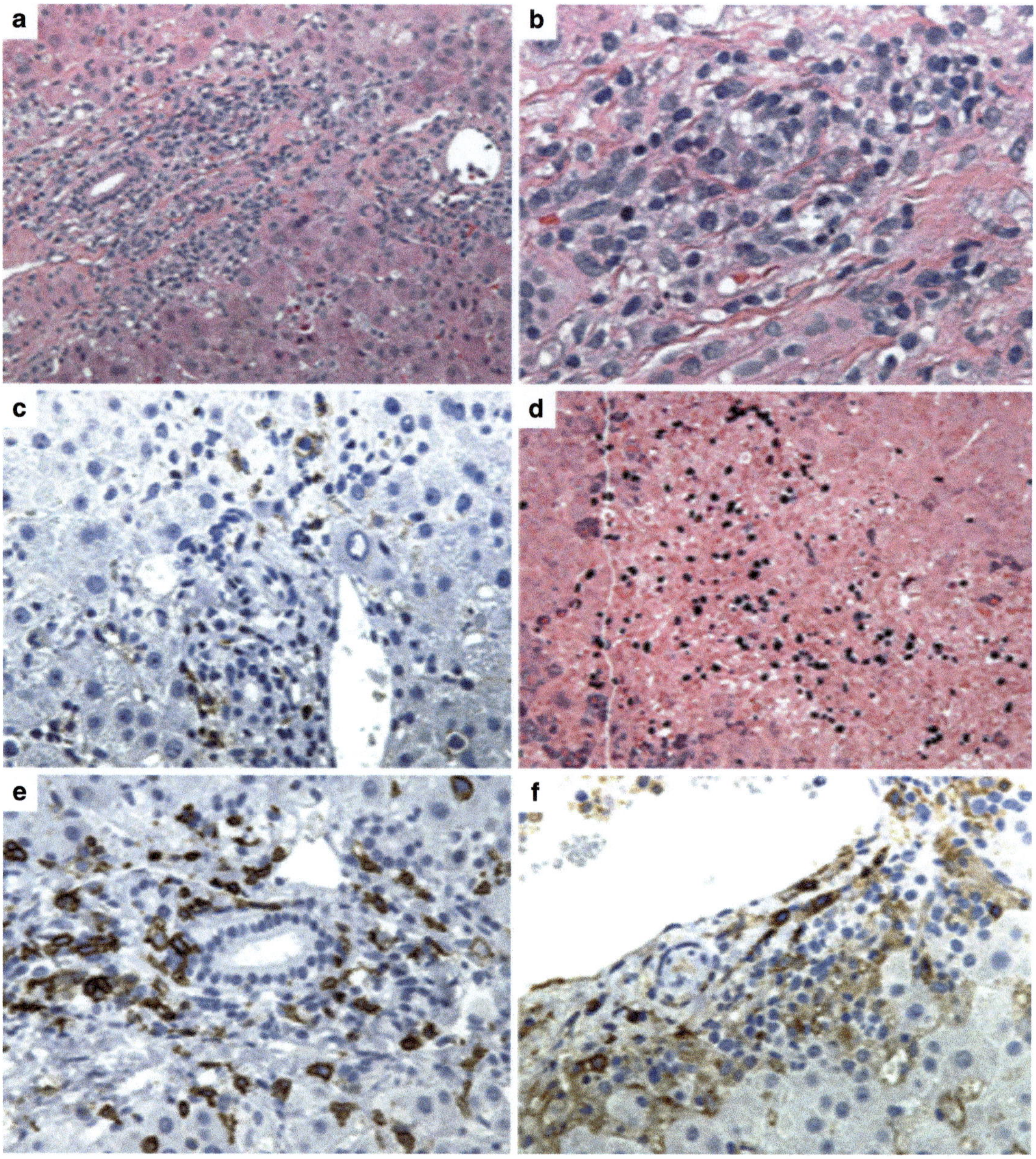

Fig. 20.6 (**a**) Atypical lymphoid cells are seen within the portal tracts and in sinusoidal spaces (Haematoxylin-eosin, ×200). (**b**) High-power magnification showing atypical medium-sized lymphocytes and small lymphocytes within the portal tracts (Haematoxylin-eosin, ×600). (**c**) The atypical cells weakly react against the NK-/T-cell marker CD56 (×400). (**d**) The same population of cells demonstrates EBV positivity by in situ hybridization (×200). (**e**) These cells are also CD8+ (shown) and CD3+ (not shown) (×400). (**f**) The small lymphocytes are predominantly CD4+ (×400)

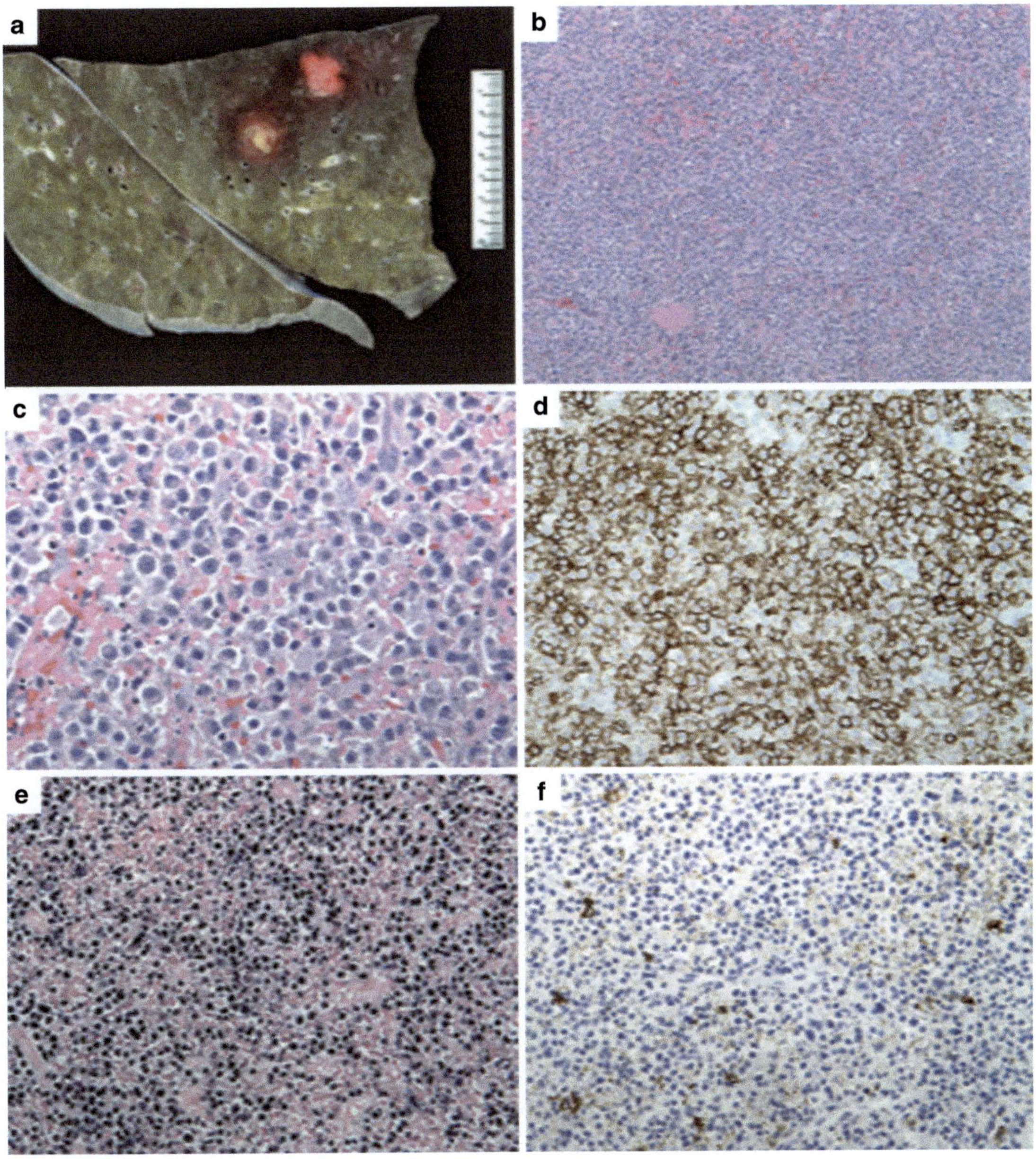

Fig. 20.7 (**a**) At post-mortem multiple discrete nodular densities were present throughout the lung fields. (**b**) The initial nasopharyngeal biopsy showing sheets of monotonous mononuclear cells infiltrating the nasopharyngeal tissues (Haematoxylin-eosin, ×100). (**c**) High-power magnification showing atypical plasma cells with variable nuclear size and shapes including binucleated forms (Haematoxylin-eosin, ×400). (**d**) Immunohistochemical staining showed strong diffuse staining for the plasma cell marker, CD138 (×400). Flow cytometry of the specimen demonstrated kappa light chain restriction (not shown). (**e**) In situ hybridization for EBER (EBV) is positive (×200). (**f**) The B-cell marker, CD20, is negative (×200)

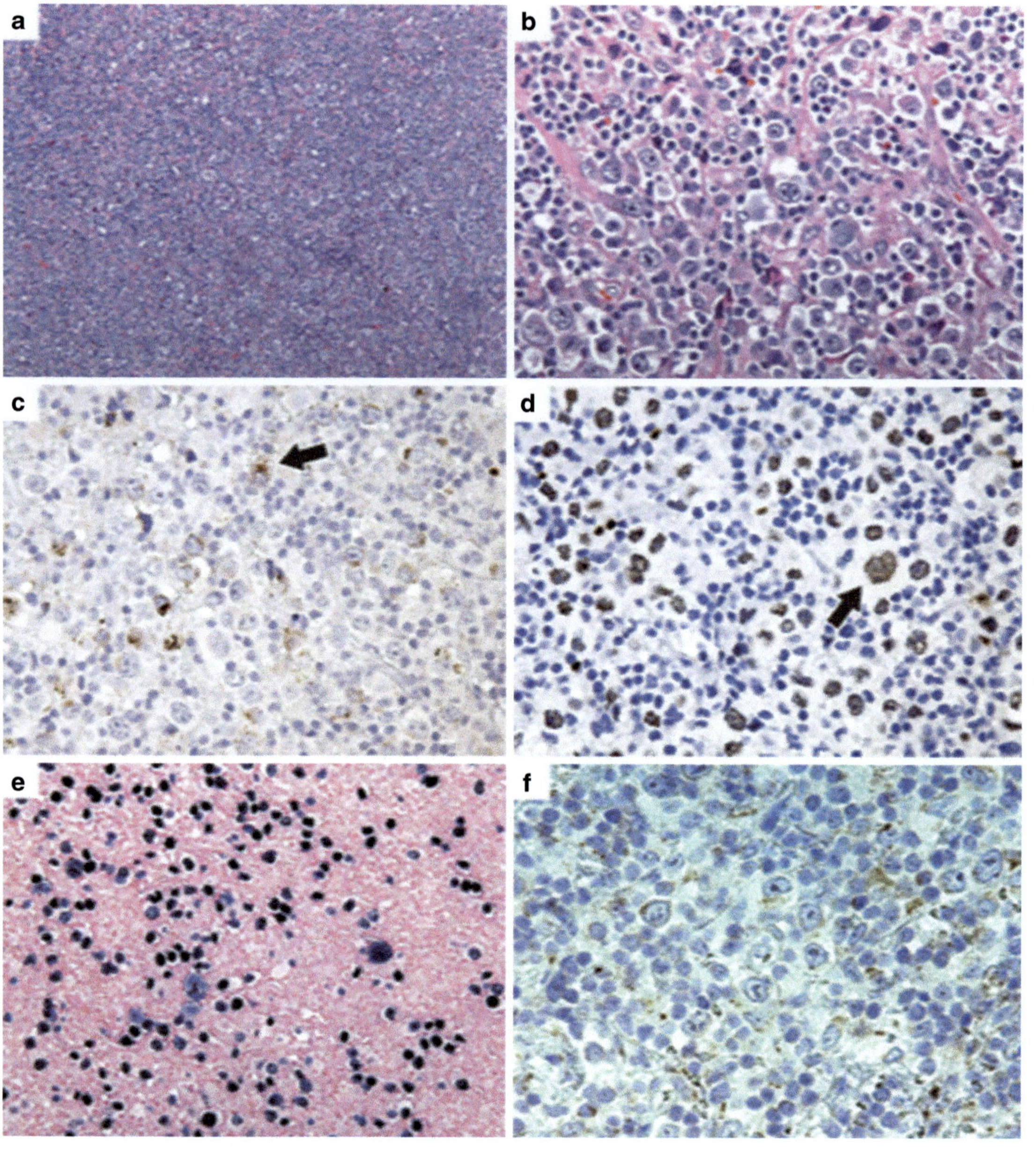

Fig. 20.8 (**a**) Effacement of the nodal architecture by a mixed cellular population (Haematoxylin-eosin, ×100). (**b**) High-power magnification showing large atypical mononuclear cells and diagnostic Reed-Sternberg (RS) cells admixed with eosinophils, lymphocytes and plasma cells (Haematoxylin-eosin, ×400). (**c**) CD15 immunoreactivity of large cells exhibiting the classic Golgi and paranuclear staining (*arrow*) (×400). (**d**) Similar staining of RS cells with PAX5 (*arrow*) (×400). (**e**) EBV in situ hybridization staining of large cells (×200). (**f**) Negative staining of RS cells with ALK (×400). The RS cells showed CD30 immunoreactivity (not shown)

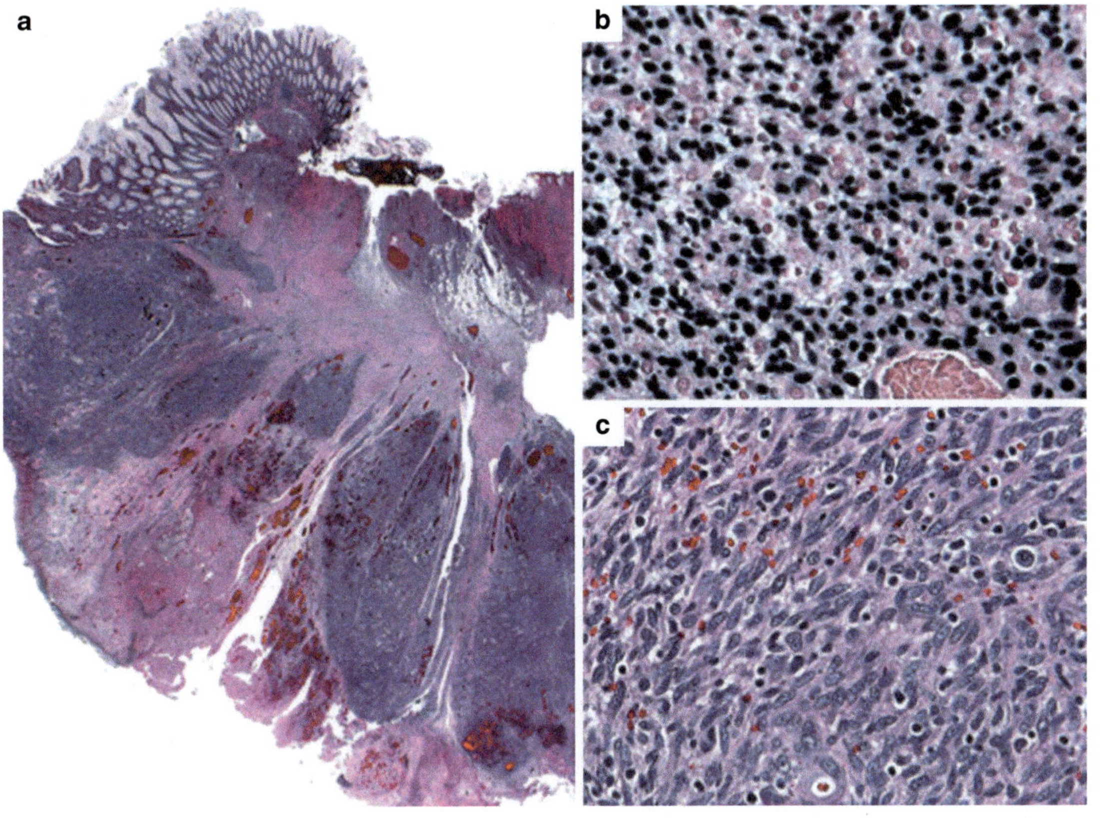

Fig. 20.9 (**a**) Low-power magnification of lesion containing a spindled cell lesion arranged in lobular aggregates (Haematoxylin-eosin, ×5). (**b**) In situ hybridization for EBV RNA (EBER) showing diffuse staining of spindled cells (×400). (**c**) Bland smooth muscle cells admixed with scattered lymphocytes. Strongly desmin and caldesmon positive (not shown) (haematoxylin-eosin, ×400)

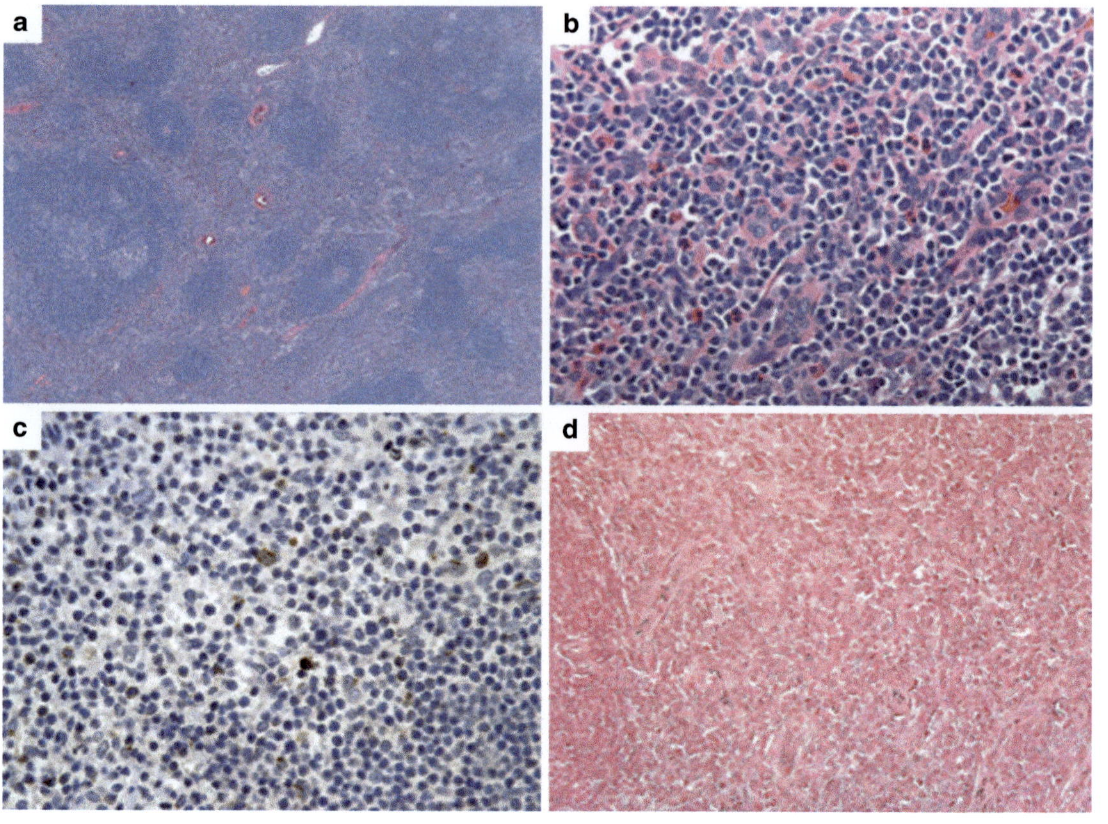

Fig. 20.10 (**a**) Low-power examination of the node shows hyperplasia of the mantle zone regions and atretic germinal centres (Haematoxylin-eosin, ×40). (**b**) The interfollicular regions contain small- to medium-sized atypical lymphocytes with irregular nuclear contains admixed with blood vessels, small lymphocytes and eosinophils (Haematoxylin-eosin, ×400). (**c**) Rare CXCL13+ cells (shown, ×400) along with a mild increase in CD21+ follicular dendritic cells and a mild increase in PD-1 follicular helper cells (not shown) was observed by immunohistochemical staining. By flow cytometry an atypical CD4+ T-cell population with dim CD3 and partial loss of CD7 was demonstrated. Clonality studies showed a T-cell clone. (**d**) EBV negative by in situ hybridization (×200)

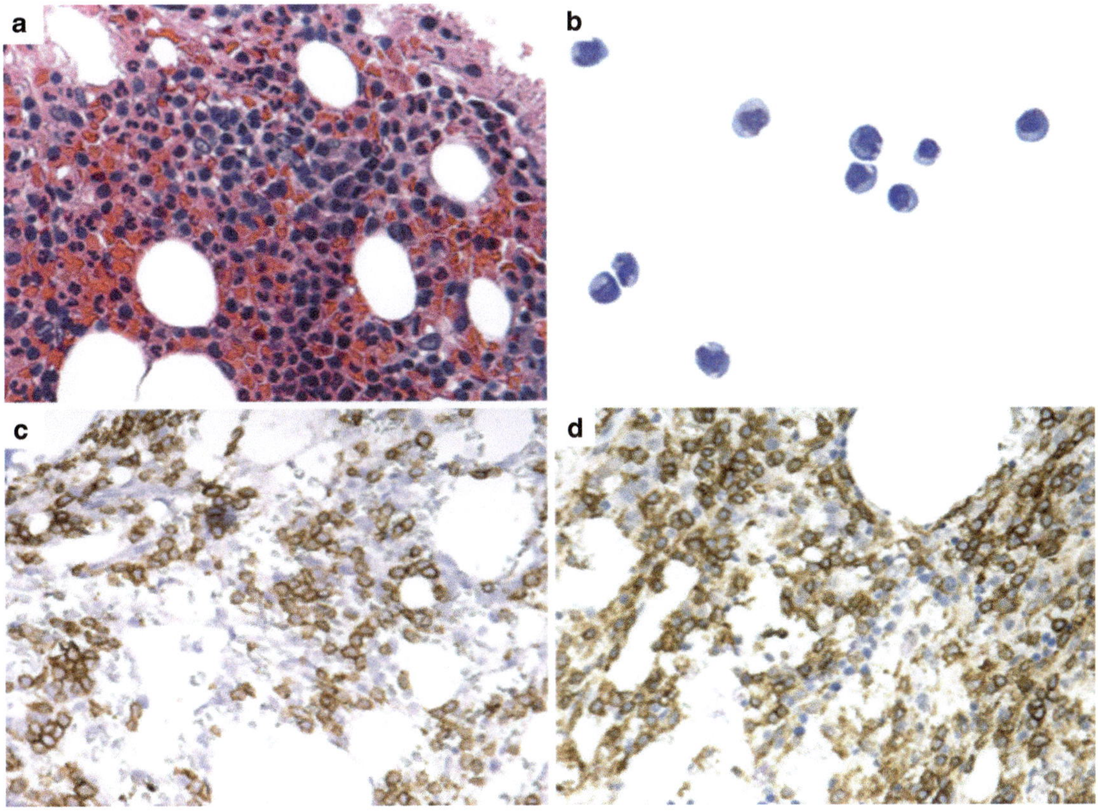

Fig. 20.11 (**a**) Bone marrow biopsy core showing a population of small lymphocytes admixed with haematopoietic elements (Haematoxylin-eosin, ×600). (**b**) The peritoneal fluid removed by paracentesis documenting recurrence after the second transplant. Numerous atypical lymphocytes with indented, eccentric nuclei, variably prominent nucleoli and abundant cytoplasm (Diff Quik ×600). (**c**) CD3 immunostaining of the bone marrow showing numerous T-cells (×400). (**d**) The majority of the T-cells are CD4+ (×400)

Key Points

- Immunosuppressive therapy is the major factor contributing to the development of malignancies (intensity and duration of immunosuppression, various and different regimens).
- Other risk factors: older patients, recipient history of neoplasm, genetic predisposition for certain tumours, usual risk factors such as smoking or ultraviolet light exposure.
- Transferring malignant tumour cells from the donor to the recipient is a rare occurrence.
- The most frequent malignancies occurring in heart transplant patients are:
  - Post-transplant lymphoproliferative disorders;
  - Non-melanoma skin neoplasms (squamous cell carcinoma, basal cell carcinoma, Merkel cell carcinoma, Kaposi sarcoma);
  - Lung cancer among solid tumours.
- Patient management is complex and should be multidisciplinary:
  - Individualized assessment of recipient risk (individual and familial history of malignancy and general risk factors, such as smoking, sun exposure, oncovirus infections, etc.);

- Pre-transplant screening for tumours or premalignant lesions and for biological markers of tumour risk;
- Early diagnosis of neoplasms and premalignant conditions after transplantation;
- Modulating immunosuppressive therapy when malignancies develop (lack of randomized studies on this issue; centre practices vary);
- Consultation and multidisciplinary collaboration is essential.

Illustrative Cases

Case 1 (Fig. 20.2): *PTLD, Early Lesion, Florid Follicular Hyperplasia.* This 10-year-old girl had undergone heart transplantation 7 years ago for hypoplastic left heart syndrome after modified Norwood procedure. Her course was complicated by EBV sero-conversion with rising EBV titres by PCR and then classical Hodgkin lymphoma type-PTLD, stage IVb 4 years after transplant. She was treated by combined chemo-radiation with complete clinical response. Three years later she underwent bilateral tonsillectomy and adenoidectomy for obstructive sleep apnoea.

Case 2 (Fig. 20.3): *Polymorphic-Type PTLD.* This 4-year-old girl with congenital biliary atresia and a failed Kasai procedure at 8 weeks of age underwent a cadaveric liver transplant at 2 years of age. Two years later she presented with cervical adenopathy that was excised. At that time her blood EBV PCR was 144,000 copies per ml. A baseline PET-CT was obtained on March 24, 2010, which showed multiple FDG-avid lymph nodes in the bilateral neck region. She was treated with four doses of rituximab with complete resolution of adenopathy.

Case 3 (Fig. 20.4): *Monomorphic-Type PTLD.* 30-year-old woman with adult-onset polycystic kidney disease had undergone living-related kidney transplant. Eight months later she developed a rapidly enlarging left neck mass along with drenching night sweats, fatigue and bone pain involving hips and femurs. An excisional lymph node biopsy yielded a 2.4×2.4 cm node. She was staged as clinical stage IVb and received four cycles of rituximab with reduced immunosuppression that produced an excellent clinical response.

Case 4 (Fig. 20.5): *EBV-Negative Monomorphic PTLD.* This 27-year-old woman had undergone living-related renal transplant 16 years previously for acute glomerulonephritis diagnosed at age 10 after presenting with proteinuria and haematuria. She was initially maintained on triple therapy with tacrolimus, prednisone and mycophenolate mofetil (MMF) but MMF was discontinued. She had an episode of acute T-cell-mediated rejection requiring intravenous methylprednisolone and a prednisone taper and re-institution of MMF. She presented with epigastric pain of 4 months duration. Upper and lower gastrointestinal endoscopy was performed with multiple biopsies of the stomach, duodenum, ampulla and colonic ulcers and polypoid lesions all showing the same morphology. Rituximab therapy was initiated with an excellent clinical response.

Case 5 (Fig. 20.6): *Monomorphic PTLD, Extranodal NK/T-Cell Lymphoma.* This 48-year-old man with end-stage liver disease secondary to alcoholic cirrhosis and haemochromatosis underwent hepatic transplantation. His post-transplant course was complicated by acute chronic renal failure, recurrent ascites, heart failure, fever and sepsis. A liver biopsy was performed within the first month after transplant.

Case 6 (Fig. 20.7): *Monomorphic PTLD, Plasma Cell Type*. This 22-year-old man with a history of aplastic anaemia received a mismatched unrelated allogeneic human stem cell transplant. His course was complicated by rejection, neutropenic fevers, EBV viremia, *Clostridium difficile* colitis, left neck lymphadenopathy and a nasopharyngeal mass. The nasopharyngeal lesion was biopsied and showed a monotonous plasma cell lesion. The patient continued to have worsening respiratory status and received five rounds of radiation to the nasopharynx. A follow-up CT scan showed persistent oedema, complete opacification of all the paranasal sinuses, persistent large soft tissue prominence filling the nasopharyngeal cavity and retropharyngeal regions and enlarging pulmonary nodules.

Case 7 (Fig. 20.8): *Classical Hodgkin Lymphoma-Type PTLD*. This 62-year-old man presented with night sweats, weight loss and supraclavicular lymphadenopathy 20 years following renal transplant. Atypical lymphoid cells were observed on fine needle aspiration smears. An excisional biopsy of a left level IV cervical lymph node was performed.

Case 8 (Fig. 20.9): *EBV-Associated Smooth Muscle Neoplasm*. This 10-year-old girl was post heart transplant (performed at 2 months of age for left ventricular non-compaction) when she presented with abdominal distension and pain. CT and MRI imaging revealed a mass in the transverse colon. A polypectomy produced a 2.0×1.8×1.6 cm polypoid lesion.

Case 9 (Fig. 20.10): *Angioimmunoblastic-Like Peripheral T-Cell Lymphoma-Type PTLD*. This 13-year-old boy underwent heart transplant at 2 years of age for heterotaxy, dextrocardia, double outlet-right ventricle, pulmonic stenosis, atrioventricular septal defect and situs inversus (with retained Glenn). He presented with generalized lymphadenopathy, shortness of breath and a left cranial nerve palsy at age 6. Lymph node biopsy showed an EBV-negative, angioimmunoblastic T-cell lymphoma. He recurred multiple times after systemic multidrug chemotherapy and underwent an autologous peripheral blood stem cell transplant in August 2015 following conditioning with multiple chemotherapy drugs. One of the excisional lymph node biopsy specimens from a left axillary nodal recurrence is presented.

Case 10 (Fig. 20.11): *PTLD, T-Cell Prolymphocytic Leukaemia Type*. This 68-year-old man was 3 years post-matched unrelated donor (MUD) non-myeloablative haematopoietic cell transplant (HCT) for high-risk chronic lymphocytic leukaemia (11q23 and 17p Del) when he developed a T-cell prolymphocytic leukaemia (PLL). Flow cytometry identified a homogeneous population of T helper cells expressing CD38, CD7 and CD2; bright CD5, CD3 and CD4; partial dim CD8 (with anomalous dual CD4/CD8); and lack of TdT expression. He underwent a second transplant following chemotherapy failure. This course was complicated by chronic graft-versus-host-disease serositis and fasciitis and then abdominal distention, nausea and vomiting.

References

AlBugami M, Kiberd B. Malignancies: pre and post transplantation strategies. Transplant Rev (Orlando). 2014;28(2):76–83.

Bajetta E, Platnia M, Catena L, et al. Merkel cell carcinoma after liver transplantation: a case report. Tumori. 2007;93:323.

Brewer JD, Colegio OR, Phillips PK, et al. Incidence of and risk factors for skin cancer after heart transplant. Arch Dermatol. 2009;147:1391.

Buell JF, Trofe J, Hanaway MJ, Lo A, Rosengard B, Rilo H, Alloway R, Beebe T, First MR, Woodle ES. Transmission of donor cancer into cardiothoracic transplant recipients. Surgery. 2001;130(4):660–8.

Caillard S, Lelong C, Pessione F, et al. Post-transplant lymphoproliferative disorders occurring after renal transplantation in adults: report of 230 cases from the French Registry. Am J Transplant. 2006;6:2735.

Campbell SB, Walker R, Tai SS, et al. Randomized controlled trial of sirolimus for renal transplant recipients at high risk for nonmelanoma skin cancer. Am J Transplant. 2012;12:1146.

Choquet S, Leblond V, Herbrecht R, et al. Efficacy and safety of rituximab in B-cell post-transplantation lymphoproliferative disorders: results of a prospective multicenter phase 2 study. Blood. 2006;107:3053.

Collett D, Mumford L, Banner NR, Neuberger J, Watson C. Comparison of the incidence of malignancy in recipients of different types of organ: a UK Registry audit. Am J Transplant. 2010;10(8):1889–96.

Costanzo MR, Dipchand A, Starling R, et al. The international society of heart and lung transplantation guidelines for the care of heart transplant recipients. J Heart Lung Transplant. 2010;29:914–56.

Crespo-Leiro MG, Alonso-Pulpón LA, Villa-Arranz A, et al. The prognosis of noncutaneous nonlymphomatous malignancy after heart transplantation: data from the Spanish Post-Heart Transplant Tumour Registry. Transplant Proc. 2010;42(8):3011–3.

Dantal J, Pohanka E. Malignancies in renal transplantation: an unmet medical need. Nephrol Dial Transplant. 2007;22 Suppl 1:i4.

David KM, Morris JA, Steffen BJ, Chi-Burris KS, Gotz VP, Gordon RD. Mycophenolate mofetil vs. azathioprine is associated with decreased acute rejection, late acute rejection, and risk for cardiovascular death in renal transplant recipients with pre-transplant diabetes. Clin Transplant. 2005;19:279–85.

Deyrup AT, Lee VK, Hill CE, Cheuk W, Toh HC, Kesavan A, Chan EW, Weiss SW. Epstein-Barr Virus-associated smooth muscle tumors are distinctive mesenchymal tumors reflecting multiple infection events: a clinicopathologic and molecular analysis of 29 tumors from 19 patients. Am J Surg Pathol. 2006;30:75–82.

Ducloux D, Kazory A, Challier B, Coutlet J, Bresson-Vautrin C, Motte G, Thalamy B, Rebibou JM, Chalopin JM. Long-term toxicity of antithymocyte globulin induction may vary with choice of agent: a single-center retrospective study. Transplantation. 2004;77(7):1029–33.

Eisen HJ, Kobashigawa J, Keogh A, et al. Three-year results of a randomized, double blind, controlled trial of mycophenolate mofetil versus azathioprine in cardiac transplant recipients. J Heart Lung Transplant. 2005;24:517.

Engels EA, Pfeiffer RM, Fraumeni Jr JF, Kasiske BL, Israni AK, Snyder JJ, Wolfe RA, Goodrich NP, Bayakly AR, Clarke CA, Copeland G, Finch JL, Fleissner ML, Goodman MT, Kahn A, Koch L, Lynch CF, Madeleine MM, Pawlish K, Rao C, Williams MA, Castenson D, Curry M, Parsons R, Fant G, Lin M. Spectrum of cancer risk among US solid organ transplant recipients. JAMA. 2011;306(17):1891–901.

Epailly E, Albanell J, Andreassen A, Bara C, Campistol GM, Delgado JF, Eisen H, Fiane AE, Mohacsi P, Shubert S, Sebbag L, Turazza FM, Valentine H, Zuckermann A, Potena L. Proliferation signal inhibitors and post-transplant malignancies in heart transplantation: practical clinical management questions. Clin Transplant. 2011;25:E475–86.

Euvrard S, Kanitakis J, Claudy A. Skin cancers after organ transplantation. N Engl J Med. 2003;348:1681.

Euvrard S, Kanitakis J, Decullier E, et al. Subsequent skin cancers in kidney and heart transplant recipients after the first squamous cell carcinoma. Transplantation. 2006;81:1093.

Geissler EK. The impact of mTOR inhibitors on the development of malignancy. Transplant Proc. 2008;40(10 Suppl):S32–5.

Geissler EK. Post-transplantation malignancies: here today, gone tomorrow? Nat Rev Clin Oncol. 2015;12(12):705–17.

Gharekhani A, Entezari-Maleki T, Dashti-Khavidaki S, Khalili H. A review on comparing two commonly used rabbit anti-thymocyte globulins as induction therapy in solid organ transplantation. Expert Opin Biol Ther. 2013;13(9):1299–313.

Higgins RS, Brown RN, Chang PP, et al. A multi-institutional study of malignancies after heart transplantation and a comparison with the general United States population. J Heart Lung Transplant. 2014;33(5):478–85.

Ho YC, Lin HJ, Tsai CH, Chang YC. Regulation of type I plasminogen activator inhibitor in human gingival fibroblasts with cyclosporine A. Oral Dis. 2010;16(4):396–401.

Jaffe ES. Hematopathology. Philadelphia: Saunders/Elsevier; 2011.

Jensen P, Hansen S, Møller B, et al. Skin cancer in kidney and heart transplant recipients and different long-term immunosuppressive therapy regimens. J Am Acad Dermatol. 1999;40:177.

Jiang Y, Villeneuve PJ, Wielgosz A, Schaubel DE, Fenton SSA, Mao Y. The Incidence of cancer in a population-based cohort of Canadian heart transplant recipients. Am J Transplant. 2010;10:637–45.

Jonigka D, Laengera F, Maegela L, Izykowskia N, Rischea J, Tiedea C, Kleinc C, Maecker-Kolhoffd B, Kreipea

H, Husseina K. Molecular and clinicopathological analysis of epstein-barr virus–associated posttransplant smooth muscle tumors. Am J Transplant. 2012;12:1908–17.

Keogh A, Richardson M, Ruygrok P, Spratt P, Galbraith A, O'Driscoll G, Macdonald P, Esemore D, Muller D, Faddy S. Sirolimus in de novo heart transplant recipients reduces acute rejection and prevents coronary artery disease at 2 years: a randomized clinical trial. Circulation. 2004;110:2694.

Khedmat H, Taheri S. Early versus late outset of lymphoproliferative disorders post heart and lung transplantation: the PTLD. Int Survey. Hematol Oncol Stem Cell Ther. 2011;4(1):10–6.

Kobashigawa J, Miller L, Renlud D, et al. A randomized active-controlled trial of mycophenolate mofetil in heart transplant recipients. Mycophenolate Mofetil Investigators. Transplantation. 1998;66:507.

Kobashigawa JA, Patel JK. Immunosuppression for heart transplantation: where are we now? Nat Clin Pract Cardiovasc Med. 2006;3:203.

Krynitz B, Edgren G, Lindelöf B, Baecklund E, Battström C, Wilczek H, Smedby KE. Risk of skin cancer and other malignancies in kidney, liver, heart and lung transplant recipients 1970 to 2008 – a Swedish population-based study. Int J Cancer. 2013;132(6):1429–38.

Krynitz B, Olsson H, Lundh Rozell B, Lindelöf B, Edgren G, Smedby KE. Risk of basal cell carcinoma in Swedish organ transplant recipients – a population-based study. Br J Dermatol. 2016;174(1):95–103.

Kuijken I, Bouwes Bavinck JN. Skin cancer risk associated with immunosuppressive therapy in organ transplant recipients – epidemiology and proposed mechanisms. BioDrugs. 2000;14(5):319–29.

Kumarasinghe G, Lavee O, Parker A, et al. Post-transplant lymphoproliferative disease in heart and lung transplantation: defining risk and prognostic factors. J Heart Lung Transplant. 2015;34(11):1406–14.

Leblond V, Davi F, Charlotte F, et al. Posttransplant lymphoproliferative disorders not associated with Epstein-Barr virus: a distinct entity? J Clin Oncol. 1998;16:2052.

LeBoit PE; International Agency for Research on Cancer; World Health Organization; International Academy of Pathology; European Organization for Research on Treatment of Cancer. Pathology and genetics of skin tumours. Lyon: IARC Press; 2006.

Martinez JC, Otley CC, Stasko T, et al. Defining the clinical course of metastatic skin cancer in organ transplant recipients: a multicentre collaborative study. Arch Dermatol. 2003;139:301.

Metchnikoff C, Mully T, Singer JP, et al. The 7th edition AJCC staging system for cutaneous squamous cell carcinoma accurately predicts risk of recurrence for heart and lung transplant recipients. J Am Acad Dermatol. 2012;67:829.

Nägele H, Bahlo M, Klapdor R, et al. Tumor marker determination after orthotopic heart transplantation. J Heart Lung Transplant. 1999;18(10):957–62.

Nair N, Gongora E, Mehra MR. Long-term immunosuppression and malignancy in thoracic transplantation: Where is the balance? J Heart LungTransplant. 2014;33:461–7.

Nelson BP, Nelesnik MA, Bahler DW, et al. Epstein-Barr virus-negative post-transplant lymphoproliferative disorders: a distinct entity? Am J Surg Pathol. 2000;24(3):375–85.

O'Donovan P, Perrett CM, Zhang X, et al. Azathioprine and UVA light generate mutagenic oxidative DNA damage. Science. 2005;309:1871.

Pandanaboyana S, Longbotham D, Hostert L, Attia M, Baker R, Menon K, Ahmad N. Transplantation of liver and kidney from donors with malignancy at the time of donation: an experience from a single centre. Transpl Int. 2016;29(1):73–80.

Rashidi A, Fisher SI. Acute myeloid leukemia following solid organ transplantation: entity or novelty? Eur J Haematol. 2014;92:459–66.

Rinaldi M, Pellegrini C, D'Armini AM, et al. Neoplastic disease after heart transplantation: single center experience. Eur J Cardiothorac Surg. 2001;19:696.

Sampaio MS, Yong W, Cho YW, Qazi Y, Bunnapradist S, Hutchinson IV, Shah T. Posttransplant malignancies in solid organ adult recipients: an analysis of the U.S. National Transplant Database. Transplantation. 2012;94:990–8.

Söderlund C, Rådegran G. Immunosuppressive therapies after heart transplantation – the balance between under- and over-immunosuppression. Transplant Rev. 2015;29:181–9.

Stallone G, Schena A, Infante B, et al. Sirolimus for Kaposi's sarcoma in renal transplant recipients. N Engl J Med. 2005;352:1317.

Stehlik J, Edwards LB, Kucheryavaya AY, et al. The Registry of the International Society for Heart and Lung Transplantation: twenty-seventh official adult heart transplant report-2010. J Heart Lung Transplant. 2010;29(10):1089–103.

Strecker T, Rösch J, Weyand M, et al. Frequency and spectrum of metachronous malignancies in heart transplant recipients: a 11-year-experience at a German heart center. Int J Clin Exp Pathol. 2013;6(3):411–2.

Swann PF, Waters TR, Multon DC, et al. Role of postreplicative DNA mismatch repair in the cytotoxic action of thioguanine. Science. 1996;273:1109.

Swerdlow SH; International Agency for Research on Cancer; World Health Organization. WHO classification of tumours of haematopoietic and lymphoid tissues. Lyon: International Agency for Research on Cancer; 2008.

Swinnen LJ, Costanzo-Nordin MR, Fisher SG, O'Sullivan EJ, Johnson MR, Heroux AL, Dizikes GJ, Pifarre R, Fisher RI. Increased incidence of lymphoproliferative disorder after immunosuppression with the monoclonal antibody OKT3 in cardiac-transplant recipients. N Engl J Med. 1990;323:1723–8.

Tsai DE, Hardy CL, Tomaszewski JE, et al. Reduction in immunosuppression as initial therapy for posttransplant lymphoproliferative disorder: Analysis of prog-

nostic variables and long-term follow-up of 42 adult patients. Transplantation. 2001;71:1076.
Valantine H. Is there a role for proliferation signal/mTOR inhibitors in the prevention and treatment of de novo malignancies after heart transplantation? Lessons learned from renal transplantation and oncology. J Heart Lung Transplant. 2007;26(6):557–64.
Veness MJ, Quinn DI, Ong CS, et al. Aggressive cutaneous malignancies following cardiothoracic transplantation: the Austrian experience. Cancer. 1999;85(8):1758–64.
Webber SA. Post-transplant lymphoproliferative disorders: a preventable complication of solid organ transplantation? Pediatr Transplant. 1999;3(2):95–9.

Chronic Kidney Disease After Heart Transplantation: Risk Factors, Clinics, and Histopathology

21

Gaia Magnani, Marialuisa Valente, and Francesco Marchini

Contents

G. Magnani
Heart Failure and Heart Transplant Program, Cardiology Unit, S.Orsola-Malpighi University Hospital, Bologna, Italy
e-mail: gaia.magnani@aosp.bo.it

M. Valente
Pathological Anatomy, Department of Cardiac, Thoracic and Vascular Sciences, University of Padua, Padua, Italy
e-mail: marialuisa.valente@unipd.it

F. Marchini (✉)
II Nephrology Unit, Azienda Ospedaliera-Universitaria Padova, Padua, Italy
e-mail: francesco.marchini@sanita.padova.it

21.1 Background

Kidney disease is a frequent and increasingly recognized complication of heart transplantation. Renal failure, in both the acute and chronic setting, increases the complexity of patient management and significantly contributes to early and late post-transplant morbidity and mortality. Chronic kidney disease in this population is associated with a four- to fivefold increased risk of death after transplant.

Although there is no uniform definition of chronic kidney disease (CKD) after heart transplantation, prevalence rates range from 10% to over 90% (Bloom and Doyle 2006). The most comprehensive assessment to date, using an estimate of kidney function, defines severe CKD as a glomerular filtration rate (GFR) of 29 ml/min/m^2 of body surface area or less.

The level of kidney function before organ transplantation is a risk factor for developing kidney insufficiency later.

O. Leone et al. (eds.), *The Pathology of Cardiac Transplantation*, DOI 10.1007/978-3-319-46386-5_21

Deterioration in kidney function typically begins within the first 6 months after transplantation and progressively declines thereafter, although it has been demonstrated that GFR at one month is the only predictive factor for the decrease in GFR seen at 24 months. The predictive value of the 1-month serum creatinine is probably related to pre-existing kidney insufficiency or to renal ischemia associated with the transplantation procedure as well as to nephrotoxic drugs administered in the peri-transplant period. In addition, the 1-month creatinine may be a marker for individuals who are more sensitive to the nephrotoxic effects of calcineurin inhibitors. Despite relatively limited life expectancies for heart transplant recipients, at least 3–10 % of these patients will ultimately go on to develop end-stage renal disease 10 years after transplant. In fact, recent Scientific Registry of Transplant Recipients analysis of 69,321 non-renal solid organ recipients surviving the first 3 posttransplant months revealed that 4 % of patients required maintenance renal replacement therapy within a median 3 years of transplantation. In the future, as survival continues to improve in heart transplant recipients, it is probable that the rate of development of end-stage renal disease will likewise increase in this population.

21.2 Pathogenesis of Renal Impairment in Chronic Heart Failure Patients

Progressive deterioration of renal function in chronic heart failure (CHF) patients occurs as a result of multiple mechanisms, including renal hypoperfusion, increased renal venous pressure, neuro-hormonal and inflammatory activation, adenosine release, and drug therapy for CHF. The kidney is sensitive to hemodynamic changes: either an increased central venous pressure ("renal afterload") or a reduced cardiac output ("renal preload") may cause renal impairment.

Although the kidneys represent less than 0.5 % of body mass, they receive 20–25 % of the total cardiac output in the normal adult. Several factors, including hypovolemia, activation of the sympathetic nervous system or the renin–angiotensin system, extrinsically administered vasopressors and vasodilators, and local neurohumoral factors, influence the distribution of cardiac output to the kidneys. As cardiac function deteriorates, renal blood flow decreases. The filtration fraction and filtered Na decrease, and the tubular reabsorption increases, leading to Na and water retention.

The renin–angiotensin–aldosterone system (RAAS) is activated: at first, angiotensin II causes preferential vasoconstriction of the glomerular efferent arteriole, favoring glomerular filtration, despite low renal blood flow; but in the long term, RAAS activation has adverse effects on the kidney including increased oxidative stress, endothelial dysfunction, and the stimulation of inflammatory pathways, leading to fibrosis formation.

Inflammation may play a pivotal role in cardiorenal interactions. In patients with CHF, C-reactive protein (CRP) levels increase with decline of left ventricular ejection fraction.

Volume overload and venous congestion cause activation of inflammatory pathways, which, among other things, leads to an increase of circulating lipopolysaccharides (LPS) which come from the mesenteric district and are a potent stimulus that activates tumour necrosis factor-α (TNF-α) and interleukin-6 (IL-6). In the tubulo-interstitial compartment, TNF-α and IL-6 promote accumulation of interstitial inflammatory cells by increasing expressions of adhesion molecules and chemokines, such as monocyte chemoattractant protein-1 (MCP-1), intercellular adhesion molecule-1 (ICAM-1), and vascular cell adhesion molecule-1 (VCAM-1). The infiltrating inflammatory cells are thought to activate the renal proximal tubular cells, which in turn are able to attract more inflammatory cells (monocytes/macrophages and lymphocytes, especially T cells) through the production of various other chemokines and cytokines.

This cytokine milieu could create a hostile microenvironment for tubular epithelial cells, rendering them adaptable to changing cell phenotype. The process known as epithelial–mesenchymal transition (EMT) is considered a process through which the differentiated injured epithelial tubular cells undergo conversion into mesenchymal cells, so giving rise to matrix-producing fibroblasts. The transition is characterized by loss of epithelial proteins, such as E-cadherin, zonula occludens-1 and cytokeratin, acquisition of mesenchymal markers including vimentin, α-smooth muscle actin, fibroblast-specific protein-1, and changes in interstitial matrix components with presence of type I collagen and fibronectin. These alterations in protein expression are usually accompanied by morphologic changes to a fibroblastoid appearance and an enhanced migratory capacity, which could contribute to the development of fibrosis in chronic renal failure. Although this mechanism is widely accepted, some studies are raising doubts about its existence in vivo (Kriz et al. 2011).

In addition inflammatory interstitial cells can also produce fibrogenetic cytokines as trasforming growth factor-β (TGB-β).

21.3 Risk Factors for Kidney Injury After Heart Transplant

21.3.1 Pre-existing Renal Failure

It could be postulated that renal function can indirectly be used as an indicator of cardiovascular status in CHF. In the early stages of CHF, kidney function is well maintained by compensatory increases in filtration fraction, but in patients with more severe CHF, glomerular filtration rate becomes more dependent on afferent arteriolar flow and the stimulation of hemodynamic and hormonal pathways. Furthermore, the fall in effective renal blood flow is relatively more pronounced and therefore disproportional to the reduction in cardiac output. Nevertheless, it was demonstrated that renal hemodynamic reserve is already impaired in patients with asymptomatic left ventricular dysfunction (Hillege et al. 2006).

Knowledge of pre-existing chronic kidney disease, cause, duration and degree of kidney insufficiency (RI), number of prior acute RI episodes, kidney congestion or low perfusion, small kidney size, and abnormal sediment may all be useful to assess irreversibility and worsening of RI.

Nowadays in some heart transplant centers, it is routine to utilize left ventricular assist device (LVAD) as a way to evaluate reversibility of organ damage in patients with end-stage heart disease: placement of an LVAD in these patients invariably improves renal function with more than half of patients with creatinine clearance (CrCl) <45 ml/min achieving a CrCl >60 ml/min 30 days after implant (Sing et al. 2001).

21.3.2 Acute Injury

Multiple factors have been implicated in increasing the risk of progressive kidney dysfunction after heart transplantation. Eligibility for nonrenal organ transplantation typically requires that potential candidates have no or minimal perturbation of underlying kidney function, with sufficient reserve to undergo transplant surgery without the need for peri- or post-operative dialysis. The risk factors for early post-operative acute renal failure following heart transplantation are generally the same as those for non-transplant patients immediately after surgery. Clinical situations that commonly contribute to acute renal failure in the post-heart-transplant setting are:

- Effective volume contraction due to severe left ventricular dysfunction caused by the severity of recipient heart failure and donor factors (surgery ischemic time, dysfunction of the right ventricle, pulmonary hypertension).
- Acute tubular necrosis secondary to sepsis worsened by immunosuppressive therapy and shock.
- Use of diuretics.
- Use of radiographic contrast, as well as nephrotoxic drugs (Ishani et al. 2002).

Less commonly, acute interstitial nephritis and athero-thrombotic disease occur.

Acute tubular necrosis (ATN) is a clinicopathologic entity characterized histologically by loss of periodic acid–Schiff (PAS)-positive brush border of proximal tubular epithelial cells, degeneration of tubular epithelial cells, and necrosis of individual cells. Tubular lumina are dilated and interstitial edema is present. In more severe cases, rupture of tubular basement membrane followed by tubular loss and interstitial inflammatory infiltrates is seen. Tubular damage occurs because during ischemia the blood bypasses the renal cortex (the Trueta renal vascular shunt), and in this way tubules of superficial and mid-cortical nephrons do not receive enough oxygen and nutrients. Peritubular capillaries arise from efferent arterioles which receive blood from afferent arterioles through the glomerular tuft; during ischemia only a negligible amount of blood goes to the afferent arterioles and to the glomeruli. Epithelial tubular regeneration may occur in cases in which tubular cell death is patchy, tubular basement membrane is intact, and there are no inflammatory infiltrates. From the clinical point of view, due to the great number of patrimonial nephrons, ATN is a reversible condition, but destruction of a variable amount of nephrons is an additional risk for posttransplantation CKD.

21.3.3 Chronic Injury

On a long-term basis, a multitude of retrospective studies, both single center and registry based, have identified factors that increase the risk of developing progressive CKD following heart transplantation. Most of these risk factors are similar to those that could be expected in non-transplant patients with underlying kidney disease. Included among these factors are the level of kidney function immediately pre-transplant as well as in the early post-operative period, increasing recipient age at the time of the transplantation, female gender, presence of diabetes mellitus, and hypertension. Hypertension occurs in the vast majority of heart recipients and usually develops in the early post-transplant period. In addition, over the past two decades, the widespread use of calcineurin inhibitors has resulted in an increase in the prevalence of chronic kidney dysfunction compared to the pre-cyclosporine era. Comorbid conditions such a chronic left ventricular dysfunction and the requirement for drugs such as diuretics, angiotensin-converting enzyme (ACE) inhibitors, and angiotensin receptor blockers (ARB) may potentiate the chronic nephrotoxic effects of calcineurin inhibitors. Occasionally, protracted pretransplant acute tubular necrosis secondary to renal hypoperfusion may be associated with persistent fibrosis and nephron loss following transplantation and may contribute to chronic kidney dysfunction.

The histopathology of CKD is non-specific and shows interstitial fibrosis (the inevitable outcome of various progressive damage), tubular atrophy, varying degrees of glomerulosclerosis, and arterio-arteriolosclerosis.

21.3.3.1 Hypertension

Hypertension, both systolic and diastolic, is commonly observed following solid organ transplantation in at least 90 % of cardiac recipients. New-onset hypertension has been attributed to multiple causes including high-dose corticosteroid use, increased body weight, and the use of calcineurin inhibitors. This effect of blood pressure on progressive kidney disease confirms similar findings observed in non-transplant patients.

Benign hypertension causes changes in all renal components (arteries, arterioles, glomeruli, tubules, and interstitium). Larger arteries present with alteration typical of arteriosclerosis, consisting in splitting and reduplication of the internal elastic lamina, fibrous intimal thickening, and lumen reduction. Intimal thickening with mucoid matrix and widely spaced cells are commonly seen in small arteries. Circumferential intimal deposition of hyaline PAS-positive material, sometimes extending toward the media, is a typical lesion of arterioles. Glomerular involvement in hypertension is focal and may occur in two patterns:

1. The first is capillary collapse evolving into glomerular sclerosis (Fig. 21.1). Early changes in affected glomeruli consist of col-

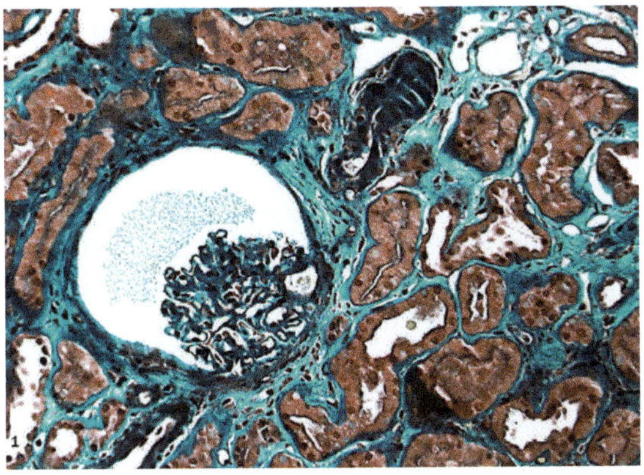

Fig. 21.1 Retraction and collapse of glomerular capillary tuft with widening of the Bowman space (Azan Mallory stain, original magnification 200×)

lapse of capillaries with lumen diameter reduction due to wrinkling of their basement membranes. Capillary shrinkage leads to tuft retraction to the vascular pole. The Bowman space becomes filled by eosinophilic material which, over time, will be replaced by collagen tissue and so usually thicken the Bowman capsule. The result is the "obsolete" glomerulus (Fig. 21.2a).

2. The second pattern of glomerular involvement consists of an increase in the PAS-positive mesangial matrix, which over time involves the entire glomerulus, without collagenization of the Bowman space, leading to what is called "solidified glomerulus" (Fig. 21.2b). There is

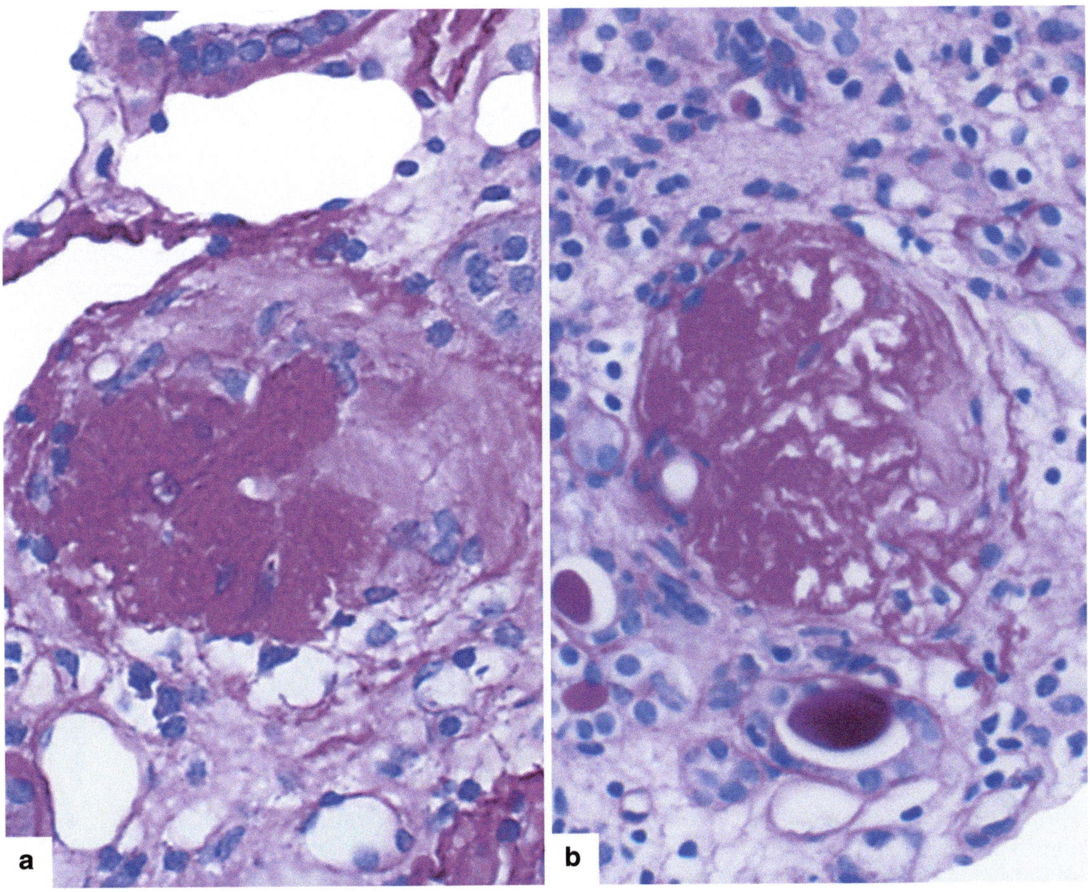

Fig. 21.2 Glomerulosclerosis due to ischemic obsolescence (**a**) and solidification (**b**) (PAS stain, original magnification 400×)

patchy tubular atrophy with tubules that are smaller and lined by fewer epithelial cells than normal; tubular basement membrane may be regular or thickened. Atrophic tubules are frequently found near an "obsolete" glomerulus, but they may also be present near less compromised glomeruli, due to the peculiar vulnerability of the tubules to the ischemia. In other fields tubules appear dilated. The interstitium is widened in correspondence to zones of tubular atrophy, due to collagen increase.

21.3.3.2 Hyperlipidemia and Diabetes

Hyperlipidemia and diabetes are frequently observed before and after heart transplant: they are major risk factors for cardiovascular disease and mortality and a recognized risk factor for progression to CKD.

"Diabetic nephropathy" is a clinical syndrome characterized by persistent macroalbuminuria (>300 mg/24 h), a steady decline in GFR, and elevated blood pressure. Kidney changes may be seen at histology and electron microscopy very early after the onset of diabetes mellitus without clinical evidence of renal dysfunction and before the occurrence of microalbuminuria, the condition which precedes overt diabetic nephropathy. These changes consist of glomerular enlargement, which causes increased filtration surface area, followed by uniform thickening of glomerular basement membrane and deposition of eosinophilic PAS-positive material within the mesangium. So, diabetic patients who undergo cardiac transplant may have histologic kidney alterations although renal function is normal. In addition diabetic patients are also hypertensive, so their kidneys have damage induced by high blood pressure.

21.3.3.3 Chronic Anemia

There is little information on chronic anemia after heart transplantation; however, up to 65 % of anemia prevalence has been reported. In this population, anemia seems to be closely associated with impaired kidney function. Besides the common association of chronic kidney disease with anemia, a multitude of other factors are implicated including anti-metabolite immunosuppression (azathioprine and mycophenolate), sirolimus, iron deficiency, dys-hemopoiesis, and relative erythropoietin deficiency.

In Table 21.1 the main factors contributing to kidney injury after heart transplantation are summarized.

Table 21.1 Factors contributing to kidney injury after heart transplantation

Acute injury	Chronic injury
Effective volume contraction	Calcineurin inhibitors
Ventricular dysfunction	Chronic effective volume contraction
Over-aggressive diuresis	Chronic diuretic use
Acute tubular necrosis	Peri-operative acute renal failure
Diabetes mellitus	Hypertension
Sepsis	Hyperlipidemia
Hypotension	Diabetes mellitus
Radiographic contrast	
Nephrotoxic drugs	
Calcineurin inhibitors	
Athero-embolism	
Acute interstitial nephritis	

21.4 Calcineurin Inhibitors

The first calcineurin inhibitor used in transplantation of solid organs was cyclosporine (CsA), a peptide derived from the soil fungus *Tolypocladium inflatum* Gams. Following reports of its immunosuppressive properties, first described in the early 1970s, CsA was approved as an anti-rejection agent in the early 1980s. A few years later, tacrolimus (TAC) was approved, a macrolactone derived from the fungus *Streptomyces tsukubaensis* discovered on Mount Fuji.

Both CsA and TAC are lipophilic prodrugs that need to bind to cytoplasmic receptors, known as immunophilins, to gain pharmacological activity. The receptor for CsA is called cyclophilin and that for TAC FK-binding protein 12. After binding to the respective immunophilin, calcineurin inhibitors (CNIs) inhibit the activity of a complex of phosphatase called calcineurin. CNI suppresses the immune response by down-regulating the transcription of various cytokine genes, of which the most significant is IL-2 which is one of the main activation factors for T cells in numerous immunological processes (Kahan and Ponticelli 2000).

As they have a similar mechanism of action, it is not surprising that CsA and TAC can exert similar side effects, including reversible acute renal insufficiency as well as chronic renal deterioration.

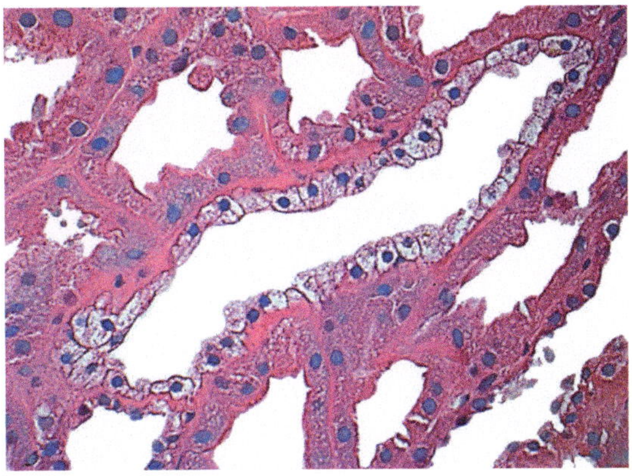

Fig. 21.3 Renal tubule lined by epithelial cells with cytoplasmic isometric microvacuolization (Hematoxylin-eosin stain, original magnification 400×)

21.4.1 Acute Renal Toxicity

Acute nephrotoxicity of CNIs may manifest with variable severity, usually dose dependent.

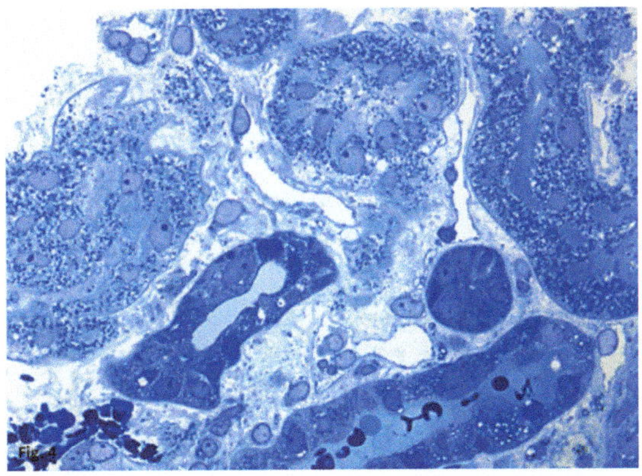

Fig. 21.4 A few tubules show cytoplasmic organelles consistent with giant mitochondria (Toluidine *blue stain*, original magnification 630×)

Tubular toxicity In the milder forms of toxicity, there is a reduction of glomerular filtration rate and renal blood flow associated with sodium retention, hypo-magnesemia, hyper-uricemia, hyper-kalemia, and hyper-chloremic acidosis. These functional changes are caused by afferent arteriolar vasoconstriction, which can be sustained by increased sympathetic nerve activity, activation of the renin–angiotensin system, increased production of thromboxane A2, impaired production of vasodilating prostaglandins, excessive renal synthesis of endothelin-1, and reduced production of nitric oxide.

Arteriolar toxicity More severe nephro-toxicity may lead to a substantial increase in plasma creatinine. Decreasing the doses of CNIs can reverse renal dysfunction and morphologic changes.

Thrombotic micro-angiopathy The most severe form of acute toxicity is thrombotic micro-angiopathy with focal glomerular and/or arteriolar thrombosis (Nizze et al. 1988), which in about 60 % of cases shows a typical picture of hemolytic uremic syndrome with acute renal failure, hypertension, micro-angiopathic hemolytic anemia, and thrombocytopenia. The precise pathogenesis of CNI-associated hemolytic uremic syndrome is unknown. Treatment should first consist of prompt withdrawal of the drug.

Histology of CNI renal damage shows different patterns, ranging from normal appearance to glomerular tuft collapse with widening of the Bowman space. Tubular epithelial changes may be present, more frequently in the form of cytoplasmic isometric vacuolization (Fig. 21.3); other early features of CNI toxic tubulopathy may be giant mitochondria (Fig. 21.4) and microcalcifications (Fig. 21.5), all features also described in renal grafts (Myers et al. 1984; Mihatsch et al. 1985). In addition CNI may induce apoptosis in tubular cells

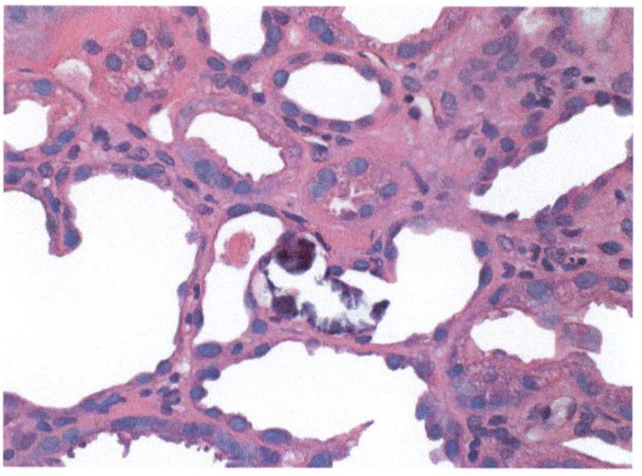

Fig. 21.5 Calcification of epithelial tubular cells (Hematoxylin-eosin stain, original magnification 500×)

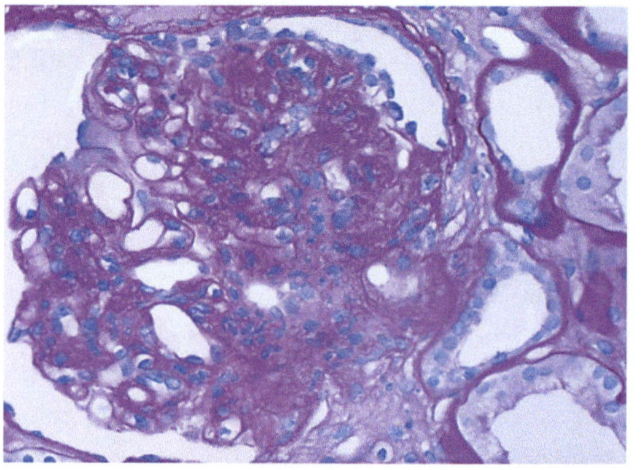

Fig. 21.6 Arteriolar hyalinosis with narrowing of the lumen due to protein insudation in the vessel wall (PAS stain, original magnification 200×)

through different pathways. Vasoconstriction of afferent arterioles is most probably due to primary endothelial damage.

21.4.2 Chronic Renal Toxicity

The main problem with the use of CNIs is the possible development of progressive nephro-toxicity.

Pathophysiology The mechanisms responsible for this chronic nephropathy have not been completely elucidated. Both CsA and TAC can cause renal and systemic vasoconstriction, through increased release of endothelin-1, activation of the renin–angiotensin system, increased production of thromboxane A2, and decreased production of vasodilators such as nitric oxide and prostacyclin. The profound vasoconstriction together with the typical arteriolar lesions may induce ischemia with consequent tubular atrophy and interstitial fibrosis. However, CNI may also increase the levels of plasminogen activator inhibitor (PAI), an inducer of interstitial fibrosis and tubular atrophy and an inhibitor of matrix degradation. PAI may favor the recruitment of interstitial cells and enhances the expression of mRNA transforming growth factor-β1 (TGF-β1), which represents a central mediator of fibrogenic remodeling process. TGF-β1 is a biologically multipotent regulatory protein implicated in functions that include the regulation of cellular growth, differentiation, extracellular matrix formation, and wound healing. This cytokine may induce trans-differentiation to myofibroblasts and extracellular matrix production either directly or through activation of the signal pathway of several intracellular proteins that play different roles in regulating cell growth, differentiation, and apoptosis (Alvarez Arroyo et al. 2002).

Clinically the chronic nephropathy caused by CNIs is characterized by slowly progressive renal dysfunction, hypertension, and mild to moderate proteinuria.

Histologically chronic CNI toxicity is characterized by nodular thickening of the afferent arteriole wall or by arteriolar hyalinosis with narrowing of the lumen. Hyalinosis is due to protein insudation in the wall, especially in the media, where it replaces dead smooth muscle cells (Fig. 21.6). Segmental and then global glomerulosclerosis occur later (Fig. 21.7), resulting in ischemic damage to the tubular interstitial compartment, with "striped" fibrosis and tubular atrophy (Fig. 21.8).

Patients should be closely monitored in order to determine the possible onset of proteinuria or a further increase in serum creatinine.

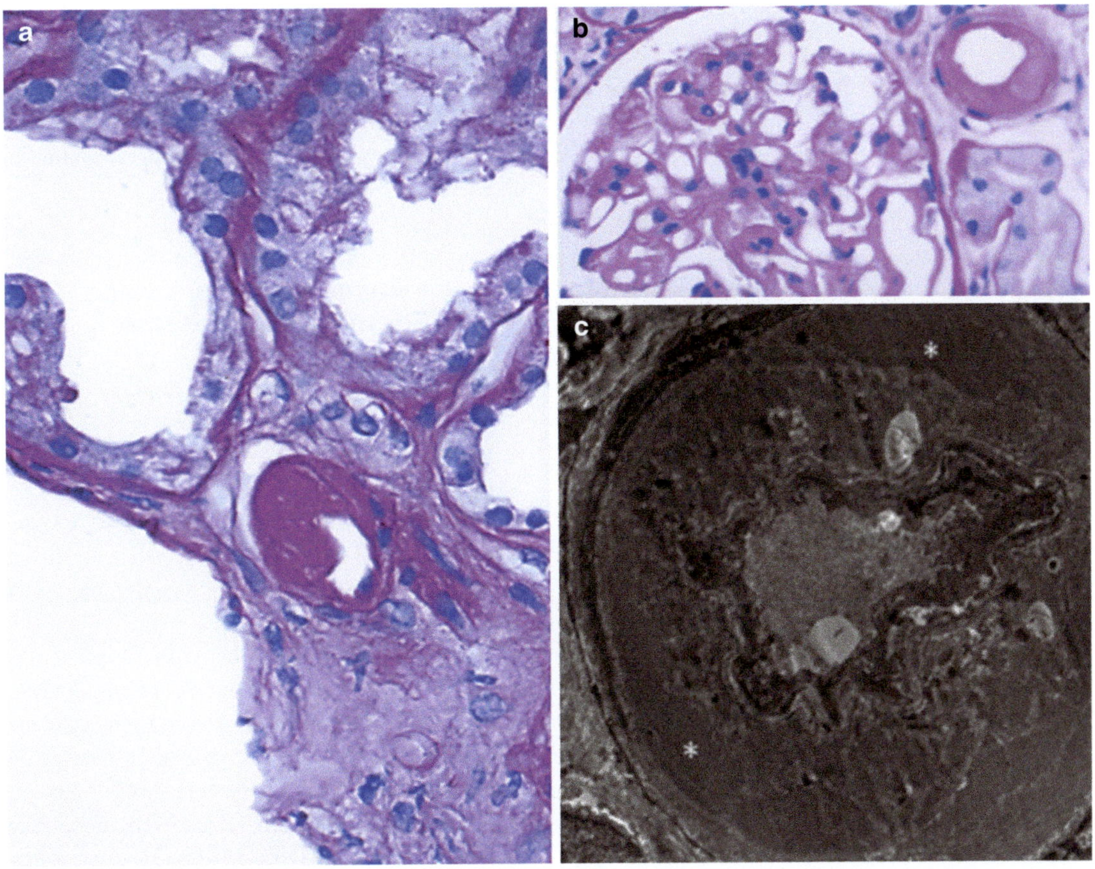

Fig. 21.7 (**a**, **b**) Afferent arterioles with nodular PAS-positive thickening. (**c**) Transmission electron microscopy showing electron dense deposits (*) in the media and adventitia of an afferent arteriole. ((a, b) PAS stain, original magnification (a) 400×, (b) 200×; (c) uranyl acetate and lead citrate-bar = 2 μm)

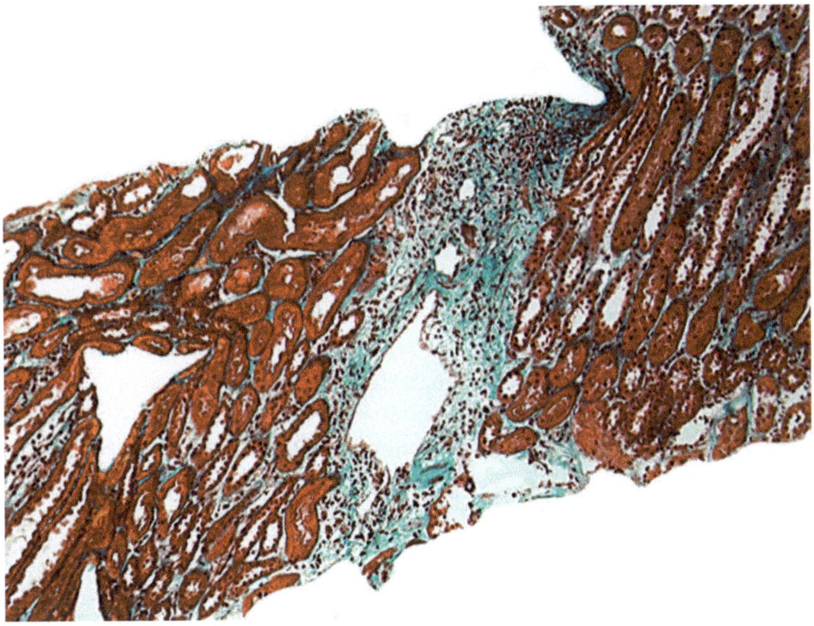

Fig. 21.8 "Striped" fibrosis (Masson trichrome stain, original magnification 100×)

21.5 Treatments

There are many possible ways to influence the outcome of CKD after heart transplantation (HTx): control and management of the main risk factors, management of CKD and CNI toxicity, renal-sparing immunosuppressive strategies, diet, and dialysis and kidney transplantation (KTx).

21.5.1 Control and Management of Main Chronic Kidney Disease Risk Factors

The first step is to obtain adequate blood pressure and glucose and lipid control.

Although there are no heart transplant-specific randomized studies, current guidelines recommend approaches similar to non-transplant patients with respect to risk factor control (Costanzo et al. 2010). Drugs like calcium channel antagonist, angiotensin-converting enzyme inhibitors (ACEI), and angiotensin receptor antagonists (ARA) are preferable for improving GFR and controlling proteinuria (Gonzales-Vilchez and Vazquez de Prada 2014). It is essential to avoid certain oral hypoglycemic drugs because of their toxicity, while repaglinide and insulin are safe. Some nephrotoxic drugs (KDIGO 2012) such as non-steroidal anti-inflammatory drugs, lithium, anti-microbial (aminoglycosides), anti-fungal (amphotericin), anti-viral agents (cidofovir), and chemotherapics (cisplatin) should also be avoided. Weight control is advisable as recipient weight is another risk factor (Gonzales-Vilchez and Vazquez de Prada 2014). Statins (no fibrates) are indicated (Gonzales-Vilchez and Vazquez de Prada 2014) for cardioprotective effects (lower cardiovascular death and cardiac allograft vasculopathy) as well as renal protective effects. Another key point is to avoid contrast medium when GFR is <30 ml/min or, when possible, to use (KDIGO 2012) a modified protocol consisting of hydration with saline solution before and after administration of contrast medium and of acetyl cysteine for 3 days. Monitoring diuresis, creatinine, and potassium after 48–96 hours should be performed. ACEI, ARA, and diuretics should be avoided the day before, the same day, and the day after contrast medium. Hepatitis C virus infection (Gonzales-Vilchez and Vazquez de Prada 2014) may also worsen renal function. Finally, prevention of recurrence of urinary tract infections with non-nephrotoxic antibiotic prophylaxis, minimization of acute kidney injury, and stopping smoking are all useful.

21.5.2 Management of Chronic Kidney Disease

The main clinical conditions to manage are:

- Hyperparathyroidism: treat with active vitamin D.
- Metabolic acidosis: treat with $NaHCO_3$ and/or $CaCO_3$.
- Anemia: treat with iron supplement, folic acid, and erythropoietin.
- High serum uric acid: treat with allopurinol (if azathioprine therapy is not already in course).
- Hypocalcemia: treat with vitamin D and calcium.
- Magnesium deficiency: treat with magnesium supplement.
- Proteinuria: treat with ACEI/ARA when GFR is >30 ml/min (KDIGO 2012).

21.5.3 Immunosuppressive-Sparing Strategies

This is the goal to improve renal function especially regarding CNI nephro-toxicity, a major clinical problem in cardiac transplanted patient management. In the near future, immunosuppressive-sparing regimes will probably improve the course of CKD itself.

Several studies propose CNI minimization strategies or avoidance to improve renal function in patients with established CKD or to prevent CKD. In this context, a major role has been played by the use of inhibitors of the mammalian target of rapamycin (mTORi). In general, CNI withdrawal studies have been conducted with the combination of sirolimus and mycophenolate, while CNI minimization strategies have been investigated by reducing CsA and adding everolimus in spite of mycophenolate or azathioprine. It has to be noted that sirolimus is not FDA (Food and Drug

Administration) or EMA (European Medicines Agency) approved for heart transplantation and that no clear evidence supports CNI avoidance over minimization (Cornu et al. 2014). In addition, some kidney transplant evidence support the concept that CNI avoidance may increase the risk for de novo donor-specific antibodies onset.

In general, reduction of the dosage of CNI may obtain reversal or stabilization of renal dysfunction in some patients. Some studies reported that about half of patients showed an improvement after introduction/conversion to mTORi, while the remaining patients had renal deterioration and the risk seems to be more elevated in patients with proteinuria (Olyaei et al. 2001; Yango et al. 2002; Potena et al. 2012; Gullestad et al. 2010).

The duration of renal dysfunction related to CNI exposure is more important than the degree of renal damage. Chances of success are therefore greater when the kidney impairment is severe but less long-standing than when the impairment is less severe but dates back longer (Gonzales-Vilchez and Vazquez de Prada 2014; Gullestad et al. 2010).

The presence of proteinuria is a negative factor for CKD outcome and is a well-known adverse event of mTORi. Their use is contraindicated if the baseline proteinuria is >0.8 g/die; if proteinuria appears "de novo," it is possible to reduce proliferation signal inhibitor dosage, augment CNI doses, and add ACEI or ARA.

A final note should be raised on the concept of complete CNI withdrawal early after transplantation. This strategy is intriguingly supported by a recent randomized study supporting CsA withdrawal at month 1–3 after HTx and subsequent therapy with everolimus and mycophenolic acid only. This strategy allowed significantly improved renal function and less coronary disease progression in the everolimus arm, at the cost of a slight increase in asymptomatic cellular rejection (Andreassen et al. 2016). Whether the advantages will overcome the side effects on long-term outcomes is still to be determined.

21.5.4 Diet

Although guidelines for diet in heart-transplanted patients with CKD are not available, looking at the KDIGO guidelines, a moderate low (0.7–0.8 g/kg)-protein diet seems reasonable for patients with severe CKD (fourth stage).

21.5.5 Dialysis and Kidney Transplantation

Hemodialysis is preferred to peritoneal dialysis because of lower infection risk. Heart-transplanted patients requiring long-term dialysis show worse survival rates than non-transplanted. The prognosis may change if a timely KTx is possible: after an initial higher mortality in the first 3 months, death risk decreases, and 5-year survival is similar to naive patients undergoing KTx (Gonzales-Vilchez and Vazquez de Prada 2014). Another option is to select patients who may benefit from a simultaneous combined heart–kidney transplantation.

Key Points

- Kidney disease is a frequent complication of heart transplantation which greatly complicates patient management and significantly contributes to early and late post-transplant morbidity and mortality.
- Chronic kidney disease in this population is associated with a four- to fivefold increased risk of death after transplant.
- Collaboration between cardiologist and nephrologist is essential both before transplantation in defining the cause of pre-heart transplant renal failure and throughout the follow-up.
- Nephro-pathologists can use renal biopsy samples to help identify the causes of renal damage after heart transplantation.
- Calcineurin inhibitor side effects may cause acute renal insufficiency as well as chronic renal deterioration. As there is no cure for CNI-linked pathology, early intervention is important to reduce CKD progression.
- "Tailored therapy" is essential for many therapies today and particularly for CKD post heart transplantation.

References

Alvarez Arroyo MV, Suzuki Y, Yague A, et al. Role of endogenous vascular endothelial growth factor in tubular cellular protection against acute cyclosporine toxicity. Transplantation. 2002;74:1618–24.

Andreassen AK, Andersson B, Gustafsson F, Eiskjaer H, Rådegran G, Gude E, Jansson K, Solbu D, Karason K, Arora S, Dellgren G, Gullestad L. Everolimus initiation with early calcineurin inhibitor withdrawal in de novo heart transplant recipients: three-year results from the randomized SCHEDULE study. Am J Transplant. 2016;16:1238–47. doi:10.1111/ajt.13588.

Bloom RD, Doyle AM. Kidney disease after heart and lung transplantation. Am J Transplant. 2006;6:671–9.

Cornu C, Dufays C, Gaillard S, Gueyffier F, Redonnet M, Sebbag L, Roussoulières A, Gleissner CA, Groetzner J, Lehmkuhl HB, Potena L, Gullestad L, Cantarovich M, Boissonnat P. Impact of the reduction of calcineurin inhibitors on renal function in heart transplant patients: a systematic review and meta-analysis. Br J Clin Pharmacol. 2014;78:24–32.

Costanzo MR, Dipchand A, Starling R, et al. The International Society of Heart and Lung Transplantation Guidelines for the care of heart transplant recipients. J Heart Lung Transplant. 2010;29:914–56.

Gonzales-Vilchez F, Vazquez de Prada JA. Chronic renal insufficiency in heart transplant recipients: risk factors and management options. Drugs. 2014;74:1481–94.

Gullestad L, Mortensen SA, Eiskjær H, Riise GC, Mared L, Bjørtuft O, Ekmehag B, Jansson K, Simonsen S, Gude E, Rundqvist B, Fagertun HE, Solbu D, Iversen M. Two-year outcomes in thoracic transplant recipients after conversion to everolimus with reduced calcineurin inhibitor within a multicenter, open-label, randomized trial. Transplantation. 2010;90:1581–9.

Hillege HL, Nitsch D, Pfeffer MA, et al. Renal function as a predictor of outcome in a broad spectrum of patients with heart failure. Circulation. 2006;113:671–8.

Ishani A, Erturk S, Hertz M, et al. Predictors of renal function following lung or heart-lung transplantation. Kidney Int. 2002;61:2228–34.

Kahan B, Ponticelli C. Immunosuppressive drugs: molecular and cellular mechanisms of action. London: Martin Dunitz; 2000. p. 314–47.

KDIGO 2012 clinical practice guideline for the evaluation and management of chronic kidney disease. Kidney Int Suppl. 2013;3(1). http://www.kidney-international.org.

Kriz W, Kaissling B, Le Hir M. Epithelial-mesenchymal transition (EMT) in kidney fibrosis: fact or fantasy? J Clin Invest. 2011;121:468–74.

Mihatsch MJ, Thiel G, Basler V, et al. Morphological patterns in cyclosporine-treated renal transplant recipients. Transplant Proc. 1985;17 Suppl 1:101–16.

Myers BD, Ross J, Newton L, Luetscher J, Perlroth M. Cyclosporine-associated chronic nephropathy. N Engl J Med. 1984;311(11):699–705.

Nizze H, Mihatsch MJ, Zollinger HU, Brocheriou C, Gokel JM, Henry K, Sloane JP, Stovin PG. Cyclosporine-associated nephropathy in patients with heart and bone marrow transplants. Clin Nephrol. 1988;30(5):248–60.

Olyaei AJ, De Mattos A, Bennett WM. Nephrotoxicity of immunosuppressive drugs: new insight and preventive strategies. Curr Opin Crit Care. 2001;7:384–9.

Potena L, Prestinenzi P, Bianchi IG, Masetti M, Romani P, Magnani G, Fallani F, Coccolo F, Russo A, Ponticelli C, Rapezzi C, Grigioni F, Branzi A. Cyclosporine lowering with everolimus versus mycophenolate mofetil in heart transplant recipients: long-term follow-up of the SHIRAKISS randomized, prospective study. J Heart Lung Transplant. 2012;31:565–70.

Singh M, Shullo M, Kormos RL, et al. Impact of renal function before mechanical circulatory support on post-transplant renal outcomes. Ann Thorac Surg. 2001;91:1348–54.

Yango A, Morrisey P, Monaco A, et al. Successful treatment of tacrolimus-associates thrombotic microangiopathy with sirolimus conversion and plasma axchange. Clin Nephrol. 2002;5:77–8.

Part VI

Special Issues in Cardiac Transplantation

Pathology of Pediatric Heart Transplantation

22

Jean-Paul Duong Van Huyen, Franck Iserin, and Claire Toquet

Contents

J.-P. D. Van Huyen, MD, PhD (✉)
Department of Pathology, University Paris-Descartes, Hôpital Necker-Enfants Malades, Paris, France
e-mail: jp.dvh@wanadoo.fr

F. Iserin, MD
Department of Pediatric Cardiology, Hôpital Necker-Enfants Malades, Paris, France

C. Toquet, MD, PhD
Department of Pathology, Hôpital Hôtel-Dieu, Nantes, France

22.1 Background

Although surgery for congenital heart disease and medical management of heart failure has dramatically improved in the last decade, cardiac transplantation remains the final option for many infants and children with end-stage heart failure. Over the past 15 years, the number of pediatric heart transplantations (HTx) reported has held remarkably at 340–390 transplantations per year, which is approximately 10 % of total heart transplantations reported to the International Society for Heart and Lung Transplantation (ISHLT) database (Kirk et al. 2012; Dipchand et al. 2013a). With advances in surgical strategies and medical therapies, the outcomes for pediatric heart transplant recipients have continuously improved (Morales et al. 2007; Ross et al. 2006).

Compared to the adult population, there are some important differences to mention in terms of epidemiology, management, and outcomes.

Here, we will focus on several issues:

1. Primary disease leading to heart failure and heart transplantation
2. Sensitization in the pediatric population
3. ABO-incompatible transplantation
4. Endomyocardial biopsy management and interpretation in the pediatric population
5. Cardiac allograft vasculopathy

O. Leone et al. (eds.), *The Pathology of Cardiac Transplantation*,
DOI 10.1007/978-3-319-46386-5_22

22.2 Indications for Pediatric Heart Transplantation

Diagnoses leading to pediatric HTx are age related and have changed during the last decades (Kirk et al. 2012; Dipchand et al. 2013a; Thrush and Hoffman 2014). These are principally congenital heart disease (CHD), cardiomyopathy (CMP), and retransplantation (Re-Tx) (Voeller et al. 2012). Approximately 90 % of pediatric heart transplantations are performed for either CMP or CHD with respective proportions varying according to the age of the recipient. In cases of CHD not amenable to correction or palliation, it is the leading indication among neonates and infants, while CMPs represent 50 % to two thirds of transplantations in children and adolescents.

Cardiomyopathy is still nowadays the most common indication for pediatric HTx, ranging from 41 % of patients <1 year of age to 65 % between 11 and 17 years. Dilated cardiomyopathy (DCM) (idiopathic or due to myocarditis, neuromuscular disease, or genetic causes) has an incidence of 0.58 cases per 100,000 children with a freedom from death or transplantation at 1 and 5 years after DCM diagnosis of 69 % and 54 %, respectively. Waiting list mortality of patients with DCM is 11 %. Hypertrophic cardiomyopathy (HCM) phenotypes (idiopathic, familial, associated with neuromuscular disorders, or syndromic) have an incidence of 0.47 cases per 100,000 children, but are a relatively rare etiology for pediatric HTx, accounting for only 5–6 %. Waiting list mortality is higher compared to those with DCM (14 % vs 11 %). Restrictive cardiomyopathy (RCM) has an incidence of 0.03–0.04 cases per 100,000 children (4.5 % of pediatric cardiomyopathies) with a frequent mixed phenotype (RCM/HCM). RCM has a poor prognosis (the evolution can rapidly be fatal) with a cumulative incidence of death of 20–28 % at 5 years from diagnosis. There is 10 % mortality in patients with RCM on the waiting list.

The pediatric population of CHD includes infants with both unrepaired and palliative complex diseases and older children with palliated CHD who either have failed palliations or have ventricular dysfunction (see also Chap. 5). Single-ventricle anatomy and failed Fontan procedure represent 60–80 % of CHD undergoing HTx. The percentage of recipients listed for HTx with CHD has decreased from 81 % in the 1990s down to 54 % in 2013 and will probably decrease further in the next few years due to advances in cardiac surgery and care, especially in single-ventricle cardiopathy. CHD still remains the most common indication for HTx in the infant age group, but is less common in older children – 23 % of the indications in 11–17-year-old recipients.

Retransplantation is an increasing cause of HTx (Conway et al. 2014; Mahle 2008). It is rare in infancy (less than 1 %), but 9 % of HTx with recipients aged 1–17 years were retransplantations. It is recognized that the majority of the children transplanted during childhood will require retransplantation in adult life: all progress in the medical care of these children aims to prolong the period before retransplantation. Most of the retransplantations (72 %) will be made beyond 3 years after primary HTx.

22.3 Sensitization in the Pediatric Population

Sensitization is a major issue in the pediatric population (Castleberry et al. 2014; Chin 2012; Girnita et al. 2006). According to the International Society for Heart and Lung Transplantation (ISHLT) registry, the percentage of sensitized patients (defined as panel-reactive antibodies >10 %) increased from 20 % in 2005 to 29 % in 2010 (Dipchand et al. 2013a). This is slightly more than in the adult population. While human leukocyte antigen (HLA) sensitization is uncommon in patients with CMP, it can frequently be seen in patients with CHD who had prior surgeries. Sensitizing events include transfusion of blood products (especially platelets), infections, and previous surgery for CHD, especially with the use of human homograft tissue. Ventricular assist device implantation dramatically increases HLA sensitization (Girnita et al. 2006; O'Connor et al. 2010). In the Pediatric Heart Transplant Study (PHTS) database and the ISHLT registry,

CHD were associated with both increased risk factors for death after transplantation and development of panel-reactive antibodies (PRA) >50 % (Dipchand et al. 2013a, b). Multiple cardiac surgery and sternotomy prior to listing, e.g., Norwood procedure, were also significant risk factors of sensitization. Studies have shown that transplantation with allosensitization increases risk of antibody-mediated rejection (AMR) and mortality (Chin 2012; Ho et al. 2011; Daly et al. 2013; Jacobs et al. 2004; Pollock-BarZiv et al. 2007; Richmond et al. 2012; Wright et al. 2007; Zeevi et al. 2013). High PRA is also associated with a twofold increase in early posttransplant mortality (Mahle et al. 2011). Elevated PRA in children listed for heart transplantation is also associated with longer waiting times for transplantation, thus increasing pretransplant mortality.

22.4 ABO-Incompatible Allografts

In very young children, the increase in pretransplantation mortality on a waiting list due to organ shortage has led to the development of strategies for ABO-incompatible (ABOi) HTx. Since 1996 when the first heart ABOi transplantations were performed on infants, there have been increasing data to support this type of transplantation in infants and young children, as a strategy to reduce waiting list mortality (Almond et al. 2010; Irving et al. 2012). Infants less than 1 year of age lack antibodies against blood group antigens since humoral immunity to carbohydrate moieties is poorly developed at this age (West 2011). Introduction of intentional ABOi HTx was based on the immaturity of the immune system in this age group, which allows transplantation across blood types. Immune tolerance to the ABO-type graft develops (accommodation), although theoretically there is the possibility of bounding the anti-ABO antibody to the graft endothelium and initiating the complement cascade, which leads to C4d positivity, but with normal histopathology and no graft dysfunction. Analysis has demonstrated persistent deficiency of antibodies toward the donor blood group in infants as well as absence of B cells with specific receptors for donor blood group antigens. The stage of immunologic maturation with regard to isoagglutinin production is the main parameter to judge suitability for ABOi transplant.

Currently, United Network for Organ Sharing (UNOS) guidelines permit ABOi HTx for infants <1 year of age with any isohemagglutinin titer and for those between 1 and 2 years of age with isohemagglutinin titers >¼. ABOi eligible infant listing increased from 0 % prior to 2002 to 53 % in 2007. It is of note that several studies have reported that ABOi listing strategy still involved more severely ill recipients (Dipchand et al. 2013b; Henderson et al. 2012). However, with increasing experience, it appears clear that, regardless of listing strategy, ABOi HTx recipients have similar outcomes to those undergoing ABOc HTx (Henderson et al. 2012; Dipchand et al. 2010). In the recent report of the PHTS centers, ABOi HTx represents 17 % of overall pediatric HTx over a 12-year period (85 ABOi HTx out of 911 pediatric HTxs). For ABOi and ABOc patients, survival at 12 months was similar (82 % vs 84 %, $p=0.7$). In a risk-adjusted analysis, ABOi was not associated with 1-year mortality (HR 0.85, 95 % CI 0.45–1.6, $p=0.61$) (Dipchand et al. 2010). Other groups have reported similar observations with good short-term outcomes. Recently, an international multicenter trial reported actuarial graft survival of 100 % at 1 year, 96 % at 5 years, and 69 % at 10 years posttransplant. The oldest recipient in this cohort at the time of transplantation was 7.5 years old.

In conclusion, there is increasing evidence showing that very young children receiving an ABOi HTx have similar outcomes as those receiving ABOc hearts (Roche et al. 2008). This is a safe and effective strategy to expand the donor pool and improve waiting list outcomes for those with the highest waiting list mortality. Although AMR has been reported in pediatric ABOi HTxs, infants who received these transplants had equivalent 1-year survival. A recent study suggested that ABOi HTx may be extended to older children (Urschel et al. 2013).

22.5 Endomyocardial Biopsies in the Pediatric Population

22.5.1 Indications for Endomyocardial Biopsy

Endomyocardial biopsy (EMB) is widely considered to be the "gold standard" for rejection surveillance in both adult and pediatric heart transplant recipients. This is particularly true in symptomatic patients of all age. However, the utility of EMB for long-term rejection surveillance in pediatric recipients has been debated (Boucek 2000; Mital 2007).

EMB also raises some problematic issues, such as the need for sedation and general anesthesia with vascular access issues and the risk of traumatic lesion of the tricuspid valve or psychological stress especially in adolescents. In addition EMB analyzes only the right ventricle. Such points have limited the development of surveillance protocol biopsies in pediatrics.

The timing of biopsies in surveillance protocols should be guided by the probability of rejection over time and by the accuracy of noninvasive procedures for the detection of rejection. According to PHTS report, in the first year post-transplantation, the incidence of rejection has declined from approximately 60 % in 1993 to 40 % in 2006, as did the number of rejection episodes per patient (Dipchand et al. 2013a; Gossett et al. 2010). Incidences of acute rejection will probably continue to decrease in the future due to improved protocols for immunosuppressive therapy. Risk factors for rejection included positive donor-specific crossmatch and older recipient age. After 1 year post HTx, the incidence of late rejection (first of recurrent) also decreased in the recent era, but late rejection was associated with poor outcomes (Ameduri et al. 2012; Webber et al. 2003). A positive EMB was most likely to be found in the first year posttransplant in symptomatic patients, in patients with a history of rejection (or recent rejection), and less likely in infants.

In the last two decades, several large studies have attempted to evaluate the performance of surveillance protocol biopsies in large pediatric series, sometimes with apparently conflicting results (Mital 2007; Levi et al. 2004; Wagner et al. 2000). In early post-HTx period (defined as from <1 month to <1 year according to the studies), EMB protocols failed to identify asymptomatic rejection in infants, but a significant proportion of subclinical cellular rejection was diagnosed in older children. All studies reported a dramatic decrease in the diagnostic rejection yield of EMB protocols after 1 year or more post HTx. A retrospective review of 1093 consecutive EMBs from 136 pediatric heart transplantations performed in a single center from January 1995 to January 2003 concluded that surveillance EMBs failed to reveal significant episodes of cellular rejection in asymptomatic patients after the first month posttransplant (Levi et al. 2004).

These studies have encouraged most pediatric centers to revise their follow-up strategies and to abandon surveillance protocols with iterated EMBs (Levi et al. 2004). The greatest limitation of these studies is that most were performed before the era of anti-HLA screening and that the pathologists did not evaluate AMR. More recent studies suggest that protocol biopsies are useful for the diagnosis of AMR associated with graft failure and mortality (Casarez et al. 2007). Although reassessment of the value of EMB protocol in the context of subclinical AMR in large pediatric series is warranted, it seems reasonable to perform EMBs in sensitized patients at high risk of humoral rejection.

At Necker-Enfants Malades Hospital, only a small number of biopsies are performed, mainly in high-risk recipients with anti-HLA DSAs for whom an annual EMB is done together with anti-HLA antibody follow-up.

22.5.2 Endomyocardial Biopsy Rejection Findings in Pediatrics

Pediatric EMBs are processed similarly to adult ones. In our center, EMBs are formalin fixed and paraffin embedded, and 3 hematoxylin-eosin-stained slides with multiple 3-µm-thick sections are performed. For all EMBs, an immunohistochemical analysis is also routinely performed on fixed sections with anti-CD3, anti-CD68, and anti-C4d antibodies.

Pediatric EMBs are characterized by a smaller size and give an impression of increased cellularity that may be misleading, particularly for the diagnosis of AMR. Diagnosis of acute cellular rejection (ACR) in the pediatric population relies on the same elementary lesions, criteria, and grading system as for adults. Both IHSLT 1990 working formulation and ISHLT 2004 for pathologic scoring of rejection severity are fully applicable in pediatrics (see Chap. 13) (Stewart et al. 2005). Figure 22.1 illustrates several aspects of ACR. Because of the smaller size of pediatric biopsies, it has been suggested that immunohistochemistry may be useful to confirm ACR (abundance of T cells and interstitial macrophages) and to avoid Quilty B lesion misdiagnosis (Levi et al. 2004).

The published prevalence of AMR in pediatric centers is higher than that reported in the majority of adult centers and ranges from 10 to 59 %, depending on whether cardiac dysfunction is required or not for AMR diagnosis (Casarez et al. 2007). The higher incidence is probably due to a combination of sensitization and medication noncompliance, particularly in adolescents. The pathological diagnosis of AMR is no different from adults and relies on the same combined histology and immunohistochemistry approach using CD68 and C4d antibodies (see

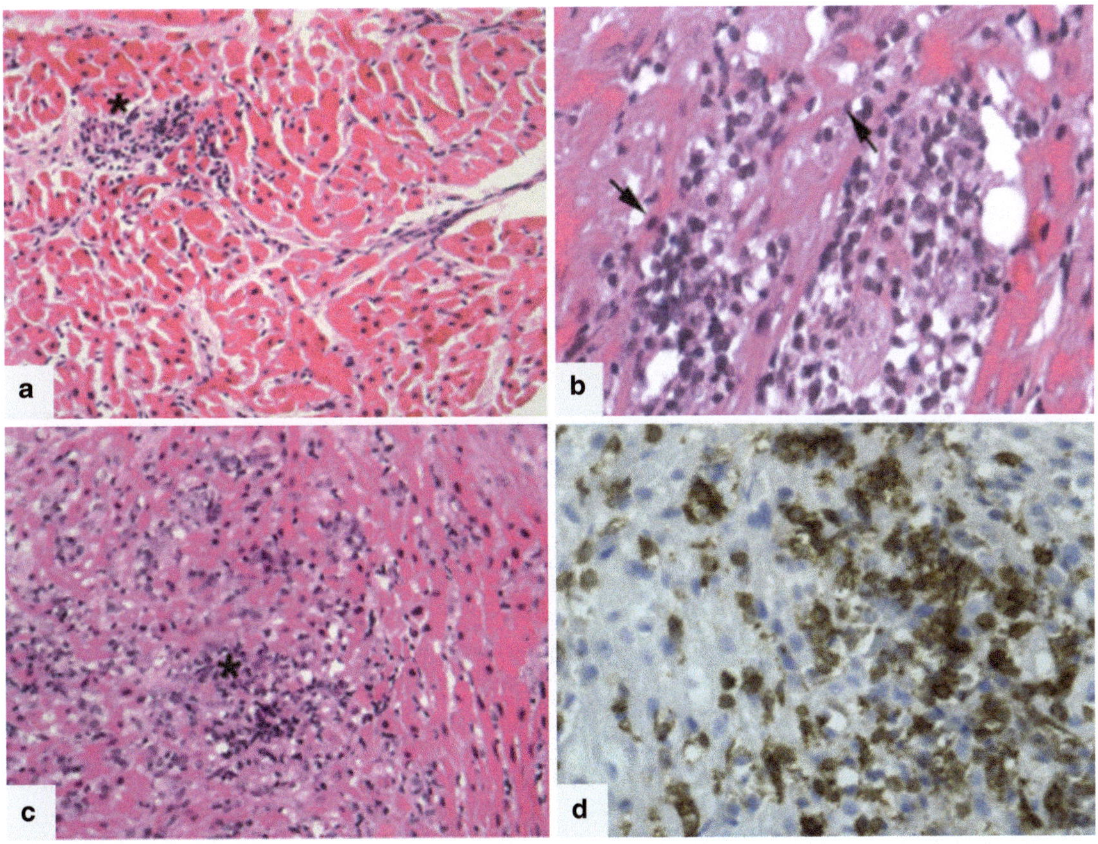

Fig. 22.1 Acute cellular rejection. (**a**) Two-month posttransplant EMB in a 7-year-old boy transplanted for CMP; no DSAs. One single focus of perivenular infiltrate (*asterisk*) in a 1R ACR rejection. (**b**) Six-year posttransplant EMB in a 12-year-old girl in a context of noncompliance; no DSAs. Perivascular and interstitial inflammation with myocyte injury (*arrows*) in a 2R ACR rejection. (**c, d**) Two-year posttransplant EMB in a 3-year-old child; DSA status at the time of biopsy unknown. Widespread interstitial cellular infiltrate (*asterisk*) in a 3R ACR rejection. Most of the cells were CD3+ T lymphocytes (**d**). C4d was negative (not shown)

Chap. 14) (Holt et al. 2008; Peng et al. 2013; Xu et al. 2013). The 2013 IHSLT pAMR classification for pathological diagnosis and scoring is also applicable to the pediatric population (Berry et al. 2013). Subclinical AMR is frequent in both the pediatric and adult populations (Everitt et al. 2012; Kfoury et al. 2009). Grade pAMR2 or higher was present in 258 (18 %) out of 1406 EMBs from the Utah cohort (45 out of 76 patients, 59 %). 6 out of 17 episodes of pAMR3 (35 %) in nine patients were subclinical. Greater age at transplantation was the only clinical factor found to predict development of pAMR3. Like cellular rejection, AMR biopsy grading seems important to delineate those at risk of adverse events: pAMR3 is associated with worse outcomes (Everitt et al. 2012). Patients with at least 1 pAMR3 episode had lower freedom from cardiovascular mortality or cardiac allograft vasculopathy within 5 years of heart transplantation than those without pAMR3 (45 % vs 91 %, $p<0.001$).

Figure 22.2 illustrates AMR in pediatric EMBs. It should be noted that at low magnification, identification and diagnosis of microcirculation inflammation (i.e., intravascular activated mononuclear cells, IAMC, according to the ISHLT working formulation (Berry et al. 2013)) may be difficult because of the overall impression of hypercellularity in pediatric biopsies. Thus, the busy pattern observed at low magnification should be interpreted with caution. At higher magnification, the presence and cellular type of IAMC do not differ from what is seen in adults. CD68 and C4d analysis and grading are also similar for pediatrics and adults, as recommended by the ISHLT pathology board (Berry et al. 2013). It is significant that diffuse positivity of C4d is a normal feature of ABOi HTx.

The incidence of mixed rejection is difficult to evaluate mainly because of the absence of a recognized pathological definition of mixed rejection (Berry et al. 2013). Nevertheless, in our experience, rejection episodes with concurrent pathological features of both ACR and AMR sometimes occur in the pediatric population, mainly in the context of noncompliance.

22.6 Allograft Vasculopathy in the Pediatric Population

Cardiac allograft vasculopathy (CAV) remains the leading cause of late mortality in pediatric heart transplant recipients (Pahl et al. 2005; Tjang et al. 2008). CAV in children exhibits some key differences compared with the adult population. The reported angiographic incidence is much lower than in adults: 17 % at 5 years, with 5 % of moderate and severe cases. In the UNOS registry, the incidence of CAV at 10 and 15 years of posttransplantation was 25 % and 54 %, respectively. Identified risk factors for CAV development include ages 1–18 years at the time of transplantation (but not infants), retransplantation, African-American recipients, and donor cigarette use. CAV seems to progress more slowly in infants and young children, but when it is diagnosed, graft survival drops to about 50 % after 5 years regardless of recipient age. One hypothesis for the age effect relates to the immaturity of the immune system in infants and the use of younger donors lacking cardiovascular risk factors for atherosclerosis. In the 2012 ISHLT registry report, only donor age but not recipient age is a risk factor for developing CAV. Various risk factors for CAV include donor cause of death, donor/recipient age difference, weight ratio, gender mismatch, number of rejection episodes, CMV infection, no induction therapy compared to the use of induction therapy, and choice of IS drugs (Kobayashi et al. 2013). HLA sensitization and AMR also emerge as important risk factors. This raises the question of the early diagnosis and treatment of AMR.

CAV diagnosis still relies on angiography, which to date remains the gold standard (Mehra et al. 2010). However, technical issues of such invasive procedure in younger children limit routine serial angiography for surveillance (concerning less than 50 % of the patients in the PHTS registry). Intravascular ultrasound (IVUS) may be more sensitive for the detection of intimal thickening as reported in adults, but faces major technical limitations in children (Costello et al. 2003). Noninvasive tests such as

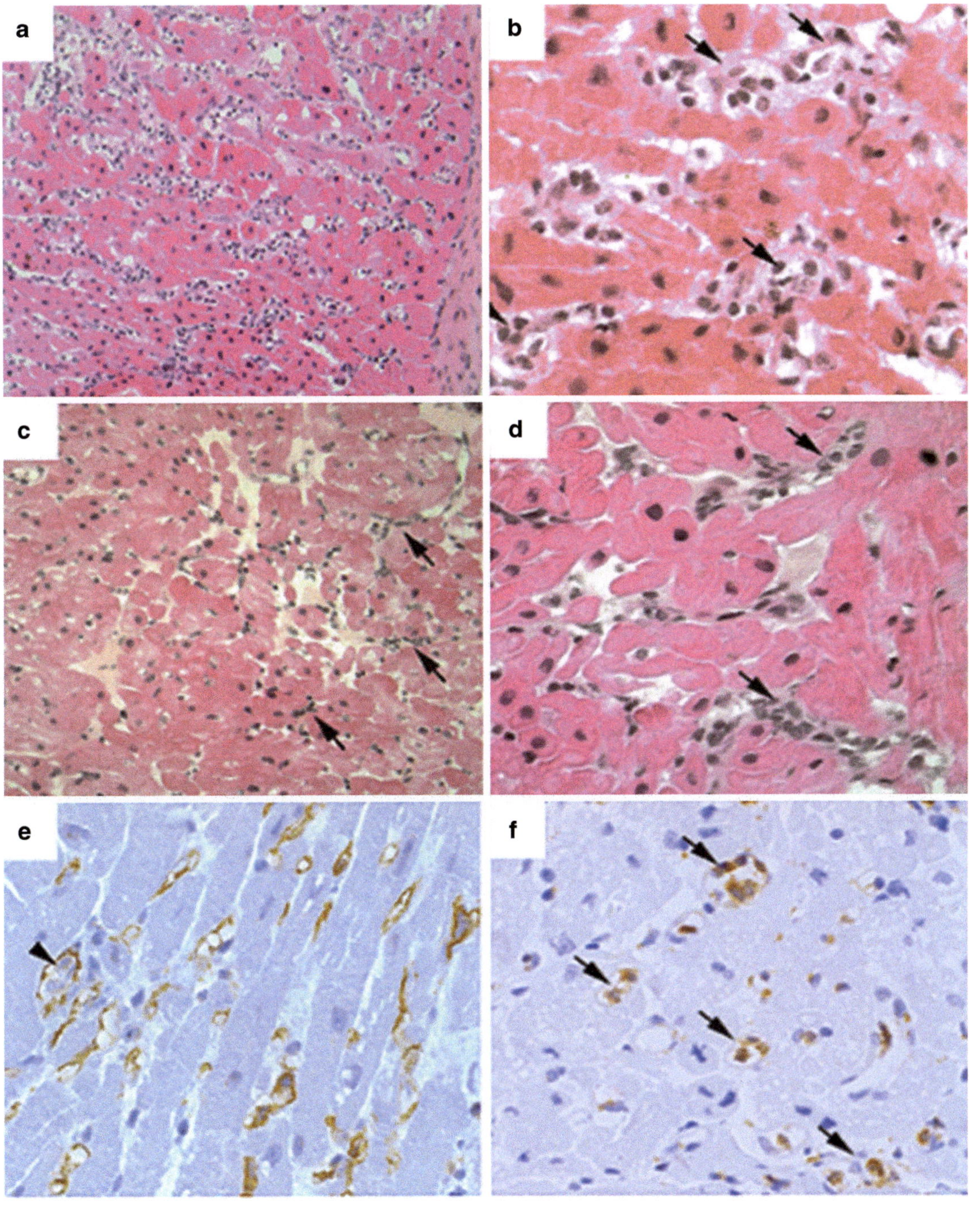

Fig. 22.2 Acute antibody-mediated rejection. (**a**, **b**) Eight-year posttransplant EMB in a 10-year-old boy transplanted for CMP; anti-HLA DSA positive (DR15, MFI = 1335; DR103, MFI = 1640; DQ5, MFI = 4901; DQ6, MFI = 5151). At low magnification, a busy pattern with the presence of numerous foci of IAMC (**b**, *arrows*) in a pAMR2 humoral rejection. (**c**, **d**) Six-month posttransplant EMB in a 5-year-old boy: anti-HLA DSA positive (DR4, MFI = 937). Near-normal biopsy except for the presence of mild microcirculation inflammation (**c**, *arrows*). At higher magnification, the presence of IAMC (**d**, *arrows*) in a pAMR1H+ humoral rejection. (**e**, **f**) Two-month posttransplant EMB in a 3-year-old boy transplanted for myocarditis; anti-HLA DSA positive (B44, MFI = 7676; A68, MFI = 5858; DR4, MFI = 1148). (**e**) Diffuse C4d capillary positivity (note the presence of IAMC, *arrows*); (**f**) intracapillary CD68+ macrophages (*arrows*) in a pAMR2 humoral rejection

dobutamine stress echocardiography (DSE) correlate reasonably with angiography findings. A negative DSE strongly supports the absence of angiographic CAV, suggesting that this test may be a good tool for monitoring and risk stratification. A coronary CT scan also seems to be a good noninvasive alternative for follow-up of patients.

Pathological reports of loss/explanted grafts in the pediatric population are limited (Lu et al. 2011; Perens et al. 2009; Seipelt et al. 2005). However, the morphological lesions of the graft vessels seem relatively similar to those reported in adults. CAV is a multifaceted disorder of the epicardial arteries with a combination of lesions including intimal fibromuscular hyperplasia, atherosclerosis, and vascular inflammation (see Chap. 18). This variety of lesions reflects the complex pathophysiology of CAV with immune and nonimmune mechanisms. Among the immune determinants of CAV, recent reports have substantiated the important role of AMR in its progression in both pediatric and adult populations (Everitt et al. 2012; Kfoury et al. 2009; Wu et al. 2009).

Conclusion

Pediatric HTx is in constant evolution. Much progress have been achieved in the last decade thus helping to move pediatric HTx from a mid- to a long-term medical procedure with good quality of life. Two major issues still remain:

- Organ shortage for children
- Late graft failure due to CAV

In the last decade, there has been increasing evidence of the implications of sensitization, DSAs, and AMR in CAV progression.

The importance of early diagnosis and treatment of cardiac asymptomatic AMR must not be underestimated in EMB pediatric surveillance.

Key Points

- Compared to the adult population, there are some important differences in terms of epidemiology, management, and outcomes.
- The main groups of primary diseases/indications for the pediatric population are congenital heart disease, cardiomyopathy (together 90 %), and retransplantations.
- Sensitization is a major issue in the pediatric population, and the percentage of sensitized patients is slightly more than that of the adult population.
- High panel-reactive antibodies are associated with longer waiting times for transplantation, thus increasing pretransplant mortality. A twofold increase in early posttransplant mortality and an increased risk for AMR are also consequences.
- Organ shortage has led to new strategies to expand the donor pool and improve waiting list outcomes for pediatric patients, such as ABO-incompatible HTx in infants (1–2 years), with similar outcomes to patients receiving ABO-compatible HTX.
- Although endomyocardial biopsy is widely considered the "gold standard" for rejection surveillance, its value for long-term rejection surveillance in pediatrics is debatable due to various limiting factors.
- Timing of biopsies in surveillance protocols should be guided by the probability of rejection over time and by the accuracy of noninvasive procedures in detection of rejection.
- EMB processing is similar for both children and adults.
- Elementary lesions, criteria, and grading systems for ACR and AMR are the same as for adults.

- Pathologists should be aware that the impression of greater myocardium cellularity in pediatric EMB may be misleading in diagnosis of ACR and especially AMR.
- Cardiac allograft vasculopathy (CAV) remains the leading cause of late mortality in pediatric heart transplant recipients.
- CAV morphological lesions of the graft vessels seem relatively similar in pediatrics and adults.

References

Almond CS, Gauvreau K, Thiagarajan RR, Piercey GE, Blume ED, Smoot LB, Fynn-Thompson F, Singh TP. Impact of abo-incompatible listing on wait-list outcomes among infants listed for heart transplantation in the United States: a propensity analysis. Circulation. 2010;121:1926–33.

Ameduri RK, Zheng J, Schechtman KB, Hoffman TM, Gajarski RJ, Chinnock R, Naftel DC, Kirklin JK, Dipchand AI, Canter CE. Has late rejection decreased in pediatric heart transplantation in the current era? A multi-institutional study. J Heart Lung Transplant Off Publ Int Soc Heart Transplant. 2012;31:980–6.

Berry GJ, Burke MM, Andersen C, Bruneval P, Fedrigo M, Fishbein MC, Goddard M, Hammond EH, Leone O, Marboe C, Miller D, Neil D, Rassl D, Revelo MP, Rice A, Rene Rodriguez E, Stewart S, Tan CD, Winters GL, West L, Mehra MR, Angelini A. The 2013 international society for heart and lung transplantation working formulation for the standardization of nomenclature in the pathologic diagnosis of antibody-mediated rejection in heart transplantation. J Heart Lung Transplant Off Publ Int Soc Heart Transplant. 2013;32:1147–62.

Boucek MM. Surveillance endomyocardial biopsy in pediatric heart transplantation: fashion or foible? Pediatr Transplant. 2000;4:173–6.

Casarez TW, Perens G, Williams RJ, Kutay E, Fishbein MC, Reed EF, Alejos JC, Levi DS. Humoral rejection in pediatric orthotopic heart transplantation. J Heart Lung Transplant Off Publ Int Soc Heart Transplant. 2007;26:114–9.

Castleberry C, Ryan TD, Chin C. Transplantation in the highly sensitized pediatric patient. Circulation. 2014;129:2313–9.

Chin C. Cardiac antibody-mediated rejection. Pediatr Transplant. 2012;16:404–12.

Conway J, Manlhiot C, Kirk R, Edwards LB, McCrindle BW, Dipchand AI. Mortality and morbidity after retransplantation after primary heart transplant in childhood: an analysis from the registry of the international society for heart and lung transplantation. J Heart Lung Transplant Off Publ Int Soc Heart Transplant. 2014;33:241–51.

Costello JM, Wax DF, Binns HJ, Backer CL, Mavroudis C, Pahl E. A comparison of intravascular ultrasound with coronary angiography for evaluation of transplant coronary disease in pediatric heart transplant recipients. J Heart Lung Transplant Off Publ Int Soc Heart Transplant. 2003;22:44–9.

Daly KP, Chandler SF, Almond CS, Singh TP, Mah H, Milford E, Matte GS, Bastardi HJ, Mayer JE, Fynn-Thompson F, Blume ED. Antibody depletion for the treatment of crossmatch-positive pediatric heart transplant recipients. Pediatr Transplant. 2013;17:661–9.

Dipchand AI, Pollock BarZiv SM, Manlhiot C, West LJ, VanderVliet M, McCrindle BW. Equivalent outcomes for pediatric heart transplantation recipients: abo-blood group incompatible versus abo-compatible. Am J Transplant Off J Am Soc Transplant Am Soc Transplant Surg. 2010;10:389–97.

Dipchand AI, Kirk R, Edwards LB, Kucheryavaya AY, Benden C, Christie JD, Dobbels F, Lund LH, Rahmel AO, Yusen RD, Stehlik J, International Society for H, Lung T. The registry of the international society for heart and lung transplantation: sixteenth official pediatric heart transplantation report--2013; focus theme: age. J Heart Lung Transplant Off Publ Int Soc Heart Transplant. 2013a;32:979–88.

Dipchand AI, Kirk R, Mahle WT, Tresler MA, Naftel DC, Pahl E, Miyamoto SD, Blume E, Guleserian KJ, White-Williams C, Kirklin JK. Ten yr of pediatric heart transplantation: a report from the pediatric heart transplant study. Pediatr Transplant. 2013b;17:99–111.

Everitt MD, Hammond ME, Snow GL, Stehlik J, Revelo MP, Miller DV, Kaza AK, Budge D, Alharethi R, Molina KM, Kfoury AG. Biopsy-diagnosed antibody-mediated rejection based on the proposed international society for heart and lung transplantation working formulation is associated with adverse cardiovascular outcomes after pediatric heart transplant. J Heart Lung Transplant Off Publ Int Soc Heart Transplant. 2012;31:686–93.

Girnita AL, Webber SA, Zeevi A. Anti-hla alloantibodies in pediatric solid organ transplantation. Pediatr Transplant. 2006;10:146–53.

Gossett JG, Canter CE, Zheng J, Schechtman K, Blume ED, Rodgers S, Naftel DC, Kirklin JK, Scheel J, Fricker FJ, Kantor P, Pahl E, Pediatric Heart Transplant Study I. Decline in rejection in the first year after pediatric cardiac transplantation: a multi-institutional study. J Heart Lung Transplant Off Publ Int Soc Heart Transplant. 2010;29:625–32.

Henderson HT, Canter CE, Mahle WT, Dipchand AI, LaPorte K, Schechtman KB, Zheng J, Asante-Korang A, Singh RK, Kanter KR. Abo-incompatible heart transplantation: analysis of the pediatric heart transplant study (phts) database. J Heart Lung Transplant Off Publ Int Soc Heart Transplant. 2012;31:173–9.

Ho EK, Vasilescu ER, Vlad G, Marboe CC, Addonizio LJ, Suciu-Foca N. Hla antibodies in pediatric heart transplantation. Pediatr Transplant. 2011;15:458–64.

Holt DB, Liapis H, Mohanakumar T, Phelan DR, Gandi SK, Huddleston CB, Canter CE. Complement fragment c4d and c3d deposition in pediatric heart recipients with a positive crossmatch. J Heart Lung Transplant Off Publ Int Soc Heart Transplant. 2008;27:1073–8.

Irving C, Gennery A, Kirk R. Pushing the boundaries: the current status of abo-incompatible cardiac transplantation. J Heart Lung Transplant Off Publ Int Soc Heart Transplant. 2012;31:791–6.

Jacobs JP, Quintessenza JA, Boucek RJ, Morell VO, Botero LM, Badhwar V, van Gelder HM, Asante-Korang A, McCormack J, Daicoff GR. Pediatric cardiac transplantation in children with high panel reactive antibody. Ann Thorac Surg. 2004;78:1703–9.

Kfoury AG, Hammond ME, Snow GL, Drakos SG, Stehlik J, Fisher PW, Reid BB, Everitt MD, Bader FM, Renlund DG. Cardiovascular mortality among heart transplant recipients with asymptomatic antibody-mediated or stable mixed cellular and antibody-mediated rejection. J Heart Lung Transplant Off Publ Int Soc Heart Transplant. 2009;28:781–4.

Kirk R, Dipchand AI, Edwards LB, Kucheryavaya AY, Benden C, Christie JD, Dobbles F, Rahmel AO, Stehlik J, Hertz MI, International Society for H, Lung T. The registry of the international society for heart and lung transplantation: fifteenth pediatric heart transplantation report--2012. J Heart Lung Transplant Off Publ Int Soc Heart Transplant. 2012;31:1065–72.

Kobayashi D, Du W, L'Ecuyer TJ. Predictors of cardiac allograft vasculopathy in pediatric heart transplant recipients. Pediatr Transplant. 2013;17:436–40.

Levi DS, DeConde AS, Fishbein MC, Burch C, Alejos JC, Wetzel GT. The yield of surveillance endomyocardial biopsies as a screen for cellular rejection in pediatric heart transplant patients. Pediatr Transplant. 2004;8:22–8.

Lu WH, Palatnik K, Fishbein GA, Lai C, Levi DS, Perens G, Alejos J, Kobashigawa J, Fishbein MC. Diverse morphologic manifestations of cardiac allograft vasculopathy: a pathologic study of 64 allograft hearts. J Heart Lung Transplant Off Publ Int Soc Heart Transplant. 2011;30:1044–50.

Mahle WT. Cardiac retransplantation in children. Pediatr Transplant. 2008;12:274–80.

Mahle WT, Tresler MA, Edens RE, Rusconi P, George JF, Naftel DC, Shaddy RE, Pediatric Heart Transplant Study G. Allosensitization and outcomes in pediatric heart transplantation. J Heart Lung Transplant Off Publ Int Soc Heart Transplant. 2011;30:1221–7.

Mehra MR, Crespo-Leiro MG, Dipchand A, Ensminger SM, Hiemann NE, Kobashigawa JA, Madsen J, Parameshwar J, Starling RC, Uber PA. International society for heart and lung transplantation working formulation of a standardized nomenclature for cardiac allograft vasculopathy-2010. J Heart Lung Transplant Off Publ Int Soc Heart Transplant. 2010;29:717–27.

Mital S. Value of surveillance biopsy in pediatric heart transplantation. Pediatr Transplant. 2007;11:233–5.

Morales DL, Dreyer WJ, Denfield SW, Heinle JS, McKenzie ED, Graves DE, Price JF, Towbin JA, Frazier OH, Cooley DA, Fraser Jr CD. Over two decades of pediatric heart transplantation: how has survival changed? J Thorac Cardiovasc Surg. 2007;133:632–9.

O'Connor MJ, Menteer J, Chrisant MR, Monos D, Lind C, Levine S, Gaynor JW, Hanna BD, Paridon SM, Ravishankar C, Kaufman BD. Ventricular assist device-associated anti-human leukocyte antigen antibody sensitization in pediatric patients bridged to heart transplantation. J Heart Lung Transplant Off Publ Int Soc Heart Transplant. 2010;29:109–16.

Pahl E, Naftel DC, Kuhn MA, Shaddy RE, Morrow WR, Canter CE, Kirklin J, Pediatric Heart Transplant S. The impact and outcome of transplant coronary artery disease in a pediatric population: a 9-year multi-institutional study. J Heart Lung Transplant Off Publ Int Soc Heart Transplant. 2005;24:645–51.

Peng DM, Law YM, Kemna MS, Warner P, Nelson K, Boucek RJ. Donor-specific antibodies: can they predict c4d deposition in pediatric heart recipients? Pediatr Transplant. 2013;17:429–35.

Perens G, Li F, Meier S, Kaur R, Alejos JC, Fishbein M. Clinico-pathologic findings in end-stage pediatric heart transplant grafts. Pediatr Transplant. 2009;13:887–91.

Pollock-BarZiv SM, den Hollander N, Ngan BY, Kantor P, McCrindle B, West LJ, Dipchand AI. Pediatric heart transplantation in human leukocyte antigen sensitized patients: Evolving management and assessment of intermediate-term outcomes in a high-risk population. Circulation. 2007;116:I172–8.

Richmond ME, Hsu DT, Mosca RS, Chen J, Quaegebeur JM, Addonizio LJ, Lamour JM. Outcomes in pediatric cardiac transplantation with a positive hla crossmatch. Pediatr Transplant. 2012;16:29–35.

Roche SL, Burch M, O'Sullivan J, Wallis J, Parry G, Kirk R, Elliot M, Shaw N, Flett J, Hamilton JR, Hasan A. Multicenter experience of abo-incompatible pediatric cardiac transplantation. Am J Transplant Off J Am Soc Transplant Am Soc Transplant Surg. 2008;8:208–15.

Ross M, Kouretas P, Gamberg P, Miller J, Burge M, Reitz B, Robbins R, Chin C, Bernstein D. Ten- and 20-year survivors of pediatric orthotopic heart transplantation. J Heart Lung Transplant Off Publ Int Soc Heart Transplant. 2006;25:261–70.

Seipelt IM, Pahl E, Seipelt RG, Mavroudis C, Backer CL, Stellmach V, Cornwell M, Crawford SE. Neointimal inflammation and adventitial angiogenesis correlate with severity of cardiac allograft vasculopathy in pediatric recipients. J Heart Lung Transplant Off Publ Int Soc Heart Transplant. 2005;24:1039–45.

Stewart S, Winters GL, Fishbein MC, Tazelaar HD, Kobashigawa J, Abrams J, Andersen CB, Angelini A, Berry GJ, Burke MM, Demetris AJ, Hammond E, Itescu S, Marboe CC, McManus B, Reed EF, Reinsmoen NL, Rodriguez ER, Rose AG, Rose M, Suciu-Focia N, Zeevi A, Billingham ME. Revision of the 1990 working formulation for the standardization of nomenclature in the diagnosis of heart rejection. J Heart Lung Transplant Off Publ Int Soc Heart Transplant. 2005;24:1710–20.

Thrush PT, Hoffman TM. Pediatric heart transplantation-indications and outcomes in the current era. J Thorac Dis. 2014;6:1080–96.

Tjang YS, Stenlund H, Tenderich G, Hornik L, Bairaktaris A, Korfer R. Risk factor analysis in pediatric heart transplantation. J Heart Lung Transplant Off Publ Int Soc Heart Transplant. 2008;27:408–15.

Urschel S, Larsen IM, Kirk R, Flett J, Burch M, Shaw N, Birnbaum J, Netz H, Pahl E, Matthews KL, Chinnock R, Johnston JK, Derkatz K, West LJ. Abo-incompatible heart transplantation in early childhood: an international multicenter study of clinical experiences and limits. J Heart Lung Transplant Off Publ Int Soc Heart Transplant. 2013;32:285–92.

Voeller RK, Epstein DJ, Guthrie TJ, Gandhi SK, Canter CE, Huddleston CB. Trends in the indications and survival in pediatric heart transplants: a 24-year single-center experience in 307 patients. Ann Thorac Surg. 2012;94:807–15; discussion 815–806.

Wagner K, Oliver MC, Boyle GJ, Miller SA, Law YM, Pigula F, Webber SA. Endomyocardial biopsy in pediatric heart transplant recipients: a useful exercise? (analysis of 1,169 biopsies). Pediatr Transplant. 2000;4:186–92.

Webber SA, Naftel DC, Parker J, Mulla N, Balfour I, Kirklin JK, Morrow R, Pediatric Heart Transplant Study G. Late rejection episodes more than 1 year after pediatric heart transplantation: risk factors and outcomes. J Heart Lung Transplant Off Publ Int Soc Heart Transplant. 2003;22:869–75.

West LJ. Antibodies and abo-incompatibility in pediatric transplantation. Pediatr Transplant. 2011;15:778–83.

Wright EJ, Fiser WP, Edens RE, Frazier EA, Morrow WR, Imamura M, Jaquiss RD. Cardiac transplant outcomes in pediatric patients with pre-formed anti-human leukocyte antigen antibodies and/or positive retrospective crossmatch. J Heart Lung Transplant Off Publ Int Soc Heart Transplant. 2007;26:1163–9.

Wu GW, Kobashigawa JA, Fishbein MC, Patel JK, Kittleson MM, Reed EF, Kiyosaki KK, Ardehali A. Asymptomatic antibody-mediated rejection after heart transplantation predicts poor outcomes. J Heart Lung Transplant Off Publ Int Soc Heart Transplant. 2009;28:417–22.

Xu Y, Galambos C, Reyes-Mugica M, Miller SA, Zeevi A, Webber SA, Feingold B. Utility of c4d immunostaining in the first year after pediatric and young adult heart transplantation. J Heart Lung Transplant Off Publ Int Soc Heart Transplant. 2013;32:92–7.

Zeevi A, Lunz J, Feingold B, Shullo M, Bermudez C, Teuteberg J, Webber S. Persistent strong anti-hla antibody at high titer is complement binding and associated with increased risk of antibody-mediated rejection in heart transplant recipients. J Heart Lung Transplant Off Publ Int Soc Heart Transplant. 2013;32:98–105.

Combined Heart Transplants

23

Martin Goddard

Contents

23.1 Background

Heart transplants have been undertaken in combination with other solid organs including the lungs, kidney, liver, and also bone marrow for many years. There are no well-established criteria or indications for these combined transplants, but the medical literature demonstrates a number of individual case studies and several series from larger single centers, and registry data show a steady increase over time of combined procedures.

The indications for combined transplants are varied and depend on the organ pairing and, however, can usually be viewed under the following criteria:

1. End-stage cardiac disease and other organ diseases because of related causes
2. End-stage cardiac disease and other organ diseases because of unrelated causes
3. End-stage cardiac with other organ transplants to correct an underlying disorder

While the outcomes of combined transplants are generally good and comparable to single-organ transplants in long-term survival, there remains the dilemma of the optimal usage of a limited donor supply and the need to use two or more organs for a single case.

23.2 Heart and Liver

The first combined heart and liver transplant was performed in 1983. As of 2014, against a background of almost 60,000 heart transplants in the USA, only 163 combined heart-liver transplants

M. Goddard
Department of Pathology, Papworth Hospital NHS Trust, Cambridge, UK
e-mail: Martin.Goddard@papworth.nhs.uk

O. Leone et al. (eds.), *The Pathology of Cardiac Transplantation*,
DOI 10.1007/978-3-319-46386-5_23

had been performed, of which 25 had been combined with a third organ transplant (13 kidney and 12 lung). Technically, the cardiac implant is usually undertaken first to reduce the ischemic time, although there are reports of the liver being implanted first in cases of recipients with high antibody titers (Cannon et al. 2012).

The most common disease indication is transthyretin (TTR)-related amyloidosis which accounts for 25–30 % of the cases in most reported series. This is a hereditary systemic form of amyloidosis caused by mutations in the gene encoding for TTR, a protein predominantly synthesized in the liver.

In this example, the rationale is to eliminate the site of the abnormal protein synthesis, stabilize or even reverse the stigmata of amyloid infiltration, and prevent the accumulation of amyloid in the transplanted organ (Llado et al. 2014).

The major metabolic indications for combined liver and heart transplants, in adults have been hemochromatosis (an iron storage disorder) and familial hypercholesterolaemia where the cardiac manifestation of the disease is accelerated atherosclerosis and ischemic heart disease (Alkofer et al. 2005).

In the unrelated causes reported, the most common is a nonischemic cardiomyopathy associated with a hepatitis C-related cirrhosis. Occasional cases have been undertaken for alcohol-related cardiac and liver disease (Befeler et al. 1999).

Prolonged and severe cardiac failure can lead to an irreversible cardiac cirrhosis of sufficient severity to merit transplantation. A degree of liver dysfunction is well recognized in cardiac failure and tends to improve post-cardiac transplantation. A few combined transplants have been undertaken but only in the presence of established liver failure. It is equally recognized that there is a degree of myocardial dysfunction in patients with cirrhosis, sometimes termed cirrhotic cardiomyopathy, with improvement of cardiac function following liver transplantation. The careful combined assessment of the patient, often with a pretransplant biopsy of the affected organ, is essential before the listing decision is made.

Outcome studies for combined heart and liver transplant have demonstrated that graft survival of both heart and liver is as good as that seen in individual organ transplantation. Published survival rates of this cohort at 1, 5, and 10 years are 83.4 %, 72.8 %, and 71.0 %.

23.3 Heart and Kidney

The first report of a combined heart and kidney transplant was published in 1978. The United Network for Organ Sharing (UNOS) has recorded from 1987 to 2013 that 910 combined heart and kidney transplants were performed although the rate has increased across time and increasing numbers of patients are being listed for combined procedures.

There are no standardized guidelines for a combined heart and kidney transplant, although certain exclusion criteria have been proposed. These include recipient age >65, history of peripheral vascular disease, ischemic origin of the heart failure, and the use of a ventricular assist device as a bridge to transplantation, but these are by no means widely agreed.

In patients presenting pretransplant with coexisting cardiac and renal disease, the presence of severe irreversible renal dysfunction is considered a contraindication for isolated heart transplant. The generally acceptable renal function for an isolated heart transplant is a glomerular filtration rate (GFR) of more than 40 ml/min following hemodynamic optimization (Banner et al. 2011; de Jonge et al. 2008). A GFR below this has been cited as an indication for combined heart and kidney transplantation.

It should be remembered that the majority of patients with heart failure will exhibit some renal dysfunction, primarily due to the lack of adequate perfusion related to poor heart function or secondary to related conditions such as hypertension and diabetes mellitus. And while renal failure has been considered a contraindication to cardiac transplantation, it is recognized that many patients will show an improvement in renal function following cardiac transplantation.

Neither the cause of the heart failure nor the level of creatinine or proteinuria can reliably

Table 23.1 Renal dysfunction following heart transplantation

Outcome	Within 1 year	Within 5 years
Renal dysfunction	22.9 %	54.6 %
Abnormal creatinine ≤2.5 mg/dl	16 %	36.4 %
Abnormal creatinine >2.5 mg/dl	5.1 %	14.5 %
Dialysis	1.7 %	3 %
Renal transplant	0.1 %	0.7 %

predict the renal pathologic diagnosis or the degree or tubular atrophy/interstitial fibrosis of the native kidneys or the degree of improvement following heart transplant.

In published series, the underlying kidney disease has included: IgA nephropathy, diabetic nephropathy, nephrosclerosis, glomerulonephritis, chronic interstitial nephritis, and polycystic kidney disease.

Graft survival for the heart and kidney is comparable to that for the individual organs with no increase in early mortality (Bacchi et al. 2011).

Chronic kidney disease following cardiac transplantation is a major cause of morbidity and mortality and reflects the presence of pre-existing renal dysfunction and the nephrotoxic effects of some of the necessary immunosuppressant drugs. The incidence of chronic renal failure (GFR of 29 ml/min/1.73 m^2 of body surface area or less), 5 years after heart transplantation, is estimated at 7–21 %. Some patients have gone on to have kidney transplants some years after their heart transplant for end-stage renal failure.

Table 23.1 shows data on renal dysfunction after heart transplantation from the International Society for Heart and Lung transplantation (ISHLT) (Yusen et al. 2014).

23.4 Heart and Lung

Combined heart and lung transplants are typically undertaken for end-stage cardiopulmonary failure. The initial disease may lie in either the heart or the lung but has led to the development of irreversible changes within the other organ and the need for a combined procedure.

End-stage cardiac and pulmonary diseases which lead to combined transplantation because of related causes are:

- Congenital cardiac anomalies with pulmonary hypertension (Eisenmenger's complex) (Hayes et al. 2013; Goldberg et al. 2014)
- Acquired heart disease with secondary pulmonary hypertension (Farber and Gibbs 2015)
- Pulmonary hypertension with irreversible right heart failure
- Other lung diseases with compromised cardiac function, e.g., bronchiectasis, chronic obstructive pulmonary disease, or idiopathic pulmonary fibrosis (rare)

Unrelated diseases are cardiomyopathy and chronic obstructive pulmonary disease.

Another disorder which can involve both the lungs and heart and requires the combined procedure, although anecdotal, is sarcoidosis (Morisse Pradier et al. 2016).

Worldwide, the number of heart-lung transplants performed has fallen from a peak of 220 per year in the early 1990s to about 80 per year. Approximately one third are performed for congenital heart disease, with the second largest indication being idiopathic pulmonary hypertension (Fig. 23.1). While historically heart-lung transplants were performed for cystic fibrosis and the explanted heart removed was used for a domino transplantation in another patient, this has become much less frequent.

More than 80 % of recipients are under 50 years of age at the time of transplantation. Long-term survival is similar to that of lung transplants with survival limited by chronic lung allograft dysfunction rather than coronary artery vasculopathy.

23.5 Heart and Bone Marrow

In a few cases of patients with acquired monoclonal immunoglobulin light-chain amyloidosis (AL), when the amyloid disease was heart

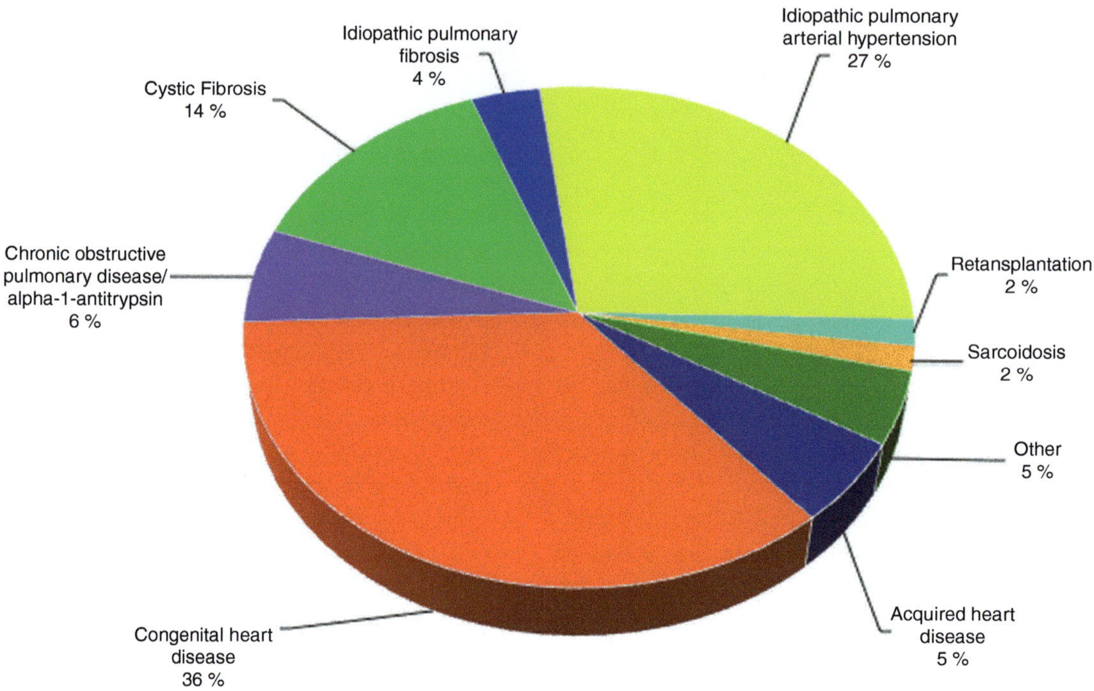

Fig. 23.1 Modified from the ISHLT 2015 Registry – heart-lung transplantation online slides: adult recipient diagnosis (January 1982–June 2013). "Other" includes cancer, lymphangio-leiomyomatosis, obliterans bronchiolitis (Yusen et al. 2014)

dominant with minimal or no other organ involvement, heart transplant has been combined with high-dose posttransplant chemotherapy and autologous peripheral blood stem cell transplantation.

In the report from Lacy et al. where 11 patients underwent sequential orthotopic heart transplantation (HT) followed by autologous peripheral blood stem cell transplantation (SCT) for treatment of AL amyloidosis, the 1- and 5-year survival for HT was 82% and 65% (Lacy et al. 2008).

More recent data show that patients with light-chain amyloidosis surviving to heart transplantation followed by autologous stem cell transplantation have a survival rate similar to other cardiomyopathy patients undergoing heart transplantation (Gray Gilstrap et al. 2014).

This approach can therefore offer an option for AL amyloidosis.

23.6 Principle Reasons for Combined Transplantation

23.6.1 Amyloidosis

Amyloidosis is a protein conformation disorder and includes a large group of diseases caused by extracellular deposition of amyloid, a pathologic proteinaceous substance, made up of abnormal insoluble fibrils of misfolded proteins, which can impair tissue structure and the function of several organs. Electron microscopy shows amyloid to be formed from non-branching fibrils with a diameter of 7.5–10 nm: these have been shown through X-ray crystallography to be arranged in a cross beta-pleated sheet, irrespective of their chemical composition; this particular conformation is at the basis of the typical green birefringence when amyloid is observed under polarized light using Congo red staining (see Chap. 5).

Amyloidosis may be systemic or localized and is currently classified according to type of precursor protein (Westermark et al. 2002).

The two most frequent types of systemic amyloidosis involving the heart, which can be considered for combined transplantation, are acquired monoclonal immunoglobulin light-chain amyloidosis (AL) and hereditary TTR-related forms (ATTR) (Walley et al. 1995), which should be considered as distinct diseases, probably characterized by different pathophysiological substrates and courses (Rapezzi et al. 2009). Cardiac localization has major clinical implications and is the main indicator of unfavorable prognosis: its presence and extent vary considerably depending on form.

In AL amyloidosis, the majority of patients have an underlying plasma cell dyscrasia, the best characterized of which is multiple myeloma, a malignant expansion of plasma cells, which produce excess amounts of a single immunoglobulin (monoclonal gammopathy). The occurrence of systemic AL amyloid in these patients is 5–15 %. These plasma cells may also produce an excess of light chains which may be detected in the urine as Bence-Jones proteins. The majority of cases with AL amyloid do not have an overt B-cell neoplasm, although monoclonal immunoglobulins or light chains are often detectable. In AL cardiac involvement is usually substantial and present in around half of cases (Falk and Dubrey 2010)

Transthyretin is a normal serum protein which transports thyroxine and retinol in the serum. In its normal form – wild-type/nonmutant – it may be deposited in the heart of elderly individuals and is referred to as senile cardiac amyloid. In familial amyloidosis, the precursor protein is a genetically mutant form of TTR, which with its fragments is deposited in tissues in a group of disorders termed the familial associated polyneuropathies (FAP) (Planté-Bordeneuve and Kershen 2013). More than 100 mutations of the gene have been described, and the type of mutation appears to influence the phenotype of the disease (Rapezzi et al. 2010).

The disease is transmitted as an autosomal dominant with high penetrance. Overall the disease typically presents in the third decade with a polyneuropathy or dysautonomia due to the deposition of the amyloid in peripheral nerves. However, some mutations such as Thr59Lys or Glu89Lys give rise to predominantly cardiac involvement (Rapezzi et al. 2010). A Thr-60-Ala amino acid substitution is also usually associated with a cardiac presentation (heart failure and conduction system disturbances and minimal neuropathy); a Val-122-Iso substitution can also present, mainly with cardiac disease, often a late-onset cardiomyopathy with progressive heart failure showing a restrictive pattern and predominant signs of right heart failure. In ATTR, the prevalence of cardiac involvement is highly variable depending on mutation type (Falk and Dubrey 2010; Shah et al. 2006).

23.6.2 Hemochromatosis

Hemochromatosis is characterized by excess iron being deposited in parenchymal organs primarily the liver and the pancreas. Humans are unable to excrete excess iron, and the total body iron store is regulated through control of absorption. Primary hemochromatosis arises from a defect in a human hemochromatosis protein known as HFE (human gene encoding a protein which regulates the intestinal absorption of iron). The disease is inherited as a homozygous recessive disorder. In Europe, approximately 9 % of the population are heterozygotes with a homozygosity frequency of 0.45 % making it one of the commonest inherited disease. However, the penetrance of the disorder is only 20 %, so not all homozygotes express the disease phenotype. The gene is expressed on the basolateral aspect of small intestinal crypt epithelial cells and facilitates the binding of transferrin to its receptor. In its absence the loss of regulation of the intracellular iron pool leads to excess absorption. Secondary hemochromatosis – hemosiderosis –

arises from blood transfusion and is associated with hemolytic anemias and ineffective erythropoiesis.

Diagnosis of iron overload is made on the finding of a transferrin saturation >55 % and elevated serum ferritin (>300 ng/ml) (Gulati et al. 2014).

The heart may be involved with other organs or may be the major site affected. Clinically the presentation is usually of cardiac failure often with a congestive or restrictive physiology. There may be atrial and ventricular arrhythmia and atrioventricular nodal block. Cardiac magnetic resonance imaging with measurement of T2* relaxation times can help quantify myocardial iron load and also monitor reduction with treatment (Murphy and Oudit 2010).

Macroscopically the heart is often enlarged and dilated and may have a brown hue to the myocardium. The hemosiderin is deposited in myocytes predominantly in the perinuclear zones and can be easily demonstrated with Perls Prussian blue stain (Fig. 23.2). Accompanying fibrosis both interstitial and perimyocytic is usually mild. The conduction system may be involved, but deposition in the sinoatrial node is said to be uncommon (Olson et al. 1987).

Average survival following diagnosis is less than a year in severe cardiac impairment; however, early identification and treatment with iron chelation and venesection to remove the excess iron can lead to improved cardiac function and improve survival rates to that of the regular heart failure population.

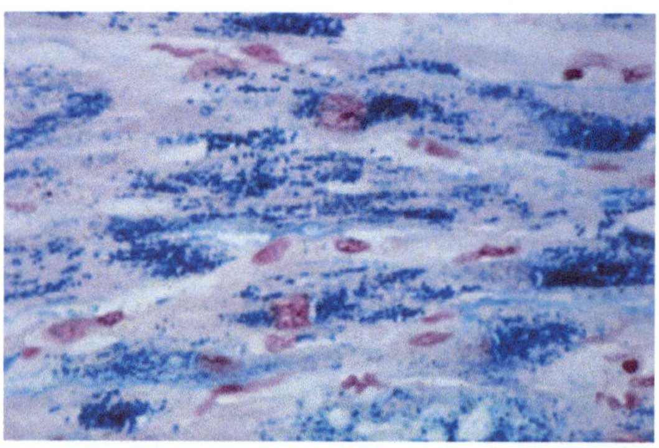

Fig. 23.2 Excess iron in myocardium in hemochromatosis. Perls *Prussian blue*, 400×

23.6.3 Eisenmenger's Syndrome

Eisenmenger's syndrome arises as a complication of congenital heart disease most commonly when there is a shunt from the left to the right side of the heart with increased blood flow resulting in pulmonary hypertension. With worsening of the hypertension, the shunt reverses with unoxygenated blood passing from the right side to the left leading to cyanosis and symptoms of breathlessness, palpitations, and syncope.

The major causes are ventricular septal defects, atrial septal defects, patent ductus arteriosus, and atrioventricular canal defects. These defects result in a hyperkinetic circulation with both a greater volume and higher blood pressure in the pulmonary circulation. In atrial septal defects, the problem is largely one of volume, and pulmonary hypertension rarely develops before middle age. With ventricular septal defects (Fig. 23.3) and patent ductuses, there is a substantial increase in pressure, and changes in the pulmonary vasculature occur much earlier (Gatzoulis et al. 2014).

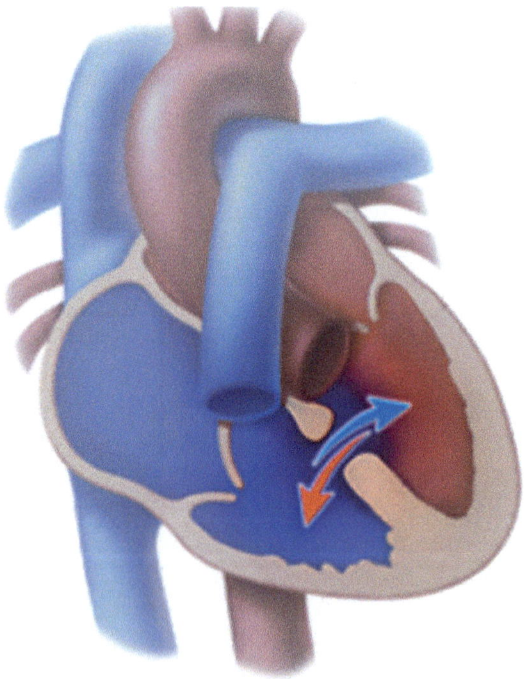

Fig. 23.3 Diagrammatic representation of a ventricular septal defect

The heart will show the underlying cardiac defect although, if surgical correction has been performed, it may be difficult to demonstrate. The major pathological changes are seen in the pulmonary vasculature. The small arteries and arterioles (40–300 um diameter) will show striking intimal thickening and medial hypertrophy, and there are characteristic plexiform lesions within small arteries. Larger vessels show intimal thickening and early atheroma.

23.6.4 Pulmonary Hypertension

The current classification of pulmonary hypertension includes five categories (Galiè et al. 2016):

1. Pulmonary arterial hypertension (PAH)
2. Pulmonary hypertension due to left heart disease
3. Pulmonary hypertension due to lung diseases and/or hypoxia
4. Chronic thromboembolic pulmonary hypertension (CTEPH) and other pulmonary artery obstructions
5. Pulmonary hypertension with unclear and/or multifactorial mechanisms

The first group comprises "different forms that share a similar clinical picture and virtually identical pathological changes of the lung microcirculation" (Galiè et al. 2016). It now includes pulmonary arteriopathy – previously known as primary pulmonary hypertension – and the subsets of pulmonary veno-occlusive disease (PVOD) and/or pulmonary capillary hemangiomatosis (PCH) and of persistent pulmonary hypertension of the newborn.

Primary or idiopathic pulmonary hypertension is largely sporadic, but up to 6 % of cases are familial with an autosomal dominant mode of inheritance, although penetrance is variable and only 10–20 % of the family members actually develop the disease. Investigations of these family groups have shown defects in the bone morphogenetic protein receptor 2 (BMPR2) and its signaling pathway. BMPR2 is part of the transforming growth factor-beta receptor super family. In vascular smooth muscle cells, BMPR2 stimulation leads to inhibition of proliferation and promotes apoptosis (Liu and Morrell 2013).

Pulmonary hypertension is a disease of the pulmonary vessels (Tuder et al. 2013): the pathological classification of vasculopathies in pulmonary hypertension drawn up at the Third World Symposium on Pulmonary Hypertension in Venice in 2003 (Pietra et al. 2004), adopted a descriptive histopathologic system of classification with four main categories and subsets (Table 23.2). Pulmonary arteriopathy affects pre- and intra-acinar arteries and is characterized by numerous elementary lesions, subdivided into constrictive (medial hypertrophy, intimal and adventitial thickening) (Fig. 23.4) and complex arterial lesions (plexiform and dilatation lesions and arteritis) (Fig. 23.5).

The main pathology of pulmonary occlusive venopathy (formerly PVOD) consists of extensive and diffuse occlusion and/or stenosis of pulmonary venules and veins of various sizes, usually intralobular and interlobular (Fig. 23.6). Pulmonary microvasculopathy (formerly PCH) is a rare condition characterized by localized capillary proliferation within the pulmonary interstitium.

Drug therapies have improved the treatment and prognosis of pulmonary hypertension, and even in severe cases where transplant is deemed necessary, bilateral lung transplant is the most common approach as the right heart can remodel after transplantation. Heart and lung transplant is only required in cases of end-stage right ventricular failure or if there is evidence of left-sided heart failure. In these cases the right side of the heart is greatly dilated and the free wall thickened with a non-trabecular wall thickness >0.8 cm. In addition, there is septal deviation with bulging of the septum into the left ventricular cavity which may impair left ventricular function. Microscopically there is myocyte hypertrophy with prominent nuclear enlargement and a variable amount of interstitial fibrosis.

Table 23.2 Pathological classification of vasculopathies of pulmonary hypertension[a]

1. Pulmonary arteriopathy (pre- and intra-acinar arteries)	Previous WHO terminology[b]
Subsets	
Pulmonary arteriopathy with isolated medial hypertrophy	Pulmonary plexogenic arteriopathy Gr. 1
Pulmonary arteriopathy with medial hypertrophy and intimal thickening (cellular, fibrotic)	
Concentric laminar	Pulmonary plexogenic arteriopathy Gr. 2, 3
Eccentric, concentric nonlaminar	Pulmonary embolic arteriopathy
Pulmonary arteriopathy with plexiform and/or dilation lesions or arteritis	Pulmonary plexogenic arteriopathy Gr. 4–6
Pulmonary arteriopathy with isolated arteritis	n.a.
1a. As above but with coexisting venous-venular changes (cellular and/or fibrotic intimal thickening, muscularization)	n.a.
The presence of the following changes should be noted	
Adventitial thickening, thrombotic lesions (fresh, organized, recanalized, colander lesion), necrotizing or lympho-monocytic arteritis, elastic artery changes (fibrotic or atheromatous intimal plaques, elastic laminae degeneration), bronchial vessel changes, ferruginous incrustation, calcifications, foreign body emboli, organized infarct perivascular lymphocytic infiltrates	
2. Pulmonary occlusive venopathy (veins of various size and venules) with or without coexisting arteriopathy	PVOD
Histopathologic features	
Venous changes: intimal thickening/obstruction (cellular, fibrotic), obstructive fibrous luminal septa (recanalization)	
Adventitial thickening (fibrotic), muscularization, iron and calcium incrustation with foreign body reaction	
Capillary changes: dilated, congested capillaries, angioma-like lesions	
Interstitial changes: edema, fibrosis, hemosiderosis, lymphocytic infiltrates	
Others: dilated lymphatics, alveoli with hemosiderin-laden macrophages, type II cell hyperplasia	
3. Pulmonary microvasculopathy with or without coexisting arteriopathy and/or venopathy	PCH
Histopathologic features	
Microvessel changes: localized capillary proliferations within pulmonary interstitium, obstructive capillary proliferation in veins and venular walls	
Venous-venular intimal fibrosis	
Interstitial changes: edema, fibrosis, hemosiderosis	
Others: dilated lymphatics, alveoli with hemosiderin-laden macrophages, type II cell hyperplasia	
4. Unclassifiable[c]	n.a.

(From Pietra et al. 2004)

Gr. grade, *n.a.* not applicable

[a] Nonvascular lung pathology needs to be listed as separate diagnosis

[b]Primary pulmonary hypertension. Report on a WHO meeting. Geneva, October 15–17, 1975. S. Hatano and T. Strasser, eds

[c]Atypical histopathological features or inadequate sampling of blood vessels

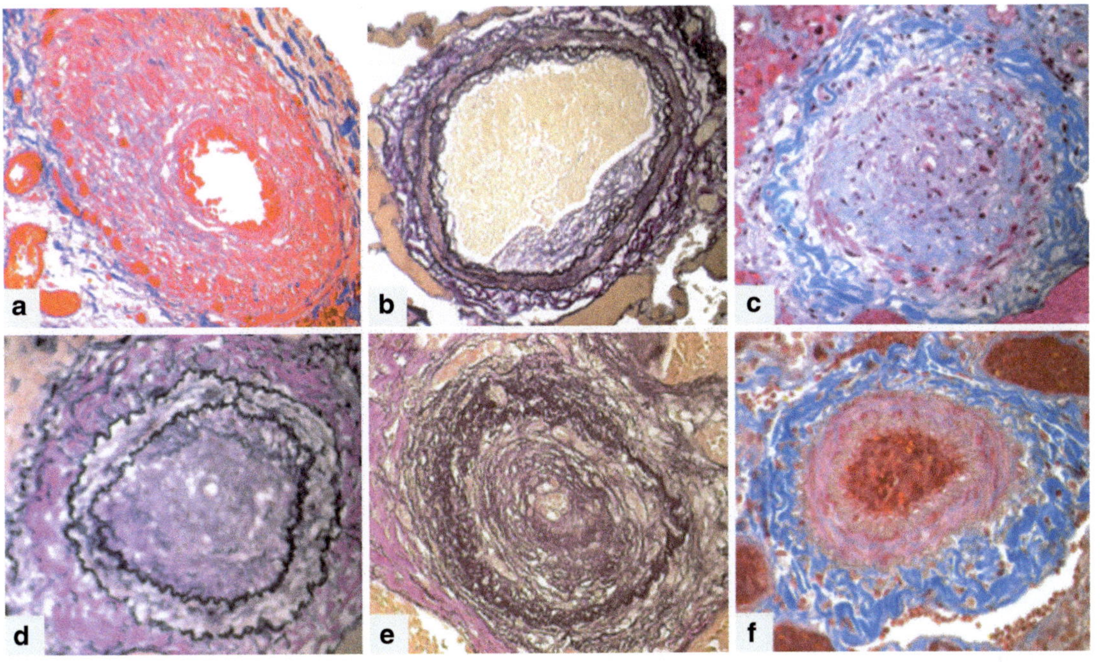

Fig. 23.4 Pulmonary arteriopathy: constrictive arterial lesions. (**a**) Medial hypertrophy (hematoxylin-eosin, 400×), (**b**) eccentric intimal thickening (Weigert-Van Gieson, 400×), (**c, d**) concentric nonlaminar intimal thickening (400×, **c** Mallory trichrome, **d** Weigert-Van Gieson), (**e**) concentric laminar intimal thickening (Weigert-Van Gieson, 400×), (**f**) adventitial thickening (Mallory trichrome, 400×) (Courtesy of Dr. O. Leone, Sant'Orsola Heart Transplant Center, Bologna-Italy)

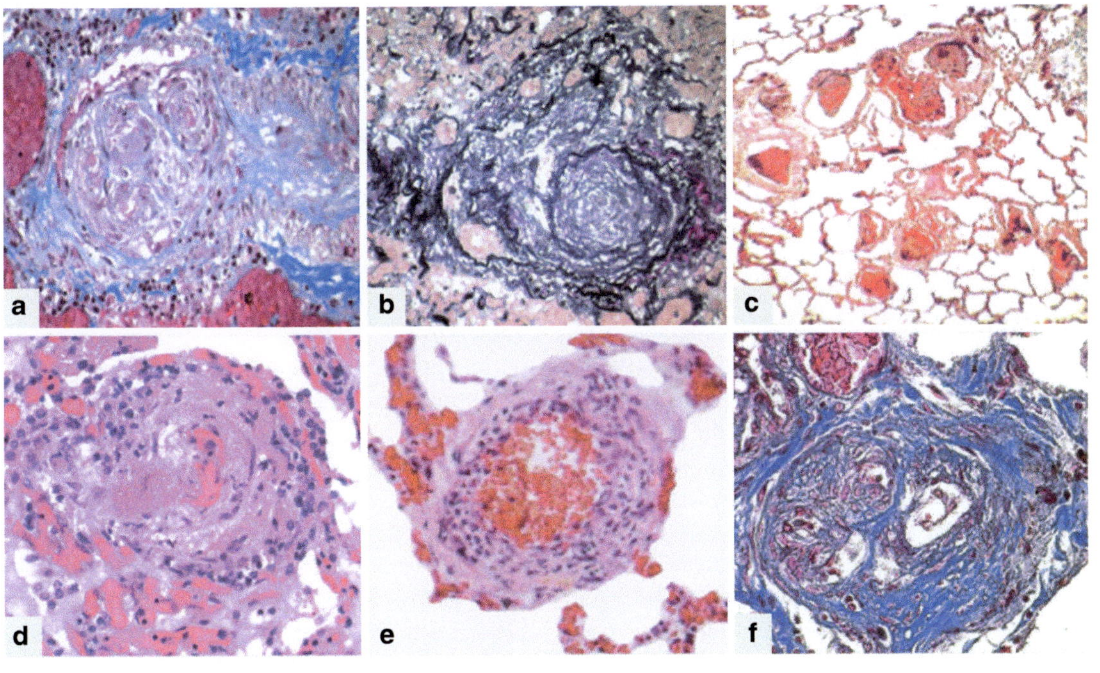

Fig. 23.5 Pulmonary arteriopathy: complex arterial lesions. (**a, b**) Plexiform lesions (**a** Mallory trichrome, 200×; **b** Weigert-Van Gieson, 200×), (**c**) dilatation (angiomatoid) lesions (hematoxylin-eosin, 200×), (**d, e**) arteritis (hematoxylin-eosin, 200×), (**f**) recanalized thrombus (Mallory trichrome, 200×) (Courtesy of Dr. O. Leone, Sant'Orsola Heart Transplant Center, Bologna, Italy)

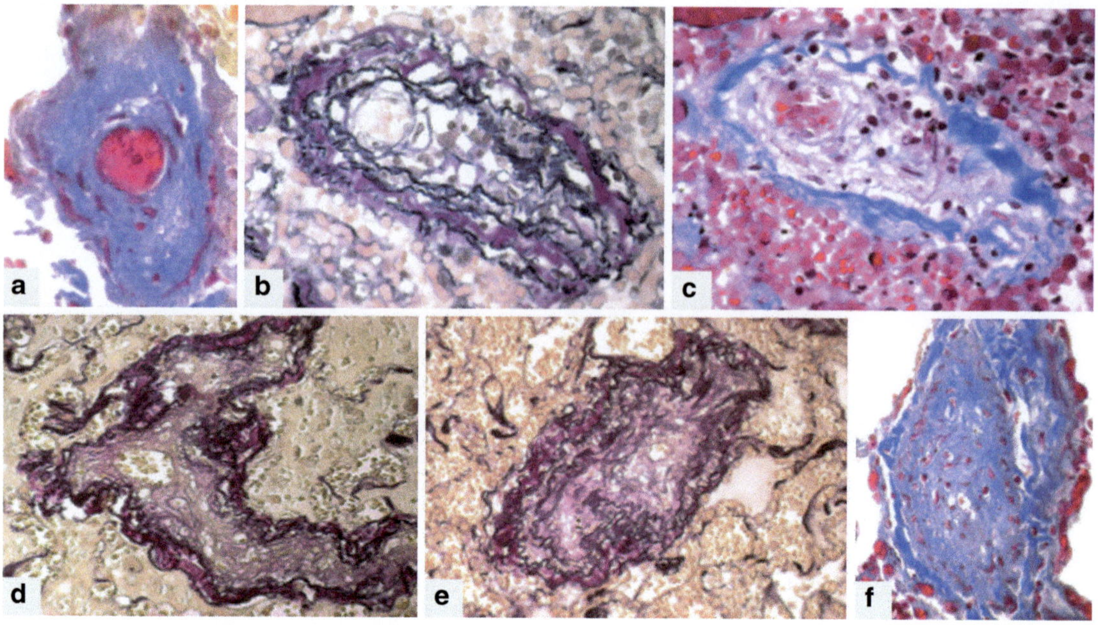

Fig. 23.6 Venous changes in pulmonary hypertension: cellular (**b**, **c**, **e**) or fibrotic intimal thickening (**a**, **d**, **f**), narrowing (**a–d**) or obstructing (**e**, **f**) the lumen of venules and little veins (Courtesy of Dr. O. Leone, Sant'Orsola Heart Transplant Center, Bologna, Italy)

23.6.5 Sarcoidosis

Sarcoidosis is a systemic disease of unknown cause, but there is growing evidence that it is a disease of disordered immune regulation in genetically predisposed individuals exposed to certain environmental factors. There is a spectrum of disease within the lung from incidental granulomas to widespread pulmonary fibrosis, and pulmonary vessels may be involved resulting in pulmonary hypertension.

Cardiac involvement in sarcoidosis has been identified in up to 30 % of all cases although less than 5 % of patients diagnosed with sarcoid in life have any cardiac symptoms. Up to half the patients present with conduction abnormalities. The sarcoidal granulomas show a predilection for certain areas of the heart particularly the fee wall of the left ventricle, atrial walls, and the conduction system. Microscopically the granulomas are well-defined non-necrotizing granulomas which include giant cells, but myocyte necrosis is typically absent and eosinophils are rare unlike giant cell myocarditis (Fig. 23.7). In healed areas there are patchy or serpiginous areas of fibrosis. In a proportion of cases, there may be involvement of the walls of the intramural coronary arteries (Silverman et al. 1978).

23.6.6 Hypercholesterolemia

Familial hypercholesterolemia is a receptor disease arising from a mutation in the gene encoding the low-density lipoprotein (LDL) receptor, which is involved in the transport of cholesterol. Elevated cholesterol leads to an early atherosclerosis and an increased risk of myocardial infarction in the second and third decades of life (Wiegman et al. 2015). The heterozygous form is common with about 1:500 carriers in the general population, and these too have a raised cholesterol level. The LDL receptor is mainly expressed on hepatocytes, and the liver is responsible for clearing approximately 70 % of the LDL from the circulation. This has been the rationale behind the few heart and liver transplants undertaken for this condition.

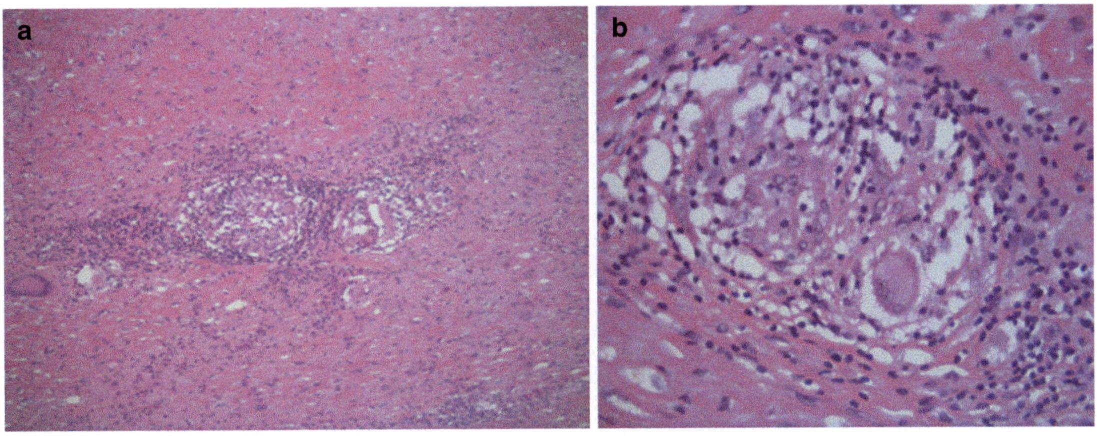

Fig. 23.7 (**a**) Myocardium containing non-caseating granulomas (hematoxylin-eosin, original magnification 100×). (**b**) High-powered view of sarcoid granuloma (hematoxylin-eosin, original magnification 400×)

23.6.7 Biopsy Protocols

Immunosuppression in cardiac transplants is generally higher than for kidney or liver transplants, and combined transplants have tended to be monitored using cardiac biopsy protocols as with isolated heart transplant. In heart and lung transplants, monitoring is through transbronchial lung biopsies according to the standard protocols.

Both liver and kidney transplants are monitored through routine blood testing, and these are used as indications for direct biopsy of the organ. Similarly, evidence of cardiac dysfunction on clinical grounds or echocardiography are used as indicators for a cardiac biopsy.

The evidence suggests that both cell-mediated and antibody-mediated rejection events are less frequent in combined transplants for reasons that are not yet understood. Furthermore, there does not appear to be a correlation between rejection episodes in the two organs.

Heart and kidney transplantation is the most frequent and the number of patients listed is increasing. The underlying kidney diseases for combined procedures are IgA nephropathy, diabetic nephropathy, nephrosclerosis, glomerulonephritis, chronic interstitial nephritis, and polycystic kidney disease.

In heart-liver transplantation, the most common indication is hereditary transthyretin-related amyloidosis (familial amyloid polyneuropathy) which accounts for 25–30 % of the cases in most reported series.

For heart-lung transplantation, congenital heart disease is the most frequent indication, with the second largest being primary pulmonary hypertension.

In a few cases of patients with AL, when amyloid disease is heart dominant with minimal or no other organ involvement, heart transplant has been combined with high-dose posttransplant chemotherapy and autologous peripheral blood stem cell transplantation.

Key Points

Indications for combined transplants depend on organ pairing and can be grouped as:

- End-stage cardiac disease and other organ diseases because of related causes
- End-stage cardiac disease and other organ diseases because of unrelated causes
- End-stage cardiac disease with other organ transplants to correct an underlying disorder

References

Alkofer BJ, Chiche L, Khayat A, Deshayes JP, Lepage A, Saloux E, Reznik Y. Liver transplant combined with heart transplant in severe heterozygous hypercholesterolemia: report of the first case and review of the literature. Transplant Proc. 2005;37(5):2250–2.

Bacchi G, Potena L, Mosconi G, Quarta C, Stalteri L, Magnani G, Feliciangeli G, Grigoni F, Branzi A, Stefoni S. Combined heart-kidney transplantation: a single centre experience. OJOTS. 2011;1:14–8.

Banner NR, Bonser RS, Clark AI, Clark S, Cowburn PJ, Gardnes RS, Kalra PR, McDonagh T, Rogers CA, Swan L, Parameshwar J, Thomas HL, Williams SG. UK guidelines for referral and assessment of adults for heart transplantation. Heart. 2011;97:1520–7.

Befeler AS, Schiano TD, Lissoos TW, Conjeevaram HS, Anderson AS, Millis JM, Albertucci M, Baker AL. Successful combined liver-heart transplantation in adults: report of three patients and review of the literature. Transplantation. 1999;68(9):1423–7.

Cannon RM, Hughes MG, Jones CM, Eng M, Marvin MR. A review of the United States experience with combined heart-liver transplantation. Transpl Int. 2012;25(12):1223–8.

de Jonge N, Kirkels JH, Klöpping C, Lahpor JR, Caliskan K, Maat APWM, Brügemann J, Erasmus ME, Klautz RJM, Verwey HF, Oomen A, Peels CH, Golüke AEJ, Nicastia D, Koole MAC, Balk AHMM. Guidelines for heart transplantation. Neth Heart J. 2008;16(3):79–87.

Falk RH, Dubrey SW. Amyloid heart disease. Prog Cardiovasc Dis. 2010;52:347–61.

Farber HW, Gibbs S. Under pressure: pulmonary hypertension associated with left heart disease. Eur Respir Rev. 2015;24(138):665–73.

Galiè N, Humbert M, Vachiery JL, Gibbs S, Lang I, Torbicki A, Simonneau G, Peacock A, Vonk Noordegraaf A, Beghetti M, Ghofrani A, Gomez Sanchez MA, Hansmann G, Klepetko W, Lancellotti P, Matucci M, McDonagh T, Pierard LA, Trindade PT, Zompatori M, Hoeper M. 2015 ESC/ERS Guidelines for the diagnosis and treatment of pulmonary hypertension: The Joint Task Force for the Diagnosis and Treatment of Pulmonary Hypertension of the European Society of Cardiology (ESC) and the European Respiratory Society (ERS)Endorsed by: Association for European Paediatric and Congenital Cardiology (AEPC), International Society for Heart and Lung Transplantation (ISHLT). Eur Heart J. 2016;69:177.

Gatzoulis MA, Beghetti M, Landzberg MJ, Galiè N. Pulmonary arterial hypertension associated with congenital heart disease: recent advances and future directions. Int J Cardiol. 2014;177(2):340–7.

Goldberg SW, Fisher SA, Wehman B, Mehra MR. Adults with congenital heart disease and heart transplantation: optimizing outcomes. J Heart Lung Transplant. 2014;33(9):873–7.

Gray Gilstrap L, Niehaus E, Malhotra R, Ton VK, Watts J, Seldin DC, Madsen JC, Semigran MJ. Predictors of survival to orthotopic heart transplant in patients with light chain amyloidosis. J Heart Lung Transplant. 2014;33(2):149–56.

Gulati V, Harikrishnan P, Palaniswamy C, Aronow WS, Jain D, Frishman WH. Cardiac involvement in hemochromatosis. Cardiol Rev. 2014;22(2):56–68.

Hayes Jr D, Galantowicz M, Hoffman TM. Combined heart-lung transplantation: a perspective on the past and the future. Pediatr Cardiol. 2013;34(2):207–12.

Lacy MQ, Dispenzieri A, Hayman SR, Kumar S, Kyle RA, Rajkumar SV, Edwards BS, Rodeheffer RJ, Frantz RP, Kushwaha SS, Clavell AL, Dearani JA, Sundt TM, Daly RC, Mc Gregor CG, Gastineau DA, Litzow MR, Gertz MA. Autologous stem cell transplant after heart transplant for light chain (Al) amyloid cardiomyopathy. J Heart Lung Transplant. 2008;27(8):823–9.

Liu D, Morrell NW. Genetics and the molecular pathogenesis of pulmonary arterial hypertension. Curr Hypertens Rep. 2013;15(6):632–7.

Llado L, Fabregat J, Ramos E, Baliellas C, Roca J, Casasnovas C. Sequential heart and liver transplantation for familial amyloid polyneuropathy. Med Clin (Barc). 2014;142(5):211–4.

Morisse Pradier H, Sénéchal A, Philit F, Tronc F, Maury JM, Grima R, Flamens C, Paulus S, Neidecker J, Mornex JF. Indications of lung transplantation: patients selection, timing of listing, and choice of procedure. Rev Pneumol Clin. 2016;72:87–94.

Murphy CJ, Oudit GY. Iron-overload cardiomyopathy: pathophysiology, diagnosis, and treatment. J Card Fail. 2010;16(11):888–900.

Olson LJ, Edwards WD, Mc Call JT, et al. Cardiac iron deposition in idiopathic hemochromatosis: histologic and analytic assessment in 14 hearts from autopsy. J Am Coll Cardiol. 1987;10:1329.

Pietra GG, Capron F, Stewart S, Leone O, Humbert M, Robbins IM, Reid LM, Tuder RM. Pathologic assessment of vasculopathies in pulmonary hypertension. J Am Coll Cardiol. 2004;43(12 Suppl S):25S–32. Review.

Planté-Bordeneuve V, Kershen P. Transthyretin familial amyloid polyneuropathy. Handb Clin Neurol. 2013;115:643–58.

Rapezzi C, Merlini G, Quarta CC, Riva L, Longhi S, Leone O, et al. Systemic cardiac amyloidoses: disease profiles and clinical courses of the 3 main types. Circulation. 2009;120:1203–12.

Rapezzi C, Quarta CC, Riva L, Longhi S, Gallelli I, Lorenzini M, et al. Transthyretin-related amyloidoses and the heart: a clinical overview. Nat Rev Cardiol. 2010;7:398–408.

Shah KB, Inoue Y, Mehra MR. Amyloidosis and the heart: a comprehensive review. Arch Intern Med. 2006;166:1805–13.

Silverman HJ, Hutchins GM, Bulkley BK. Cardiac sarcoid: a clinicopathologic evaluation of 84 unselected patients with systemic sarcoidosis. Circulation. 1978;58:1204–11.

Tuder RM, Stacher E, Robinson J, Kumar R, Graham BB. Pathology of pulmonary hypertension. Clin Chest Med. 2013;34(4):639–50.

Walley VM, Kisilevsky R, Young ID. Amyloid and the cardiovascular system: a review of pathogenesis and pathology with clinical correlation. Cardiovasc Pathol. 1995;4:79.

Westermark P, Benson MD, Buxbaum JN, Cohen AS, Frangione B, Ikeda S, Masters CL, Merlini G, Saraiva MJ, Sipe JD. Amyloid fibril protein nomenclature – 2002. Amyloid. 2002;9(3):197–200.

Wiegman A, Gidding SS, Watts GF, Chapman MJ, Ginsberg HN, Cuchel M, Ose L, Averna M, Boileau C, Borén J, Bruckert E, Catapano AL, Defesche JC, Descamps OS, Hegele RA, Hovingh GK, Humphries SE, Kovanen PT, Kuivenhoven JA, Masana L, Nordestgaard BG, Pajukanta P, Parhofer KG, Raal FJ, Ray KK, Santos RD, Stalenhoef AF, Steinhagen-Thiessen E, Stroes ES, Taskinen MR, Tybjærg-Hansen A, Wiklund O. Familial hypercholesterolaemia in children and adolescents: gaining decades of life by optimizing detection and treatment. European Atherosclerosis Society Consensus Panel. Eur Heart J. 2015;36(36):2425–37.

Yusen RD, Edwards LB, Kucheryavaya AY, Benden C, Dipchand AI, Dobbels F, Goldfarb SB, Levvey BJ, Lund LH, Meiser B, Stehlik J, International Society for Heart and Lung Transplantation. The registry of the International Society for Heart and Lung Transplantation: thirty-first adult lung and heart-lung transplant report-2014; focus theme: retransplantation. J Heart Lung Transplant. 2014;33(10):1009–24.

The Autopsy in Heart Transplantation

24

Annalisa Angelini, Marny Fedrigo, and Margaret Burke

Contents

A. Angelini (✉)
Pathology of Cardiac Transplantation and Regenerative Medicine Unit, Department of Cardiac, Thoracic and Vascular Sciences, University of Padua, Padua, Italy
e-mail: annalisa.angelini@unipd.it

M. Fedrigo
Cardiovascular Pathology Unit, Department of Cardiac, Thoracic and Vascular Sciences, Azienda Ospedaliera Padua, Padua, Italy
e-mail: marny.fedrigo@unipd.it

M. Burke
Department of Histopathology, Harefield Hospital, Royal Brompton and Harefield NHS Trust, London, UK
e-mail: M.Burke@rbht.nhs.uk

24.1 Background

The outcome after heart transplantation has improved considerably in recent years with a survival rate of up to 85 % reported at 1 year, 72.5 % at 5 years and 57 % at 10 years (Lund 2014). The major drop in survival is in the first 3 months after transplantation with a more gradual decrease thereafter. Accurate identification of the cause of death represents an important step in the management of heart transplant recipients with the potential to influence clinical diagnosis and therapy in subsequent recipients and to identify unexpected pathologies of donor and recipient origin.

A full clinical, or hospital autopsy remains the gold standard for identification of the cause of death. In recent years we have seen a steady drop in the rate of hospital autopsies worldwide often for cultural and economic reasons, with some detractors questioning its cost-benefit ratio. In some countries the autopsy rate has fallen to about 10 % of all deaths in teaching hospitals, reaching 5 % or less in general hospitals. There has also been a change in the levels

O. Leone et al. (eds.), *The Pathology of Cardiac Transplantation*,
DOI 10.1007/978-3-319-46386-5_24

of autopsy-detected diagnostic errors over time (Shojania et al. 2003). The failure to glean information from the hospital autopsy can affect medical standards of care and scientific validation of public health measures introduced to reduce morbidity and mortality and improve quality of life. The falling autopsy rates nowadays extends even to heart transplant centers where, in contrast to experience in the eighties and nineties, transplant physicians are now more confident in the management of their patients, many of whom are followed up in peripheral centers far from the Transplant Unit which "owns" them and where an ever-increasing number may die unexpectedly. However we consider that the autopsy procedure still has an important role to play in the medicine of the new millennium.

Although substantial data have been reported on causes of death in the transplant population (Rose et al. 1992; Sanroman et al. 2004; Graham 1992; Gallo et al. 1997), most autopsy-based studies were confined to initial experience gained in cardiac transplantation and date back 10 or 20 years. Starting with the early studies of Alan Rose in early nineties (Rose et al. 1992), these papers highlighted the need for the autopsy mainly in reporting epidemiological data on the cause of death from single institutions and focusing on differences in causation of early and late death or on the mode of death and its underlying causes (Chantranuwat et al. 2004; Alexander and Steenbergen 2003; Patel et al. 1996; Vaseghi et al. 2009; Zuppan et al. 2009) (Table 24.1). A very important aspect has been the issue of sudden unexpected death. Among others, Chantranuwat et al. (2004) looked at sudden, unexpected death in a cohort of cardiac transplant recipients and found acute cellular rejection and coronary artery disease to be the most frequent cause (39 % each), with no anatomic cause demonstrated in a further, significant number of cases (32 %). A recent paper from a Brazilian group reported that, in their experience, about one third of autopsies showed discrepancies between clinical and autopsy findings which may have impacted on management of their recipients (Valette et al. 2014).

Regardless of the experience of individual transplant programmes the autopsy can still reveal unexpected pathology and often sheds light on details of the final illness. Hence it is important to discuss the pathological findings with the clinician in order to reach a correct final diagnosis that is helpful for both clinician and families.

24.2 Role of Autopsy in Transplantation

The autopsy remains a key investigation in the integration of medical knowledge in cardiac transplantation with several well-defined roles (Table 24.2). Its key role is *diagnosis* and *identification of the cause(s) of death*; this requires assessment of the technical aspects of the transplant and any subsequent surgical procedures and interventions, and the identification of medical complications of transplantation and of immunosuppression. It is essential to identify all graft-related and systemic comorbidities. A comprehensive report should include the cause of death, expressed according to international norms (e.g. World Health Organisation 2015, ICD10) and a full clinicopathological correlation. Before signing out the final report the case should be reviewed and discussed with the clinician to ensure that all questions have been addressed.

In modern medicine *clinical governance* systems should be in place to facilitate quality assurance and clinical audit. This applies no less to the autopsy than to diagnosis, management and treatment of the patient in life. Pathologists should ensure that the quality of the autopsy procedure and report is subject to audit internally and through quality assurance schemes and peer review. Regular mortality review meetings should be held with the compulsory presence of all clinicians and ancillary staff involved in the management of the transplant recipients.

The third role is *education* for undergraduate and postgraduate medical students and experts from other professions. The autopsy provides an opportunity to educate and train clinicians and pathologists through its unrivalled impact and immediacy, presenting educational opportunities through case review and audit as well as attendance at and involvement in the procedure itself.

The fourth role is *research* which can be generated through the collection of tissues during the autopsy. This can be for individual ongoing projects using stored tissue left over from diag-

Table 24.1 Reviews reporting significant number of autopsy in heart transplantation

Authors	Journal and year	No. autopsy	Key points
Rose AG	*Arch Pathol Lab Med.* 1992;116(11):1137–41.	81	Infection, together with acute and/or chronic rejection, is still the major causes of death in HTX pts.
Graham AR	*Am J Clin Patrol.* 1992;97(3):369–75.	44 (80 % rate)	25 % autopsy had gastrointestinal and/or pancreatic abnormalities (mucosal inflammation, erosions or hemorrhage and pancreatitis). 64 % pts with rejection had had an episode of rejection 3 weeks after Tx and/or one episode of severe rejection
Patel VS	*Circulation.* 1996;94:II273–7.	13/25 SD (incidence for all death of 9.7 %)	20 % died < or = 12 months, 80 % died after > 12 mo, and 20 % died after > or = 60 months. CAD in 92 % and rejection in 15 % autopsy (grade > 3A). Of the deaths, 64 % occurred within 3 months from last EMBs, 96 % had normal EMBs, and the only rejection was without hemodynamic compromise.
Gallo P	*J Heart Lung Transplant.* 1997;16(11): 113–21	97 (1985–1995) with >2years follow-up	In late death Graft vasculopathy was the main cause (40 %). Tumors ranked second (23 %). Emergence of disease recurrence was confined to longer follow-up (>5years).
Alexander RT	*Am J Clin Pathol.* 2003;119(5):740–8.	39	SD in 27 % of cases. Pulmonary hypertensive arteriopathy was associated with early death and right-sided heart failure.
Chantranuwat C	*J Heart Lung Transplant.* 2004;23(6):683–9.	28/79 SD (37.8 %)	SD is common (37.8 % of all deaths). ACR, in the first year, and CAV, afterwards, are associated with SD. Cardiac hypertrophy is not increased and coronary thrombosis is not more frequent in pts who died suddenly.
Sanromán Budiño B	*Transplant Proc.* 2004;36(3):787–9.	76	Infections are the main cause of death <1 year, 30 % of other pathologies were represented by pulmonary embolism, central nervous system pathology, acute pancreatitis, digestive hemorrhage and acute myocardial infarction.
Zuppan C	*J Heart Lung Transplant.* 2009;28:579–84	128 autopsy/168 death (pediatric experience)	Early death: Acute graft dysfunction and technical issues. Late deaths : acute rejection and CAV. A significant number of late SD due to Acute rejection
Valette TN	*Arq Bras Cardiol.* 2014; 102(5):505–509	48 (10 years interval)	Discrepancies between clinical diagnosis and necroscopic findings do exist. 29 (60.4 %) had concordant clinical and necroscopic diagnoses, 16 (33.3 %) had discordant diagnoses and three (6.3 %) had unclear diagnoses. Among the discordant ones, 15 (31.3 %) had possible impact on survival and 1 (2.1 %) had no impact on survival

Table 24.2 Role of the autopsy in cardiac transplantation

1. Diagnosis and identification of the cause of death
Assessment of technical aspects of the transplant procedure
Identification of the complications of transplantation and of immunosuppression
Identification of comorbidities (other graft-related, systemic and iatrogenic pathology)
2. Clinical governance
Quality control
Transplant-related clinical audit
3. Education
Undergraduate, postgraduate and clinical teaching
4. Research
Collaborative retrospective studies using material surplus to diagnosis (bioarchives)
Regenerative medicine
Validation of imaging techniques
Biobanking
5. Public health monitoring

nosis (the diagnostic *bioarchive*) or by donation of tissue samples for the primary purpose of research to an institutionally or regionally regulated *biobank* with appropriate staffing, facilities and procedures for authorized tissue collection, storage and release for ethically approved research studies.

The fifth role is data collection for *public health monitoring*. This includes feedback of appropriately anonymized autopsy data to each country's Office of National Statistics or equivalent organization. For transplantation there should also be feedback to the relevant transplant coordinating center, e.g., the National Italian Transplant Centre (http://www.trapianti.salute.gov.it) and the UK's NHS Blood and Transplant (http://www.nhsbt.nhs.uk) for purposes of monitoring transplant program activity. Likewise input of coded autopsy data to Registries such as that managed by the International Society for Heart and Lung Transplantation (ISHLT, http://www.ishlt.org) ensures access to the latest data when establishing and evaluating new transplant programmes, devising collaborative research studies and updating international protocols of practice.

24.3 Types of Autopsy

Hospital autopsies are usually performed by a pathologist and their main aim is to identify cause(s) of death and patient's disease(s). Usually this is a full autopsy, which typically includes the removal and examination of all/main internal organs, with or without the brain.

A full autopsy is desirable because it allows the complete inspection of all/main organs and offers a greater guarantee that all diseases present, cause(s) of death and concurrent factors are recorded. It also allows tissue sampling for histology, further investigation when necessary and research (see below).

It can happen that for a number of reasons, an objection to a full autopsy is raised: by express wish of the patient, by the family – at times because of how or when the request is made – for religious or cultural reasons, lack of information on the autopsy procedure, etc. Alternatives can be proposed. These include *limited autopsies*, ranging from exclusion of examination of the brain to removal, examination and sampling of the transplanted heart only and *minimally invasive autopsies*, such as percutaneous needle biopsies of specific organs (Van der Linden et al. 2014; Kang et al. 2014). Restricted autopsies, however, imply the risk of missing or underdiagnosing clinically significant conditions, thus limiting the value of autopsy to the family, to physicians, to quality assurance and to medical statistics and science. However even autopsies confined to dissection of the graft, only, through a limited incision, can carry "added value", permitting correlation of the findings with imaging studies as well as pathological evaluation of the graft and its complications (Michaud et al. 2015). An example is cardiac magnetic resonance imaging (CMRI) performed antemortem for tissue characterization of underlying structural abnormalities. These can be correlated with the findings in corresponding histological sections of myocardium of both ventricles and thus contribute to our understanding of the pathological substrates for the *in vivo* images. Experience combining CT or

MR imaging with biopsy sampling as a means to limit or prevent body dissection is still limited, with significant drawbacks preventing its application in routine clinical practice (Michaud et al. 2015; Thayyil et al. 2013; Weustink et al. 2009; Ross et al. 2012; Arthurs et al. 2014).

There is increasing support for the "added value" of what is called the *molecular autopsy* regardless of the extent of the dissection. In the molecular autopsy fresh tissue samples, including blood, are collected from all organs, DNA and RNA is extracted and is then stored at −80 °C for future diagnostic testing, e.g., detection of viruses in the differential diagnosis of myocarditis, detection of infections in other organs or evaluation of malignancy and its possible donor or recipient origin (Calabrese et al. 1999; Basso et al. 2010). Future molecular studies may be important for current and future family members if there is a potentially inheritable genetic cause for the disease that led to the transplant procedure. The completeness of tissue investigation using molecular investigation regardless of the extent of the dissection represents a unique method of reaching a diagnosis and can contribute important information for detailed clinical audit (Van der Linden et al. 2014). However technology has now improved to the extent that DNA and RNA can be extracted from formalin fixed paraffin embedded blocks in a high percentage of cases with excellent results (Carturan et al. 2008; Fedrigo et al. 2013).

24.4 Preparing for the Autopsy

24.4.1 Consent Issues

Before commencing the autopsy two important aspects to be considered are consent and the extent of the examination permitted. Often, provision of an information leaflet for families about their options is helpful in aiding discussions, as is the help of a dedicated Bereavement Officer acting as liaison between the family and the hospital or Coroner's/Medical Examiner's office.

Certain categories of death such as perioperative and peri-intervention deaths and sudden death early or late after transplantation may fall under the jurisdiction of the Coroner/Medical Examiner and a full medicolegal autopsy may be required. Sudden deaths, which are particularly traumatic to families, typically occur at home or in the community, represents a challenge for the pathologists and should be performed according to published national or international standards (Basso et al. 2008). In all these cases communication between the officers of the coroner/medical examiner, the family and the clinical team or pathologist is important to ensure that consent is sought through the appropriate channels from the family for retention of any material beyond his requirements and authority.

The alternative – the hospital, or consent autopsy in all its forms – may be done at the request of the clinician in some countries but in others it cannot take place without the witnessed written consent of the family or legal representative of the deceased, who are entitled to limit its extent. Thus, before starting the procedure it is mandatory to check the consent paperwork to see what restrictions, if any, apply. Consent should cover retention of tissue and organs and also all uses to which these samples may be put, e.g., diagnosis, clinical audit, education and research. Separate consent must be obtained before retaining samples for RNA/DNA extraction and storage for possible future analysis. Often limiting the autopsy may be related to religious or personal beliefs about body dissection and families' perception of death, especially in paediatric cases, when consent is often limited to inspection of the thoracic cavity and the dissection and retention of the cardiac allograft.

It is important to note here that in the UK, in general, consent is not required for the recording and use of digital images or video recordings of organs and pathology slides providing that before use the recordings are anonymized by the removal of identifying recipient data (General Medical Council 2015). However nowadays many peer-review journals may require documented consent from the patient or family for use of images in publication.

24.4.2 Autopsy Facilities, Staffing and Health & Safety Issues

In all jurisdictions, the facilities provided for the conduct of autopsies must conform to national or regional accreditation standards for ensuring health and safety in autopsy suites, including prevention of infections and for electrical safety, manual handling, radiological hazards and chemical substances hazardous to health. Importantly, there should be an assessment of risk on a case-by-case basis, including checking that any pacemakers and defibrillators have been deactivated. The presence of premortem infections should be checked from the notes and there should be protocols for dealing with more commonly encountered infections and with rare but dangerous pathogens. The pathologist has a responsibility to notify the local consultant in communicable disease control of certain infections where these were not suspected prior to the autopsy. Autopsies must be conducted either by specialist senior cardiac pathologists with experience in the pathology of transplantation or by trainee pathologists supervised by them and assisted by a trained anatomic pathology technician (mortician) who should be skilled at opening and evisceration of the body and at its reconstruction afterwards to a high standard.

24.4.3 Review of Clinical Notes

The pathologist should have access to the clinical notes prior to the autopsy and optimally should speak to the clinician who cared for the patient. He/she should know key details of the donor and recipient at the time of transplantation, including the disease for which the transplant was done (Calabrese et al. 1999; Melacini et al. 2010; Melacini et al. 2001), details of the transplant procedure, significant complications thereafter, the clinical events leading to death and the mode of death. If the patient dies in the community or in a hospital remote from the Transplant Centre where the procedure was done, the local pathologist should be advised to contact the Transplant Centre's pathologist or transplant coordinator for relevant clinical information and advice and, where relevant, for advice about aspects of conducting the autopsy and/or referral of the transplanted heart for expert examination. Otherwise the referring clinician should provide a full clinical history for the pathologist and, where possible, should attend the autopsy. This is of particular importance in postoperative deaths.

24.4.4 The Autopsy Procedure

The pathologist must be present at the start of the autopsy to check the identity and external appearance of the deceased. He/she must note all surgical and other scars and placement of all lines and devices, including pacemakers and defibrillators which must be deactivated prior to removal. A standard approach to cadaveric dissection and tissue sampling is essential to ensure that valuable information is not missed. This is especially important when examining postoperative and postintervention deaths, when often it might be advantageous to have the operator assist in the dissection. A similar approach should be adopted when dealing with the long-term systemic complications of transplantation and of the recipient's original disease. Several published general autopsy protocols are available and one specifically for heart transplantation is given in the Appendix. It may need to be modified as appropriate to each case. Today's autopsy should include extensive tissue sampling for histology, which is still the pathologist's main instrument, for documentation and to allow a more detailed diagnosis. Appropriate samples for biochemical, microbiological and molecular investigations should also be taken. Digital imaging of relevant findings is important for clinicopathological correlation afterwards, especially if the autopsy takes place off site or the clinicians are unable to attend the autopsy.

24.5 Interpretation of the Findings and the Cause of Death

The first major objective of the autopsy is to establish the final diagnoses, or cause of death – which may not be as straightforward as one might at first anticipate. In a typical case much comorbidity may contribute to the final illness and death. Determining which comorbidity is responsible can be difficult and often requires detailed discussion with the clinician at several stages before the final report is signed.

24.5.1 Mode of Death

The immediate cause of death is often ascribed to end-organ or multiorgan failure – and reflects the mode of death but not its underlying cause. Despite this it is often cited on death certificates as the cause of death. Death after transplantation may be sudden in up to 30 % of cases, mainly in long-term survivors, and in such instances is often the result of cardiac allograft vasculopathy or humoral and/or acute cellular rejection (Chantranuwat et al. 2004; Alexander and Steenbergen 2003). Immediately after transplantation death due to right heart failure is usually due to high lung vascular resistance and vasculopathy. Early graft failure can be due to diffuse ischemic injury resulting from poor graft quality or preservation, complicated by the side-effects of sustained, high levels of inotrope support, a prolonged ischemic time ≥ 4 h or technical complexity of the operative procedure because of previous cardiac surgery or ventricular assist device placement. In severe cases insertion of an intra-aortic balloon pump or a temporary right ventricular assist device may be required after transplantation to sustain output. Multiorgan failure may be the end-result of a range of other factors such as blood loss/hypovolemia, systemic infections and poor end-organ function such as renal or hepatic insufficiency. Death may also follow gradual long-term clinical deterioration resulting from immunosuppressant drug-related chronic nephropathy, cardiac allograft vasculopathy, malignancy, rejection and recipient disease recurrence in the allograft or its systemic effects.

24.5.2 Cause of Death

The main causes of death in heart transplantation are listed in Table 24.3 in decreasing order of frequency. It is important to remember that at any stage the cause of death could be unrelated to transplantation and its pharmacological therapy. Cerebrovascular events leading to haemorrhage or infarction could be due to other recipient pathologies such as vascular malformations causing rupture and intracranial bleeding. Native atherosclerosis may affect the large vessels such as the aorta and lead to aneurysm formation and subsequent rupture. Pretransplant risk factors may contribute to the development of atheroma complicating late cardiac allograft vasculopathy (CAV) and resulting from metabolic or hemodynamic factors acquired as a result of transplantation and its treatment. Under the term "others" we refer to conditions that, unrecognized and unsuspected, could cause death, such as severe traumatic accidental injury producing splenic rupture and catastrophic haemorrhage.

Table 24.3 Complications of transplantation and of immunosuppression

1. Perioperative complications
2. Postoperative myocardial ischaemic injury
3. Acute cellular and antibody-mediated rejection
4. Chronic allograft macro and microvasculopathy
5. Infections
6. Drug-related side-effects
7. Recurrence of disease in the graft
8. Neoplasia (NB lymphoproliferative disease)
9. Systemic effects of underlying disease, e.g., atherosclerosis and its complications

It is important to know the time interval between transplantation and death, as well as the history of the terminal illness, in order to consider likely causes of death at a given time point. There are three helpful time frames: *postoperative deaths*, which include those occurring up to 30 days after transplantation, usually referred to as in-hospital deaths; *early deaths*, which include those occurring between 30 days and 12 months; and *late deaths*, which include those occurring after 12 months (Table 24.4 and Fig. 24.1).

24.5.2.1 Postoperative Deaths <30 Days Posttransplant)

Less than 10 % of recipients die within the first 30 days after transplantation. There are often several contributing factors mainly graft failure,

Table 24.4 Likely causes of death according to time after transplantation

Time since transplantation	Cause of death
Post-operative cause of death (within 1 month, in-hospital death)	Technical aspects of surgical procedures Perioperative myocardial damage (poor quality of the graft, diffuse ischemic injury due to poor preservation of the graft, prolonged high inotrope therapy, long ischemic time) Multiorgan failure Infections Others
Early death (between 1 and 12 months)	Infections Acute rejection Recurrence of disease Others
Late death (after 12 months)	Cardiac allograft vasculopathy Malignancy Recurrence of disease Renal failure Others

infections and multiple organ failure. *Technical aspects* related to the surgical transplant procedure, especially the atrial and great vessel anastomoses should be always carefully evaluated both in the postoperative period and in the longer term, even up to 3 months after transplantation. They are usually confined to in-hospital deaths. Regardless of the cause the final common denominator is usually a longer transplant surgical procedure, with early allograft failure almost inevitable due to an unavoidable increase in ischemia and cardiopulmonary bypass times.

Care in opening the chest and in initial dissection of the mediastinum is advised in the setting of previous cardiac or mediastinal surgical procedures, ventricular assist device (VAD) implantation and congenital structural pathologies, whether or not these have been surgically corrected. In complex congenital heart disease there may need to be adjustments to the often-used bicaval transplant surgical technique, as in the

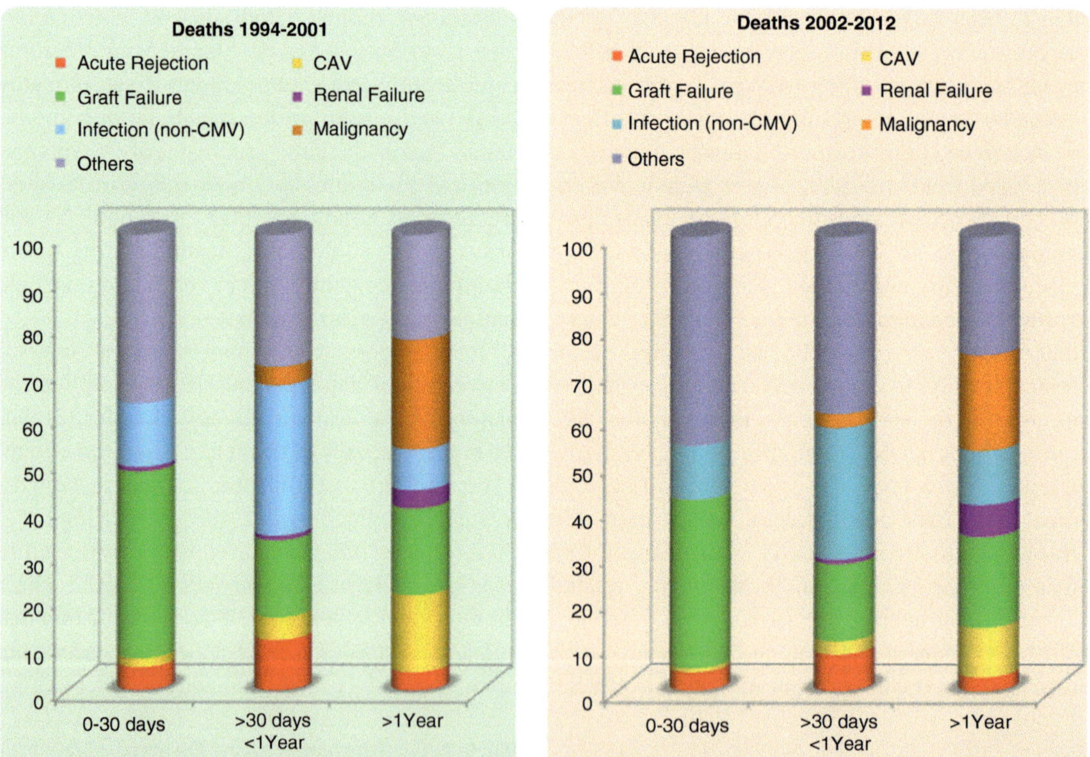

Fig. 24.1 Histogram with distribution of causes of death according to time post-transplantation and era (adult recipients-1994-2012) (Data from the ISHLT registry. Lund et al. 2013)

case of recipients with a failing Fontan procedure, when it will be necessary to adopt a hybrid procedure, to include stenting of the pulmonary vessels because of stenosis of branches of the pulmonary artery near the site of graft implantation (Fig. 24.2). There are usually dense adhesions between the right ventricle and the inner surface of the sternum with obliteration of the anterior pericardial space. Hence careful dissection of the inner surface of the sternum at autopsy is very important.

When evaluating the right atrial anastomosis it is important to know that different techniques have been used over the years. The original technique employed for cardiac transplantation – the *biatrial* anastomosis – leaves *in situ* the sinus part of the recipient right atrium to which the donor right atrium will be anastomosed, thus preserving the recipient's sinoatrial junction with the crista terminalis and the sinus node. The donor sinoatrial junction is also preserved and is anastomosed to that of the recipient after suturing closed the donor superior vena cava. With this standard technique there remain two sinus nodes, one from the donor and one from the recipient. The recipient's sinus node will undergo coagulative necrosis because of transection of the sinus nodal artery – a branch of the right coronary artery – during resection of the heart. Although the donor sinus node together with its blood supply is left intact with, hopefully, preservation of a regular pacemaker function the donor sinoatrial junction may undergo ischaemic damage when anastomosed to the recipient's right atrium. The anastomotic technique results in folding of the donor crista terminalis, with a horseshoe-shaped distortion of the sinus nodal artery. This, together with suture-related trauma may lead to iatrogenic damage of the sinus node, with irreversible ischaemic necrosis, thus leaving the recipient without any atrial pacemaker function. In the more physiological *bicaval* technique the recipient right atrium is resected in its entirety, with suturing of the donor atrium at the level of the superior and inferior vena cava. This results in removal of the recipient sinus node while leaving intact the donor sinoatrial junction with the crista terminalis and sinus node. The bicaval technique is now commonly employed, evidence suggesting that it leads to improved post-operative haemodynamics compared to the biatrial technique, with reduced right atrial pressure, less tricuspid regurgitation, an increased chance of recovering sinus rhythm and a reduced need for pacing (Schnoor et al. 2007).

Perioperative myocardial injury is a broad term encompassing different aspects of early allograft failure. Several factors may affect the condition of the donor organ during and after transplantation, most of them leading to severe myocardial ischemia-reperfusion injury with allograft failure and, often, death of the recipient. They include poor quality of the allograft, poor preservation of the allograft, prolonged treatment with high doses of inotropes and prolonged allograft ischemia time. The resultant ischemia-reperfusion injury is characterized by severe edema with flaccidity of the heart, biventricular dilatation and variegated, hemorrhagic myocardium. The histology shows multifocal, diffuse myocyte coagulative necrosis associated with contraction band necrosis at the interface with normal myocardium and, occasionally, a "spotty" distribution of clusters of necrotic myocytes with focal/multifocal extension. Sometimes there may also be clusters of vacuolated myocytes. The inflammatory response is typically less severe than the myocyte necrosis and is characterized by leucocyte infiltration with a prevalence of macrophages. It is impossible to differentiate between the different causes of ischemic-reperfusion injury based on pathology (World Health Organization 2015). Various initiatives to improve the condition of the donor heart have been instituted, the most promising being the recently introduced *ex vivo* normothermic preservation of the beating heart between harvesting and implantation (see Chap. 8, 9).

The use of *marginal donor hearts*, introduced in countries with falling donation rates, can increase the risk of intra- or postoperative death. Clinical information on donor age, sex, inotropic support and cause of death should be collected before the autopsy. Marginal donor hearts at harvesting may show coronary artery disease with subobstructive atherosclerotic lesions that may

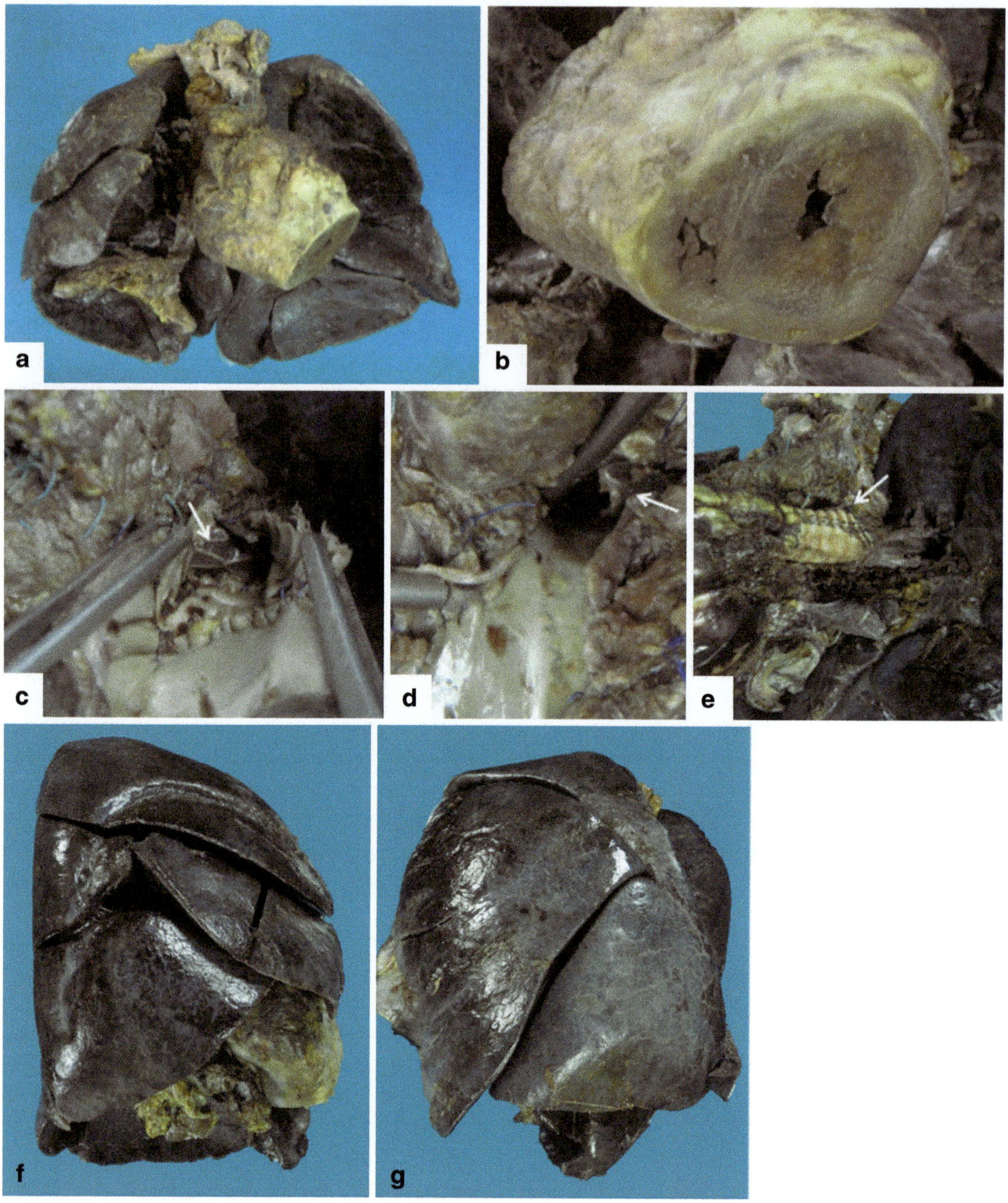

Fig. 24.2 Complex congenital heart disease in a 17-year-old boy with a Fontan procedure. The transplantation procedure was lengthy due to reconstruction of the right ventricle outflow tract. A covered stent was inserted percutaneously due to persistence of peripheral pulmonary stenosis. The patient died postoperatively of pulmonary hemorrhage. (**a**) Frontal view of the heart and lung block removed at autopsy. (**b**) A cross section of the heart at midventricle with discoloration of the ventricular wall suggestive of perioperative ischemic injury. (**c**) The right ventricle outflow tract is reconstructed: note the presence of the covered stent in the pulmonary arteries (*arrow*). (**d**) Posterior view of the left pulmonary artery, which has been opened, and shows the stent (*arrow*) at the pulmonary trunk bifurcation. (**e**) Frontal view of the reconstructed main pulmonary artery (vascular graft, *arrow*) and vein. (**f, g**) Macroscopic view of the right (**f**) and left lung (**g**) with signs of extensive hemorrhage

require coronary artery by-pass grafting before implantation. They may also show left ventricular hypertrophy. Their use has been confined to marginal recipients. Thus during autopsy particular attention should be given to evaluation of the degree of native coronary artery disease and left ventricular hypertrophy for subsequent clinicopathological correlation. Such data may guide future assessment of allograft adequacy with adjustment and updating of donor selection criteria.

Right ventricular failure may occur in the setting of borderline pulmonary hypertension and raises the important question of sensitivity of techniques to evaluate pretransplant pulmonary wedge pressure during the assessment of potential transplant recipients. Even a mild increase of pulmonary vascular resistance has been reported as an independent predictor of perioperative/early mortality after heart transplantation. In the setting of poor preservation of the allograft ischemia-reperfusion injury of the myocardium may lead to right ventricular failure even in the presence of normal or borderline pulmonary hypertension. Very occasionally, unexpected pathology of the allograft right ventricle may be found. In the early years of the Padua experience a donor allograft with extensive fibrofatty replacement of the right ventricle led to allograft failure due to inability to cope with borderline pulmonary hypertension in the recipient. Extensive sampling of lungs for histology should normally be done to identify changes suggestive of increased pulmonary vascular resistance.

Multiorgan failure accounts for approximately one in five deaths in the postoperative period (Lund 2013) and may be given as the cause of death in some instances as it may be difficult to attribute death to a single underlying clinical or pathological entity. It is important to consider the "knock-on" effect on other organs such as the kidney and liver of prolonged end stage cardiac failure, perhaps worsened by a long time on the waiting list and the additional operative risks posed by extended pretransplant mechanical circulatory support. Intraoperative complications leading to a prolonged cardiopulmonary bypass time may exacerbate subclinical prerenal or congestive hepatic failure or lead to coagulopathy with prolonged bleeding at the operative site or elsewhere, for example, intracerebral haemorrhage.

Infections, often multiple and systemic, may complicate the picture (see below). Therefore it is important that a complete autopsy is done to ensure extensive tissue sampling for both histology and microbiological investigation and that the final cause of death reflects the outcome of multidisciplinary case conference discussions (Fig. 24.3). Rarely, unexpected donor-related infections are identified (Calabrese et al.1999). In this instance communication with the appropriate organ donor registry is important as other recipients from the donor will be at risk.

24.5.2.2 Early Deaths (30 Days – 12 Months Posttransplant)

Infections continue to be a significant risk in the longer term follow-up of transplant recipients, overall accounting for about 10–12 % of all deaths except in the early period when they may be responsible for up to one third of deaths (Lund et al. 2013). A broad spectrum of infections may be encountered, including viral, bacterial, fungal and parasitic agents. The heart may be involved either in isolation or as part of multiorgan involvement in the clinical setting of sepsis or septic shock.

Early infections within the first few weeks of transplantation may localize to the surgical wound site, vascular or pacemaker access sites, urinary tract or lung. They may be donor-related (Calabrese et al. 1999) or acquired *de novo* after transplantation. Identification of the site of primary infection can be challenging in the context of multiorgan involvement. At autopsy sampling for microbiological investigation should be done of catheter or cannula tips, together with any adherent thrombotic material and tissue from their insertion sites, as well as of potentially involved organs and fluid from tissue cavities such as the pleural and posterior pericardial sacs.

Mediastinum is a possible site of infection following sternotomy. It is easy to identify when the sternum is still open, but may be more difficult when the wound site has healed and superficially

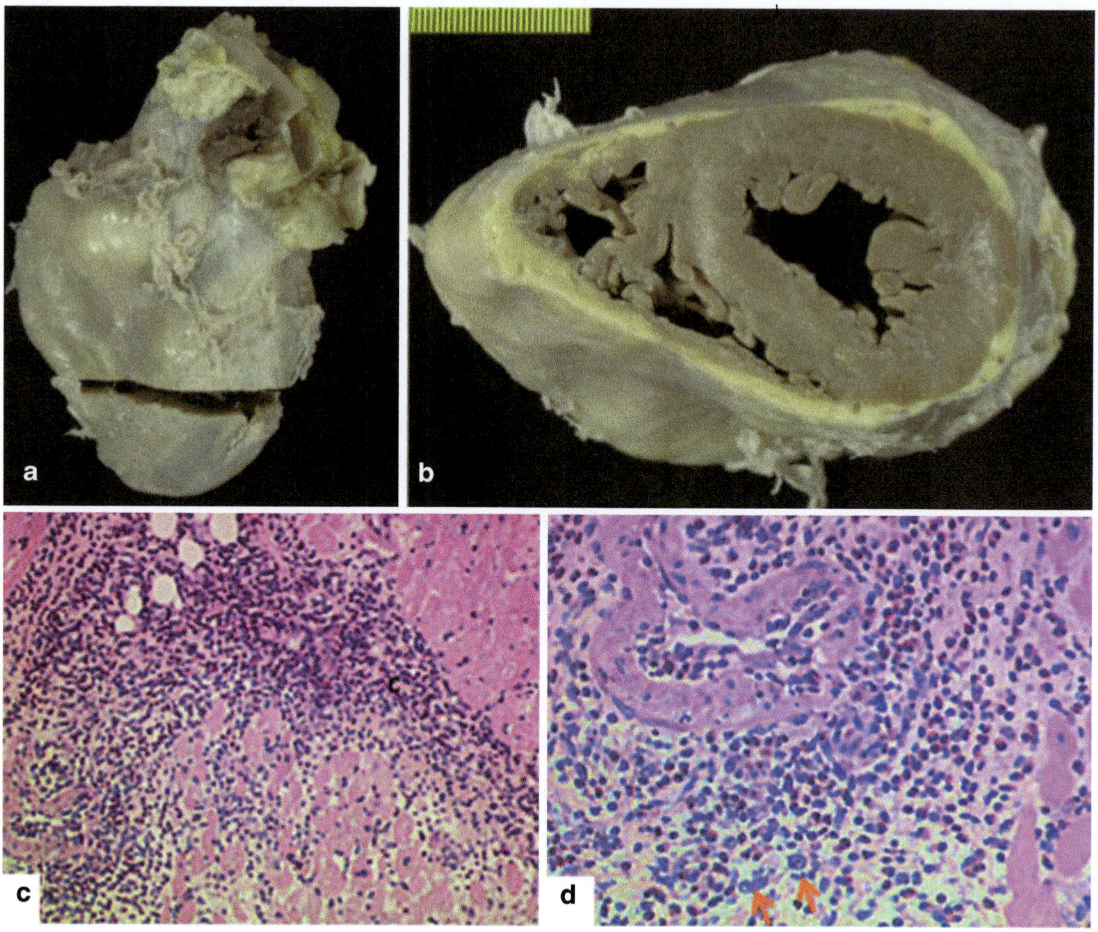

Fig. 24.3 CMV myocarditis in the early phase after transplantation. A 17 year old male affected by dilated cardiomyopathy was successfully transplanted, but developed CMV myocarditis and died suddenly while still in hospital. (**a**) Macroscopic frontal view of the heart removed at autopsy with fibrinoid pericarditis. (**b**) Cross section of the heart at midventricle with nondilated ventricles. The myocardium shows spotty discolorations suggestive of myocarditis. (**c**) Diffuse inflammatory infiltrates associated to myocyte necrosis. Haematoxylin-eosin staining, original magnification ×100. (**d**) High power view of **c** with evidence of vasculitis and intravascular thrombosis. Note the monomorphic type of inflammation with numerous plasmacells and eosinophils and the presence of CMV cytopathic features of a few cells (*arrows*). Haematoxylin Eosin staining, original magnification ×200. Molecular analysis was positive for CMV in the tissue

lacks typical signs of infection. Even in the immediate postoperative period the immunosuppressed transplant recipient has an increased susceptibility to infection and delayed healing with development of wound dehiscence and mediastinitis. There may be subsequent difficulties in chest closure, even after the infection has been successfully treated. Everolimus, a potent mTOR inihibitor, can delay wound healing. Postsurgical infections and pneumonia are common in in-hospital recipients while, opportunistic infections are more common later on, especially after increasing immunosuppression to treat an episode of acute rejection. Cardiac allograft endocarditis should be excluded. Closed-space fungal infections such as Candida, Histoplasma, Coccidia, Nocardia, Toxoplasma gondii and Mycobacteria have been encountered.

There is a significant risk of primary allograft involvement by Toxoplasma gondii and cytomegalovirus (CMV) in cases of serological mismatch i.e. a heart from a seropositive donor transplanted

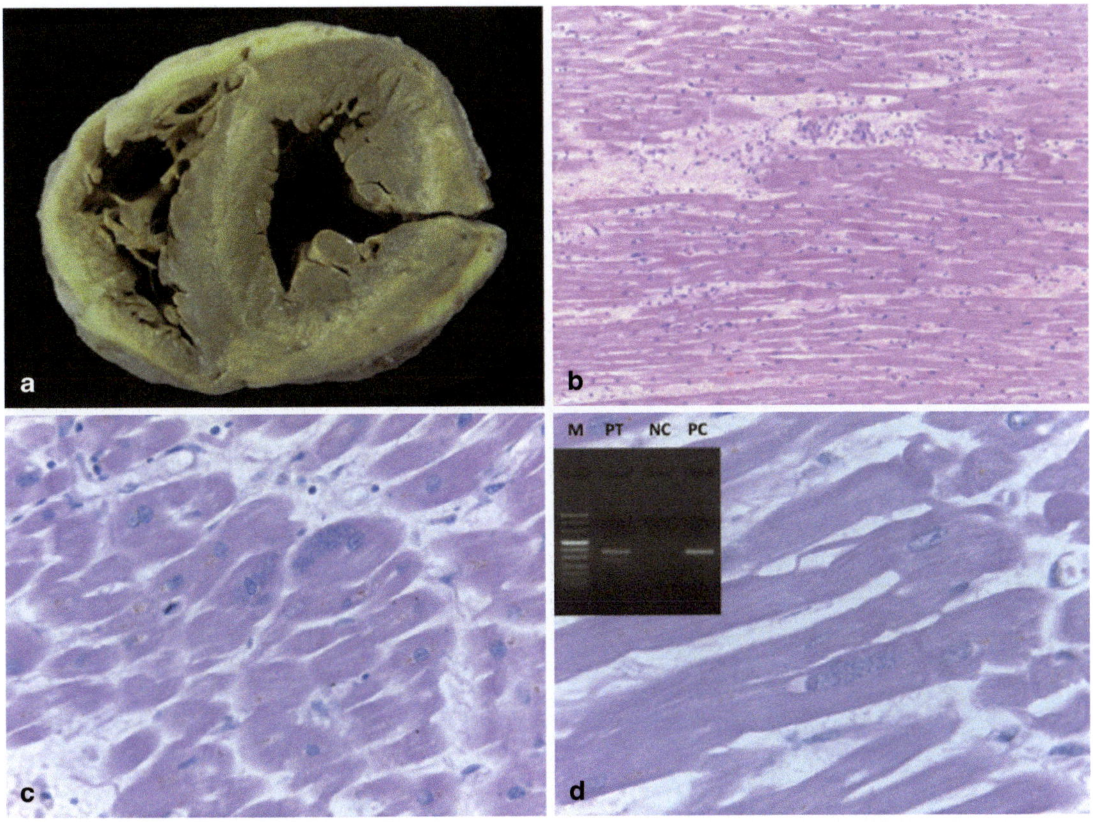

Fig. 24.4 An 18-year-old man was successfully transplanted because of myocarditis. After a few months he developed fever and astenia. He died shortly afterwards with congestive heart failure refractory to conventional therapy. The diagnosis of toxoplasma gondii myocarditis was made on the day of death. There was a mismatch between a positive toxoplasma donor and a negative recipient. (**a**) Midventricle cross section of the transplanted heart removed at autopsy with a yellowish appearance of the lateral and posterior walls of the left ventricle. (**b**) Histologic section of the lateral wall of the left ventricle showing edema and inflammatory infiltrates. Haematoxylin-eosin staining, original magnification ×100. (**c**, **d**) Histologic section of the left ventricle with evidence of bradizoites inside the cysts in cardiomyocytes, not in proximity to inflamed areas. Haematoxylin-eosin staining, original magnification ×400. In **d** there is an insert of the Toxoplasma gondii PCR analysis performed in the tissue from the left ventricle. (*M* marker, *Pt* patient, *NC* negative control, *PC* positive control)

into a seronegative recipient. While serological monitoring and sometimes prophylactic treatment of recipients at risk is necessary, a *de novo* diagnosis may be made on endomyocardial biopsy or at autopsy. Microscopic involvement of the cardiac allograft by *T. gondii* may be suspected if there is a diffuse interstitial granulomatous inflammatory infiltrate with sparse multinucleated giant cells. The cysts of *T. gondii* may be seen in myocytes but are often very sparse and trophozoites themselves are often only seen at magnification × 100 under oil immersion (Fig. 24.4). In CMV myocarditis the diffuse lymphocytic infiltrate may resemble that of acute cellular rejection (see below) with repercussions for the recipient if the CMV inclusions are not identified, the appropriate serological or molecular tests are not done and enhanced immunosuppression for an erroneous diagnosis of acute rejection is given. This is of particular importance as CMV infection may, itself, precipitate acute rejection, necessitating treatment for both disorders in cases where the diagnostic dilemma cannot be resolved. Immunohistochemical staining and molecular studies such as *in situ* hybridization, PCR or RT-PCR should be done to identify

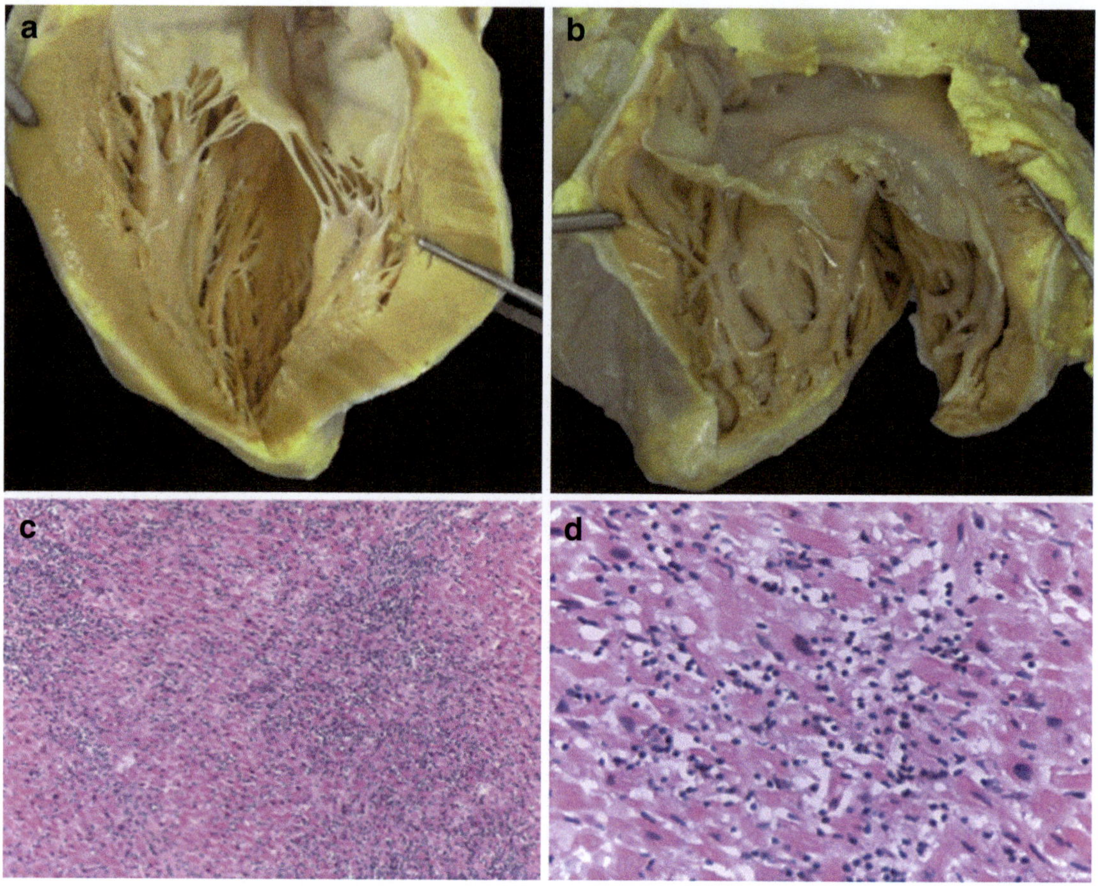

Fig. 24.5 Acute cellular rejection 10 years post transplantation in a 24-year-old woman who spontaneously withdrew from immunosuppressive therapy. (**a**, **b**) The autoptic heart, opened along the obtuse margin in **a** and acute margin in **b** shows both ventricular cavities dilated. (**c**, **d**) Histologic section of the left ventricle with diffuse inflammatory infiltrates and myocyte necrosis (Haematoxylin-eosin staining. **c**: original magnification ×10; **d**: original magnification ×200)

or confirm the suspected pathogens. Both infections may also be systemic.

Acute rejection accounts for about 11 % of deaths in the first year (Lund et al. 2013). However acute and chronic immune injury are likely important contributors to graft failure early and late after transplantation and remain leading cause of death throughout follow-up. Hence at any time post-transplantation acute cellular rejection should be considered as a possible cause of death, including that known to the clinicians to be the consequence of noncompliance with treatment (Fig. 24.5). The acutely rejecting allograft shows the typical macroscopic appearance of a streaky haemorrhagic endocardium and blotchy discoloration of the myocardium. Typically the recipient's right and left atrial myocardium at the site of the anastomosis, is macroscopically pale, being spared by inflammation, whereas the donor side is blotchy and haemorrhagic. Acute rejection involves the conduction system with equal severity to working myocardium, with the exception of the bundle of His, which appears insulated and protected within the surrounding fibrous tissue. During an acute rejection episode, the sudden appearance of first-degree AV block may suggest involvement of the conduction system with impending cardiac arrest. When evaluating cases of sudden cardiac death in allograft recipients it is important to study the conduction system to assess severity of involvement as a possible mode of death (Chantranuwat et al. 2004; Alexander and Steenbergen 2003; Patel et al. 1996; Vaseghi et al. 2009). Humoral rejection may lead to death through various mechanisms: it may be present in isolation or coexist with acute cellular rejection (mixed rejection) and/or cardiac allograft vasculopathy. Hence it should be always assessed by both histological and immunohistochemical investigation in the autopsied allograft.

Disease recurrence in the allograft is uncommon but can occur at any time after transplantation depending on the diagnosis. The knowledge of native pathology such as *lymphocytic myocarditis* leading to transplantation is important in the interpretation of cases with an inflammatory infiltrate where the macroscopic appearance of myocardial involvement as well as the microscopic features do not distinguish between acute cellular rejection and either recurrent or de novo lymphocytic myocarditis. In this instance molecular detection of viral genomes and sequencing analysis of the viral strands enables differentiation of acute rejection from myocarditis. This is a more frequent occurrence in the pediatric population. *Giant cell myocarditis* may recur early after transplantation or within the first year. Its diagnosis in the allograft at autopsy is confirmed by the presence of giant cells and possibly eosinophils in the inflammatory cell infiltrate on histology. Usually recurrence in this setting has already been confirmed in life on routine endomyocardial biopsy monitoring. *Sarcoidosis* may also recur in the cardiac allograft, the granulomas showing more fibrosis and less lymphocytic infiltration than in the other forms of granulomatous myocarditis. A systemic disorder, it may be found in tissue sections from other organs such as lymph nodes, liver and lungs. Recurrent *amyloid* deposits may produce pallor and firmness of myocardium, if extensive. It is often diagnosed in life on routine endomycardial biopsy monitoring but may not lead to clinical problems until the volume of deposited amyloid is sufficiently high. Recurrence may involve other organs and may occur many years after transplantation.

24.5.2.3 Late Deaths (>12 Months)

With increasing time post-transplantation *cardiac allograft vasculopathy* (CAV) becomes a leading cause of death through ischaemic cardiomyopathy and/or acute myocardial infarction. It accounts for about 11 % of deaths from one to 15 years and beyond after transplantation (Lund 2013). The heterogeneity in clinical symptoms from silent ischemia to severe congestive heart failure and sudden death is paralleled by heterogeneity in the pathological features of CAV. It is important to remember that the identification of CAV at autopsy does not necessarily correspond to identification of the cause of death although it could be a comorbidity which could have influenced the final illness and death of the recipient from another cause.

CAV is a rapidly progressive form of atherosclerosis characterized by an accelerated progressive, diffuse intimal hyperplasia of the vascular tree that leads to insidious vessel narrowing and eventually to allograft ischemia (Fig. 24.6). There are many features that are peculiar to CAV compared to classical native atherosclerotic lesions (ATS). One of these is the involvement of the venous and postcapillary vascular bed in CAV which can be assessed easily on histology.

There are two components of CAV of clinicopathological importance to be considered at autopsy. The first is epicardial coronary involvement with heterogeneous lesions ranging from early diffuse intimal thickening, often with endotheliality which can lead to thrombosis (Fig. 24.7), to complicated atheroma, often with superimposed acute coronary thrombosis and myocardial infarction (Fig. 24.8). The second is microvasculopathy with involvement of small intramyocardial coronary arteries, arterioles and capillaries, in life leading to reduction in microvascular density with reduction of coronary flow reserve and progressive heart failure (Fig. 24.8). The myocardial remodelling process, with patchy or diffuse interstitial fibrosis, could represent the substrate for arrhythmic events leading to death. It is also important to check if there is obstructive vasculopathy of the allograft sinus node artery which could lead to a terminal arryhthmia.

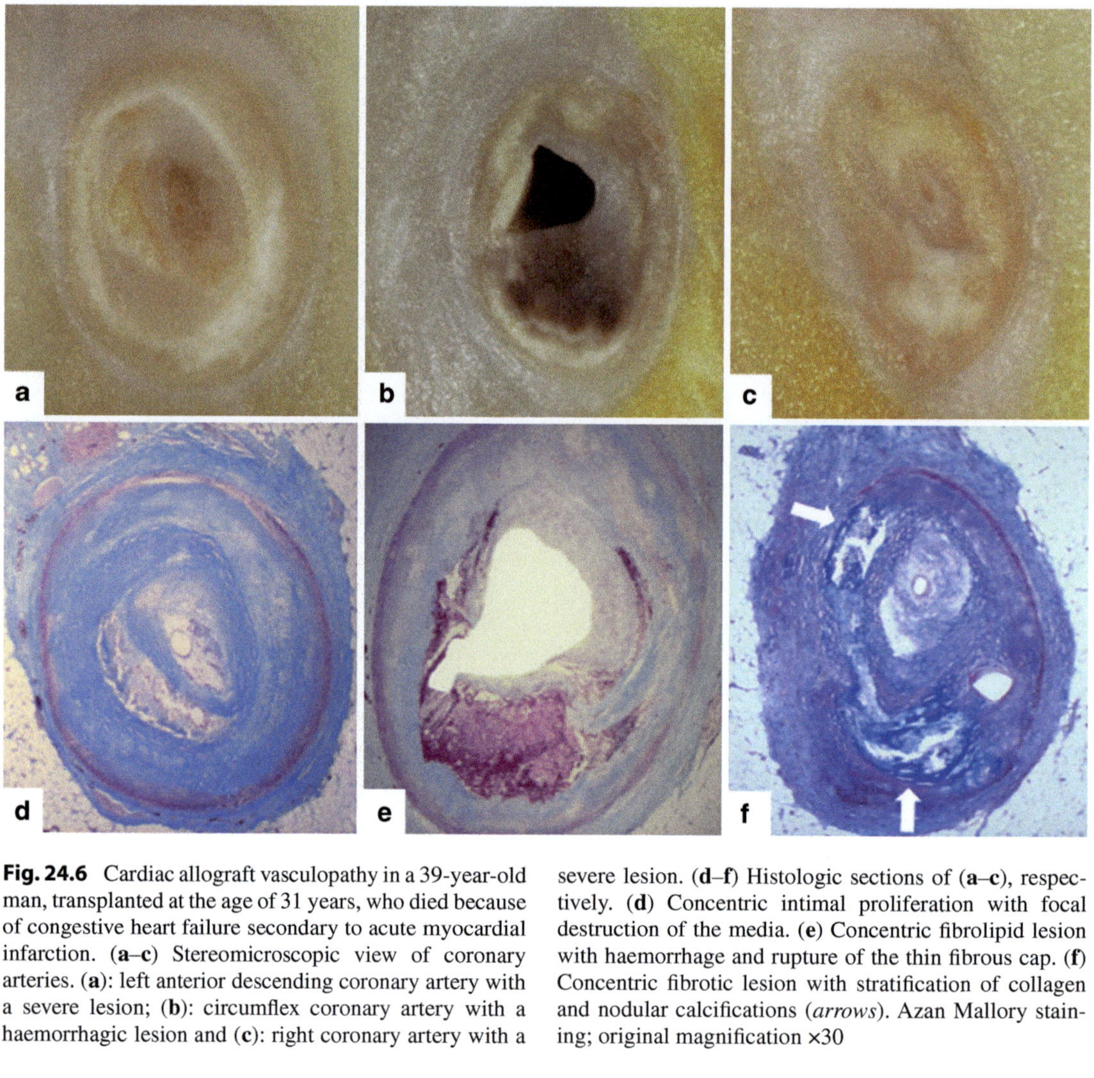

Fig. 24.6 Cardiac allograft vasculopathy in a 39-year-old man, transplanted at the age of 31 years, who died because of congestive heart failure secondary to acute myocardial infarction. (**a–c**) Stereomicroscopic view of coronary arteries. (**a**): left anterior descending coronary artery with a severe lesion; (**b**): circumflex coronary artery with a haemorrhagic lesion and (**c**): right coronary artery with a severe lesion. (**d–f**) Histologic sections of (**a–c**), respectively. (**d**) Concentric intimal proliferation with focal destruction of the media. (**e**) Concentric fibrolipid lesion with haemorrhage and rupture of the thin fibrous cap. (**f**) Concentric fibrotic lesion with stratification of collagen and nodular calcifications (*arrows*). Azan Mallory staining; original magnification ×30

The pathologist should thoroughly evaluate the epicardial vessels to identify the culprit lesion. These vary from the 'classical' CAV fibrocellular intimal proliferation, characterized by concentric diffuse intimal thickening of epicardial and intramyocardial coronary arteries, to classical ATS-like lesions characterized by atheroma with focal eccentric plaques and a lipid pool (fibrolipid plaques). Histological evaluation may also show transmural vasculitis of epicardial and intramyocardial vessels or more selective intimal involvement with endothelialitis. Fibrocellular lesions are present in about two-third of CAV cases in the first few years after transplantation, but their incidence drops markedly in the long term when fibrolipid plaques are more frequently detected. The remodelling process of CAV is time-dependent. One might expect a dramatic reduction in the numbers of fibrocellular plaques over the years because of their transition into fibroatheromas, in part due to exposure to atherosclerotic risk factors such as hypercholesterolemia or diabetes mellitus. However, analysis of lesions from longer term survivors shows that about half of the plaques remain fibrocellular in nature.

Malignancy accounts for about 20 % of deaths after the third year post-transplant (Lund et al. 2013) The identification of de-novo or previously unrecognized/undetected tumors can occur during postmortem. If this should happen early after

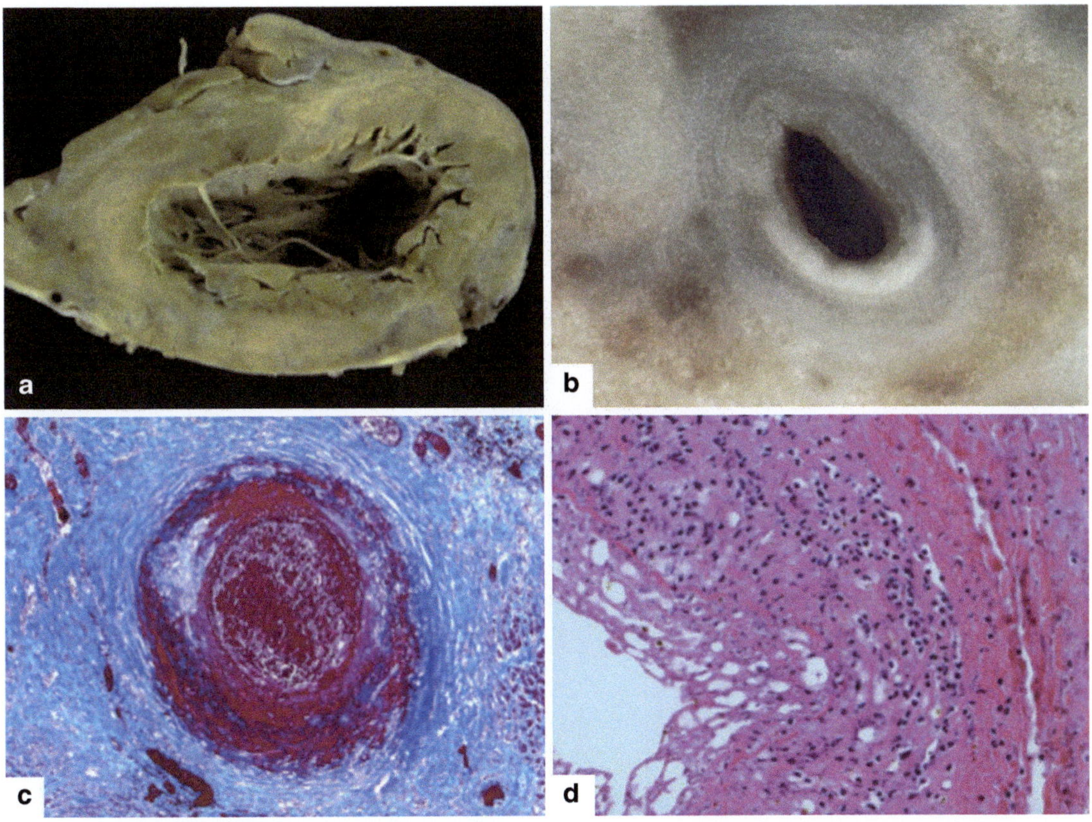

Fig. 24.7 Cardiac allograft vasculopathy in a 53-year-old man. (**a**) Apical cross section of the transplanted autoptic heart with whitish fibrotic areas. (**b**) Cross section of the left descending coronary artery seen under a stereomicroscope. (**c**) Corresponding histologic section of the coronary artery with acute occlusive thrombosis (Azan Mallory staining, original magnification ×30). (**d**) Histologic section of an artery with intimal smooth muscle cell proliferation and inflammation (Haematoxylin-eosin staining, original magnification ×200)

transplantation, especially in the graft, molecular investigation should be done to attempt to differentiate between donor and recipient origin (Fig. 24.9), of significance for other potential recipients of organs from the same donor. The most common neoplasm after cardiac transplantation is skin cancer, mainly squamous cell carcinoma often with numerous lesions requiring resection. Other solid tumours, such as carcinomas of lung or gastrointestinal tract may occur with increased frequency. Regardless of site and cell type the main issue confronting both recipient and clinician is the unpredictable course of malignant tumours in the context of long-term iatrogenic immunosuppression.

In post-transplant lymphoproliferative disorders (PTLDs) autopsy is critical to refine a definitive diagnosis in late allograft failure and to enhance our understanding of the natural history of these group of diseases and the impact of potentially cardiotoxic chemotherapy in advanced disease. PTLDs show a spectrum of pathologies ranging from early lesions characterized by plasmacytic hyperplasia or infectious mononucleosis-like pathology to polymorphic PTLD to monomorphic PTLD (see Chap. 20). Monomorphic lesions almost invariably show a B-cell phenotype (>80 %) although less frequently T-cell or Hodgkin-like lymphomas are seen. Late PTLDs are more likely to be negative for EBV. Detection of EBV by in situ hybridization is a useful tool in the differential diagnosis between PTLD and rejection in the allograft. Early PTLD is more common in children and

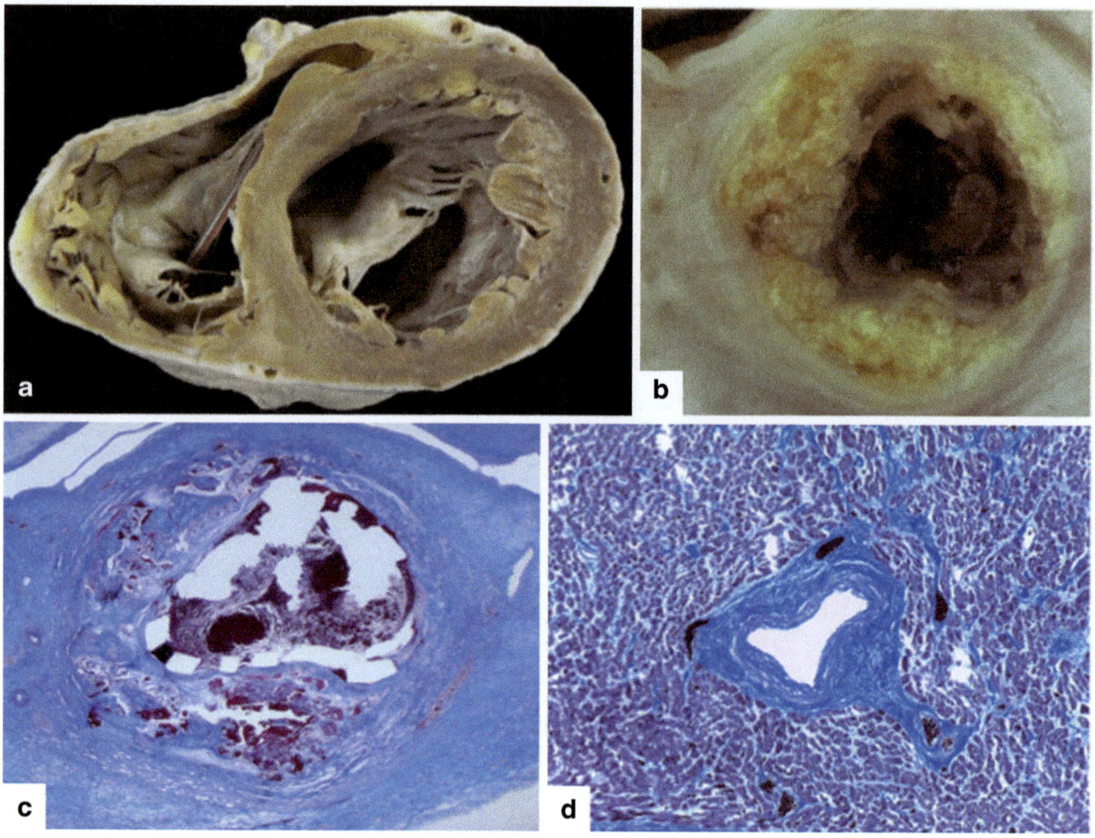

Fig. 24.8 Cardiac allograft vasculopathy in a 39-year-old man, transplanted at the age of 17 years for dilated cardiomyopathy secondary to myocarditis. (**a**) Basal cross section of the transplanted autoptic heart. (**b**) Stereomicroscopic view of anterior descending coronary artery showing the occlusive atherothrombotic lesion. (**c**) The histologic section shows the atherosclerotic plaque with haemorrhage, occlusive thrombosis and periadventitial fibrosis (Azan Mallory staining, original magnification ×30. (**d**) Histologic section of the left ventricle with microvasculopathy affecting a small intramyocardial artery (Azan Mallory staining, original magnification ×100)

young adults and is more frequently EBV-positive than PTLD in older recipients or occurring late after transplantation (Fig. 24.10). Molecular genetic studies are important to show clonal rearrangement of immunoglobulin genes and or EBV genomes. The majority of PTLD are of recipient origin, reflecting escape of recipient EBV-positive cells from immune surveillance. Only a minority are of donor origin, as a result of lymphoid donor cells transplanted with the graft. Many PTLDs are extranodal, often affecting the gastrointestinal tract. Rarely, they involve the cardiac allograft, usually as part of secondary dissemination. Primary involvement of the cardiac allograft is very rare. The cellular infiltrate of cardiac involvement by PTLD requires differentiation from lymphocytic myocarditis and acute rejection and requires application of immunohistochemical and molecular techniques.

24.5.2.4 Other Graft-Related and Systemic Pathology

The evaluation of the cardiac allograft should identify the presence of other pathologies which may not be related to the cause of death, but represent comorbidities. For example, cardiac allograft macro or microvasculopathy may be detected on histology in a recipient dying from another cause. We have already alluded to the impact of systemic disorders such as generalized atherosclerosis in a recipient transplanted for

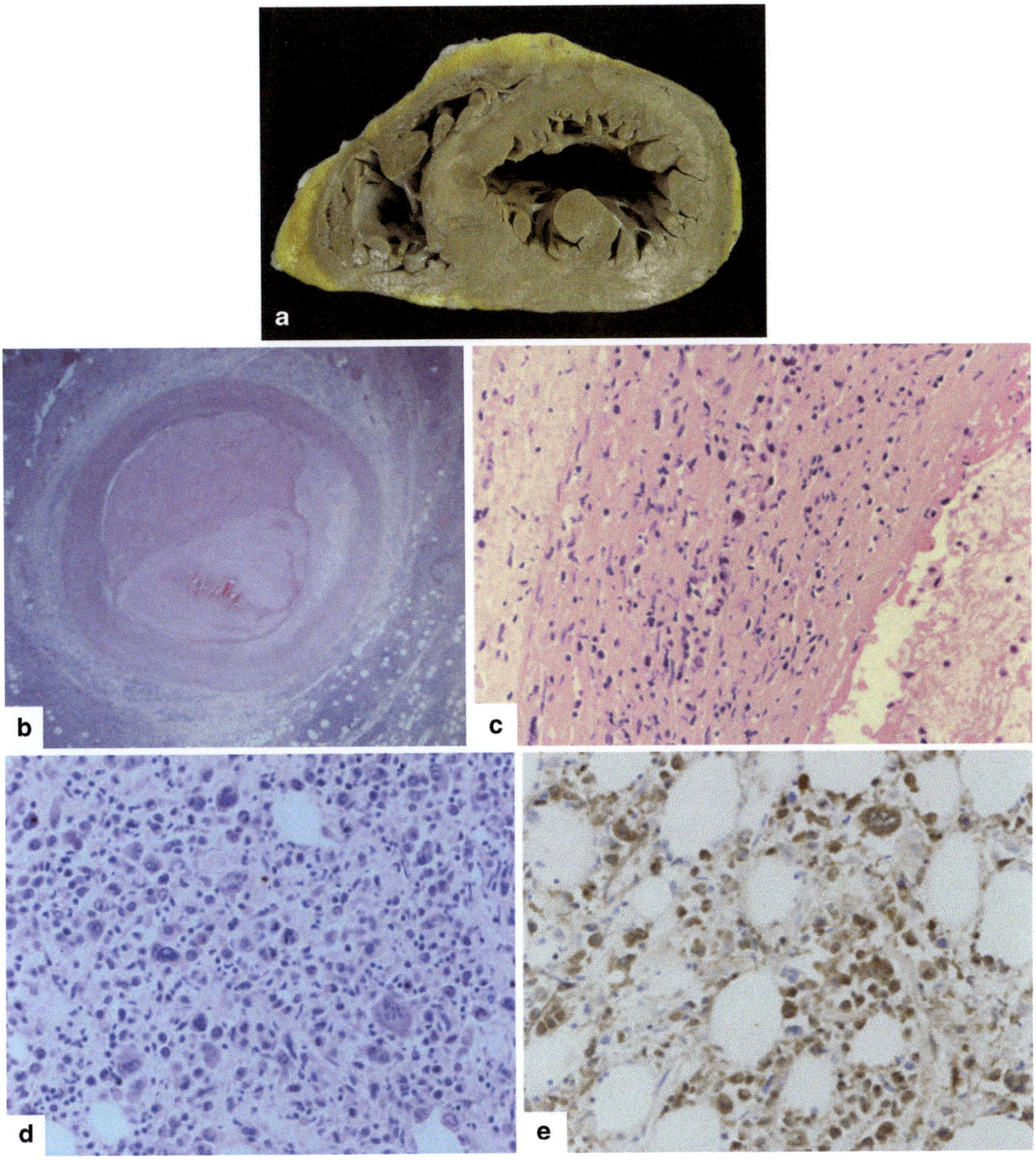

Fig. 24.9 *PTLD* early after transplantation in a young woman who presented with acute myocardial infarction due to vasculitis and occlusive thrombosis of the anterior descending coronary artery. (**a**) Midventricle cross section of the transplanted autoptic heart. (**b**) Histologic section of the culprit lesion with thrombosis (Haematoxylin-eosin staining, original magnification ×30. (**c**) High power view of **b** showing the vascular wall infiltrated by the lymphoblastic cells. Haematoxylin-eosin staining, original magnification ×200. (**d**) High power view of the epicardial perivascular fat infiltrated by neoplastic cells with pleomorphic appearance and giant and bizzare nuclei (Haematoxylin-eosin staining, original magnification ×400. (**e**) EBV Immunostaining showing positivity of the neoplastic cells with anti-EBV antibody (original magnification ×400)

ischaemic heart disease. Other systemic disorders such as the muscular dystrophies, amyloidosis, sarcoidosis and autoimmune disorders may complicate management of recipients and cause significant comorbidity and death even in the face of a normally functioning allograft. Drug-related side-effects may involve specific organs such as the liver and kidney, both of which may be target organs of immunosuppression. Chronic renal failure may account for 10% of deaths in long term recipients, the kidney manifesting either the nephrotoxic effects of calcineurin inhibitors with tubular damage and vascular arteriolopathies and/or secondary damage from glomerulopathy or vasculopathy due to diabetes secondary to corticosteroids therapy (Lund et al. 2013).

24.6 The Autopsy Report and Clinicopathological Correlation

The quality of the autopsy is reflected in the quality of the information given in the final autopsy report and its contribution to clinical audit; it should conform to national or international standards (TRAGEDY 2015; Royal College of Pathologists, 2015; Basso et al. 2008).

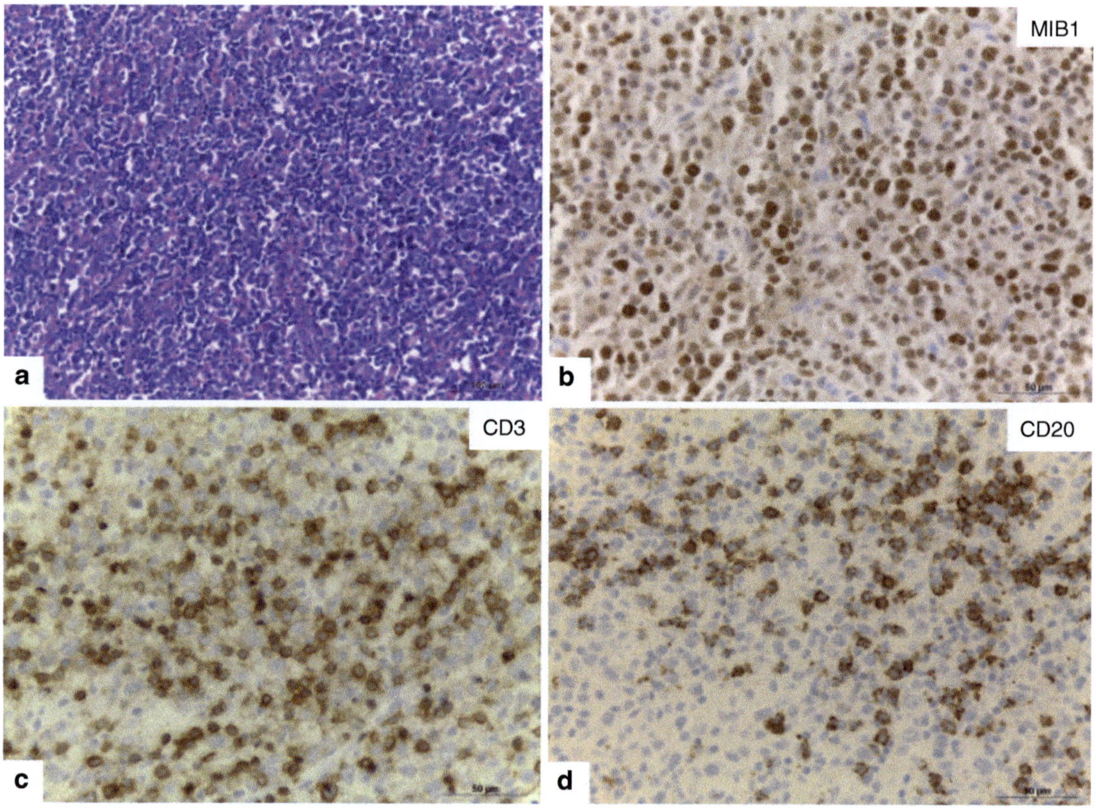

Fig. 24.10 A 20-year-old woman, who died of sepsis following chemotherapy for recurrence of monomorphic PTLD (large B cell type, rich in T-lymphocytes), which first developed 6 years previously. (**a**) Histology of the PTLD within a lymph node with large neoplastic cells and high mitotic index (Haematoxylin-eosin staining, original magnification ×100. (**b**) Immunohistochemistry with MIB1 antibody showing a high number of proliferating neoplastic positive cells (original magnification ×400). (**c**) CD3 immunohistochemistry revealing the presence of T-lymphocytes (original magnification x400). (**d**) CD20 immunohistochemistry showing B-lymphocytes. EBV molecular analysis of the tissue was negative (original magnification x400). (**e**) Cross section of the transplanted autoptic heart at basal level. (**f**) Histology of the left ventricle wall shows edema, myocyte necrosis, aspergillus hyphae and scarce inflammation (Haematoxylin-eosin staining, original magnification ×100. (**g**) High power view of **f** with fungal aspergillus hyphae (Haematoxylin-eosin staining, original magnification ×200. (**h**) High power view of **g** with lymphoblastic cells (*arrow*) and hyphae (Haematoxylin-eosin staining, original magnification ×400)

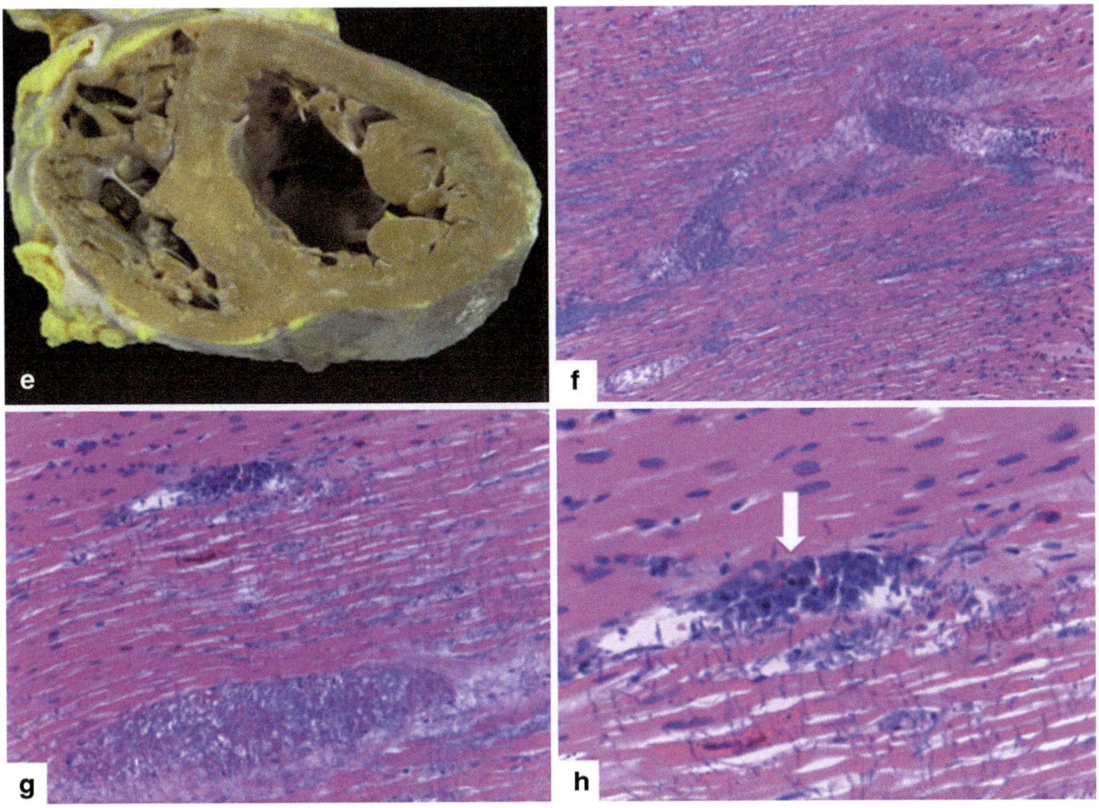

Fig. 24.10 (continued)

The report should include a clinical history of sufficient detail to highlight key issues and any concerns of the clinician and family, then a systematic description of the macroscopic, microscopic and other findings. The conclusion of the report should include the following:

1. The summary of findings in order of priority
2. A recommended cause of death
3. A conclusion comprising a clinicopathological correlation of the key findings contributing to the recipient's demise
4. A brief review of pertinent literature with citations, if relevant
5. A note of organs and tissues which have been retained, including the uses to which they may be put and if any digital images or video recordings were done (and anonymized)

If the autopsy examination fails to resolve all the clinical questions, the final report may provide a ranked differential diagnosis.

As a rule the final report should not be completed until the pathologist has discussed the case with the clinicians as clinical information could have a bearing on the cause of death. The next-of-kin should also receive a copy if they request it, although this is best done in the context of a face-to-face meeting with the clinician after mortality case review has been completed. It should be remembered that information gleaned from high-quality autopsies and reports will help families in the aftermath of the death of their loved one and, in the wider context, has the potential to regain public and professional support for the procedure.

24.7 Clinical Audit

Clinical audit is a core component of clinical governance and should be done by all HealthCare organizations to systematically analyze the quality of care given to their patients. The use of autopsy data contributes to this process by ensuring comparison between the autopsy findings and the clinical cause of death and enabling identification of previously unrecognized nonfatal conditions. Thus to be an effective clinical tool the autopsy should be of a high standard, be performed with competence and care according to validated protocols and be reported in a timely fashion. The pathologist must ensure a high standard of autopsy performance and reporting through ongoing laboratory quality assurance, including audit of the autopsy report. He/she should also participate in external quality assurance schemes and peer review.

Autopsies can provide an opportunity to assess the standard of care not just in cases of sudden unexpected deaths and postoperative deaths but also in cases in which there appear to be no clinical uncertainties. This applies no less to the transplant recipient than to any other patient. Ideally the autopsy should be a compulsory part of clinical audit, not just an option. Discrepancies between clinical diagnosis and pathological diagnosis should be highlighted in the final report, differentiating between major and minor discrepancies and between those which could have an impact on patients' management and those with no impact on treatment and outcome (Valette et al. 2014; Burton and Underwood 2007; Horowitz and Naritoku 2007). Mortality meeting and/or clinicopathological conferences should be routinely scheduled after autopsy of heart transplant patients with the presence of clinicians from the key specialties such as surgeons, physicians, intensivists, immunologists, microbiologists, pathologists and all clinical staff involved in transplantation. The autopsy findings can contribute to furthering our understanding of the pathophysiology of organ transplantation and ongoing diagnosis and therapeutic management of complications and their outcome.

24.8 Education and Training

The autopsy examination of the transplant recipient is an important means of teaching undergraduate and postgraduate students and doctors, including trainee pathologists and clinicians, about the pathology of heart transplantation and its complications. As in other organs heart transplantation is nowadays no longer an experimental option but a standard therapeutic procedure. However the consideration of the autopsy procedure as a valid teaching instrument in the perception of students has paralleled the drop in autopsy rate (Burton 2002; Burton and Underwood 2007; Horowitz and Naritoku 2007). A survey among undergraduate medical students before approaching autopsies in the pathology course during their fourth year in the University of Padua Medical School showed that more than 70 % would have refused to give consent to an autopsy on one of their relatives and about 40 % would have declined one on one of their patients, confirming the widespread impression held of the autopsy as a devastating, unpleasant and disrespectful procedure. After completion of the autopsy component of their pathology course, this figure fell to 20 %.

Even though pathologists have been slow in applying modern imaging tools for recording and storing autopsy images, it is our experience in Padua that recording the autopsy procedure is a powerful tool which guarantees that at any time the results can be reviewed by the surgeon or clinician who could not attend the procedure in person. The recordings can be used very effectively for clinical audit and serve to improve understanding of the pathology underlying the last illness and death of recipients. They are of value for clinicopathological conferences, clinical audit, meetings to review deaths or even in cases of medicolegal investigation. Constructing a video archive of autopsies is also an invaluable teaching tool. As part of an interactive autopsy teaching session a brief presentation of the clinical history should be followed by the presentation of the main findings, the organs and tissues being cleaned beforehand which will favour a more positive acceptance of the procedure by students. The subsequent discussion of the findings can lead students to a greater understanding of the pathological substrates of diseases and their pathophysiology.

24.9 Research and Biobanking

The availability of tissue samples from the allograft removed at autopsy for ethically approved research studies and to contribute to a biobank is of fundamental importance for research studies into the complications of transplantation. Obtaining consent from bereaved families for this to be done can be viewed as an opportunity for them to contribute positively to the well-being of future recipients despite the loss of their loved one.

Among the many examples of such research is that carried out about 10 years ago in the field of regenerative medicine. The revolution in this field changed our thinking from the traditional concept in medicine that some organs in the body were fully differentiated without the capacity to regenerate, among them the heart. This doctrine has been questioned through study of the transplanted heart removed at autopsy (Quaini et al. 2002). Using cardiac tissue from sex-mismatched heart transplants, in which a female donor heart had been implanted into a male recipient they showed, using fluorescence in situ hybridization that the allograft was colonized by recipient stem cells which could differentiate into cardiomyocytes, smooth muscle cells and endothelial cells. This set the scene for the development of regenerative medicine with evidence of existence and trafficking of pluripotent stem cells of bone marrow origin which could migrate into solid organs and terminally differentiate. Samples from the allografts were evaluated with molecular tests that identified the Y-chromosome and antigens on cell surfaces to identify their origin from donor or recipient. Other groups used the same model to confirm or disprove their results but nonetheless this model represents an example of proof of concept which derived from the availability of autopsied sex-mismatched allograft tissue. These and similar studies using different technologies have been used to further our understanding of the pathophysiology of cardiac allograft vasculopathy and the contribution of recipient and donor cells to development of this disease which ultimately leads to allograft failure and the death of the recipient.

The possibility of retrieving and sampling the heart allograft during an autopsy and to sample all the organs is of fundamental importance in setting up a bioarchive or biobank. A bioarchive, or diagnostic archive, is any collection of tissue and biological materials left over after diagnosis, which can subsequently be used in anonymized form for the secondary purposes of teaching and research studies. A biobank represents a collection of tissue or biological material such as serum, plasma or extracted DNA or RNA, obtained specifically for research with appropriate consent from recipients in the case of material obtained in life, or families in the case of autopsy material (Shickle et al. 2010). Biobanks are licensed and more strictly regulated compared to a bioarchive. There are stringent rules focusing on fundamental issues such as ethical approval and informed consent for all donated tissue samples under conditions of anonymization to be stored in optimum, safe and secure conditions with controlled access (Shickle 2006; Asslaber and Zatloukal 2007). However it is beyond the scope of this chapter to discuss all these aspects in detail. With increasing knowledge of molecular genetics, proteomics and investigations using molecular technology in general, it is important to obtain, according to local practice, informed consent from the family to keep the cardiac allograft and tissue samples for teaching and for future research, including molecular studies using stored DNA and RNA.

Conclusion

Autopsy remains the gold standard for identification of the cause of death in allograft recipients. To be an effective clinical tool it should be of a high standard, performed with competence and care and reported in a timely fashion. Completeness of the diagnostic procedure, including molecular investigation, is irreplaceable even in the era of digital technology because of the possibility of conserving and analyzing biological samples for diagnosis, audit and teaching and for current and future research studies. Contact with specialists looking after the transplant recipient is essential before and after the autopsy to help correctly diagnose the final cause of death and any contributing comorbidities and so close the chapter of the recipient's extended life. Clinical and pathological quality control and audits are important to ensure a high standard of service. Regular mortality review conferences should be held to discuss death taking place in the Transplant Unit and elsewhere, including in the community. Even in the best regulated centers a percentage of the cases will defy identification beyond reasonable doubt of the cause of death. In such cases the death certificate should include a ranked list of possible causes of death. Last but not least the important educational and research potential of the autopsy must always be kept in mind.

Key Points

- The complete autopsy is still the gold standard for investigating death in transplant recipient.
- The autopsy should be performed or supervised in a validated and accreditated laboratory by specialist cardiovascular pathologists assisted by trained anatomic pathology technicians and using standard protocols for dissection, tissue sampling and histopathological investigations.
- A key role is identification of mode and cause of death and significant comorbidities which may have a bearing on the death. It is essential to involve clinicians in discussions and case review in order to establish an agreed cause of death and prioritizing of comorbidities.
- Completion of the final report should await the outcome of formal multidisciplinary mortality review which may include additional clinical information and thus amend interpretation of the findings.
- Photographic documentation and video recordings of the procedures should be done for further evaluation with key clinicians involved in the management of the patient.
- The autopsy represents an opportunity to collect and store blood and tissue samples, with appropriate consent and according to each country's legislation, for diagnosis and related activities, education, research and biobanking, including RNA and DNA extraction and storage for future ethically approved research.
- Ensure relevant anonymized data on the autopsy is made available to each country's national and transplant data audit organizations

References

Alexander RT, Steenbergen C. Cause of death and sudden cardiac death after heart transplantation. An autopsy study. Am J Clin Pathol. 2003; 119(5):740–8.

Arthurs OJ, Thayyil S, Olsen OE, Addison S, Wade A, Jones R, et al. Diagnostic accuracy of post-mortem MRI for thoracic abnormalities in fetuses and children. Eur Radiol. 2014;24(11):2876–84.

Asslaber M, Zatloukal K. Biobanks: transnational, European and global networks. Brief Funct Genomic Proteomic. 2007;6(3):193–201.

Basso C, Burke M, Fornes P, Gallagher PJ, de Gouveia RH, Sheppard M, et al. Guidelines for autopsy investigation of sudden cardiac death. Virchows Arch. 2008;452(1):11–8.

Basso C, Carturan E, Pilichou K, Rizzo S, Corrado D, Thiene G. Sudden cardiac death with normal heart: molecular autopsy. Cardiovasc Pathol. 2010;19(6):321–5.

Burton EC. The autopsy: a professional responsibility in assuring quality of care. Am J Med Qual. 2002;17(2):56–60.

Burton JL, Underwood J. Clinical, educational, and epidemiological value of autopsy. Lancet. 2007;369(9571):1471–80.

Calabrese F, Valente M, Thiene G, Angelini A, Testolin L, Biasolo MA, et al. Enteroviral genome in native hearts may influence outcome of patients who undergo cardiac transplantation. Diagn Mol Pathol. 1999;8(1):39–46.

Carturan E, Tester DJ, Brost BC, Basso C, Thiene G, Ackerman MJ. Postmortem genetic testing for conventional autopsy-negative sudden unexplained death: an evaluation of different DNA extraction protocols and the feasibility of mutational analysis from archival paraffin-embedded heart tissue. Am J Clin Pathol. 2008;129(3):391–7.

Chantranuwat C, Blakey JD, Kobashigawa JA, Moriguchi JD, Laks H, Vassilakis ME, et al. Sudden, unexpected

death in cardiac transplant recipients: an autopsy study. J Heart Lung Transplant. 2004;23(6):683–9.
Fedrigo M, Poli F, Esposito G, Feltrin G, Toscano G, d'Agostino C, et al. HLA-DRB1 typing by micro-bead array assay identifies the origin of early lymphoproliferative disorder in a heart transplant recipient. Am J Transplant. 2013;13(3):802–7.
Gallo P, Agozzino L, Angelini A, Arbustini E, Bartoloni G, Bernucci P, et al. Causes of late failure after heart transplantation: a ten-year survey. J Heart Lung Transplant. 1997;16(11):1113–21.
General Medical Council. Making and using visual and audio recordings of patients - Deceased patients. 2015. Ref Type: Online Source.
Graham AR. Autopsy findings in cardiac transplant patients. A 10-year experience. Am J Clin Pathol. 1992;97(3):369–75.
Horowitz RE, Naritoku WY. The autopsy as a performance measure and teaching tool. Hum Pathol. 2007;38(5):688–95.
Kang X, Cos T, Guizani M, Cannie MM, Segers V, Jani JC. Parental acceptance of minimally invasive fetal and neonatal autopsy compared with conventional autopsy. Prenat Diagn. 2014;34(11):1106–10.
Lund LH, Edwards LB, Kucheryavaya AY, Benden C, Christie JD, Dipchand AI, et al. The registry of the International Society for Heart and Lung Transplantation: thirtieth official adult heart transplant report – 2013; focus theme: age. J Heart Lung Transplant. 2013;32(10):951–64.
LundLH, Edwards LB, Kucheryavaya AY, Benden C, Christie JD, Dipchand AI, et al. The registry of the International Society for Heart and Lung transplantation: thirty-first official adult heart transplant report-2014; focus theme: retransplantation. J Heart Lung Transplant. 2014;33(10):996–1008.
Melacini P, Basso C, Angelini A, Calore C, Bobbo F, Tokajuk B, et al. Clinicopathological profiles of progressive heart failure in hypertrophic cardiomyopathy. Eur Heart J. 2010;31(17):2111–23.
Melacini P, Gambino A, Caforio A, Barchitta A, Valente ML, Angelini A, et al. Heart transplantation in patients with inherited myopathies associated with end-stage cardiomyopathy: molecular and biochemical defects on cardiac and skeletal muscle. Transplant Proc. 2001;33(1–2):1596–9.
Michaud K, Grabherr S, Faouzi M, Grimm J, Doenz F, Mangin P. Pathomorphological and CT-angiographical characteristics of coronary atherosclerotic plaques in cases of sudden cardiac death. Int J Legal Med. 2015;129(5):1067–77.
Patel VS, Lim M, Massin EK, Jonsyn GP, Ates P, Abou-Awdi NL, et al. Sudden cardiac death in cardiac transplant recipients. Circulation. 1996;94(9 Suppl):II273–7.
Quaini F, Urbanek K, Beltrami AP, Finato N, Beltrami CA, Nadal-Ginard B, et al. Chimerism of the transplanted heart. N Engl J Med. 2002;346(1):5–15.
Rose AG, Viviers L, Odell JA. Autopsy-determined causes of death following cardiac transplantation. A study of 81 patients and literature review. Arch Pathol Lab Med. 1992;116(11):1137–41.
Ross SG, Thali MJ, Bolliger S, Germerott T, Ruder TD, Flach PM. Sudden death after chest pain: feasibility of virtual autopsy with postmortem CT angiography and biopsy. Radiology. 2012;264(1):250–9.
Royal College of Pathologists. Guidelines on autopsy practice scenario 1: sudden death with likely cardiac pathology. 2015. Ref Type: Online Source.
Sanroman BB, Vazquez ME, Pertega DS, Veiga BA, Carro RE, Mosquera RJ. Autopsy-determined causes of death in solid organ transplant recipients. Transplant Proc. 2004;36(3):787–9.
Schnoor M, Schafer T, Luhmann D, Sievers HH. Bicaval versus standard technique in orthotopic heart transplantation: a systematic review and meta-analysis. J Thorac Cardiovasc Surg. 2007;134(5):1322–31.
Shickle D, Griffin M, El-Arifi K. Inter- and intra-biobank networks: classification of biobanks. Pathobiology. 2010;77(4):181–90.
Shickle D. The consent problem within DNA biobanks. Stud Hist Philos Biol Biomed Sci. 2006; 37(3):503–19.
Shojania KG, Burton EC, McDonald KM, Goldman L. Changes in rates of autopsy-detected diagnostic errors over time: a systematic review. JAMA. 2003;289(21):2849–56.
Thayyil S, Sebire NJ, Chitty LS, Wade A, Chong W, Olsen O, et al. Post-mortem MRI versus conventional autopsy in fetuses and children: a prospective validation study. Lancet. 2013;382(9888):223–33.
TRAGEDY – Trans-Tasman Response AGAinst Sudden Death in the Young, 2008. Best Practise Guidelines for post-mortem investigation of sudden unexpected death in the young. 2015. Ref Type: Online Source.
Valette TN, Ayub-Ferreira SM, Benvenuti LA, Issa VS, Bacal F, Chizzola PR, et al. NHETS–Necropsy Heart Transplantation Study. Arq Bras Cardiol. 2014;102(5):505–9.
Van der Linden A, Blokker BM, Kap M, Weustink AC, Riegman PH, Oosterhuis JW. Post-mortem tissue biopsies obtained at minimally invasive autopsy: an RNA-quality analysis. PLoS One. 2014;9(12), e115675.
Vaseghi M, Lellouche N, Ritter H, Fonarow GC, Patel JK, Moriguchi J, et al. Mode and mechanisms of death after orthotopic heart transplantation. Heart Rhythm. 2009;6(4):503–9.
Weustink AC, Hunink MG, van Dijke CF, Renken NS, Krestin GP, Oosterhuis JW. Minimally invasive autopsy: an alternative to conventional autopsy? Radiology. 2009;250(3):897–904.
World Health Organisation. International statistical classification of diseases and related health problems 10th revision. 2015. Ref Type: Online Source.
Zuppan CW, Wells LM, Kerstetter JC, Johnston JK, Bailey LL, Chinnock RE. Cause of death in pediatric and infant heart transplant recipients: review of a 20-year, single-institution cohort. J Heart Lung Transplant. 2009;28(6):579–84.

25 Examination of Native Hearts with Implantable Mechanical Circulatory Support Systems

Klaus Aumayr and Katharina Wassilew

Contents

K. Aumayr, MD (✉)
Clinical Institute for Pathology,
Medical University of Vienna,
Vienna, Austria
e-mail: klaus.aumayr@meduniwien.ac.at

K. Wassilew, MD, DScmed
Department of Pathology,
Rigshospitalet, University of Copenhagen,
Blegdamsvej 9, Copenhagen 2100, Denmark
e-mail: katharina.wassilew@regionh.dk

25.1 Background

Mechanical circulatory support systems (MCS) are now widely used as a treatment option to bridge the failing heart to transplantation. The 2015 annual report of the Registry of the International Society for Heart and Lung Transplantation states that MCS devices were used as short and long-term treatment option in up to 35 % of heart recipients at time of transplantation (Lund et al. 2015). However, serious life-limiting complications may occur in this patient group whether or not they proceed to transplantation (Kirklin et al. 2015).

There are a number of descriptions in the literature of how best to dissect the heart depending on the underlying pathology (Houser 2009; Billingham 1997; Gilbert-Barness et al. 2014; Devine et al. 1991). In recent decades the number of end-stage heart failure patients and, within this group, those treated with mechanical circulatory support systems is growing. However, the literature on cardiac examination in this patient group is very limited, apart from reports referring to implantation techniques used for different MCS systems, which could in turn be used as guidance for opening the heart.

The dissection method described below supplements dissection techniques of the heart already in widespread use.

O. Leone et al. (eds.), *The Pathology of Cardiac Transplantation*,
DOI 10.1007/978-3-319-46386-5_25

25.2 Components of Mechanical Assist Devices

Before proceeding to the dissection of the heart, the pathologist should be familiar with the components of the implanted MCS system (Fig. 25.1a) and its anticipated location in the heart with regard to the supported ventricle (left, right, or both, Fig. 25.1b). The components of implantable left ventricular assist devices (LVAD) usually encountered at autopsy are the inflow cannula, which is inserted into the ventricular apex or into the left atrium and is connected to the pump itself (Fig. 25.2a); the outflow cannula, extending from the apex to the ascending or descending aorta, where it is anastomosed above the valves (Fig. 25.1a, b); and the driveline (Fig. 25.3a), an insulated electrical cable which exits the body from the device through an opening in the skin in the upper abdomen (Fig. 25.2b). The exception is the Jarvik device, in which the driveline exits via a retroauricular skull pedestal.

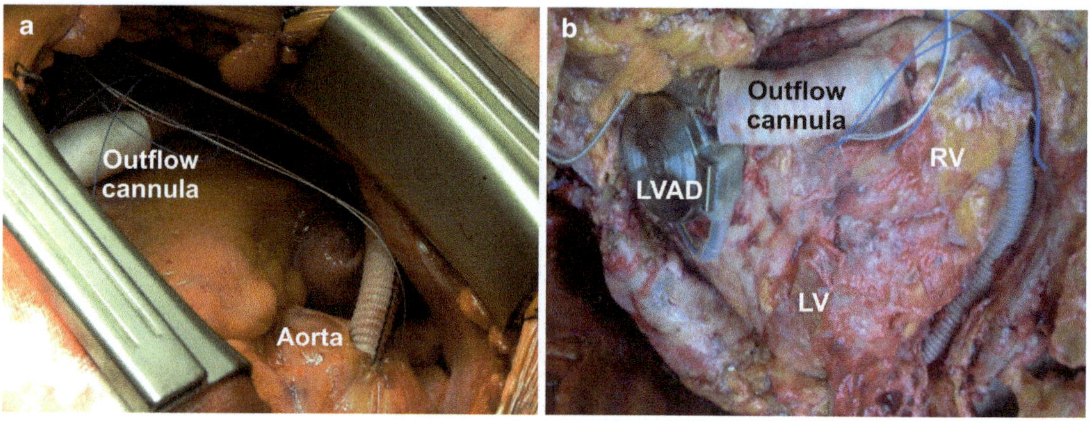

Fig. 25.1 (**a**) Situs after implantation of left ventricular assist devices (LVAD). The outflow cannula is seen at the apex, at the base of the heart, and at its anastomosis with the aorta. (**b**) Situs at autopsy. The pericardial sac has been opened. The MCS device with outflow cannula extending along the lateral wall of the right ventricle (RV) is observed. *LV* left ventricle

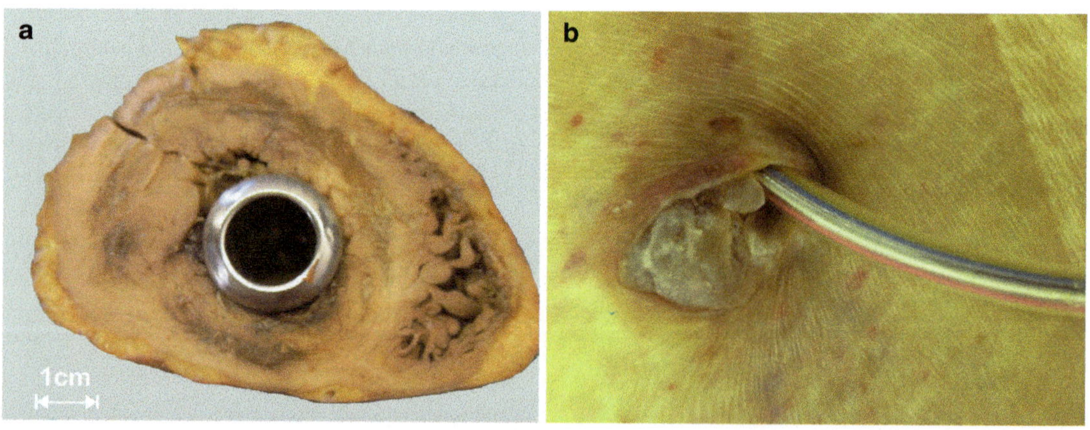

Fig. 25.2 (**a**) Cross section through short axis of both ventricles in a severe case of myocarditis. The apical cannula and its location in the narrow left ventricular cavity are demonstrated. (**b**) Transcutaneous exit site of driveline cable. Note in the surroundings the histologically confirmed focal hemorrhage and granulation tissue

In patients with an isolated right ventricular assist device (RVAD) or those supported with biventricular implantable systems (BVAD), the inflow cannula is implanted into the right ventricle or right atrium, while the outflow cannula in most cases connects to the pulmonary trunk.

Patients supported with a total artificial heart (TAH) will have had their native heart removed at supravalvular level at the time of device implantation. The residual native atria are connected by cuffs to the two ventricles of the artificial heart, which are in turn connected to the great arteries by Dacron tubes. The pneumatic driver (compressor) is extracorporeal and is connected with the TAH by two tubes penetrating the skin below the xiphisternum. TAHs are rarely encountered at autopsy. In the case of heart transplantation, only the explanted atria are received for histopathological examination.

25.3 Examination Prior to Removal of the Heart and Device

The area around the transcutaneous driveline exit site represents one of the main entry points for bacterial and fungal infections, which may spread along the driveline into the mediastinum. These are responsible for a major proportion of deaths related to sepsis in MCS patients. This area should therefore be carefully examined (Fig. 25.2b). Ancillary techniques to identify specific pathogens, such as taking swabs from this area, may be appropriate in the clinical setting. Usually the driveline is cut off before sending explanted hearts from heart transplant patients for histopathological examination.

At autopsy, on opening of the chest wall, the likelihood of encountering dense adhesions between the chest wall and anterior mediastinum increases with time after MCS implantation and

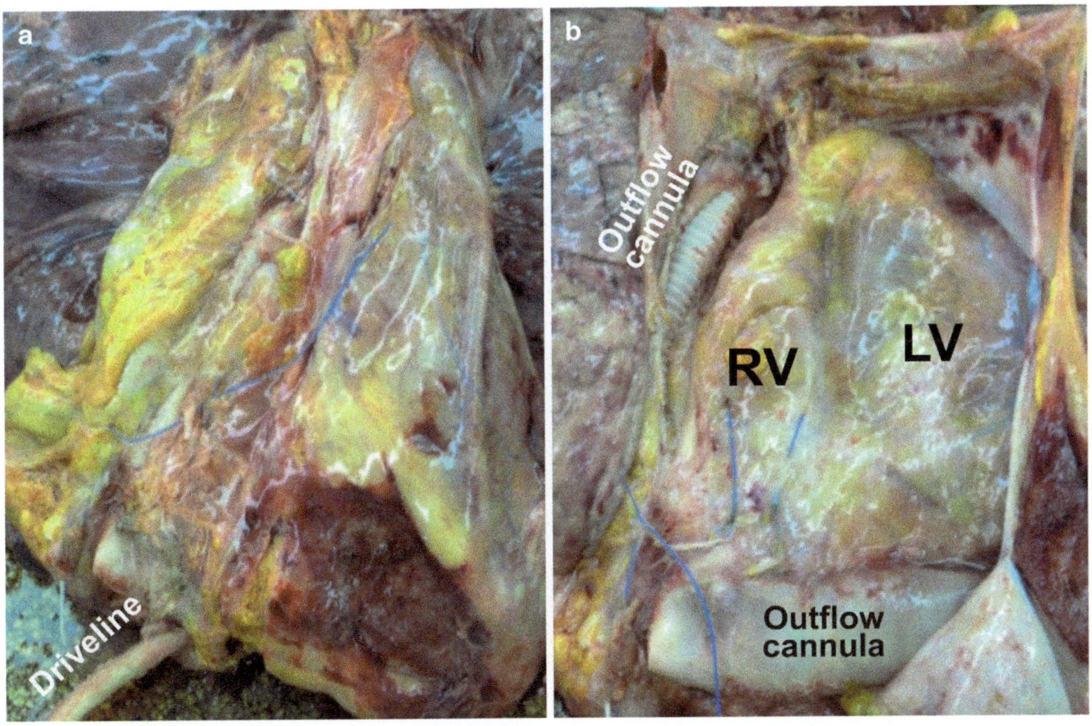

Fig. 25.3 (**a**) Eviscerated thoracic organs with the driveline extending distally from the closed pericardial sac. (**b**) Anterior view into the opened pericardial sac. The epicardial surface of both heart chambers is exposed; the course of the outflow cannula along the lateral right ventricular wall is seen. *LV* left ventricle, *RV* right ventricle

each episode of thoracic infection. These often cannot be separated by blunt dissection. As in the presence of mammary artery bypass grafts, the anterior rib cage and sternum should be lifted carefully and separated from the adhesions with short-length cuts along the internal surface of the sternum and ribs in order to avoid cutting through the outflow cannula of the LVAD. This is usually positioned on the anterior epicardial surface of the right ventricle, anterior to the level of the left ventricle (Fig. 25.3b). The driveline cable should be pulled in its entirety through the skin into the chest cavity and then checked for macroscopically visible defects. The pericardial sac may be adherent to much of the epicardial surface of the heart, obliterating the pericardial cavity. However, the two layers of pericardium may be separated, beginning with a small cut into the pericardial sac posteriorly, where the adhesions are not as pronounced as on the anterior surface. From there, the adhesions can be loosened manually, working forward from the posterior surface.

When the thoracic cavity and the pericardial sac lie open (see Fig. 25.3b), the presence and quantity of liquid and/or clotted blood should be recorded. There is a risk of oozing of blood due to obligatory anticoagulation treatment, especially from the great arteries at the site of anastomoses with the graft.

The different components of each MCS system, their location, and their correlation to the anatomic structures should be recorded. The outflow cannula should be evaluated with regard to length, signs of tension, and kinking. Photographic documentation of the site before and after removal of the MCS may be useful to illustrate the position of each component and any complications encountered.

If blood cultures are required for microbiological examination, samples should be submitted from the right ventricle or inferior vena cava.

25.4 Removal and Examination of the Heart and MCS Device

The heart can then be lifted from the pericardial sac and separated from all its vascular connections, well above the anastomoses between the MCS outflow graft component and the great arteries and at least 2 cm above the annuli of the atrioventricular valves (Fig. 25.4a, view from posterior) or, if possible, at the level of the vena cava and pulmonary veins. The pathologist should be aware that the anastomoses of the outflow cannula may be located in the descending aorta. Adhesions between outflow cannula and epicardial surface, which are present from a few weeks after implantation, should, whenever possible, be separated manually along the epicardial surface. The cardiac circumference is measured at the valvular level on the exposed epicardial surface. The coronary arteries can now be examined as appropriate. Preliminary assessment of the aortic valve with regard to the presence of commissural fusion and thrombosis can be made.

To open the heart, a single transverse section is made through the anterior and posterior ventricular walls, parallel to the base of the heart, below the valvular apparatus of the mitral valve but above the apical cannula, tunneling between outflow cannula and epicardial surface (Fig. 25.4b). The proximal part of the apical cannula can be easily palpated from the pericardial surface, as the mechanically unloaded ventricle remains in diastole. The bisected heart exposes the apical cannula to view so its position in relation to the septum and inflow tract and its distance to the (mitral) valve leaflets can be assessed. The presence of antemortem thrombus, within and on the luminal surface, fibrous tissue, and, in rare cases, anatomic structures obstructing the lumen of the apical cannula, is recorded. The endocardial surface, mostly over the ventricular septum, is assessed for signs of suction from the device in cases of suboptimal positioning of the inflow cannula (Fig. 25.5). In addition, measurements of the wall thickness of ventricles and interventricular septum and left ventricular diameter can be taken. The top half of the heart is now further opened from the atria along the inflow tracts at the lateral wall of the ventricles through the mitral and tricuspid valves and then along the outflow tracts parallel and in proximity to the interventricular septum through the pulmonary and aortic valves. The atrial appendages are opened and examined for the presence of thrombi.

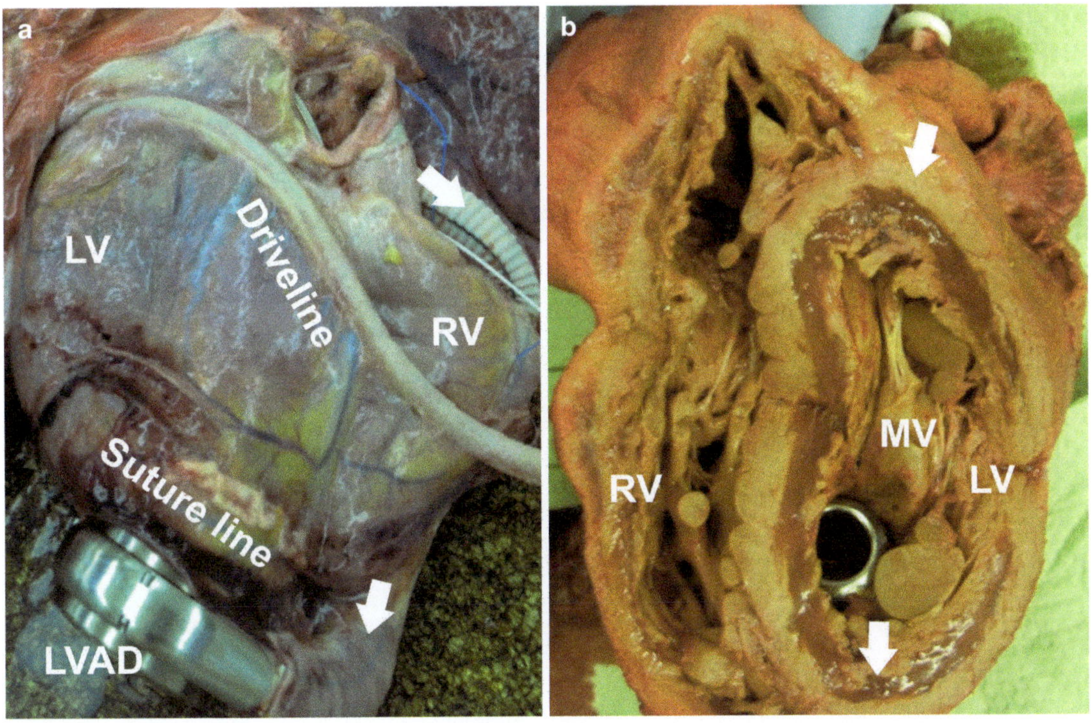

Fig. 25.4 (**a**) View of the posterior surface after severing of the vascular connections. The LVAD, its connection with the left chamber, the outflow graft (*arrow*), and the driveline are evaluated. (**b**) Opened heart with a section across the short heart axis above the LVAD inflow cannula. The ventricular chambers and the tension apparatus of the mitral valve (MV) are exposed. *LV* left ventricle, *LVAD* left ventricular assist devices, *MV* mitral valve, *RV* right ventricle

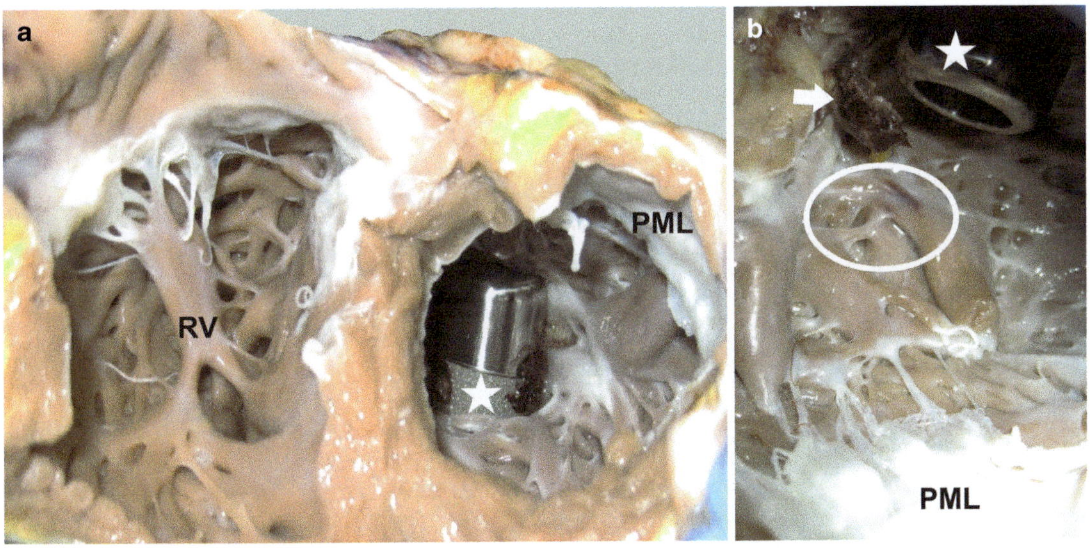

Fig. 25.5 (**a**) Suboptimally positioned apical cannula of HeartWare device (*asterisk*), which is directed toward the posterior wall of the left ventricle, below the posterior mitral leaflet (PML). (**b**) There is a thrombus (*arrowhead*) between the apical cannula (*asterisk*) and the ventricular wall. Just above the opening of the apical cannula, there is hemorrhage of the thickened endocardium (*encircled*). *PML* posterior mitral leaflet, *RV* right ventricle

The valves are now exposed. The commissures of the aortic cusps are examined for thrombosis and presence and length of commissural fusion (Fig. 25.6). The mitral valve is assessed for thickening of leaflets as well as for shortening and fusion of the chordae tendineae. The distance between the opening for the apical cannula and the free margin of the anterior mitral valve leaflet is assessed. The circumference of each valve is measured. Endocardial thickening below the valvular ring is regarded as a sign of valvular insufficiency. The suture ring at the site of anastomosis of the outflow cannula is carefully evaluated (Fig. 25.4a). The distance to the valve annulus is recorded.

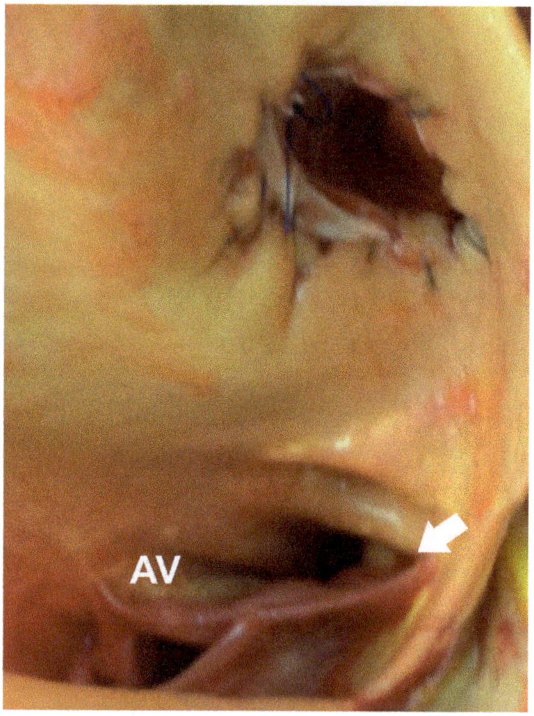

Fig. 25.6 Site of anastomosis of outflow graft with the aorta, above the aortic valve (*AV*). Note the commissural fusion involving the free margin of two cusps (*arrow*)

In rare cases in which the patient had been weaned from the device, the tissue defect remaining after removal of the apical cannula will have been closed with a plug (Fig. 25.7). The position of the plug and the degree of endothelialization should be assessed (Fig. 25.7).

The heart may now be weighed after removal of the different device components, if their weight has not been communicated by the clinicians. Usually a technician from the MCS team is present at autopsy, to photograph the relevant macroscopic findings for documentation purposes. The motor component will be sent back to the manufacturer, who will examine the rotor for signs of malfunction or thrombus.

Further serial sectioning at 1–2 cm intervals along the short axis of the heart is advised in

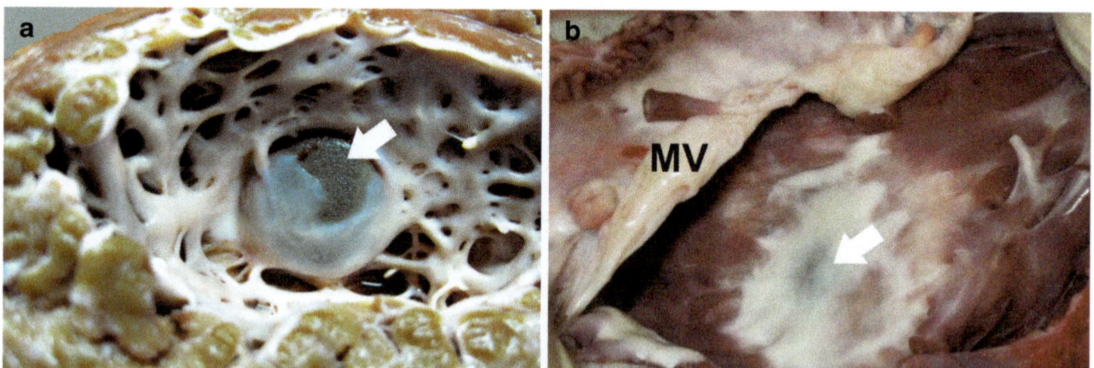

Fig. 25.7 (**a**) Partially endothelialized plug in the former position of the inflow cannula of the LVAD (*arrow*). (**b**) Fully endothelialized plug in the former position of the inflow cannula of the LVAD (*arrow*). *MV* mitral valve

order to examine the cut surface of myocardium for areas of scarring, hemorrhage, or infarction. Whenever possible, besides sampling the altered macroscopic areas, additional full thickness samples from the ventricular myocardial walls and the interventricular septum should be obtained for histopathological examination. The same can be done for the myocardial tissue around the apical inflow cannula. The sinoatrial and atrioventricular nodes should be examined in cases of arrhythmia of any kind. When vasculitis is suspected, the aorta and pulmonary trunk should be investigated as should be the valves in cases of endocarditis or structural damage relating to MCS therapy.

The above described method of examination and dissection can also be applied mechanically unloaded hearts explanted at time of heart transplantation.

CAVE The diagnosis of decompensated heart failure as the immediate cause of death should be avoided for ventricles supported with MCS, as the heart chambers will have been mechanically unloaded by the device. In exceptional cases of technical impairment or insufficient blood flow through the device, signs of failure of the VAD-supported ventricle, for instance, lung edema in acute left-sided heart decompensation, may be encountered. Only in the presence of manifest severe findings that could only be explained by acute cardiac decompensation may signs of impaired ventricular function be attested. In the majority of cases, the pathological findings in the rest of the autopsy support a diagnosis of multi-organ failure. On the other hand, diagnosis of acute failure of the contralateral ventricle, as, for instance, acute right ventricular decompensation in an LVAD patient, is regularly found.

Key Points

- Be sure you know what you are looking for – familiarize yourself with the device type used.
- Identify all relevant device components before dissecting, and open the heart along the inflow and outflow tracts after sectioning across both ventricles parallel to its base above the level of the apical cannula.
- Be aware of the main complications of MCS therapy, infection and bleeding, and document them as appropriate.
- To complete the pathology study, sampling for histology should be as extensive as possible.
- Avoid autopsy diagnosis of acute failure of the ventricle supported with the VAD.

References

Billingham ME. Dissection method for an adult heart. In: Sternberg SS, editor. Histology for pathologists. 2nd ed. Philadelphia: Lippincott Williams & Wilkins; 1997.

Devine WA, Debich DE, Anderson RH. Dissection of congenitally malformed hearts, with comments on the value of sequential segmental analysis. Pediatr Pathol. 1991;11(2):235–59.

Gilbert-Barness E, Spicer DE, Steffensen TS. Handbook of pediatric autopsy pathology. 2nd ed. New York: Springer Science Business Media; 2014.

Houser SL. The operated heart at autopsy. Dordrecht/London: Springer Science Business Media; 2009.

Kirklin JK, Naftel DC, Pagani FD, Kormos RL, Stevenson LW, Blume ED, et al. Seventh INTERMACS annual report: 15,000 patients and counting. J Heart Lung Transplant. 2015;34(12):1495–504.

Lund LH, Edwards LB, Kucheryavaya AY, Benden C, Dipchand AI, Goldfarb S, et al. The registry of the international society for heart and lung transplantation: thirty-second official adult heart transplantation report-2015; focus theme: early graft failure. J Heart Lung Transplant. 2015;34(10):1244–54.

Appendix

Worksheet: Endomyocardial biopsy	
1. Pre-transplant for diagnosis	
Specimen procurement and triage	*Light microscopic examination:* At least three, preferably four, endomyocardial fragments, each 1–2 mm^3 in size, should immediately be fixed in 10% buffered formalin at room temperature. When there is a suspicion of myocardial lesions, possibly characterized by focal distribution, additional sampling is recommended. *Molecular tests or specific stains (when required):* One or two specimens may be snap frozen in liquid nitrogen and stored at minus 80°C. Fragments may also be stored in RNAlater at room temperature. *Ultrastructural tests (when required):* One fragment fixed in 2.5% glutaraldehyde or Karnowsky solution. A sample of peripheral blood (5–10 ml) in EDTA or citrate from patients with suspected myocarditis allows molecular testing for the same viral genomes sought in the myocardial tissue.

O. Leone et al. (eds.), *The Pathology of Cardiac Transplantation*,
DOI 10.1007/978-3-319-46386-5

Worksheet: Endomyocardial biopsy	
1. Pre-transplant for diagnosis	
Pathological analysis	*Light microscopic examination* is routinely performed on formalin-fixed and paraffin-embedded tissue using: Multiple, numbered haematoxylin-eosin section examination. Additional histochemical, histomorphological, histoenzymatic and immunohistochemical stains performed on paraffin-embedded fragments or on frozen sections. *Additional stains on formalin-fixed and paraffin-embedded sections (when required)* *Histomorphological and histochemical stains:* Masson or Mallory trichrome, Movat pentachrome and Weigert-Van Gieson for collagen and elastic fibres and small vessel evaluation. PAS with and without diastase for glycogen storage (better on frozen sections). Congo red for amyloid (modified sulfated alcian blue or thioflavin T may also be used although the first choice is Congo red). Perls' iron stain. *Immunohistochemical stains:* CD45, CD20, CD3, CD4, CD8, CD68/PGM1 for inflammatory and cellular infiltrate assessment (some centres also evaluate HLA-DR and HLA-ABC expression in suspected cases of myocardial inflammatory disease). Transthyretin, kappa and lambda chains, apolipoprotein and amyloid A component for amyloid typing. Dystrophin, lamin A/C, emerin, desmin, plakoglobin and N-cadherin for some genetic cardiomyopathies. *Additional stains on frozen sections:* Sudan black, oil red and PAS with and without diastase for storage disease. Histoenzymatic stains (succinate dehydrogenase, SDH, and cytochrome oxidase, COX) for mitochondrial disease. Immunofluorescence stains. Many immunostains listed above, including HLA-DR and HLA-ABC, amyloid subtypes and desmosomal proteins, may also be done on frozen tissue according to centre practice. *Molecular analysis (when required):* Polymerase chain reaction (PCR), quantitative or qualitative, and reverse transcriptase-PCR on the fragments frozen in liquid nitrogen or stored in RNAlater for viral detection in myocarditis. Protein sequencing and mass spectroscopy on formalin-fixed and paraffin-embedded fragments or fragments frozen in liquid nitrogen to subtype amyloid deposits. *Transmission electron microscopy examination (when required):* Fragments fixed in glutaraldehyde or Karnowsky solution and embedded in resin.

Worksheet: Endomyocardial biopsy	
2. Post-transplant monitoring	
Specimen procurement and triage	*Light microscopic examination:* At least three, preferably four, endomyocardial fragments, each 1–2 mm^3 in size, should immediately be fixed in 10% buffered formalin at room temperature. Samples should be obtained from different ventricle sites and not divided once procured. One specimen should be snap frozen in liquid nitrogen in centres performing immunofluorescence for AMR. One more specimen may be snap frozen in liquid nitrogen and stored at minus 80°C or stored in RNAlater at room temperature for research. *Preparation* Biopsies are usually rapidly processed using microwave oven or pressure cooker and then paraffin embedded.
Pathological analysis	*Light microscopic examination* is routinely performed on formalin-fixed and paraffin-embedded tissue using: At least three slides at three levels through the tissue samples, each including a minimum of three sections, stained with haematoxylin-eosin with spare sections between levels kept for more detailed assessment as required. There is no common practice among various centres: most institutions evaluate from three to six haematoxylin-eosin slides at different levels of the paraffin block – optimally to a max of sixty sections; the number of sections on each slide may vary from three to eight. *Biopsy adequacy* An adequate sample should contain at least 50% of myocardium free of previous biopsy sites, scar, adipose tissue and blood clots.
Pathological evaluation of acute cellular rejection (ACR)	ACR is usually assessed on haematoxylin-eosin stained sections: no routine special stains are required.
Pathological evaluation of antibody-mediated rejection	*Paraffin sections for immunoperoxidase:* A minimum of two slides (for C4d and CD68) and more for further stainings according to centre routine. *Frozen sections for immunofluorescence:* A minimum of two slides (for C4d and C3d) and more for further stainings according to centre routine. Some centres include anti-HLA-DR in the primary panel to identify capillaries.
Rare conditions	*Suspected myocarditis:* Immunohistochemistry for Cytomegalovirus. Polymerase chain reaction for viral detection on paraffin-embedded sections or preferably on frozen sample if centre usually stores it. *Suspected Post-transplant lympho-proliferative disorders:* Appropriate immunohistochemistry. In situ hybridization for Epstein Barr virus. Clonality studies and mutation analysis. *Suspected amyloid recurrence:* Congo red stain.

Template for Acute Cellular Rejection (ACR) Pathology Report

The pathology report should include the features listed below, either tabulated or as a descriptive report, and a final diagnosis.

Description/Tabulated Features

- Number of samples specifying number of any inadequate
- Adipose tissue (if any)
- Pericardium (when present)
- Oedema (if any)
- Interstitial haemorrhage (if any)
- Previous biopsy sites – recent, intermediate, old (if any)
- Findings related to peritransplant injury (if any):
  - Type
  - Degree (mild, moderate, severe)
  - Distribution (focal, multifocal, diffuse)
- Thrombus (if any)
  - Recent/organising
- Fibrosis (if any):
  - Type: endocardial, perivascular/perimyocyte interstitial, replacement
  - Degree (mild, moderate, severe)
  - Distribution (focal, multifocal, diffuse)
- Inflammatory infiltrates
  - Not present
  - Present
  - Site: perivascular interstitial, perimyocyte interstitial, subendocardial (extended or not to myocardium)
  - Type (lymphocytic or other)
  - Degree (mild, moderate, severe)
  - Distribution (focal, multifocal, diffuse)
- Myocyte damage (if any)
  - Type
  - Associated or not to inflammatory infiltrates
  - Degree (mild, moderate, severe)
  - Distribution (focal, multifocal, diffuse)
- Arteritis/arteriolitis (if any)
- Chronic microvasculopathy related to graft vasculopathy (if any)
  - Type (intimal, medial, mixed)
  - Severity in terms of stenosis (mild, moderate, severe)

Diagnosis

ACR Rejection Grade

- Grade 0R
- Grade 1R (can also specify if 1A, 1B or 2 by 1990 grading scheme)
- Grade 2R/3A
- Grade 3R (can also specify 3B or 4 by 1990 grading scheme)

In case of inadequate biopsy: No evidence of rejection in inadequate biopsy.

Should also be mentioned:

- Evolution in relation to previous biopsy
- Perioperative damage when significant
- Quilty lesions (optional)
- Degree of chronic microvasculopathy (when present)

Template for Antibody-Mediated Rejection (AMR) Pathology Report

The pathology report should include the histopathology features related to microvascular inflammation listed below, either tabulated or as a descriptive report, results of immunopathology findings and the final diagnosis.

Histopathology

- Features absent
- Features present:
  - Swollen activated endothelial cells (endothelial cells with prominent large nuclei and expanded cytoplasmic projections narrowing or occluding the lumens)
  - Intravascular activated mononuclear cells (more than occasional focal aggregates or scattered isolated foci)
  - Interstitial oedema (found in AMR but may be a nonspecific finding)
  - Severe AMR features (haemorrhage, endothelial cell pyknosis/karyorrhexis, capillary fragmentation, mixed inflammatory infiltrates, extensive myocyte damage/necrosis)

Ischaemic injury area, healing biopsy site, Quilty lesions and myocardial scars must be excluded from evaluation.

Immunopathology

Paraffin immunohistochemistry

C4d

- Negative staining: 0–10%
- Focal staining (10–50%) weak or strong
- Multifocal/diffuse staining (>50%), weak or strong.

The percentage refers to the surface of evaluable myocardium. Positive C4d result: multifocal/diffuse (>50%) weak or strong staining.

CD68 (intravascular macrophages)

- Negative staining: 0–10%
- Focal staining (10–50%)
- Multifocal/diffuse staining (>50%)

Positive CD68 result: focal (>10) or multifocal/diffuse (>50%) intravascular macrophages

Secondary panel

List the antibodies used (for C3d use the same mask as C4d)

Frozen immunofluorescence

C4d

- Negative staining: 0–10%
- Focal staining (10–50%) weak or strong
- Multifocal/diffuse staining (>50%) weak or strong

The percentage refers to the surface of evaluable myocardium. Positive C4d result: multifocal/diffuse (>50%) weak or strong staining.

C3d

- Negative staining: 0–10%
- Focal staining (10–50%) weak or strong
- Multifocal/diffuse staining (>50%) weak or strong

HLA- DR is used by some centres to identify capillary structures

The percentage refers to the surface of evaluable myocardium. Positive C4d result: multifocal/diffuse (>50%) weak or strong staining.

Secondary panel

List the antibodies used and patterns observed

Diagnosis and Grading

- *pAMR 0:* Negative for pathological AMR (Both histological and immunopathological findings negative)
- *pAMR 1:* Indicative of possible pathological AMR
  - *pAMR 1 (H+):* Histopathological AMR alone (histological findings present and immunopathological findings negative)
  - *pAMR 1 (I+):* Immunopathological AMR alone (histological findings negative and immunopathological findings positive) (CD68+ and/or C4d+)
- *pAMR 2:* Positive for pathological AMR (both histological and immunopathological findings present)
- *pAMR 3:* Severe pathological AMR

Worksheet: Native hearts	
Common to Each type	
Appropriate photographic documentation of both the intact and the sectioned hearts should be made	
Handling of the native heart	**Fresh heart** Wash out to remove blood clots. Put crumpled paper towels or gauze soaked in formalin in ventricle cavities to allow fixation without distortion. Take small ventricle pieces to be frozen or be fixed in glutaraldehyde (for graft harvest, research and when appropriate for diagnosis). Put the heart in an appropriately sized container with sufficient 10% formalin to cover. **Formalin-fixed heart** When a distorted heart is received: Put crumpled paper towels soaked in formalin in ventricle cavities to allow fixation without further distortion. Make sure that container is appropriately sized with sufficient 10% formalin to cover.
Gross examination before sectioning the heart	Specify if formalin-fixed or unfixed heart. Describe the completeness of the heart (pieces previously removed for research or one or more valves for use as homografts). Detail any wires, catheters or devices present. Weigh the heart. Measure: Longitudinal length (distance from the crux cordis to the apex on the posterior aspect) Transverse breadth (distance from the obtuse to the acute margin along the posterior atrioventricular sulcus) Describe general shape: Normal Globular Conical Altered volumetric ratio between the ventricles at external examination Possible aneurysms Describe amount and distribution of epicardial fat. Examine the atrial cuffs and atrial appendages for size, endocardial lesions and thrombi. Examine atrioventricular valves from the atria and the semilunar valves from above and note any abnormalities.

Worksheet: Native hearts	
Sectioning, internal gross examination and sampling for histology according to disease groups	
1. Ischaemic heart disease	
Native coronary arteries	Check the number, position, size of coronary arteries and patency of the coronary ostia. Assess the size, course and dominance of the major coronary arteries. Make a series of transverse cuts at 3 mm intervals in the main epicardial branches (left anterior descending, left circumflex artery, diagonal and obtuse marginal branches, right coronary artery) and for each indicate atherosclerotic plaques and degree of stenosis. In the presence of severely calcified atherosclerotic lesions, dissect the segment and section it after decalcification. Sample representative specimens from stenotic segments of coronary arteries.
Coronary artery stents	Remove the stented vessel by cutting it proximally and distally to the device, fix it in formalin and then process appropriately alternatively. Cut across the stented vessel with sharp scissors to check patency. Sample representative specimens (when appropriate processing is available).
Coronary artery by-pass grafts	Carefully dissect the coronary artery by-pass grafts (internal mammary arteries, saphenous veins, radial arteries, etc.) from the pericardial adhesions. Examine the removed specimen(s) with transverse cuts as for native vessel. Take representative specimens from the anastomotic area (one proximally, one at the anastomotic level and one distally).
Heart	Cut a transverse slice of the heart at mid-ventricular level and then parallel slices of the ventricles, working towards the apex at 1 cm intervals. Describe chamber sizes (normal, small, dilated). Document scars as subendocardial or transmural and describe their radial (anterior, lateral, posterior and septal) and longitudinal (base, mid-ventricle and apex) location. Measure thickness of free wall of both ventricles and the interventricular septum (parietal compact myocardium excluding trabeculae) at basal, medium and apical levels. Describe wall thinning and aneurysm formation (bulge at transmural scar) and any other alterations of myocardium.
Sampling for histology	A complete section of the heart at mid-ventricular level, including infarcted and non infarcted myocardium. One sample from the right ventricle, one from the left ventricle and one from the interventricular septum at both basal and apical segments.
Staining	Haematoxylin-eosin. When warranted by Haematoxylin-eosin, stains for collagen and elastic fibres (Masson or Mallory trichrome, Movat pentachrome, Weigert-Van Gieson, etc.) and additional stains or immunohistochemistry.

Worksheet: Native hearts	
Sectioning, internal gross examination and sampling for histology according to disease groups	
2. Myocardial disease	
Sectioning	Echocardiographic short axis cut (see Chap. 5, Fig. 5.11a, b). Make serial transverse sections (i.e. perpendicular to the long axis of the heart) from the apex to the mid-ventricular level or the base as far as the apex of papillary muscles at 1 cm intervals. Section the cardiac basal segment along its longitudinal axis (optional). Echocardiographic four-chamber cut (see Chap. 5, Fig. 5.11c, d). Make an entire cut from the base to the apex along the acute and obtuse edges and the atrioventricular valves.
Gross examination	Describe chamber sizes (normal, small, dilated). Measure thickness of free wall of both ventricles and the interventricular septum (parietal compact myocardium excluding trabeculae) at basal, medium and apical levels. When walls differ significantly in thickness, detail points of difference for each. Detail gross appearance of myocardium: recent lesions, scars or fibrosis and fatty or fibro-fatty replacement, specifying their extent and site (transmural, subendocardial, mediomural, subepicardial) and location (anterior, lateral, posterior at basal, medium and apical levels).
Sampling for histology	A complete section of the heart at mid-ventricular level in the most altered area (see Chap. 5, Fig. 5.12). One sample from the right ventricle, one from the left ventricle and one from the interventricular septum at both basal and apical segments (the most altered areas).
Coronary arteries	Although significant coronary atherosclerosis is not usually present in native hearts with cardiomyopathies, it is still good practice (especially in idiopathic dilated cardiomyopathy where an occult coronary artery disease might concur) to: Check the number, position and size of coronary arteries and patency of the coronary ostia. Assess the size, course and dominance of the major coronary arteries. Make a series of transverse cuts at 3 mm intervals in the proximal sites of the main epicardial branches (left anterior descending, left circumflex artery, diagonal and obtuse marginal branches, right coronary artery). Take representative/randomised specimens.
Staining	Haematoxylin-eosin. When warranted by Haematoxylin-eosin, stains for collagen and elastic fibres (Masson or Mallory trichrome, Movat pentachrome, Weigert-Van Gieson, etc.) and additional stains or immunohistochemistry.

Worksheet: Native hearts	
Sectioning, internal gross examination and sampling for histology according to disease groups	
3. Heart valve disease	
Sectioning	Echocardiographic short axis cut (see Chap. 5, Fig. 5.11a, b). Make serial transverse sections (i.e. perpendicular to the long axis of the heart) from the apex to the mid-ventricular level or the base as far as the apex of papillary muscles at 1 cm intervals.
Gross examination	*Prosthetic valves or annuloplasty rings and mitral-clip* Evaluate in situ in order to recognise type and note any complication. When in atrioventricular position: examine both from the atrial view and, after sectioning, from the ventricular view. When in aortic position: examine from the aortic view and from the ventricular side by opening the outflow tract of the left ventricle basal segment along the anterior surface. *Heart* Describe chamber sizes (normal, small, dilated). Measure thickness of free wall of both ventricles and the interventricular septum (parietal compact myocardium excluding trabeculae) at basal, medium and apical levels. When walls differ significantly in thickness, detail points of difference for each. Detail gross appearance of myocardium: recent lesions, scars or fibrosis and fatty or fibro-fatty replacement, specifying their extent (transmural, subendocardial, mediomural, subepicardial) and location (anterior, lateral, posterior at basal, medium and apical levels).
Sampling for histology	A complete section of the heart at mid-ventricular level in the most altered area (see Chap. 5, Fig. 5.12). One sample from the right ventricle, one from the left ventricle and one from the interventricular septum at both basal and apical segments (the most altered areas).
Staining	Haematoxylin-eosin. When warranted by Haematoxylin-eosin, stains for collagen and elastic fibres (Masson or Mallory trichrome, Movat pentachrome, Weigert-Van Gieson, etc.), and additional stains or immunohistochemistry.

Worksheet: Native hearts	
Sectioning, internal gross examination and sampling for histology according to disease groups	
4. Congenital heart disease	
Non-operated congenital heart disease	
Sectioning	Before dissection, check whether the heart is biventricular or univentricular: with univentricular physiology, it is essential to identify the rudimentary ventricle. Dissect the heart following blood flow (a transverse cut at mid-ventricle is not usually recommended).
Gross examination	Use the *sequential segmental approach* whose main steps are: Definition of atrial situs. Morphologic identification of atria, ventricles and great arteries. Recognition of atrioventricular and ventriculo-arterial connections.
Sampling for histology	Histology is not usually required in non-operated congenital heart disease except for specific cases or research.
Operated congenital heart disease	
General recommendations	Assess any devices and patches or biological grafts relating to previous surgical or interventional procedures. Check for any catheters within the cavities and any epicardial leads. As the structure and morphology of the heart can be very altered, before sectioning it is advisable to have a clear idea of the primary disease and subsequent surgery, if possible with the surgeon or cardiologist present.
Sectioning	The echocardiographic short axis cut with serial transverse sections, each of 1–2 cm, from the apex to the medium third of the heart is the most frequently used.
Coronary arteries	In adult patients it is advisable to evaluate coronary arteries in order to identify atherosclerotic lesions superimposed on the congenital heart disease: Make a series of transverse cuts at 3 mm intervals in the main epicardial branches (left anterior descending, left circumflex artery, diagonal and obtuse marginal branches, right coronary artery), and for each indicate any atherosclerotic plaques and degree of stenosis.
Sampling for histology	A complete section of the heart at mid-ventricular level in the most altered area (see Chap. 5, Fig. 5.12). One sample from the right ventricle, one from the left ventricle and one from the interventricular septum from both basal and apical segments (the most altered areas) Samples from main coronary artery branches.
Staining	Haematoxylin-eosin. When warranted by Haematoxylin-eosin, stains for collagen and elastic fibres (Masson or Mallory trichrome, Movat pentachrome, Weigert-Van Gieson, etc.) and additional stains or immunohistochemistry.

Worksheet: Autopsy	
Issues related to consent according to national legislation	
Clinical information relevant to the postmortem	*Mismatches* Human leukocyte antigens (HLA). Infections (especially Cytomegalovirus, *Toxoplasma*). *Recipient data:* Details of underlying disease and its treatment, pre-operative renal and hepatic function. *Donor and donor heart data:* Sex, age, cause of death. Events preceding harvesting (e.g. inotropic drugs, arrhythmias, infections, duration of intubation). Preservation technique after harvesting (including if ex vivo circuit used for myocardial protection). *Transplant procedure:* Date of transplant, type of transplant, details of surgical procedure (including assist device and removal details), total ischaemia time, total cardio-pulmonary by-pass time. *Post-transplant events* Post-operative bleeding, renal and hepatic function, cerebro-vascular episodes. Drug therapy, right and left ventricular function including details of ventricular support, if needed. Rejection episodes/treatment. Complications (infection, malignancy, disease recurrence, allograft vasculopathy, etc.). Terminal event and mode of death.
Autopsy procedure	
It is usually a full autopsy including removal and examination of all/main internal organs and brain (this last especially in sudden death cases). Autopsy is performed according to standard autopsy protocols. Particular attention should be given in cases of mechanical circulatory support (see below).	
Alternative autopsies (in limited cases, generally by specific request of family)	*Limited autopsies* (ranging from exclusion of examination of the brain to removal, examination and sampling of the transplanted heart only). *Minimally invasive autopsies* (such as percutaneous needle biopsies of specific organs).
General recommendations	Ample photographic documentation, including video. Check all scars, sutures, devices and drain sites. Be careful when removing the sternum because of possible adhesions of the heart after surgery.

Focusing on the grafted heart	Check the pericardium, which is usually left open, dissect it from the rest of the mediastinum, explore the pericardial cavity and note the volume and type of any fluid present. Check the great arteries and the transplant suture lines in the atria before transecting them above the suture lines. Open the right atrium from the inferior vena cava to the apex of the appendage. Open the left atrium between the pulmonary veins and then to the atrial appendage. Inspect the atrial cavities. Examine the mitral and tricuspid valves from above and check the integrity of the papillary muscles and chordae tendineae. Inspect the aorta, the pulmonary artery and the aortic and pulmonary valves from above. *Coronary arteries* Check the number, position, size of coronary arteries and patency of the coronary ostia. Assess the size, course and dominance of the major coronary arteries. Make multiple transverse cuts at 3 mm intervals along the course of the main epicardial arteries and branches and check patency. Heavily calcified coronary arteries can sometimes be opened with sharp scissors. If this is not possible, they should be removed intact, decalcified and then opened transversely. Identify the presence of possible cardiac allograft vasculopathy, its type and the presence of any culprit lesions. Coronary artery segments containing a metallic stent should be referred intact to laboratories with facilities for resin or other embedding and cutting; otherwise it might be possible to open the stent transversely with scissors and to inspect its position and contents. Coronary artery by-pass grafts should be carefully examined using serial sections. *Heart* Make a complete transverse (short axis) cut of the heart at the mid-ventricular level and then parallel slices of ventricles towards the apex. Dissect the basal half of the heart in the flow of blood and complete the examination. Describe chamber sizes (normal, small, dilated). Measure thickness of free wall of both ventricles and of the interventricular septum (parietal compact myocardium excluding trabeculae) at basal, medium and apical levels. Assess slices carefully and detail any myocardial recent lesions, scars or fibrosis specifying their extent and location.
Other organs	All other organs should be carefully assessed bearing in mind: Cause of death is not necessarily related to transplantation and its pharmacological therapy. Timing of death post-transplant is an important guide to examining cause of death (see Table 24.4, Chap. 24).
Tissue sampling	
Heart graft	Sample any altered myocardial areas. If no lesions are evident, sample a complete section of the heart at mid-ventricular level and other random samples from the right and left ventricle and the septum. Sample (if indicated) the sinus node and atrioventricular node of the conducting system as for the standard approach. Sample of the main epicardial coronary arteries widely according to lesions detected at macroscopic examination or randomly for evaluation of non macroscopically evident allograft vasculopathy. Sample any alterations/lesions in the presence of coronary artery stents or by-pass grafts. At least one sample from atrial suture line including both donor and recipient myocardium. *Stains* Haematoxylin-eosin, connective tissue stain such as Elastic Van Gieson or Masson/Mallory's trichrome.

Other organs	All/main organs (lung, liver, kidney, pancreas, bowel, bone marrow, brain) should be sampled: According to macroscopic findings. Randomly if no macroscopic alterations evident.
Sampling for microbiology and molecular analysis	Collect fresh tissue samples (heart, liver, spleen) and blood sample for DNA and RNA extraction. Spleen tissue could be used as substitute for blood samples, if these are unavailable.
Particular issues in patients with mechanical cardiac support (MCS)	
Components of mechanical assist devices	The components of left ventricular assist devices (LVAD) usually encountered at autopsy are: The inflow cannula, inserted into the ventricular apex or into the left atrium and connected to the pump. The outflow cannula, extending from the apex to the ascending or descending aorta, where it is anastomosed above the valves. The driveline, an insulated electrical cable which exits the body from the device through an opening in the skin in the upper abdomen. In patients with right ventricular assist device (RVAD) or biventricular systems (BVAD), the inflow cannula is implanted into the right ventricle or right atrium, and in most cases, the outflow cannula is connected to the pulmonary trunk.
Some general points	When removing the anterior rib cage and sternum, be careful with adhesions in order to avoid cutting through the outflow cannula of the LVAD, which is usually positioned on the anterior epicardial surface of the right ventricle. *MCS systems:* Record component position and relation to the anatomic structures. Evaluate length, signs of tension and kinking of the outflow cannula. Pull the driveline cable entirely through the skin and check for macroscopic alterations.
Special points concerning the heart	Lift the heart from the pericardial sac and separate it from its vascular connections, well above the anastomoses between the MCS outflow graft component and the great arteries and at least 2 cm above the annuli of the atrioventricular valves or, if possible, at the level of the vena cava and pulmonary veins. Open the heart with a single transverse section at mid-ventricular level below the mitral valvular apparatus but above the apical cannula, tunnelling between outflow cannula and epicardial surface. Cut further serial sections at 1–2 cm intervals along the short axis of the heart in order to examine the myocardium for any scarring, haemorrhage or infarction. Cut the top half of the heart following blood flow. Measure the wall thickness of ventricles and of interventricular septum and left ventricular diameter. Assess coronary arteries, as usual. Examine valve cusps for thrombosis and any other alteration. *Apical cannula:* Examine position in relation to the septum and the inflow tract and distance from the free margin of the anterior mitral valve leaflet. Check any thrombus, fibrous tissue or anatomic structures obstructing lumen. Carefully evaluate the suture ring at the site of anastomosis. *Sampling for histology:* Take samples from the altered macroscopic areas and whenever possible additional full thickness samples from the ventricles and interventricular septum. Sample myocardial tissue around the apical inflow cannula. *Stains* Haematoxylin-eosin, connective tissue stain such as Elastic Van Gieson or Masson/Mallory's trichrome. *NB: This method of examination and sectioning of the heart can also be applied to native hearts with these devices still in situ.*

Template for Autopsy Report

The pathology report should include a descriptive section and the final diagnosis.

Descriptive section should include:

- A sufficiently detailed clinical history
- Systematic description of the macroscopic findings
- Systematic description of the microscopic findings
- Description of any additional tests

Final diagnosis should include:

- Cause(s) of death
- Other pathologic findings in order of priority
- Epicrisis or clinico-pathological correlations and comments

Index

O. Leone et al. (eds.), *The Pathology of Cardiac Transplantation*,
DOI 10.1007/978-3-319-46386-5

C

D

CPI Antony Rowe
Chippenham, UK
2017-09-04 22:33